Emotions, cognition, and behavior

The activities of the Social Science Research Council's Committee on Social and Affective Development During Childhood have been supported primarily by the Foundation for Child Development, a private foundation that makes grants to educational and charitable institutions. Its main interests are in research, social and economic indicators of children's lives, advocacy and public information projects, and service experiments that help translate theoretical knowledge about children into policies and practices that affect their daily lives.

Emotions, cognition, and behavior

*Based, in part, on workshops sponsored by the
Committee on Social and Affective Development During
Childhood of the Social Science Research Council*

Edited by

CARROLL E. IZARD, JEROME KAGAN,
and ROBERT B. ZAJONC

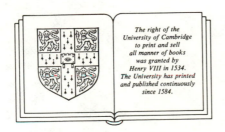

The right of the
University of Cambridge
to print and sell
all manner of books
was granted by
Henry VIII in 1534.
The University has printed
and published continuously
since 1584.

CAMBRIDGE UNIVERSITY PRESS

Cambridge
London   New York   New Rochelle
Melbourne   Sydney

Published by the Press Syndicate of the University of Cambridge
The Pitt Building, Trumpington Street, Cambridge CB2 1RP
32 East 57th Street, New York, NY 10022, USA
10 Stamford Road, Oakleigh, Melbourne 3166 Australia

First published 1984
First paperback edition 1985

Printed in the United States of America

Library of Congress Cataloging in Publication Data
Main entry under title:
Emotions, cognition, and behavior.
1. Developmental psychology. 2. Emotions.
3. Cognition. 4. Emotions in children. 5. Cognition in
children. I. Izard, Carroll E. II. Kagan, Jerome.
III. Zajonc, Robert B. (Robert Boleslaw), 1923–
[DNLM: 1. Emotions. 2. Cognition. 3. Behavior. BF 531
E538]
BF713.E47   1984   153.4   83-7765
ISBN 0 521 25601 1 hard covers
ISBN 0 521 31246 9 paperback

Contents

List of contributors   *page* vii
Foreword   ix
Peter B. Read
Introduction   1
Carroll E. Izard, Jerome Kagan, and Robert B. Zajonc

Part I   Theoretical issues in emotions and cognition

1   Emotion-cognition relationships and human development   17
    Carroll E. Izard
2   The idea of emotion in human development   38
    Jerome Kagan
3   Affect and cognition: the hard interface   73 ✳
    R. B. Zajonc and Hazel Markus
4   Interaction of affect and cognition in empathy   103
    Martin L. Hoffman
5   Emotion, attention, and temperament   132
    Douglas Derryberry and Mary Klevjord Rothbart
6   An attributional approach to emotional development   167
    Bernard Weiner and Sandra Graham
7   Cognition in emotion: concept and action   192
    Peter J. Lang

Part II   Emotion and cognition in early development

8   Toward a new understanding of emotions and their
    development   229
    Joseph J. Campos and Karen Caplovitz Barrett
9   The cognitive-emotional fugue   264
    Michael Lewis, Margaret Wolan Sullivan, and Linda
    Michalson
10 The role of affect in social competence   289
    L. Alan Sroufe, Edward Schork, Frosso Motti, Nancy
    Lawroski, and Peter LaFreniere

11 Affect, cognition, and hemispheric specialization   320
    Richard J. Davidson
12 Theoretical and empirical considerations in the investigation
    of the relationship between affect and cognition in atypical
    populations of infants   366
    Dante Cicchetti and Karen Schneider-Rosen

Part III Language, memory, and emotion

13 Children's understanding of emotions   409
    Reid M. Schwartz and Tom Trabasso
14 Children's and adults' understanding of the causes and
    consequences of emotional states   438
    John C. Masters and Charles R. Carlson
15 Emotion, self, and others   464
    Bert Moore, Bill Underwood, and D. L. Rosenhan
16 The role of emotion in moral socialization   484
    Richard A. Dienstbier
17 Thinking and feeling in Woolf's writing: from childhood to
    adulthood   515
    Jeannette M. Haviland
18 Cognitive consequences of emotional arousal   547
    Stephen G. Gilligan and Gordon H. Bower

Author index   589
Subject index   601

Contributors

Karen Caplovitz Barrett
University of Denver

Gordon H. Bower
Stanford University

Joseph J. Campos
University of Denver

Charles R. Carlson
Institute for Public Studies
Vanderbilt University

Dante Cicchetti
Harvard University

Richard J. Davidson
State University of New York at
    Purchase

Douglas Derryberry
University of Oregon

Richard A. Dienstbier
University of Nebraska-Lincoln

Stephen G. Gilligan
Stanford University

Sandra Graham
University of California at Los
    Angeles

Jeannette M. Haviland
Livingston College
Rutgers University

Martin L. Hoffman
University of Michigan

Carroll E. Izard
University of Delaware

Jerome Kagan
Harvard University

Peter LaFreniere
Institute of Child Development
University of Minnesota

Peter J. Lang
University of Florida

Nancy Lawroski
Institute of Child Development
University of Minnesota

Michael Lewis
University of Medicine and
    Dentistry of New Jersey
Rutgers Medical School

Hazel Markus
Institute for Social Research
University of Michigan

John C. Masters
Institute for Public Studies
Vanderbilt University

Linda Michalson
University of Medicine and
    Dentistry of New Jersey
Rutgers Medical School

Bert Moore
University of Texas at Dallas

Frosso Motti
Institute of Child Development
University of Minnesota

D. L. Rosenhan
Stanford University

Mary Klevjord Rothbart
University of Oregon

Karen Schneider-Rosen
Harvard University

Edward Schork
Institute of Child Development
University of Minnesota

Reid M. Schwartz
University of Chicago

L. Alan Sroufe
Institute of Child Development
University of Minnesota

Margaret Wolan Sullivan
University of Medicine and
    Dentistry of New Jersey
Rutgers Medical School

Tom Trabasso
University of Chicago

Bill Underwood
University of Texas at Austin

Bernard Weiner
University of California at Los
    Angeles

R. B. Zajonc
Institute for Social Research
University of Michigan

Foreword

In 1975 the Social Science Research Council established a Committee on Social and Affective Development During Childhood. With funds from the Foundation for Child Development and the Bush Foundation, this interdisciplinary group of scholars has sponsored a series of workshops and conferences focused on noncognitive aspects of children's development. The emphasis on social and emotional factors stemmed from a concern that an understanding of development in these domains appeared meager when compared with the growing knowledge of cognitive growth. Despite this concern, in its various considerations of child development the committee could never successfully separate the domains of emotion, cognition, and social behavior. They came to accept the fact that the connections are intrinsic to development, probably from the first day of life. Furthermore, they also concluded that the advancement of knowledge in one domain often relies upon a researcher's ability to discern critical interactions with the other domains.

In 1979 and 1980 the SSRC committee devoted a number of meetings to an examination of the relationships between emotion and cognition. Two workshops with invited research presentations were held in San Francisco in November 1979 and June 1980. Emerging research on this topic was provocative and the discussions were lively. Childhood seemed a particularly rich period in which to investigate the nature and origins of affect-cognition interactions. This was clearly a research frontier. Cognitive scientists were beginning to take a hard look at how emotions were or were not incorporated in existing models of cognition and behavior. Scholars studying emotions realized the inadequacy of many of their postulates regarding links to cognitive processing. The ferment present in those early committee discussions is reflected in the growing empirical research on the relations between affect, cognition, and behavior.

This volume includes recent reports on some of the research originally discussed in the SSRC committee's workshops. Yet it was Carroll Izard, a member of the committee from 1976 to present, who perceived the need to push further on this topic. He approached other scholars, many of whom had not begun to explore systematically the implications of their work for understanding the relationships between emotion and cognition. His vision of a volume that would document innovative empirical and theoretical work is realized here.

ix

Although there have been several major conferences and a growing number of publications on this topic in recent years, this volume contains an impressive array of challenging articles that go well beyond the careful reporting of empirical findings. The authors do not hesitate to approach difficult theoretical questions and, although the evidence is still just trickling in, these chapters attest to the undeniable importance of the questions asked.

This volume reflects primarily the insights and energy of its editors and authors. One would be remiss, however, not to acknowledge the more indirect contributions of those members of the SSRC Committee on Social and Affective Development During Childhood who are listed at the beginning of this volume and those scholars who joined them in early discussions of this topic, including: Gordon Bower, Mihaly Csikszentmihalyi, Robert N. Emde, Richard S. Lazarus, Howard Leventhal, George Mandler, Donald Meichenbaum, Ulric Neisser, Donald A. Norman, Elinor Ochs, and Bambi Schieffelin.

Finally, the committee and editors of this volume wish to express their gratitude to Susan Milmoe and her colleagues at Cambridge University Press who have been so supportive of the SSRC's work in the area of child development and who have made the publication process comfortable and rewarding.

Peter B. Read
Social Science Research Council

Introduction

Carroll E. Izard, Jerome Kagan, and Robert B. Zajonc

This volume brings together contributions to the study of emotions from several areas: cognitive psychology, developmental psychology, social psychology, psychophysiology, and personality-clinical psychology. Contributors within and across these areas share some common concerns despite differences in theoretical orientation and special interests. All contributors agree that emotion concepts can be operationally defined and investigated as both independent and dependent variables. These definitions vary in some degree among contributors, but all of them have made clear their definition. The problem of definition is the first of several theoretical issues dealt with in the chapters of Part I.

All the chapters in this volume illustrate the enormous progress that has been realized recently in our understanding of emotions. It is not clear why emotion is returning to the legitimate status it occupied in nineteenth-century discussions of psychological functioning in animals and humans. It is too simple to regard the renaissance as an example of the regular cycling of interest in major themes. Rather, it is more likely that the return is due to the current vitality of evolutionary biology and neurophysiology, both of which have focused on the commonalities between animals and humans, and the exciting findings of neurochemistry, which seem to have more relevance for mood than for thought.

However, the questions are more sophisticated this time around than they were when scholars last examined emotions. There is a sensitivity to the issues surrounding levels of analysis as well as a concern with such important differences as those bodily changes detected by the individual and those that do not enter awareness. Second, modern scholars recognize that their constructs are not independent of the procedures that gave them life. Ever since the famous conference of physicists at the Solvay Congress during the first decade of this century, scientists have appreciated the contribution of their procedures to the meaning of invented explanations. This is a new idea for naturalists who now acknowledge the intimate relation between concepts and data. It makes a difference if a *statement* about a person's fear state is based on self-report, heart-rate acceleration, concentration of cortisol in the urine, or a patterned change in facial muscles. Each factor may index something different about the same phenomenon or each factor may index it imperfectly.

Theoretical issues in emotion and cognition

A most profound issue in this volume and one that applies to investigators in several areas asks whether it is theoretically useful to regard discretely different patterns of neurophysiological activity, independent of cognitive appraisal, as capable of generating emotions. Some contributors believe that it is. Although they acknowledge that cognition (appraisal, remembering, anticipation) is a sufficient (though not necessary) cause of the neural processes that produce emotion, they affirm that afferent information can be transformed directly into emotion without cognitive mediation. The behavior of young infants and the unconscious or preconscious processing of affective stimuli may be fertile areas for investigating the validity of this proposition.

Other contributors believe that the generation of emotions is always dependent on appraisal or evaluative processes. They prefer to view all emotion as an emergent phenomenon derived from the interaction of physiological changes and psychological processes in the same way that physicists talk of radiation emerging from the interaction of an electric charge in a magnetic field.

The problem of definition is not confined to emotions. It applies to cognition as well. This is particularly so when considering the question of the interface or interaction of emotion and cognition, and when considering the question of emotion activation or the sequence of events involved in a "cause-emotion consequence." It is important to be as specific as possible regarding the emotion and cognitive processes that are implicated. Very broad definitions as well as very narrow ones may need to be carefully scrutinized. For example, if we define cognition as information processing in its broadest sense, we may be putting the neural messages of reflex action and symbolic processes in the same basket. Likewise, if we define emotion as any type of motivational arousal, we are placing the need for elimination and the joy of discovery side by side. Arguments can be made for such broad definitions, but we question their utility as a guide for experimentation.

A way of analyzing definitions of emotions

Dictionary definitions as well as common conceptions of emotions are dominated by reference to feelings or subjective states. The most common meaning in the etymological antecedents of the term *emotion* are "to stir up or excite." While we are inclined to think of emotions in terms of their effects on our conscious states, a moment's reflection or a probing question will often reveal some awareness of physiological changes.

Major theories of emotion generally agree that there are three aspects or components of an emotion: neurophysiological-biochemical, motor or behavioral-expressive, and subjective-experiential. The contributors to this volume differ in the degree to which they make these components explicit and in the way in which they define them. Defining characteristics of the neurochemical component relate to neurotransmitters and to autonomic and somatic nervous system activities. In examining the various definitions of emotion one can ask whether the emphasis is more on the biochemical substrates, autonomic nervous system involvement, somatic nervous system activity, or some combination of these. For example, traditionally psychophysiological indices of affect have been based on autonomic nervous system activity. In the past decade, following the publication of robust evidence for the innateness and universality of a limited set of facial expressions of emotions, there has been increasing interest in indexing functions of the somatic nervous system, particularly via facial electromyography.

The motor or expressive component of emotions is in some respects the most clearly understood, particularly if one accepts facial expression as the best single index of this component. There are now several anatomically based systems for measuring the facial movements that signal emotion, and although much remains to be learned, there has been considerable progess in this area. Still, there are a number of problems in relying on facial expression as a sole index of emotion. Emotion can and does express itself in postural, gestural, and instrumental acts, as well as in vocal intonation. And with the acquisition of language, emotion is verbalized as well as vocalized. The key question in considering the meaning and usefulness of an index from any of these spheres of motor expression may be that of specificity. In terms of the quantity of current empirical evidence, the evidence for the specificity of facial signals is the most abundant, that for acoustic characteristics of vocal expression is second, and that for postural, gestural, and instrumental acts is last. This suggests that context and convergent data are relatively more important in conjunction with some of these indices than with others when identification of a specific emotion is attempted.

Definition of the third component of emotion, the subjective or experiential aspect of emotion in consciousness, is controversial. Some understanding of the differences in definition of this component is important in gaining perspective on the differences among the contributions to this volume. The central question is whether the third component of emotion is basically a *feeling state*, a special type of *cognitive process* (e.g., "hot cognition"), or a *combination* of feeling and cognition. We do not consider it a trivial question. For those who consider the third component as consisting solely of a feeling state, there is a large and relatively unexplored territory of emotion-cognition relationships. How do feelings become associated or bonded with images and symbols? The view of the third component of emotion as a feeling state also requires a definition of subjective experience that includes emotion (represented as feeling) and images, concepts, memories, and all the other products of information processing and consciousness. For those who view the third component of emotion as basically cognitive in nature, there is the problem of sorting out the cognitive component of emotion from other products of cognitive processes. These differing definitions of the subjective-experiential component have different implications for the study of emotion in lower animals and in young infants with limited cognitive capacities. Those who see emotion experience as essentially cognitive in nature need to confront the question as to the difference between cognition about emotion and the cognition that is a component of emotion. How does the labeling and the symbolization of emotion relate to the subjective experience of emotion? These concerns and questions regarding the nature of the third component of emotion are relevant in reading not only the contributions in Part I on theoretical issues but also those in Part II on emotion and cognition in early development and those in Part III on understanding emotion experiences and their effects.

Although definition is a current issue, we recognize that at some stages of development a given discipline may well refrain from setting up strict formal demands upon its definitions. The more specific the definition, the sharper the boundary it draws among phenomena. And at some stages of knowledge it isn't always clear where these boundaries should be. Therefore, when knowledge is lacking, formal definitions may sometimes do more harm than good. They may, for example, eliminate from analysis some aspects of phenomena that may eventually turn out to be essential to the understanding of the entire process. For example, if one defines emotion so as to exclude interest, we might have difficulty in dealing with surprise and boredom. The urgent need in a growing field, such as emotion, is less for strict and formal definitions (although we do wish to have some common agreement about what we mean by "emotion") and more for insight into what are the essential and fundamental processes that are necessarily implicated in all emotions.

Emotion activation and the sequence problem

Although the generation or activation of emotion is a topic discussed explicitly by only a few of the contributors, it is a background question in many chapters. Some authors treat emotions as though they are temporary and transient. In this framework, emotion experience is an episode in an otherwise affectless consciousness. The activation of a particular emotion is generally considered to be independent of any other emotions. Other theorists consider emotion experience as a continuing aspect of consciousness. For them the problem of emotion activation is more a question of how one emotion replaces, combines with, or otherwise relates to the emotion already present. If emotion in awareness consists of temporally discrete units, then it is possible to explicate the antecedents of emotion in strictly cognitive terms. On the other hand, if some emotion is always present in consciousness (at some level of intensity or awareness), then the activation of any different or "new" emotion is always a function in part of the ongoing emotion process. The impact of the ongoing emotion would be a function of its intensity, the degree to which it is focal in awareness, and the way in which it relates to the new emotion.

A number of theorists have formulated the emotion activation issue as a sequence problem. Is some cognitive process (appraisal, evaluation) always an antecedent of emotion? There is no argument as to whether cognition is a sufficient cause of emotion; the question is whether it is a necessary cause. Considering it as a necessary cause is consistent with a linear model of event-emotion-effect relationships. Considering cognition as a sufficient, but not necessary, antecedent of emotion is consistent with a feedback-feedforward loop model of emotion-event-emotion-effect relationships. The linear model is compatible with the typical approach to setting up an experiment, but the loop model can also guide research.

The emotion-cognition interface

One of the greatest challenges relating to the emotion-cognition-behavior complex is the specification in greater detail of the relationship of emotion and cognition, especially the development of this relationship. There is a unanimous voice throughout this volume that cognitive factors participate heavily in the emotion process. While we do not agree fully or know whether cognitive factors are always necessary, it is clear that under most circumstances cognitive factors contribute heavily to every aspect of the emotion process. They are present as sufficient conditions in the generation of emotion; they participate as necessary processes in the symbolization and labeling of the emotion; and they influence emotion expression. The arousal of guilt, for example, and of all complex emotions, such as jealousy and pride, sometimes requires the appreciation of a host of subtle circumstances – an appreciation that is not possible without a great deal of tacit knowledge. Finally, the expression of emotion involves cognitive factors, especially when the expression occurs in a social context, which is the case more often than not. Thus, for example, the child must gauge the possible reaction of the parents should he cry, scream, or throw a veritable fit when he is refused an ice cream cone. There is not only an appraisal at the point of the generation of emotion; there is also quite often an appraisal at the point of discharge and expression.

The readiness of the study of emotion to proceed toward a greater elaboration and explication of cognitive mediators and correlates is now a conspicuous fact. The enormous sophistication that has been developed in the experimental study of information processing and generally in the growth of cognitive science speaks loudly to this readiness. What is terribly surprising is that the theoretical sophistication reached by cognitive science, the new technical and methodological developments in mental chronometry and story analysis, have not yet been absorbed formally into the study of emotion. Throughout this volume there are numerous affirmations of the role of cognitive factors in emotion. Yet the empirical research and theoretical analysis of this participation does not avail itself fully of the wealth of concepts in cognitive science, of their methods, and of the empirical material that has been accumulated. No doubt, it is only a matter of time when cognitive science will enter more completely into the study of emotion, and the contributions of cognitive psychologists to this volume promise a solid beginning in this direction.

Our discussion of the problem of definition is very relevant to the issue of emotion-cognition relationships. Before we can talk about the relationships we have to establish some kind of definitional boundary for the two concepts. All the contributors have done this for emotion and some have done it for cognition. There is of course the option of defining either of the terms sufficiently broadly to incorporate the other, and indeed some theorists propose just this. Although definitions that subsume one concept to the other may be appealing as part of the superstructure of a general systems theory or a systems theory approach, we do not believe that such definitions are the most fruitful for guiding empirical research. Most of the research reported in this volume seems to assume either implicitly or explicitly that some differences in emotion and cognitive processes are operationally definable. Hence we have studies in which cognitive sets or instructions are used as independent variables and some in which the indices of emotion are used as dependent variables. In some experiments a cognitive process is used to induce emotion, which then becomes the independent variable and some index of cognitive functioning, the dependent variable. Likewise, the contributors from developmental psychology assume that cognitive development paves the way for emotional development, that emotional development motivates and facilitates cognitive development, or that the two types of processes develop through interaction. So regardless of varying theoretical orientation many investigators are defining and measuring emotion variables and cognitive variables separately.

Stronger statements on the issue of the relationship between emotion and cognition would be that there is one system (though with measurably different functions) or that there are two separate systems (which are highly interactive or perhaps interdependent). Both viewpoints are represented in this volume. The one-system view generally subsumes emotion as a factor in information processing and cognition. The two-system view argues that a separate emotion system can process "affective information" and influence behavior independent of cognitive process, when the latter is defined in terms of representational memory and symbolization derived from learning and experience.

Emotions in learning, temperament, and personality

For most of the past two decades learning theory and cognitive psychology in general, as well as social-psychological and personality theory, was largely devoid of emotion concepts. Partial exceptions were psychodynamically oriented personality theories that gave some role to affects (sex, aggression) or temperament. One could argue that some learning theories remain concerned with affects, defined broadly to include survival needs. For the most part, however, none of these areas produced empirical research dealing with emotion concepts (e.g., joy, sadness, anger, shame, fear) as they are dealt with in some chapters of this volume. In this respect this book marks an early phase of theory and research that attempts to integrate emotion concepts into a number of relatively well established approaches in several different domains of behavioral science.

What is most remarkedly different about the present volume is that many of its contributors, representing several disciplines, are unabashedly investigating the emotions of human experience. Although the editors applaud and participate in this movement, we do not see it as problem-free. As we have already indicated, a serious problem exists in the definition of emotion terms, and the movement is growing so rapidly that there are very likely to be contradictory or controversial findings regarding the antecedents, concomitants, and consequences of emotions, a result in part of inconsistencies in conceptualization. It is for this reason that we urged contributors to specify what they meant by emotion or the particular emotions they discuss.

In retrospect (we are writing this after our final comments to contributors), we feel remiss in not requesting the authors to specify what they mean by cognition. Perhaps it is a sign of the times or our proximity to the cognitive psychology era that allowed our tacit assumption that everyone knows what cognition means. In our effort to place this volume in some perspective, however, we feel that definitional boundaries for cognitive processes are open for discussion and that a clear understanding of them will become more important as a central theme of this volume – emotion-cognition interaction and relationships – becomes more prominent in psychological research.

The definitions of cognitive processes are explicit in some chapters, but their absence in others leads us to caution the reader to examine each contribution with some criteria in mind for placing implicit definitions in perspective.

Just as overly general definitions of emotion will prove faulty in the lab, so will such definitions of cognition. Take, for example, the general definition of cognition as any information processing that influences or guides behavior. Can one argue well that information processed in viral DNA does not ultimately influence the behavior of the virus? And what about hormonal information processing in which the development of synapses is influenced as well as behaviors ranging from song acquisition in the canary to aggression in primates? In any case, information processing at the neurochemical level differs from symbolic processing on many dimensions. Even when we consider the more conventional aspects of cognition, none of them seem altogether simple any more, especially when we consider them in the context of cognition-emotion interaction. In discussing perception, we must be aware of the possibilities of preconscious processes that bear unknown relationships to affect. In thinking of learning we have to consider biological preparedness, emotion thresholds, and temperament as possible modulating variables. There is substantial evidence that emotion can influence memory, and some investigators have inferred from their data that there is a type of affective memory. And finally, representational processes may not necessarily live or die on the basis of images and symbols. They may also thrive on feeling states or other affective phenomena.

We think it may be useful to hold open the possibility that there may be one ultimate integratory system that is on the order of self or personality and that at this level one may fruitfully conceptualize human activities as a function of the integration of perceptual, cognitive, motor, and emotion processes. We also feel that we should hold open the possibility that each process – emotion, perception, cognition, and motor activity – has some systemic properties and some independence that make system-specific concepts and variables noteworthy in psychological experimentation.

Social factors in emotion

Social constraints, like mediators and correlates, enter at every aspect of the emotion process: evocation, experience, and expression. Of course, the most powerful effects are at the output side. The expression of emotion is regulated socially, an aspect that is repeatedly emphasized throughout this volume, especially in the study of socialization and development.

However, social controls over expression are not more important to the understanding of the emotion process than to the communication of emotion. That emotions are a subject matter of interpersonal communication is acknowledged. Yet what has been studied most extensively in the communication of emotion has been the receiving aspect, that is, the ability of perceivers to recognize and identify the emotions of others or their ability to empathize, matters that are considered extensively in this volume.

But there is another side to the communication of emotion and that is the side of the communicator. Emotion expression may well be under severe social control, but emotion itself is a means of social control that is seen over and over again in our everyday encounters. The example given earlier of a child gauging his outburst by the consequences it might have represents a means of social control over the parents. And the emotion states of lovers, relatives, subordinates and their supervisors – in short, people who stand in more than superficial social relationships to each other – serve as a means of influence and social control. The mood of a lover is used to bring about the acquiescence of a reluctant partner, the affability of an acquaintance might result in a later favor, the overt disappointment expressed by a supervisor may increase the efforts of the subordinate. There is very little systematic work in this area, and the study of the emotion-cognition-behavior system would benefit substantially by our understanding of how and under what circumstances various emotions serve to influence the behavior of others. Much emotion acts to reinforce others' behavior. Our joy and sadness, fear and anger, shame and contempt, if they follow another person's responses, are not without effects, which are yet to be well understood in the broader context of social interaction.

An overview of the volume

In Chapter 1, Izard frames his discussion of theoretical issues in the context of a definition of personality as a set of systems. In this framework the emotions are conceived as a system that interacts with the cognitive and motor systems. Even an individual emotion such as joy or sadness is viewed as having systemic properties such that its various components (neurophysiological, expressive, experiential) interact with and influence each other in a kind of feedback-feedforward loop. Emotions influence cognition and vice versa. Arguments for a separate emotion system and for conceiving of each individual emotion as having unique motivational and adaptive characteristics are placed in an evolutionary-developmental perspective.

In Chapter 2, Kagan argues that different constructs must be used for emotions that follow from detected or undetected physiological changes. Further, he believes that the currently popular names for emotions should be replaced with a new set of constructs that specify target and occasion and uses cross-cultural data to support this idea. Finally, he urges a temporary period of Baconian empiricism in which empiricists hold in abeyance the currently popular words and see whether new, robust relations among physiological and psychological events require a different set of affect names.

In Chapter 3, Zajonc and Markus bring new insights to the old issue of the role of the motor system in emotion and cognition. They argue that the motor system is pivotal in affect-cognition relationships. Accordingly, the representation of emotion is discussed in terms of different levels and processes, with soft representation mediated by the cognitive system and hard representation by the motor system. They review the theory and evidence consistent with the notion of soft and hard representations of emotion, as well as the literature relating to "cognitive hardware." The authors discuss the possible role of motor cues in mood-dependent learning and describe some research approaches to this problem. In their concluding section they confront the major criticisms of the idea that the motor system serves representational functions.

Hoffman, in Chapter 4, extends his theory of empathy by examining the processes of interaction of affect and cognition in the development of empathic behavior. He describes a developmental sequence of six modes of empathic arousal and then delineates the cognitive attainments required for different arousal modes. Arousal modes range from the primary circular reaction (distress-induced distress in the newborn) to symbolic association and role taking, and the associated cognitive capacities vary from something like pattern recognition or simple perceptual discrimination to the ability to imagine one's self in the other's place. Of particular importance is the development of the cognitive sense of the other, levels of which are determinants or at least correlates of four increasingly complex levels of empathic response. Finally, Hoffman's concerns overlap those of Weiner and Graham and of Dienstbier as he discusses the role of language, semantic processing, and causal attribution in empathic experiences.

In Chapter 5, Derryberry and Rothbart suggest that attentional mechanisms may provide a key for understanding emotion-cognition relationships. Their focus is on temperament and they review concepts of temperament in the context of a number of current theories of emotion and motivation. They discuss the possibility of some independence between "arousal" and "affective-motivational systems" and suggest that some emotions are indexed more readily by measures of arousal and others by measures of attentional processes. Because they define temperament "as constitutional differences in reactivity and self-regulation," they are particularly concerned with the sources and mechanisms of regulatory processes and with the relationships between the reactivity component of temperament and affective-motivational processes. A case is made for the regulation of affective-motivational systems by means of attentional processes, such as attention shifting and attention focusing. They report a number of interesting findings from their own temperament research with adults and infants. After reviewing the theory and research on temperament and related concepts, they conclude that ability to shift and focus attention is positively related to the affective regulation of negative emotions.

In Chapter 6, Weiner and Graham make it clear that their approach to the study of emotional development is guided by their interest in attributional processes. Their theory and research tell us a great deal about what kinds of attributional thoughts are linked to specific emotions. They focus on three dimensions of causality: locus, stability, and controllability. They show, for example, that attribution of one's failure to lack of effort or to others may identify the emotion experience as guilt or anger. They found similarities and differences in linkages between attributions and emotions across age groups. Finally, they present a thoughtful discussion of some "vexing problems," including the emotion-cognition sequence issue, emotions versus thoughts *about* emotions, and the origin of attribution-emotion linkages.

Chapter 7 presents an impressive body of empirical findings and insights on cognition-emotion-action relationships that Peter Lang has gathered through his experience as a clinician and psychophysiologist. He presents convincing arguments for his concept of the "emotion prototype": a conceptual network of coded information that is activated by information matching that in the network and that has as functional output a visceral and somatomotor program. The focus is on the fear prototype (phobia), which is used to illustrate a number of principles relating to the stimulus, meaning, and response propositions constituting the conceptual network of the prototype. Lang advances our knowledge of fear activation and fear-related behavior by demonstrating differences in effects obtained in activating fear with good and poor imagers and with focus on stimulus and response information. His work has implications for theory relating to the formation, storage, and retrieval of "emotion prototypes," a concept similar in some respects to Izard's concept of affective-cognitive structure.

In Chapter 8, Campos and Barrett conceive emotions as having motivational and organizational functions, and they highlight the role of emotions as "crucial regulators of social and interpersonal behavior." They include a review of some of the exciting research on the infant's use of "social referencing," accessing and using emotion information in mother's facial expressions to guide behavior. An infant will or will not cross the deep side of the visual cliff depending, for example, on whether the mother is displaying a happy or fearful expression. This result raises the interesting question of whether the mother's facial expression serves simply as a conditioned stimulus (signal) or induces emotion (intrapsychic motivation) in the infant or does both. Finally, Campos and Barrett propose five postulates for describing the most important features of emotional development.

In Chapter 9, Lewis, Sullivan, and Michalson accept the reality of emotional phenomena and the interdependence of cognition and emotion. They insist that both sets of processes must be viewed as continual and "interwoven in highly complex ways such that to separate them is to distort the phenomenon." In support of their belief, they report a study of contingency awareness in infants. As an infant learns a contingency, he shows an increase in positive facial expression, suggesting that the orienting reflex is emotional, not cognitive, in nature. Along with most investigators, they are forced to assume a one-to-one correspondence between the behavioral expressions of emotion and some internal emotional state, an issue that is still of serious debate.

In Chapter 10, Sroufe and his colleagues present empirical studies of affect in social interaction. They developed observational measures for assessing general categories of positive, negative, and inappropriate affect expression in preschool children. They found, for example, that affect plays a significant role in initiating, regulating, and animating social exchanges and that the frequency of positive affect expression in social interactions minus the frequency of negative affect expression was highly correlated with social competence as indexed by teacher ratings and sociometric status. They interpret their findings as supporting the view that emotions are motivators and organizers of individual behavior and social interaction.

In Chapter 11, Richard Davidson argues that the cerebral hemispheres play different roles in the regulation of emotions and moods. Adopting the ancient division between pleasant and unpleasant affects, he uses his evidence to argue that the frontal region of the left cerebral hemisphere participates in the more pleasant emotions, whereas the frontal region of the right hemisphere participates in unpleasant emotions. Relying on data from Sroufe, Campos, and Izard he suggests that the fear behavior that emerges in the second half of the first year of life, as evidenced by avoidance of the deep side of the visual cliff and the stranger response, depends upon interhemispheric communication.

Cicchetti and Schneider-Rosen, in Chapter 12, are influenced by "the organizational perspective" in their discussion of the development of relationships between emotion and cognition in atypical infants. They discuss the reasons for the paucity of research on this topic and in doing so they place some major developmental theories and research approaches in perspective. They discuss some of the issues in the development of emotion expressions and elucidate some of the problems by reference to work on expression development in atypical populations. They note some important differences in affective-cognitive interactions of normal and atypical mother–infant dyads. For example, their own research and that of other investigators show that the decreased affective and dampened emotion expressions of Down's syndrome infants create decoding or interpretive difficulties for care givers and that the care givers' response in turn affects the infant. Such disruptions in socioemotional communication may contribute to psychological problems for both the infant and the care giver. They summarize evidence suggesting that the emotion expressions and response of care givers to infants' affective signals influence the quality of the attachment or relationship of mother and infant. They review studies on the development of a number of different deviant populations and discuss how differences between normal and deviant development can increase our understanding of the relationships between emotion and cognition. For example, the finding that Down's syndrome babies, matched on mental age with normal infants, show less positive and negative emotion to a variety of stimuli was interpreted as evidence for separate developmental systems for emotion and cognition.

Schwartz and Trabasso, in Chapter 13, deal with the relation between the language of emotion and emotional phenomena. In investigating what children know about certain emotions, they verify the assumptions of Sroufe and Davidson that children make a basic distinction between pleasant and unpleasant feeling states and among a number of discrete emotions. They present evidence of considerable similarity in the understanding of some fundamental emotions by 3-year-olds and adults. Their experiments examine the relative ease with which children and adults distinguish several characteristics of emotions – valence, direction, and self–other orientation – and interpret emotion cues with and without contexts.

In Chapter 14, Masters and Carlson are also concerned with the child's understanding of the causes and consequences of emotional states. Adopting a pragmatic, commonsense definition of an emotion as a shared concept among children and adults in the society, they contend that children under 7 years of age cannot grasp the causal relationships of emotions. They demonstrate that children as young as 3 years share some understandings that adults have about the relationships between events and emotions. With age, there is increasing complexity of the understanding of emotional terms and an awareness that people vary in their emotional response.

Moore, Underwood, and Rosenhan, in Chapter 15, review the literature relating to the effects of induced joy and sadness on a variety of behaviors. The authors take the position that the relationship between emotions and cognition is bidirectional, or, in effect, that it can be described as a kind of feedforward-feedback loop. They discuss the evidence for emotion as an influence in self-attribution and self-description or "transient self-concept." Their own research and that of others show substantial effects of emotions on a variety of tasks, attention, self-reward, and the delay of gratification. For example, they conclude that emotion relates differentially to contingent self-reward and noncontingent self-reward and that the mechanisms underlying noncontingent self-reward may differ for positive and negative emotions. They suggest that the differential effects of positive and negative emotions on altruism are explainable in terms of attention focusing: negative affects are more likely to diminish attention to external cues and to the needs of others. Their own research showed that experimental manipulation of the focus of attention can change the effects of the negative emotion of sadness on altruism.

In Chapter 16, Dienstbier examines the role of emotions in the socialization of moral behavior and in moral decision making. He presents an incisive review of theory and research on the functions of autonomic arousal and of cognition about the source and meaning of such arousal in emotion and behavior. The chapter is replete with interesting findings from a series of five experiments with children and adults. For example, he found a new kind of evidence to support the notion that gentle psychologically oriented techniques of moral socialization are more effective than punitive interventions. Of special interest is his demonstration of how imperfect theory guides research that, in turn, alters and improves the theory. In particular, the data lead him to modify his emotion-attribution theory away from the "classical" notion that one's understanding of the causes of one's arousal symptoms determines the quality of emotion. He concludes that the emotion experiences of anxiety, fear, shame, and guilt profoundly influence responses to temptation. Like Weiner and Graham, he believes that those emotion states and their impact on behavior depend in large measure on attributions about their meaning and origin.

In Chapter 17, Haviland examines biographical and literary material in search of affective-cognitive continuity in the life of Virginia Woolf. She combines intuitive and objective analysis to demonstrate the emergence, waxing, and waning of a number of affective themes that are evident from childhood through young adulthood. She argues that distress/sadness is so central to Woolf's personality that it clarifies the meaning of various life situations, provides continuity, and organizes the self-image. Haviland's approach and her conclusions have implications for studying and theorizing about personality development.

In Chapter 18, Gilligan and Bower present an extensive series of empirical investigations on the effects of hypnotically induced emotions on learning and memory. Their overall conclusion is that emotion or mood has significant measurable effects on what is learned and remembered. The effects of the emotion experience vary with the type of material (input), the match between the emotion and the emotion connotation of the material, and the intensity of the emotion. They show that emotions affect a wide range of cognitive processes including free associations, fantasies, and social judgments. They interpret their findings in terms of their associative network model that begins ontogenetically with a limited set of innate emotion-arousal-expression connections and expands throughout a lifetime of learning and acculturation.

Part I

Theoretical issues in emotions and cognition

1 Emotion-cognition relationships and human development

Carroll E. Izard

A decade ago I defined personality as a set of interrelated systems: the homeostatic, motor, emotion, perceptual, and cognitive systems (Izard, 1971). I postulated several characteristics of this set of systems. Of most relevance for the present discussion is the assumption that though interrelated and typically interdependent, the systems have separate functions, and they can and do, under certain conditions, operate independently. I believe that distinctions among these systems and the primacy of emotions can be most clearly seen in early development. Emotion processes have to be primal in human behavior if the central postulate of differential emotions theory – that the emotions system is the primary motivational system for human beings – is true.

Emotion-cognition interactions

The assumption of separate organismic systems such as emotion and cognition is alarming to some people, but it does not imply Cartesian dualism or parallelism. Systems that interact do not run on parallel circuits. In the cases of the various organismic systems, they necessarily share neural circuits or interconnecting neural pathways to allow the systems to develop as the organized holistic set that we identify as the individual, autonomous person. Thus postulating separate organismic systems implies the consequent postulate that human development can be described as the growth processes whereby the separate organismic systems become an effectively organized set – an autonomous integrated whole, capable of adapting as an individual and of forming social bonds. Another consequent postulate is that dysadaptive development results from failure of biosocial growth processes to produce effective organization of the organismic system.

The assumption of separate systems for emotion and cognition creates no more of a Cartesian dichotomy than the division of the brain and central nervous systems into functional complexes such as sympathetic system and parasympathetic system, somatic system and autonomic system. The heuristic value of these divisions for the neurosciences has ample documentation. Yet

Preparation of this chapter was supported by NSF Grant BNS 811832.

17

no neuroscientist would argue that any one of these systems alone accounts for very much in the way of integrated adaptive behavior. Rather, these brain and neural systems interact in intricate and complex fashion. Similarly, the emotion system and the cognitive system interact in intricate and complex ways in facilitating the integration of the super system, or individual person, and in the bonding of person to person in social relationships.

The survival of the individual requires that its systems produce actions (sometimes with great rapidity) that adapt it to its environment or ecological niche. In evolutionary perspective it seems reasonable to assume that early forms of life adapted on the basis of simple sensory-affective processes long before complex cognitive phenomena emerged. In early life forms, the function of emotion, or affect, was to motivate approach and avoidance behaviors that provided nurturance and escape from harm. To survive, unicellular or very simple organic structures needed only two affects, one to subserve approach and nurturance and the other, avoidance or defense. By the time evolutionary processes produced human beings, there were many emotions. Even in young infants we have observed expressive behaviors that signal many different emotions, each having inherently adaptive functions that relate both to the individual and to the social group (Izard et al., 1980).

The function of an emotion for the individual is evidenced in the motivational value and action tendency that stem from the quality of consciousness that characterizes the "felt emotion." The primary social functions of emotion are (a) signaling something of the expressor's feelings and intent, (b) providing a basis for certain inferences about the environment, and (c) fostering social interactions that can facilitate the development of interpersonal relationships. Each emotion that emerged over the course of human evolution added a different quality of motivation and new behavioral alternatives that increased adaptive prowess. For example, *interest*, a very important positive emotion, motivates cognitive and motor search and exploratory behaviors, and *anger* mobilizes energy for physical action as well as confidence in one's powers (Izard, 1977). Both interest and anger, like each of the emotions, are significant determinants of selective attention and hence of the contents of perception and cognition.

Zajonc (1980) has also argued that it is necessary to modify the typical information-processing model because it neglects affective phenomena. He suggests that new models need to allow for important occasions wherein affect precedes what is typically described as cognition, or information processing, based on discriminanda. Norman (1980) does not argue for a principle of affective primacy, but he sees emotion as one of twelve "issues," or "topic matters," essential to cognitive science, and he maintains that the "pure cognitive sciences" of the past two decades have taught us little about how we learn to converse or read and write or to remember what we said or how we forget it.

A central issue for contemporary psychology is the question of whether the emotions constitute a separate system that requires the use of noncognitive concepts and variables to study it. Put another way, is it fruitful to think of emotion processes and the emotion system as sources of significant independent variables that are important predictors of human development? As Norman's (1980) discussion of the state of cognitive science makes very clear, studying cognition without considering emotion variables led to a science of "pure cognition" that shed little light on learning, thought, and memory as experienced outside the laboratory. Zajonc (1980) suggests that we need to examine the possibility of emotion-cognition interactions at different levels. I strongly support this view and would like to comment briefly on possibilities for interaction within each of the three levels or components of emotion.

Interaction of the neurophysiological substrates of emotion and cognition

The case for considering emotions as a separate system seems fairly well established at the neurophysiological-biochemical level. At this level it is well known that some brain structures, neural pathways, and neurotransmitters are relatively more involved than others with emotion expression, emotion experience or feelings, and emotion-related behaviors. The limbic system is sometimes referred to as the "emotional brain," and that at least one limbic structure, the hippocampus, has been strongly implicated in information processing (Simonov, 1972) and memory (O'Keefe & Nadel, 1979) suggests the existence of brain mechanisms, specially adapted for mediating emotion-cognition interactions. It is plausible that the hippocampus forms part of the neural substrate of the emotion of interest, which in turn can be considered as the motivational basis for selective attention, a cognitive process that is critical in providing focus for learning and memory. Tucker's (1981) recent review of the experimental and clinical literature on lateral brain functions led him to conclude that the two hemispheres are differentially involved in emotion and cognition and that without the neurophysiological processes that give rise to emotion there is no cognition.

Interaction of emotion and cognition at the behavioral-expressive level

Consistent with differential emotions theory and the separate-systems view, the behavioral-expressive component of emotion is a direct function of sensory processes that do not require cognitive mediation. Surely this is true for the discrete emotion expressions that infants produce prior to the emergence of the first level of object permanence or short-term *cognitive* memory.

Perhaps the statement that young infants' emotion expressions do not require cognitive mediation will be clearer if we draw a distinction between the concepts of information processing and cognition. The term cognition as typically used by psychologists is a narrower concept than information processing. The latter term as used in the various life sciences includes neural coding and the transmission of messages by genes, hormones, and enzymes. Because information processing in its generic sense occurs continuously in living organisms, any discussion of the sequencing of emotion and cognition requires some specification of what is meant by emotion *and* by cognition, and the latter has to be defined more narrowly than information processing.

Just as genes contain neurochemical information that can be processed without cognition (in the usual sense), so too preprogrammed motor patterns (facial expressions) contain affective information that can be processed without cognition. It is reasonable to assume that processing of the sensorimotor information in preprogrammed facial expressions is mediated by the neural substrates of the emotions. Such processing is basically *affective processing* mediated by the *affective* structures associated with the motor patterns of the fundamental emotions.

Some additional affective structures relating preprogrammed affective information to other phenomena are acquired before the infant has the capacity to develop cognitive structures that involve representational memory. In ontogenesis these preprogrammed and early acquired affective structures associated with the motor patterns of emotion expressions are the foundation for the life-span development of a network or open system of *affective-cognitive* structures.

The motor pattern we call the "social smile," displayed by the 1½- to 5-month-old infant indiscriminately to strange and familiar people, illustrates one type of affective information processing. Any nodding face or facelike object can provide the affective information (input), and a preprogrammed affective structure mediates the patterned neuromuscular activity of the social smile. One could argue that the infant is at least discriminating "faceness" from "nonfaceness," but one can also argue that this level of information processing is affective in nature: the sensing and perceptual registration of a particular affect-eliciting pattern. The infant at this age is incapable of the comparison or matching of perceptual input and stored schema that is typically associated with cognitive processing. Yet this simple smiling response is highly adaptive in fostering social bonds. The ethological concepts of innate releaser and innate releasing mechanism provide an analogy to affective information and affective structure, but the latter in comparison with innate releasers in lower animals are conceived as less rigid in nature and more amenable to change as a function of learning and experience.

Although the emotion expressions of young infants (and the uninhibited ones of any age group) are automatic-reflexive, the principal mechanism of expression, the superficial musculature of the face, is innervated by the somatic nervous system and is under voluntary control. Thus, at the expressive level, too, the stage is set for emotion-cognition interactions. Perception of a need to appear calm or brave or a decision to acquiesce to a cultural rule can lead to voluntary expressions that simulate, albeit imperfectly, the facial patterns of emotion without the activation of the corresponding emotion feeling. There is considerable evidence that supports the hypothesis that these cognitively instigated or voluntarily simulated expressions can be used, as Darwin (1872/1965) and James (1890/1950) suggested, to regulate or even activate genuine emotions (Duncan & Laird, 1977; Laird, 1974; Laird et al., 1982; Rhodewalt & Comer, 1979; Zuckerman et al., 1981). In view of the cognitive and motor capability of instigating simulated emotion expressions, it is reasonable to hypothesize that cognitive processes can be used to reduce the intensity or duration of the innate expressions of a genuine emotion and hence to regulate the neurophysiological and subjective-experience components of the emotion. Indeed, Lanzetta, Cartwright-Smith, and Kleck (1976) and Lanzetta and Orr (1980) have confirmed this hypothesis with adult subjects.

Interaction of emotion and cognition at the experiential level

In an early study of the emotion-cognition interface, some of my students and I (Izard, Wehmer, Livsey, & Jennings, 1965) studied the effects of induced enjoyment and anger on selective perception. Enjoyment was induced by warm, friendly interactions and compliments, and anger by cold, hostile interactions and insults. One set of stimuli consisted of photographs of 26 people, each portraying joy in one pose and anger in another. The second set of stimuli were photographs of 22 pairs of people portraying a friendly interaction and a hostile interaction. The photographs of contrasting happy and angry faces and interpersonal scenes were mounted in pairs and presented in a stereoscope. The stereoscope exposes the contrasting stimuli (happy, angry) to different visual fields, and the subject resolves binocular rivalry by perceiving either the right or left photograph or a fusion. Special procedures were used to eliminate problems of illumination and focus and to control for differential acuity, convergence, and eye dominance. The data for the two sets of stimuli – facial expressions and interpersonal scenes – were analyzed separately.

The interpersonal induction of joy and anger had a strong effect on selective perception. Subjects in the joy-induction condition resolved the binocular rivalry significantly more frequently in favor of the joy expression and friendly interpersonal scenes. Subjects in the anger-induction condition perceived significantly ($p < .01$) more angry expressions and hostile scenes in the stereoscope. The results clearly supported the differential emotions theory postulate that emotion influences basic cognitive processes, even determining the content of perception.

A second experiment examined the effects of self-esteem and induced emotion on interpersonal perception, opinion change, and performance on cognitive tasks. Subjects were divided into four levels of self-esteem based on their scores on the Tennessee Self-Concept Scale (Fitts, 1954). Positive and negative emotion induction was accomplished by structured role playing similar to that in the preceding experiment except that the confederate was an experienced actor. The dependent measures were the subjects' perceptions of the experimenter, the experiment, amount of opinion change relating to the choice of treatment for a juvenile offender, and performance on three cognitive tasks: naming multiple uses for common objects, digit span, and problem solving. The predicted effects were obtained for both induced emotion and level of self-esteem. Induced positive emotion resulted in more favorable perceptions of experimenter and experiment, a greater amount of opinion change, and better performance on all three cognitive tasks. A predicted interaction effect for induced emotion and self-esteem on intellectual performance was supported by the data on the cognitive tasks of multiple uses and problem solving.

The second experiment demonstrated the breadth and pervasiveness of the influence of emotion on a variety of cognitive processes. The affected responses ranged from affective-cognitive phenomena like preferences and attitudes to intellectual performance on tasks assessing rote memory and creativity. A recent study of Hettena and Ballif (1981) extended these findings by showing a similar main effect for naturally occurring emotion states.

We conducted several other experiments on the influence of positive and negative affective stimuli on learning and recall (Izard, Nagler, Randall, & Fox, 1965; Izard, Wehmer, Livsey, & Jennings, 1965). Independent variables in the different studies included interpersonal treatment or role-play, electric shock, and attractive and aversive pictures. The dependent variable was retention or memory, measured on a variety of paired associate learning tasks. The results were consistent with our prediction that induced emotion significantly affects learning and recall. Stimuli of different affective valence elicited different rates of learning and amounts of material recalled. Both intensity and quality of emotion significantly influenced these processes, and the relevance of the affect-inducing stimuli was important in determining the influence of emotion on cognition.

Fifteen years after these early experiments – which were buried under an avalanche of cognitive psychology – Bob Zajonc (1980) made an eloquent case for separate systems for affect and cognition and for the primacy of emotion in matters of mind. He summarized numerous ingenious experiments showing that affective processing and affective judgment of objects were independent of and prior to basic cognitive processes involved in feature discrimination. The next year Gordon Bower (1981) presented excellent data demonstrating the influence of various discrete emotions on learning and recall. Bower reported the results of several well-designed experiments emphasizing particularly the mood-congruency effect on memory. For example, anger during recall facilitates recall of material learned in an angry mood, sadness improves recall of unpleasant events in childhood, and so forth (Gilligan & Bower, Chapter 18, this volume).

A paper by Laird and his associates (1982) extends our findings and those of Zajonc, Bower, and their colleagues in a very interesting way. First, they reviewed the evidence supporting the facial feedback hypothesis of emotion activation – different versions of which have been detailed in differential emotions theory and by Laird (1974). The evidence suggests that under certain conditions even blind experimental manipulation of facial muscles into patterns of emotion expression produce emotion feelings or experiences corresponding to the patterns. This was true at least for certain subjects. According to Laird, they were those who favored self-produced cues over situational cues in the experimental situation. Empirically, they were divided into these two types based on whether they reported emotion experience changes corresponding to manipulated facial patterns.

In Study 1, subjects were told that the study was concerned with muscular activity during cognitive tasks. The requested facial muscle movements actually produced either the smile of joy or the frown of anger. The procedure was in three parts: (a) subjects received four trials of the muscle manipulation procedure to determine which subjects would experience emotion as a result of the self-produced cues, (b) subjects read a happy or angry passage, (c) subjects were manipulated into a happy or angry expression and asked to write down as much of the passage as could be recalled. The results confirmed the hypothesis that the self-produced cue group recalled significantly better when their happy or angry expression matched the happy or angry passage. Since the expression manipulation had no effect on recall in the situational cue group, the investigators attributed the improved memory in the self-produced cue group to the emotion experience generated by the manipulated expression. I think this is accurate inference, but there are alternative explanations of the generation of emotion experience by facial expression. Laird follows a Bemian (Bem, 1967) type self-inference view in which the subjects somehow infer their emotion experience from their own facial behavior. Differential emotions theory holds that limbic-cortical integrative processing of the sensory feedback from the face generates emotion experience without self-inference or any other cognitive-attributional process. Attribution explains or describes some phenomena very well, but it is not needed in the basically neurosensory process of generating emotion feeling.

I do not want this difference in conception of the mechanism generating emotion feeling to detract from the empirical finding of Laird and his associates (1982). They have shown convincingly that expression-generated emotion experience can guide memory and influence the quantity and the affective quality of material recalled.

The point I want to emphasize here is that although emotion and cognition are in large measure *interdependent*, another body of evidence suggests as well that emotion processes and cognitive processes have a significant degree of *independence*. Thus there is a heuristic advantage in maintaining a distinction between emotion as we feel it and experience it in consciousness and the accompanying cognitive processes in consciousness, which we do not feel. Thus emotion at the conscious level is a special kind of awareness (cf., Levy, 1982) that generates motivational cues for cognition and behavior and provides a sense of attachment and engagement with the social and physical world. Support for the concept of emotion experience or emotion feeling as motivating and cue-producing comes from the studies on emotion, memory, and perform- ance just reviewed. That emotion feeling connects and engages the individual in the social and physical world is supported in part from the evidence that emotion motivates, in particular from the evidence that empathic emotion fosters prosocial behavior (see Hoffman, Chapter 4, this volume). Further, Bowl- by's (1969) intensive observations of the first social relationship – mother–infant attachment – led him to describe it as basically an emotional phenomenon. Finally, the evidence described by Sroufe and his associates (Chapter 10, this volume) makes a case for the role of emotion and emotion expression in the development of social competence and peer relationships.

On the assumption that emotion at the conscious level is a special kind of awareness or *feeling*, one can argue that emotion has no cognitive component. I maintain that the emotion process is bounded by the feeling that derives directly from the activity of the neurochemical substrates. In this framework, then, emotion-cognition relationships develop as emotion feeling and cognitive processes interact in consciousness to form affective-cognitive structures, which by definition have both an emotion and a cognitive component. These affective- cognitive structures, products of the interaction of biological and sociocultural phenomena (learning and experience), become the more and more predominant structures of mind with increasing age.

The theoretical arguments and empirical data favoring the assumption of primacy of emotions in human development and human behavior recognize that cognition, in turn, influences emotion processes. Cognition is a highly important source of events that activate and regulate the emotions. However, other emotions and physiological needs also serve these functions. Fatigue can lower the threshold for anger, interest can attenuate sadness, and severe depression can demolish interest. Such changes in emotion states are changes in the quality of consciousness that account for the selectivity of attentional processes and hence the content of cognition and the direction of behavior.

Emotions in human development

The concept of emotional development has so many possible meanings that it is of rather limited value in a scientific vocabulary. In addition to meaning different things to different investigators, the term has not been carefully delineated in relation to developmental processes. The first requirement for a discussion of this topic is a definition of an ;motion. A given emotion is defined as the integration of a particular set of neurochemical, motor, and mental processes (Izard, 1977). It is assumed that the neurochemical process of a given emotion has some underlying structural features that distinguish it from any other emotion, and evidence for this comes from its unique motoric and mental representations. The motoric representation, facial expression, is innate and universal, for at least a limited set of emotions (Ekman, Friesen, & Ellsworth, 1972; Izard, 1971). In early life the motoric representation is encoded in a visible configuration of facial (and sometimes bodily) movements (Izard et al., 1980; Hiatt, Campos, & Emde, 1979). With socialization (the enculturation of norms for emotion expression) and the development of self-regulation, the motoric representation may create changes in muscle potential (sufficient for sensory feedback to participate in the activation of emotion feeling) without changes in observable facial patterns (cf., Schwartz et al., 1974). Evidence supporting the universality of the motoric representation of a given emotion suggests that its mental representation, or feeling component, is also cross-culturally constant, that is, people in different cultures label the motoric representation, or facial expression, with semantically equivalent terms.

Our definition of emotion might suggest to some that the interfacing of emotions and developmental processes is an easy process. Certainly there are well-recognized developmental processes in the biological, social, and experiential-motivational domains. But the emotions pose some special and infrequently considered problems. First, several of the emotions are fully functional at birth (e.g., interest, distress, disgust), at least at the motor-expressive (or social signaling) level (see Izard, 1978). The question remains as to whether the other components of these emotions must go through a course of development before emotion can be felt or experienced. There is no evidence bearing directly on this issue, but differential emotions theory assumes that in normal infants the essential quality of the feeling component of any basic emotion is activated whenever the facial-movement pattern of that emotion is spontaneously displayed. It also assumes that the emotion-specific feeling is invariant over the life-span and that it is, in fact, a central ingredient in selfhood and in the sensing of self as active and continuous across time and situations.

The postulate of invariance in emotion feelings is a radical departure from cognitively oriented theories, which hold that emotions change as a function of cognitive development (see Kagan, Chapter 2, this volume). In weighing the tenability of the postulate, three things should be considered. First, it is the invariance of emotion feeling that is postulated, not the invariance of event-emotion, emotion-cognition, or emotion-behavior relationships. All the latter follow a developmental course; they are a large part of the subject matter of emotional development.

Second, emotion feeling as defined here – a direct derivative of certain neurochemical-sensory processes not requiring cognitive transformation or cognitive representation – is very basic to animal adaptation, providing cues that guide approach and avoidance and a variety of other environmental interactions. The survival value of emotions as motivations for goal-directed behaviors requires invariance of their basic cue-producing function.

Third, in view of the considerable overlap in neural mechanisms subserving both the sense of taste and the emotions, it is possible to argue by analogy that feeling states, like taste discrimination, are invariant across the life-span.

For many species the ability to discriminate and experience the basic tastes – sweet, salt, sour, bitter – develops prenatally and those that do not have the ability at birth develop it within a few weeks, apparently independent of experience. Thus experience can shape a wide variety of taste preferences and aversions, but learning and experience are not required for the development of the basic taste discriminations (Scott, 1981). What I am proposing is that the fundamental emotion feelings are analogous to the basic gustatory experiences and like them are mediated by phylogenetically old subcortical structures.

In the course of evolution, animals developed a gustatory system that serves both protective and body-maintenance functions relative to sound nutrition. It is noteworthy that gustation is not independent of affect or motivation. The gustatory system is so intimately bound to taste hedonics that its capacity to recruit the positive and negative affects of sensory pleasure and disgust is critical to its effectiveness. Thus gustation plus the sensory pleasure of delectables can challenge and overcome cognitive decisions to diet and avoid obesity (Scott, 1981; Scott, personal communication, 1982).

Gustatory information is processed primarily in the medulla and pons, and taste discrimination is apparently complete at, or caudal to, the midbrain (Scott, 1980). Of special interest for emotion researchers, Grill and Norgren (1978) have shown that taste reactivity can be determined by observation of orofacial mimetic responses. They found that decerebrate and normal rats show virtually identical taste reactivity (Grill & Norgren, 1978a, 1978b).

The work of Steiner (1973, p. 254; 1974, p. 229) suggests that taste discrimination in humans is also largely a function of brainstem mechanisms. He found that anencephalic neonates responded to sweet, sour, and bitter substances (sucrose, citric acid, quinine) with appropriate acceptance–rejection responses and with different facial-affective responses. They sucked, swallowed, and smiled to sucrose, and they spit or vomited and cried to quinine. The presence of these affective responses suggests that at least some rudimentary emotion-expressive behavior (probably the endogenous smile and physical distress) is processed in the brainstem but, following the taste analogy, that an intact limbic system is probably necessary for the generation of motivational-feeling states. Although the brainstem mediates taste discrimination in decerebrate rats, such animals are not capable of developing conditioned taste aversions. For the latter, it seems reasonable to assume that some kind of association mechanism and motivation substrates not resident in the brainstem would be required.

Differential-emotions theory proposes that the quality of a given emotion feeling is as invariant as the processes that determine taste hedonics (sensory pleasure and disgust) and that emotion feelings like sensory pleasure and disgust are essential for the effective operation of the cognitive and motor systems. In contrast, however, to the specificity of the relationship of taste hedonics to gustation, emotion feelings have great generality and flexibility and can become, through learning and experience, motivation for a virtually endless variety of thoughts and actions.

There is one other aspect to the analogy between the development of taste and the development of emotions. Sensory biopsychologists who study taste have not yet considered the broader concept of flavor. This is so, in part, because flavor is not simply a function of the gustatory sense but is probably influenced as well by the olfactory, haptic, and visual senses and countless cultural factors. I suggest that in some respects the development of an affective-cognitive structure – the interaction or bonding of emotion and cognition in values, attitudes, and traits – is similar to the development of flavor appreciation.

If we accept the analogy between the development of the four basic gustatory sensations and the development of the basic emotion feelings, then it is reasonable to assume that the invariance of the feeling state of a fundamental emotion goes back through eons of evolutionary time (cf., Izard, 1982; Panksepp, 1982). To assure survival and adaptation, emotions, as motivations for coping behaviors, had to retain an invariant and unerring directional impact on awareness and behavior. The anger and fear mechanisms generate defensive-attack or escape-avoidant behaviors that facilitate survival in hares and hominids alike.

Still, the theoretical position sketched here must deal with the objection from cognitively oriented theories of development that in early infancy there is no subjective consciousness and no emotion (Kagan, Chapter 2, this volume). My answer to this objection begins with reference to my definition of emotion at the subjective-experiential level as *feeling* that can exist in consciousness without being symbolized or represented cognitively. A feeling is by definition a conscious process, a part of awareness. The credibility of the assumption that young infants experience emotions hinges on the further assumption that feelings can exist as a product of neurochemical processes independent of their cognitive representation. To deny this is to say that neurochemical activity resulting from trauma or tickling that leads to a motor representation or facial expression of emotion neuromuscularly identical to the adult expression (Izard et al., 1980) does not lead to a mental-affective representation or emotion feeling. Surely there is sensory feedback from the motor-expressive movements to the brain, and this neural input must affect the brain in some way. That its effect is the integration of the sensory data into a discrete feeling seems consistent with the premise that emotions are inherently motivational and adaptive. It seems important for even the young infant to experience the motivational aspect of emotion feeling even though it cannot represent the feeling cognitively.

What is certainly not present in consciousness in early infancy is any cognitive (imaginal, symbolic) representation of emotion feeling, for the young infant is incapable of this.

My argument for emotions in young infants calls for two types of conscious processes or awareness. The first is a function of sensory data being transformed directly into feeling, which is considered as the mental or affective representation of emotion. This contrasts with processes by which sensory data are transformed into images, schema, or symbols, the cognitive contents of consciousness. I propose that both the affective and cognitive contents of consciousness can and do exist at different levels of awareness. The level of awareness for feelings varies with the intensity of the feelings, with low-intensity feelings operating more in terms of filtering and focusing percpetual-cognitive processes and high-intensity feelings dominating consciousness by gating out information irrelevant to the emotion and the related coping behaviors.

Not all emotion expressions are present at birth. Anger is thought to emerge at about 4 months, fear at 7 or 8 months, and guilt in the second year. Do these emotions, unlike those present at birth, undergo something more than biologically programmed developmental changes? Do they have precursors, pass through stages, or undergo modifications? Evidence of any kind relating to these questions is scant (see Sroufe, 1979), and evidence showing the development of an anger or fear expression by the gradual addition of components or by the modification of an earlier expression is totally absent.

Although evidence for developmental changes in these emotions is scarce, various developmental antecedents can nevertheless be demonstrated. At least this is true for certain event-cognition relationships. For example, the infant apparently does not show fear of strangers before about 8 months of age and the attainment of some level of immediate memory (object permanence) (Emde, Gaensbauer, & Harmon, 1976), fear of heights before some locomotor experience (Campos et al., 1978), or anger at separation from mother until after social attachment (Shiller & Izard, 1981). But these responses are event-specific and tell us little about the emergence of these emotions in the infant's repertoire. Thus attachment is an antecedent to anger during mother–infant separation, but attachment is not a prerequisite of anger expressions. The infant of 4 months, and well before object permanence or attachment, expresses anger at arm restraint (Stenberg, Campos, & Emde, 1981).

I suspect that the later appearing emotions, like those present at birth, are preprogrammed on a biological clock and that their time of emergence is largely a function of the maturation of their underlying neural substrates and of the substrates of the cognitive and motor functions that subserve the motivational component of these emotions. Of course, even a biological clock can be speeded up, slowed down, or rendered defective by trauma, deprivation, and many less dramatic circumstances. Still, under reasonably normal circumstances, all the emotions emerge on schedule, and on emergence, each one is prepared to respond to a limited set of incentive events without any conditioning or learning experience. Thus, not only emotions but a circumscribed set of event-emotion relationships are part of our evolutionary-biological heritage.

Is it possible or fruitful, then, to characterize the concept of emotional development in such a way as to make it understandable and useful? Let us examine this possibility by considering emotional development in terms of each of its components and in terms of emotions as systems interacting with other organismic systems, in particular the motor and cognitive systems.

Emotional development at the neurophysiological level

I have proposed that the development of the brain mechanisms and pathways of the emotions is largely a matter of biological growth processes that begin in the embryo and produce functional mechanisms for most of the fundamental emotions by the end of the first nine months postpartum and for the rest by midway the second year. That this is mainly biological development does not mean that it is unalterable. It has been well established that radical environmental events and conditions can modify neural structures (Dennenberg, 1981). Most of the hard data come from animal research, but there is suggestive evidence that the fear mechanism becomes functional much earlier than usual in abused infants (Gaensbauer, 1980). What we do not know is how much the development of the emotion circuitry is influenced by less dramatic events and circumstances, by frequent use or disuse, or by subtle but pervasive social influences.

I have argued that the biological development that is required for the basic emotion expressions and feelings occurs prenatally or in the early months of life. This does not mean that the neural substrates do not continue to develop after the individual is capable of expressing and experiencing the fundamental emotions. Biological development is necessary for the establishment of inhibiting processes and self-regulating capacities. Thus, with biological development of emotion substrates, changes occur in emotion responsiveness or emotion thresholds for particular incentive events. Changes also occur in the intensity and duration of emotions in relation to particular events. For example, young infants display the physical distress expression in response to inoculation longer than do older infants. Further biological development of the neural substrates of emotion, together with development in motor and cognitive capacities, may account for the greater amount of anger that older infants show as a result of inoculation (Izard et al., 1983). In summary, there is some evidence that patterns of emotion expression in relation to specific events change with increasing age. Yet, although the direct evidence is lacking, emotional responsiveness in general or emotion thresholds determined by a broad spectrum of incentive events probably show continuity or traitlike characteristics. There is indirect support in the research on temperament (see Derryberry & Rothbart, Chapter 5, this volume).

Adamec's (1978) experimental alteration of the temperament of cats is suggestive of possibilities in this domain. Adamec conceived the amygdala, a structure in the limbic system, as a source of emotional biasing. He used a variety of threatening stimulus situations to sort cats into groups according to their natural affective disposition or temperament, ranging from bold rat killers to fearful nonattackers that withdrew to a sheltered location even in the face of a mild threat. Adamec found that the threshold for production of an after discharge upon stimulation of the amygdala varied inversely with the cats' sensitivity to threat. In other words, the cats with the lowest after-discharge thresholds, indicative of a tendency to become neurally overactive, were also the most fearful. Where Adamec used kindling techniques to lower the after-discharge threshold of the fearless killer cats, they became more fearful in the threatening stimulus situations.

Viewing the experiential component of emotion as a feeling state that derives directly from activity of the neurochemical substrates makes it reasonable to assume that emotion in human beings is analogous to that in other animals. Thus Adamec's study, like differential emotions theory, suggests that emotional disposition or temperament in human and nonhuman animals can be conceived in terms of emotion thresholds. The concepts of temperament and emotion thresholds as determinants of personality have not received the attention they deserve in experimental psychology.

Emotional development at the expressive level

Involuntary or spontaneous emotion expression is tied to the neurophysiological component of the emotion. Research across cultures and with the born blind and other deviant populations has shown that the basic patterns of facial expression are preprogrammed for at least a limited set of emotions (Darwin, 1872/1965; Eibl-Eibesfeldt, 1970; Ekman et al., 1972; Izard, 1971). I have labeled these the fundamental emotions and maintained that all emotion experiences derive directly from them, either separately or from blends and interactions among them.

That fundamental emotions have innate expressions does not mean that there is no variability in expressive patterns. Individual variation is basic to the evolutionary process, and biology accounts for some of the variability in expressions. Izard and his associates (1983) studied developmental changes in 2- to 19-month-old infants' affect expressions following the acute pain of inoculation. They found that with increasing age there was a significant decrease in the physical distress expression and a significant increase in the anger expression. Although only a few of our 2-, 4-, and 6-month-old infants expressed anger, most of our 19-month-olds did. Data from a study of Campos and Stenberg (1981) suggest that the sharp increase in anger expression between 6 and 19 months was not due simply to changes in the ability to express anger.

They found that 4-month-old infants regularly expressed anger in response to arm restraint.

A study of Huebner and Izard (1983) suggests that the younger infants' relatively greater use of the compelling social signals of the distress expression following acute pain is adaptive. They found that the distress expression, more than the anger expression, elicited care-giver tendencies to minister to the physical needs of the infant. On the other hand, an anger response to pain might be more adaptive in the 19-month-old, who is more capable of using anger-mobilized energy in organized defensive behavior.

Two other findings indicated the meaningfulness of individual differences in anger expressions following pain. Duration of objectively coded anger expression following DPT inoculation at 19 months correlated significantly with mothers' ratings of the infants' anger expressiveness in daily life. And mothers' ratings of their infants' anger expressiveness at 12 months correlated highly significantly with mothers' own self-reported anger experiences when their infants were 19 months old. There was a lower, though significant, correlation between mothers' self-reported anger experiences when their infants were 12 months old and their ratings of the infants' anger expressiveness at 19 months of age. These data show that relationships between events and emotion expressions undergo development and that these changes can index important developmental phenomena in the infant and the infant–mother relationship (Izard, Huebner, & Hembree, 1983).

The foregoing findings leave open the possibility that culture and social learning as well as biology can influence emotion expression in a number of ways, varying from the modification of a basic pattern to the structuring of rules regarding the time and place for expression (Ekman, 1972; Izard, 1971). At the same time that culture is influencing involuntary expression it is shaping the development of voluntary expressions such as the social smile, which may bear no relation, or even an inverse relation, to underlying emotion experience. All five of the mechanisms or processes of development described by Flavell (1972) may operate here.

It should be noted in this discussion of expressions that the cultural shaping of expressions may be tantamount to the cultural shaping of emotion experiences. There is a growing body of evidence that supports the facial feedback hypothesis of emotional activation (see Laird et al., 1982; Zuckerman et al., 1981). Most of the evidence has come from studies using various techniques to manipulate facial muscles into emotion expression patterns. Although this technique seems intrusive and subject to demand characteristics and confounding, it has proved repeatedly effective in well-controlled experiments in producing predicted emotions in subjects who remain sensitive to self-produced cues in the experimental situation (Laird et al., 1982).

To the extent that the facial-feedback hypothesis is valid, modifications in expressive patterns as well as culturally determined inhibition or the facilitation of expression or expressive style can be expected to alter the flow of emotion experiences and by implication personality development. Precisely how and to what extent learned modifications in expressions and expressive styles affect social, cognitive, and personality development are problems for future research.

Emotional development at the subjective-experiential level

One way to understand the issues in emotional development at the subjective-experiential level lies in the definition of this third component of emotion as a feeling state, distinct from cognitive processes. It is assumed that some emotion feeling is present in consciousness all the time. The notion that emotions are transient phenomena arose largely as a result of the rapid onset and frequently micromomentary duration of certain expressions and the pervasiveness in early animal research of experimentation involving the eliciting of emotions with intense stimulation or under emergency conditions. The duration of emotion experience cannot be judged by expression. The most significant functions of expression relate to emotion activation and social communication. The duration of a given emotion feeling in consciousness is a function of several variables including cognition and the level of particular hormones and neurotransmitters in the brain and nervous system. Fortunately, under most circumstances, emotions do not remain at high intensities for very long, but a decrease in intensity does not necessarily mean a decrease to zero or nonexistence. Whenever a particular emotion feeling does exit consciousness, one or more of those waiting in the wings immediately enters.

If we assume that the third component of emotion is a *feeling*, not an image, symbol, or thought representing a feeling, then a central issue of emotional development is immediately obvious: In the course of development emotions must be effectively linked with cognitive processes and instrumental behaviors. In this conceptual framework, emotional development can be viewed as the development of integrative processes and mechanisms that adaptively organize emotion, cognition, and action.

A somewhat more concrete conceptualization can be achieved by considering the transition from the prelingual infant to the verbally accomplished child. In the early months of life social communication is primarily accomplished by facial and vocal expression (Emde et al., 1976; Malatesta & Izard, in press; Sroufe, 1979). Empirical evidence suggests that these expressive signals have some specificity of meaning for the care giver (Izard et al., 1980; Scherer, 1982). Care-giver responses are differentially influenced by these signals (Huebner & Izard, 1983; Malatesta, 1981a, 1981b), and infants, in turn, are influenced by the care giver's expressive behavior (Tronick et al., 1978).

Beginning usually in the second year of life after many important social transactions have occurred (e.g., attachment), the child adds language to its repertoire of communication skills. But as important as language is to development, it does not replace the nonverbal signal system; for as Zajonc (1980) and others have noted, verbal communication may always be in second place in significant social interactions. Nevertheless, the process of adding language to the already existing nonverbal communication system is of monumental importance in human development.

The central questions for the interested developmental psychologist are how do emotion-feeling processes and linguistic-symbolic processes relate, and how does the addition of these great new capabilities affect the child? The child who was once capable only of experiencing a given emotion directly as a feeling becomes capable of representing that feeling in consciousness, with or without that particular feeling being present. What is the differential impact of existential feeling as sense impression and the symbolic representation of feeling on cognition and behavior?

In any case it is undoubtedly a landmark in emotional development when feeling and thoughts about feeling are able to exist in consciousness simultaneously. The child can, in fact, have one feeling in consciousness while dealing with others symbolically. This is of great consequence for the development of emotion regulation, empathy, and prosocial behavior (cf. Hoffman, 1978, and Chapter 4, this volume).

In the course of development, particular feelings and patterns of feelings become associated with particular classes of images, symbols, and actions, resulting in the development of affective-cognitive structures and networks. In such networks, emotion feelings constitute the main organizing and motivational forces, influencing what we perceive (Izard et al., 1965), what we remember (Bower, 1981; Laird et al., 1982), and what we think and do.

Summary

I have argued for a systems conception of personality and for the assumption that emotions operating separately and in combination or patterns constitute the chief motivational system, the most important wellspring of human behavior. A corollary of this assumption is that emotions subserve the growth processes and thus allow the separate organismic systems to become an effectively organized, integrated whole.

Emotions and cognition are considered as separate but interrelated, interactive systems. A growing body of empirical evidence now exists indicating that different emotions and patterns of emotions affect perceptual and cognitive processes differentially.

There is some reason to believe that there is interaction between the neural substrates of emotion and cognition. They share common structures in the limbic system. Emotion and cognition interact in numerous ways at the motor-expressive level. Emotion expression by means of sensory feedback (Izard, 1977) or self-perception (Laird et al., 1982) leads to emotion ᵢₑ ling/experience, which in turn influences perceptual and cognitive processes – attention focusing, learning, memory.

Several experiments have shown that cognitive processes (verbal instructions, imagery, hypnosis) can induce emotion, which in turn significantly influences cognition in specific ways. In the experiment conducted by Laird and his colleagues (1982), induction of a specific emotion *expression* led to the corresponding emotion *experience* that produced specific effects on learning and memory.

This chapter presents a discussion of several assumptions relating to emotions in human development: (a) Emotion conceived as motivation for cognition and behavior can also be conceived as primal in development, facilitating the functioning and organization of the various organismic systems. (b) The invariance of emotion feelings over the life-span provides a sense of continuity and contributes to the development of the self-image or concept of self. (c) Feeling is the mental representation of emotion, and it is important to distinguish between emotion experience as *felt* and as *symbolized*. The young infant who can represent emotion only as *motor expression* and *feeling* eventually becomes capable of feeling one emotion while symbolizing and verbalizing another.

That the core emotion feeling is invariant over time does not indicate a lack of emotional development. On the contrary, the invariance of emotional feeling states serves a stabilizing and organizing function in development. Emotional development at the neurophysiological level produces the inhibitory and self-regulatory capacities so essential to effective adaptation amid increasingly complex social and environmental demands. Development at the motor-expressive level brings children increasing command over their emotion expressions, including expression regulation (and also expression inhibition, fragmentation, masking, etc.) and the use of voluntary expressions in social interactions. Research on the development of emotion expressions, or expressive styles, must be concerned with the possibility that the regulations or shaping of emotion expression or expression style through socialization may be tantamount to shaping emotion experiences.

Emotional development at the subjective-experiential level is best understood when this level is conceived as a feeling state, a noncognitive phenomenon. Emotion feeling states are the motivational aspect of experience, and through development they become linked to images, symbols, and thoughts. This process results in affective-cognitive structures and orientations that shape personality and behavior.

References

Adamec, R. E. Normal and abnormal limbic system mechanisms of emotive biasing. In. K. E. Livingston & O. Hornykiewicz (Eds.), *Limbic mechanisms*. New York: Plenum, 1978.
Bem, D. Self perception: An alternative interpretation of cognitive dissonance phenomena. *Psychological Review*, 1967, *74*, 183–200.

Bower, G. H. Emotional mood and memory. *American Psychologist*, 1981, *36*, 129–148.

Bowlby, J. *Attachment and loss* (Vol. 1). New York: Basic Books, 1969.

Campos, J. J., Hiatt, S., Ramsay, D., Henderson, C., & Svejda, M. The emergence of fear on the visual cliff. In M. Lewis & L. Rosenblum (Eds.), *The development of affect*. New York: Plenum, 1978.

Campos, J. J., & Stenberg, C. *An appraisal process crucial for infant emotional development*. Paper presented at the Meeting of the Society for Research in Child Development, Boston, 1981.

Darwin, C. R. *The expression of emotions in man and animals*. London: Murray, 1965. (Originally published, 1872.)

Dennenberg, V. H. Hemispheric laterality in animals and the effects of early experience. *Behavioral and Brain Sciences*, 1981, *4*, 1–49.

Duncan, J., & Laird, J. D. Cross-modality consistencies in individual differences in self-attribution. *Journal of Personality*, 1977, *45*, 191–196.

Eibl-Eibesfeldt, I. *Ethology: The biology of behavior*. New York: Holt, 1970.

Ekman, P. Universals and cultural differences in facial expressions of emotion. In J. K. Cole (Ed.), *Nebraska symposium on motivation* (Vol. 19). Lincoln: University of Nebraska Press, 1972.

Ekman, P., Friesen, W. V., & Ellsworth, P. *Emotion in the human face: Guidelines for research and an integration of findings*. New York: Pergamon Press, 1972.

Emde, R. N., Gaensbauer, T. J., & Harmon, R. J. *Emotional expression in infancy*. New York: International Universities Press, 1976.

Fitts, W. H. *The role of the self concept in social perception*. Unpublished doctoral dissertation, Vanderbilt University, 1954.

Flavell, J. H. An analysis of cognitive-developmental sequences. *Genetic Psychology Monographs*, 1972, *86*, 279–350.

Gaensbauer, T. Anaclitic depression in a 3½-month-old child. *American Journal of Psychiatry*, 1980, *137*(7), 841–842.

Grill, J. H., & Norgren, R. The taste reactivity test. I. Mimetic responses to gustatory stimuli in neurologically normal rats. *Brain Research*, 1978, *143*, 263. (a)

Grill, J. H., & Norgren, R. The taste reactivity test. II. Mimetic responses to gustatory stimuli in chronic thalamic and chronic decerebrate rats. *Brain Research* 1978, *143*, 281–297. (b)

Hettena, C., & Ballif, B. Effect of mood on learning. *Journal of Educational Psychology*, 1981, *73*(4), 505–508.

Hiatt, S. W., Campos, J. J., & Emde, R. N. Facial patterning and infant emotional expression: Happiness, surprise, and fear. *Child Development*, 1979, *50*(4), 1020–1035.

Hoffman, M. L. Empathy, its development and prosocial implications. In H. E. Howe, Jr., & C. B. Keasey (Eds.), *Nebraska symposium on motivation* (Vol. 25). Lincoln: University of Nebraska Press, 1978.

Huebner, R. R., & Izard, C. E. *Mothers' responses to infants' facial expressions of sadness, anger, and physical distress*. Unpublished manuscript, 1983.

Izard, C. E. *The face of emotion*. New York: Appleton-Century-Crofts, 1971.

Izard, C. E. *Human emotions*. New York: Plenum, 1977.

Izard, C. E. On the development of emotions and emotion-cognition relationships in infancy. In M. Lewis & L. A. Rosenblum (Eds.), *The development of affect*. New York: Plenum, 1978.

Izard, C. E. From stimulus-bound emotive command systems to drive-free emotions. Commentary on J. Panksepp's "Toward a general psychobiological theory of emotions." *Behavioral and Brain Sciences*, 1982, *5*(3), 433–434.

Izard, C. E., Hembree, E. A., Dougherty, L. M., & Spizzirri, C. C. Changes in 2- to 19-month-old infants' facial expressions following acute pain. *Developmental Psychology*, 1983, *19*(3), 418–426.

Izard, C. E., Huebner, R. R., & Hembree, E. A. *Anger in infants and mothers*. Manuscript in preparation, 1983.

Izard, C. E., Huebner, R. R., Risser, D., McGinnes, G., & Dougherty, L. The young infants' ability to produce discrete emotion expressions. *Developmental Psychology*, 1980, *16*(2), 132–140.

Izard, C. E., Nagler, S., Randall, D., & Fox, J. The effects of affective picture stimuli on learning, perception and the affective values of previously neutral symbols. In S. S. Tomkins & C. E. Izard (Eds.), *Affect, cognition and personality*. New York: Springer-Verlag, 1965.

Izard, C. E., Wehmer, G. M., Livsey, W., & Jennings, J. R. Affect, awareness, and performance. In S. S. Tomkins & C. E. Izard (Eds.), *Affect, cognition, and personality*. New York: Springer-Verlag, 1965.

James, W. *The principles of psychology*. New York: Dover, 1950. (Originally published, 1890.)

Laird, J. D. Self-attribution of emotion: The effects of expressive behavior on the quality of emotional experience. *Journal of Personality and Social Psychology*, 1974, *29*, 475–486.

Laird, J. D., Wagener, J. J., Halal, M., & Szegda, M. Remembering what you feel: The effects of emotion on memory. *Journal of Personality and Social Psychology*, 1982, *42*, 646–657.

Lanzetta, J. T., Cartwright-Smith, J., & Kleck, R. E. Effects of nonverbal dissimulation on emotional experience and autonomic arousal. *Journal of Personality and Social Psychology*, 1976, *33*(3), 354–370.

Lanzetta, J. T., & Orr, S. P. Influence of facial expressions on the classical conditioning of fear. *Journal of Personality and Social Psychology*, 1980, *39*(6), 1081–1087.

Levy, R. I. *On the nature and functions of the emotions: An anthropological perspective*. Unpublished manuscript, 1982.

Malatesta, C. Z. *Determinants of infant affect socialization: Age, sex of infant and maternal emotional traits*. Unpublished doctoral dissertation, Rutgers University, 1980.

Malatesta, C. Z. Affective development over the lifespan: Involution or growth? *Merrill-Palmer Quarterly*, 1981, *27*, 145–173. (a)

Malatesta, C. Z. Infant emotion and the vocal affect lexicon. *Motivation and Emotion*, 1981, *5*, 1–23. (b)

Malatesta, C. Z., & Izard, C. E. Human social signals in ontogenesis: From biological imperative to symbol utilization. In N. Fox & R. J. Davidson (Eds.), *Affective development: A psychobiological perspective*. Hillsdale, N.J.: Erlbaum, in press.

Norman, D. A. Twelve issues for cognitive science. In D. A. Norman (Ed.), *Perspectives on cognitive science: Talks from the LaJolla Conference*. Hillsdale, N.J.: Erlbaum, 1980.

O'Keefe, J., & Nadel, L. Précis of O'Keefe and Nadel, "The hippocampus as a cognitive map" (and open peer commentary). *Behavioral and Brain Sciences*, 1979, *2*(4), 487–533.

Panksepp, J. Toward a psychobiological theory of emotions. *Behavioral and Brain Sciences*, 1982, *5*(3), 407–467.

Rhodewalt, F., & Comer, R. Induced compliance attitude change: Once more with feeling. *Journal of Experimental Social Psychology*, 1979, *15*, 35–47.

Scherer, K. R. The assessment of vocal expression in infants and children. In C. E. Izard (Ed.), *Measuring emotions in infants and children*. Cambridge: Cambridge University Press, 1982.

Schwartz, G. E., Fair, P. L., Greenberg, P. S., Freedman, M., & Klerman, J. L. Facial electromyography in the assessment of emotion. *Psychophysiology*, 1974, *11*, 237.

Scott, T. R. Taste and hedonics: A neural assessment. In H. van der Starre (Ed.), *Olfaction and taste VII*. London: IRL Press, 1980.

Scott, T. R. Brain stem and forebrain involvement in the gustatory neural code. In Y. Katsuki, R. Norgren, & M. Sato (Eds.), *Brain mechanisms of sensation*. New York: Wiley, 1981.

Scott, T. R. Personal communication, University of Delaware, May, 1982.

Shiller, V. M., & Izard, C. E. *Patterns of emotion expression during separation*. Unpublished manuscript, University of Delaware, 1981.

Simonov, P. V. On the role of the hippocampus in the integrative activity of the brain. *Acta Neurobiologiae Experimentalis*, 1972, *34*, 33–41.

Sroufe, L. A. Socioemotional development. In J. D. Osofsky (Ed.), *Handbook of infant development*. New York: Wiley, 1979.

Starr, A., McKeon, B., Skuse, N., & Burke, D. Cerebral potentials evoked by muscle stretch in man. *Brain*, 1981, *104*, 149–166.

Steiner, J. E. The human gustofacial response. In J. F. Bosma (Ed.), *Fourth symposium on oral sensation and perception*, pp. 254–278. Rockville, Md.: U.S. Department of Health, Education and Welfare, 1973.

Steiner, J. E. Discussion paper: Innate discriminative human facial expressions to taste and smell stimulation. *Annals of the New York Academy of Science*, 1974, *237*, 229–233.

Stenberg, C., Campos, J., & Emde, R. *The facial expression of anger in seven month old infants.* Unpublished manuscript, 1981.

Tanaka, T., & Asahara, T. Synaptic actions of vagal afferents on facial motoneurons in the cat. *Brain Research*, 1981, *212*, 188–193.

Tronick, E., Als, H., Adamson, L., Wise, S., & Brazelton, T. B. The infant's response to entrapment between contradictory messages in face-to-face interaction. *Journal of the American Academy of Child Psychiatry*, 1978, *17*, 1–13.

Tucker, D. M. Lateral brain function, emotion, and conceptualization. *Psychological Bulletin*, 1981, *89*(1), 19–46.

Zajonc, R. B. Feeling and thinking: Preferences need no inferences. *American Psychologist*, 1980, *35*(2), 151–175.

Zuckerman, M., Klorman, R., Larrance, D., & Spiegel, N. Facial, autonomic, and subjective components of emotion: The facial feedback hypothesis versus the externalizer-internalizer distinction. *Journal of Personality and Social Psychology*, 1981, *41*(5), 929–944.

2   The idea of emotion in human development

Jerome Kagan

Most theoretical essays on human emotion written by Western philosophers or psychologists begin by assuming a limited set of discriminable experiential qualities, each associated with broad but boundaried classes of events and named by words, like fear or anger, that contain no reference to the originating context or target of the experience (Rorty, 1980). Although scientists do not agree on the quintessential events that define emotion (some award origin and centrality to the limbic lobe, others attribute those qualities to the patterned discharges of facial muscles), they all agree that a necessary feature of the class of phenomena called emotional is a change in internal state. For William James, the change in internal state was the central event and the immediate cause of an emotion (James, 1981).

James's position implies that it is both empirically possible and theoretically useful to separate the patterned bodily changes – no matter what their source – from any accompanying or subsequent psychological events. The chain of reasoning, which is not intellectually taxing, assumes that different classes of external incentives or thoughts are lawfully linked to special biological events that are the fundamental elements in emotion. Theorists favoring this view wish to award a name to the internal state while acknowledging that it should be different from the name given to the combination of the change in state and its subsequent detection and cognitive appraisal. This is a reasonable strategy, even if the two experiences are not always separate for the subject. Garner (1981) has noted that even though scientists acknowledge that the perception of a flower is immediate, holistic, and unanalyzed, the experimental psychologist analyzes into separately named mechanisms the unity that was unanalyzed by the perceiving subject.

Independent of the eventual utility of this epistemological position, I believe that the universally popular emotional labels – for example, fear, sadness, joy – are used most often to refer to the combination of a detected change in

Preparation of this chapter was supported in part by grants from the Foundation for Child Development and the John D. and Catherine T. MacArthur Foundation. I thank Joseph Campos for his comments on an original draft and informal conversations during preparation of the final manuscript and J. S. Reznick for his collaborative wisdom in the empirical work to be described.

38

internal state and an appraisal, rather than to the raw, unevaluated physiological changes, even if we grant the possibility that "raw feels" exist without any cognitive participation whatsoever (Rorty, 1979). However, under either frame, the variety in potential feeling states is enormous; hence, James suggested that the number of emotions was limitless.

If one should seek to name each particular one of them [emotions] of which the human heart is the seat, it is plain that the limit to their number would lie in the introspective vocabulary of the seeker, each race of men having found names for some shade of feeling which other races have left undiscriminated (James, 1981, 2:1097).

This conclusion has never appealed to most empiricists who have selected for study a very small proportion of the total number of possible internal states and treated them as biologically more fundamental than the rest. The so-called primary emotions studied by Western psychologists – most often fear, anger, contempt, joy, sadness, disgust, excitement, surprise, guilt, and shame – omit many emotions that some cultures would regard as equally fundamental derivatives of potentialities inherent in the human genome. Thirteenth-century Japanese Buddhists claimed that the state of enlightenment was the most significant affective mood to attain; modern Japanese regard the emotion of *amae* (the feeling of mutual interdependence with another) as primary (Doi, 1973). The Utku Eskimo of Hudson Bay believe *naklik* (the feeling that accompanies wanting to nurture and protect another) is a primary emotion (Briggs, 1970); the Ifalukians of Micronesia treat *song* (the feeling that accompanies noting that another person has violated a community norm) as a basic human feeling (Lutz, 1982).

Reflection on the emotions Western psychologists designate as primary suggests that this status may be due to their significant pragmatic consequences. They are perceptually salient events that often interfere with sustained, difficult thought, accompany or follow successful coping with a challenge, communicate to others information on how to behave, or lead to symptoms that interfere with the capacity for love and work. These are good reasons for studying these particular states, but they are not a persuasive rationale for regarding them as more significant or fundamental than others. The feeling state that accompanies a lovely sunset and the mood that follows strenuous physical exercise, although perceptually distinct, are rarely named as primary, perhaps because neither seems to have obvious pragmatic consequences, for successful problem solving, communication, or mental health.

The controversies surrounding the classification of emotional states resemble the disagreements over the last three centuries among naturalists and biologists regarding the proper way to classify living forms. Hence, a brief consideration of those nodes of debate may clarify comparable themes in the study of emotions. First, because it is so easy to find shared qualities among objects and events, it is possible to invent many classification schemes that place the same objects or events in different categories. For example, classifications of the apes and hominids vary depending on whether one uses similarities in the structure of the cerebral cortex or physiological macromolecules, like hemoglobin (Mayr, 1982). It is necessary, therefore, to select a criterion that can guide the choice of features to be given special weights in the classification scheme.

The evolutionary biologists chose phylogenetic descent as the central criterion, and its application serves to eliminate many qualities that are irrelevant to that criterion, like economic value, habitat, or social relationship to man. Unfortunately, psychologists have not yet achieved consensus on a criterion for the classification of emotions. Those who make communicative potential the criterion concentrate on affect states that are accompanied by visible gestures and facial expressions. Hence, when the face of a crying infant assumes the same morphology as that shown by a husband yelling at his wife (squared mouth, narrowed eyes, and eyebrows drawn together), it is assumed both organisms are experiencing the state of anger. Investigators who make the phenomenological feeling states of pleasure–displeasure a major axis of classification are tempted to place a display of justified anger at a rival in the same category with smiling at the attainment of a goal, if both make the agent "feel better." Scientists who choose similarities in physiology as the basis for classification occasionally assume that an acceleration of heart rate or a decrease in skin resistance in response to an incentive event indicates the presence of an emotional state, often called arousal (Mandler, 1975). Finally, those who are interested in the relation of motives to emotions are prone to focus on the intensity of feeling, for perceptually salient feeling states are most likely to alter motive hierarchies and maintain in ascendance those wishes that are associated with intense feelings. None of these schemes is wrong or muddleheaded. Each is correct given the criterion selected, just as it is not incorrect to classify deer, oysters, and frogs in a common category because all are expensive cuisine.

A major advance in biological taxonomy occurred in the early part of the nineteenth century when the strategy of classification changed from the dichotomous splitting of superordinate categories into subunits to a more profitable inductive strategy in which the investigator detected similarities in morphology at the level of individual organisms and moved up to higher taxa by combinations of shared features. I suspect this inductive plan will also be useful in the study of emotions. Currently many investigators begin their work by assuming the reality of abstract categories, like fear, joy, and sadness, and create subcategories within each by noticing subtle distinctions in incentive and response. But it may be more profitable, as it has been for taxonomists, to begin at the level of real events and synthesize new affect categories. That is why I suggested in an earlier paper (Kagan, 1978) that emotion is a superordinate term representing the varied relations among external incentives, thoughts, and detected changes in internal feeling states, as weather is a superordinate term for the relations among wind velocity, humidity, temperature, barometric pressure, and form of precipitation. We do not ask what weather means but determine, instead, the relations among the measurable phenomena and name the discrete coherences. Similarly, it may not be useful to debate the meaning of emotion; rather, the task is first to detect and then to name the coherences. We should, for example, agree on a label for the combination of seeing a dangerous animal in an unfamiliar place, expecting physical harm, and perceiving a sudden increase in heart rate. But the name for that coherence should be different from the one applied to seeing a frown on the face of a loved one, expecting a sign of rejection, and noticing a similar sudden rise in heart rate because I suspect complete profile of physiological reactions to the two incentives is different and because the behavioral consequences are rarely similar. However, one problem with this position is that it awards too little significance to the changes in internal state that are not perceived, even though one contemporary philosopher restricts the meaning of emotional state to only those occasions when a person's evaluation of an incentive leads to a physiological change (Lyons, 1980).

Issue 1: the significance of detection of feeling tone

The importance assigned to the subject's conscious detection of a change in feeling state is one of the three major nodes of controversy (the other two pertain to the naming of affect states and the empirical indexes used to infer emotional states). Put plainly, how shall we classify the reliable state changes that are not recognized?

Most adults react to an unexpected event they are mentally set to evaluate with a positive, event-related potential that occurs at about 300 msec following the stimulus and, less regularly, a cardiac deceleration that reaches its trough at about 5 sec after the onset of the unexpected stimulus. I doubt that adults in such a situation detect any distinct feeling at 300 msec after the presentation of the incentive. Similarly, eye blinks and/or pupil dilation often accompany presentation of a difficult problem, but most persons would not report a change in feeling state while these reactions were occurring.

The presence or absence of detection of internal changes is of extreme importance for the subsequent emotional state. I do not suggest that the undetected biological changes are unimportant, only that the evaluation that follows detection often changes the affect experienced. Years ago I experienced after each meal a headache that lasted from 5 to 15 minutes. I evaluated the throbbing feeling as a possible sign of a serious organic illness and named my affect anxiety whenever the headache occurred. After a doctor reassured me it was due to psychological factors, I began to analyze its relation to my mood and decided, whether valid or not, that it was most likely to occur when I felt sad. From that time forward, whenever the symptom appeared, or when I anticipated its appearance, I experienced an affect of sadness, not anxiety.

My headache had not changed, but my emotion had, solely because of the change in evaluation.

Every event occurs in a larger frame, and the consequence of the event is always dependent on the frame in which it is inserted. This principle holds even at the level of the individual cells of the motor cortex. Depending upon the animal's set to act, the neurons of the motor cortex respond in dramatically different ways to the same stimulus, namely, an imposed flexion of the paw. In one experiment a monkey was trained to make a pulling action at the appearance of a red light and a pushing reaction in response to a green light. When the monkey was set to issue a pull response, because it had just seen a red light, the motor neurons displayed one pattern of reaction to the flexing of the paw. When the animal was set to push, because it had seen a green light, the identical neurons displayed a different pattern of discharge to the same imposed flexion of the paw (Tanji & Evarts, 1976). Schwartz (1982, p. 91) notes that an "emotion cannot be equated with a particular behavioral expression, a particular subjective experience, or a particular underlying physiological response. Rather, all of the above are incomplete manifestations, at different levels, of a complex process that can be inferred only from the convergence of the pattern of such responses."

I prefer to call the undetected physiological changes "internal tone" and the detected ones "feeling states." The perceptual dimensions of the changes in feeling state include rise time, perceived origin, intensity, and hedonic quality. The perceived change in feeling state, unlike the change in internal tone, is a discrepant event that invites an interpretation of cause, a name, and a behavioral plan. Hence, perceived changes in state might be regarded as motivational and predictive of changes in thought and action. These consequences are missing when physiological changes are undetected.

However, many believe that the core of an emotion is inherent only in the biological changes that define feeling tone, and they award secondary significance to the cognitive judgment that follows detection, or to the combination of detection and appraisal, although they do not disregard these subsequent states completely. I suggest that the states are different and should be awarded different category names. The state defined by an undetected ten-beat change in heart rate to a mild insult should be treated as different from one in which the same cardiac change to the insult was detected; the afferent patterns created by the smiles of a sleeping newborn should not be classified with the smile of a 5-year-old on seeing his mother return from a holiday. Although the constructs that name patterns of undetected bodily changes – whether in facial muscles, heart, palm, or stomach – are legitimate, they should be distinguished from those that name detected and evaluated changes. Both classes of phenomena can be regarded as belonging to the superordinate category of emotional.

It might be helpful to treat the physician's distinction between disease and illness as analogous to the differences between the undetected changes in internal tone and the evaluated feeling state. Human biologists posit a set of lawful relations between specific pathogens and subsequent changes in tissues and metabolic functions. These coherences are given disease names, like cancer or tuberculosis, whether or not the patient has any conscious recognition of the change in internal function. Indeed, prophylactic medical examinations are intended to find these undetected physiological changes.

However, on occasion, the diseased individual becomes aware of the biological changes created by the disease, and if he or she evaluates them as resulting from a pathogenic process, the person regards the self as having an illness. The recognition typically has nontrivial consequences. It creates a novel psychological state that can either exacerbate or reduce the symptoms of the disease, depending upon the coping mechanisms implemented. In some cases, the realization that one is ill leads both to new symptoms, because of disturbances in eating and sleeping, and to special reactions from those to whom the patient communicates his state of illness.

This state of affairs seems analogous to emotional phenomena. An impending responsibility can produce a change in biology that, although undetected by the subject, is detected by an observer. If the person eventually detects the change in tone and evaluates his state, let us say, as anxious, a new feeling state is created that alters the original one and has communicative implications for others. The differences between the states before and subsequent to appraisal pose a serious quandary with respect to the classification of the two states. Should the scientist regard the evaluated state simply as a gloss on the original, undetected one created by the impending responsibility or treat the new unity as a different emotional state? Human biologists usually prefer the former frame. If a woman who learned she had a malignant tumor became an insomniac and, as a result, became seriously fatigued and developed new symptoms, her new physiological state would be diagnosed as an addition to, not a replacement of, the original cancerous state.

Although many investigators prefer the medical strategy, it is not obvious that it is the correct frame for classifying acute emotional states, in part, because of the transient and dynamic nature of acute affect states. When the immune system recognizes a small number of pathogens, it destroys them before the biologist would classify the person as having a disease. It is likely that both positions are reasonable, with the choice depending on the theoretical interests of the investigator, another example of the wisdom of Bohr's principle of complementarity. If the investigator wishes to explain the coping behavior that follows evaluation of a change in feeling tone, it is probably more useful to assume that detection and evaluation produce a new and different emotional state. However, if the investigator was more interested in explaining the changes in facial musculature or cardiac responses that follow an incentive, it would not be an error to treat the state subsequent to the evaluation as a gloss on the original change in feeling tone.

Issue 2: the naming of feeling states

The differences among acting, thinking, and feeling are so compelling phenomenologically that most scholars have assumed these distinctions must represent fundamentally different psychological functions. But classifications based on intuition are often misleading. Our intuitions also insist that ice, snow, fog, and water are fundamentally different substances and that the sun moves around the earth. Humans invented emotional terms to describe the fact that on occasion, an action, external event, or thought seems to produce a perceptible change in feeling state. Even though children and adults in a particular culture agree on the meaning of some emotional terms, the names for those states should not be regarded as referring to fixed material entities that can be defined intrinsically, as we do for trees and robins. Rather, most often they are names for the less than perfect covariation that exists among classes of external incentives, thoughts, and detected changes in feeling states. The popular emotional words, like the terms *witch*, *phlogiston*, or *quark*, are constructs. This position is not less defensible because children and adults agree on the feelings they believe accompany hypothetical but stressful situations (Shields & Stern, 1979).

Although most scientists are ready to admit that the words they use to name human motives are arbitrary and intended only as constructs, many do not extend this frame to emotions. Motives and emotions are classes of internal states linked to classes of incentives, and, occasionally, they are detectable in behavior. Because the maturation of cognitive competences probably changes the nature of a motive – the 15-year-old's desire for recognition is not the same as the 2-year-old's – it is also likely that the 2-year-old's emotional reaction to a mother's sneer is different from that of a 15-year-old. But, unfortunately, because we use the same language to name emotions in 2- and 15-year-olds but more often use different motive labels for the two age groups (we do not say the 6-month-old has an affiliative or a power motive), many investigators write as if the experiences were the same, not unlike the sixteenth-century herbalists who classified wheat (a grass) with buckwheat (a dicotyledon) because both had *wheat* in their name (Mayr, 1982). Darwin went further and assumed that insects were capable of anger, terror, jealousy, and love (Darwin, 1965, p. 349). The view that emotional experience does not change with growth assumes that the central nervous system's reaction to salient incentives remains constant over ontogeny. But this premise ignores the major changes that occur in brain structures and functions during the early years of life. If the brain's pattern of discharge to an emotionally relevant incentive is a major basis for the emotion, it is likely that the emotions of infants and adults are not identical, and indeed may be far less similar than has been supposed.

Because each emotional name is a classification category, the extraordinary diversity among cultures in presuppositions and values should be accompanied by differences in how feeling states are categorized (we do not know how they are experienced). Hence, there should not always be consensus across societies in the envelope of referents to which particular emotional words are applied. Indeed, the variation across societies in the classification of emotions may be greater than the variety of categories used to name plants and animals. (Berlin, Breedlove, & Raven, 1973, have reported that the names for plants and animals used by certain tribes in New Guinea are close to Linnean groupings.) The influence of culture on the choice of emotional terms is nicely illustrated in a study of emotional words used by the approximately 500 people living on the small isolated atoll of Ifaluk, located in the Western Caroline Islands of Micronesia (Lutz, 1982).

Fago, one of the most frequently used emotional words on Ifaluk, has no clear synonym in English. *Fago* is applied to that feeling provoked by individuals who need help, have suffered illness, death in the family, or misfortune, have subordinate status, or surprisingly, possess qualities that are in accord with the ego ideal of the society, which includes a state of calm and generosity. Sympathy or compassion comes close to capturing the meaning of *fago* for the first five examples, but no English-speaking adult would use the word sympathy to name the feeling aroused by a person who is respected and admired. The fact that the Ifalukians do implies a symbolic parsing of emotional experience different from our own. The Ifalukians believe that a child under age 7 cannot experience *fago* because of immaturity in mental capacity. It is likely that the ability to appreciate a state of misfortune in another across a variety of situations is one basis for the Ifalukian belief. A Piagetian would be pleased by this hypothesis, for the child under age 7 is presumed to be too egocentric to appreciate subtle states of need in other persons, although the young child can empathize with obvious distress.

Song, another frequently used term, is best translated as "justified anger." The primary incentive for applying *song* to experience is improper behavior by another person, often a violation of the community norm regarding false gossip or the sharing of resources with another. But *song* is also used when misfortune befalls a person to whom one feels *fago*. There is no comparable word in English that covers both situations. The Ifalukians use a different term, *nguch*, for states of frustration or annoyance that are less justifiable. Thus, the Ifalukians make a linguistic distinction between two forms of anger, which is less clear in English, for we use angry, irritated, or mad to name either class of incentive.

The importance of context in the application of Ifalukian affect terms is also apparent in the use of *rus* and *metagu*. *Rus* names the feeling that arises when an agent is in a situation of potential physical harm – a typhoon, a violent fight – and experiences a salient internal reaction. *Rus* seems close in meaning to the English term *fear*, but not quite, for the sudden death of a person also elicits *rus*. Thus, a mother would say she felt *rus* if her child died, while

English speakers would be less likely to declare they felt fear to that event. *Metagu* refers to situations that have the potential to cause *rus* – a future interaction with a stranger, possible encounter with a ghost, or anticipation of the anger of, or rejection by, another person. *Metagu* comes close to what we might call social anxiety, but this is not a perfect translation.

Lutz analyzed 31 Ifalukian affect words using multidimensional scaling techniques. The resulting space suggests that Ifalukians were likely to group emotions on the basis of similarities in their incentives. For example, *song* (justified anger), *tang* (grief), and *fago* (compassion), which were grouped together, are typically generated by the properties or actions of other people. By contrast, the incentive conditions for *metagu* (anxiety), *kamayaya* (indecision), and *fileng* (incapability), which were grouped in a cluster distant from the first set, require prolonged reflective thought.

A comparable analysis of the groupings of English emotional words by Americans would probably reveal that a similarity in the intensity and evaluation of feeling states would be more significant than a similarity in incentives. English affect terms typically focus on the quality of the agent's feeling experience and, unlike the language of the Ifalukians, do not contain a sharp differentiation with respect to the psychological origin of the feeling. Thus, anxiety and anger, which are intense, unpleasant feelings, would be closer in English than *song* and *metagu* are in Ifaluk. This suggestion is supported by the fact that when American college students rated 717 concepts for their emotionality, the resulting factor analysis revealed that evaluation was the first factor and degree of arousal was the second. None of the factors implied classifications based on context or situation; all involved the quality of the agent's feelings, evaluations, and sense of control (Averill, 1980).

The affect terms of the Utku (Briggs, 1970) are also differentiated by context. For example, different terms are used to name the desire to be with another, to kiss or touch another, or to be under the covers with another. The Gururumba, a New Guinea group, ascribe an emotional term meaning "wild pig" only to men between about 25 and 35 years of age who lose control of socialized behavior, because during this age interval men assume marital and social responsibilities that are anxiety arousing. Similar behavior in a 15- or a 60-year-old would not be awarded the same affect label (Newman, 1960).

For the Ifalukians, the Utku, and the Gururumba, other people are significant incentives for emotional states, and motives and emotions associated with people are awarded a special status they do not have in English. We might speculate that individual mastery and achievement in Western society have the same degree of salience that relations with other people do in non-Western cultures. English terms for emotions are Platonic. Like the cognitive competences we call memory, perception, inference, or reasoning ability, emotional words are names for events minimally constrained by the specific situation that provokes them. This attitude is not of recent origin. When David Hume declared that pride and humility were the basic emotions, he ignored completely the contexts in which those passions occurred.

Although English affect words do not map exactly on those used by members of other cultures, some might reply that this linguistic relativism is unimportant for the understanding of emotion. The central fact, it is argued, is that beneath the language there are universal relations among certain incentive events, physiological reactions, and experiential outcomes. This position has not been refuted by any set of empirical data. But if we are interested primarily in the class of evaluated changes in feeling states, it is reasonable to assume that the imposition of an interpretive label on the evaluation of a situation-cum-feeling will have psychological consequences. Hence, the private experience of an Ifalukian who has witnessed a violation of a community norm on gossiping may not be identical to that of an American who has seen an adolescent maliciously tease an old woman.

There is, of course, a way out of the counterintuitive suggestion that my experience to a coiled, venomous snake is not like that of the Ifalukian. Identity of experience is probably too strong a criterion to impose. Let us borrow the biological distinction between species and variety and suggest that there are classes of emotions defined by the quality of feeling associated with the evaluation of a thought or incentive event. The feelings following loss of hope in attaining a goal, danger to one's body, violation of a standard, and threat from a rival represent some basic classes. But within each of these classes individuals from different age and cultural groups will have different varieties of emotional experience because of variation in the symbolic evaluation of the union of feeling, thought, and incentive.

The need for new names

Because most empirical inquiry in this domain uses a limited number of indexes (most often self-report, changes in facial expression, decreased skin resistance, or increases in heart rate) to a limited number of incentives in young adult subjects, it is usually possible to assimilate the data to the popular emotional terms. But when the investigator studies different parameters in infants, where evaluation is less likely, the imprecision in available emotional terms is revealed, as long as the investigator avoids the temptation to impose a priori emotional categories and accommodates to the special combinations of behavioral and autonomic reactions that occur to certain events.

In a recent experiment in our laboratory 45 infants, 14 months old, were habituated to a series of chromatic slides of physically different exemplars of *dogs* and *women*. Following habituation, the children saw, in random order, three different transformations on each category, each separated by a representation of a new member of the familiarized category. The three transformations were a dog (or a woman) without a head, without limbs, or without

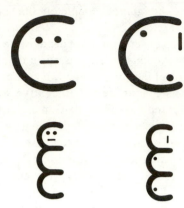

Figure 2.1. The four stimuli shown to 8-, 14-, and 20-month-old infants for a single trial.

a body. When each child's heart rate to each transformation was compared with its heart rate to an exemplar of the familiarized category on the immediately previous trial, the picture of "woman without a head" produced a distinctive cardiac reaction while the children were looking at the stimulus. More children showed their least variable heart rate (defined by the standard deviation of the interbeat intervals) to that stimulus than to either of the other two transformations on the woman, whereas for the category *dog*, most children showed a minimally variable heart rate to the dog "without limbs." Of the 17 children who showed their lowest heart rate variability to woman "with no head," 14 had their lowest variability to the dog with either no body or no limbs ($p < .05$). Significantly more children showed their lowest heart rate variability to "no head" when *woman* was the familiarized event than when *dog* was the familiarized category.

It is reasonable to assume that removing the head from such a familiar event as a woman would produce a special psychological state in the 1-year-old infant that might not occur to the same change in the less familiar dog. But what word should we award to the psychological state, probably unevaluated, that accompanies this cardiac reaction in this context? It is not obvious that the popular emotional terms, like fear, interest, or surprise are appropriate. The child's face and posture revealed no signs of wariness or anxiety, and interest and surprise are usually accompanied by a cardiac deceleration and, therefore, an increase in heart rate variability.

A different experiment on children 8, 14, and 20 months old provides a similar result. At the end of a series of episodes in which infants were habituated to chromatic slides of animals and people, each of 48 infants was shown only one of four black-white stimuli for a single 20-second trial (12 infants in each group). The stimuli are illustrated in Figure 2.1. Duration of fixation time, heart period, and the standard deviation of all the interbeat intervals were quantified. Heart period increased linearly with age and equally for all groups (that is, the heart rate decreased with age). Fixation times were equal to the four stimuli at 8 months, but slightly higher to the two figures composed of a single circle than to the figures composed of three circles at 14 and 20 months. But the key observation held for heart-rate variability. Despite equal variability values for all four figures at 8 months, heart-rate variability decreased with age only for the three-circled figure without a face, and by 20 months it evoked significantly lower heart-rate variability values than the other three stimuli. If we assume that this stimulus was the most difficult event to assimilate to the child's schema for a human, it is reasonable to conclude that when 1- to 2-year-old infants are having difficulty assimilating an event, they are in a special state that is not always revealed by duration of fixation time.

Consider a related example in which similar evidence invites the invention of a less popular emotional term. The story begins with the discovery of a relation between extreme behavioral inhibition to the unfamiliar in 2-year-old children and a tendency to show a rise and stabilization of heart rate while processing visual and auditory information that is not immediately assimilable (Garcia Coll, 1981). Briefly, out of a group of 117 children, 21 months old, preselected by a telephone interview with their mothers to be behaviorally inhibited or uninhibited in unfamiliar places or with unfamiliar people, about one-half of the children were, indeed, extremely inhibited or uninhibited when they were observed on two occasions in a laboratory setting following confrontation with unfamiliar adults, a brief separation from the mother, and a large robot figure that lit up and spoke to the child. Some children stopped playing, became extremely quiet, withdrew to their mothers, and clung to the parent for several minutes. The uninhibited children, by contrast, approached the unfamiliar adults or object with little or no wariness. The children were taken to another laboratory where they saw slides of events ranging from moderately familiar (women and dogs) to completely unfamiliar (abstract patterns), and they listened to recordings of environmental sounds and human speech. The children who had been behaviorally inhibited with the unfamiliar people and the robot showed higher heart rates to all the information and significantly more stable heart rates to the more unfamiliar stimulus events.

One way to interpret this association is to assume that children become sympathetically aroused when they sustain a mental set to assimilate discrepant information that is not immediately comprehensible. We chose the term *vigilant* as a descriptive label for this state. Others may prefer phrases like *sustained mental effort*, *cognitively aroused*, *confused*, *puzzled*, or *uncertain*. Obrist, Light, & Hastrup (1982) note that sympathetic influences on the heart (which typically lead to slight acceleration and stabilization) are most likely to occur when the subject has an opportunity to try to cope with an aversive event. One prediction implied by these terms is that children who adopt this mental set consistently will be perceptually more analytic when they are trying to relate a discrepant event in their perceptual field to their acquired knowledge.

Reznick (1982) familiarized 48 infants, 8 months old, on physically different exemplars of four categories: women, dogs, infants, and butterflies. When the children had habituated to these categories (or saw them for a maximum of 18 trials), each child was shown, in random order, a stimulus that was very similar to the familiarized category (e.g., a cat for the category *dog*; a bee for the category *butterfly*); a stimulus moderately discrepant from the familiarized category (a frog for *dog*, a bird for *butterfly*); and a novel stimulus that had no relation to the familiarized category (a truck, car, set of keys). The dependent variable of interest was the relative degree of dishabituation of attention to each of the three classes of discrepant events within each child – an ipsative analysis.

The children who showed both the highest and the least variable heart rates during the base-line period, before the familiarization began (the cardiac pattern we use to infer a vigilant mental set), were significantly more likely to show maximal dishabituation of fixation time to the stimuli that were most similar to the familiarized category; the least vigilant children were most likely to show maximal dishabituation of attention to the novel events.

These results have implications for our theoretical attitude to the naming of emotions. We have discovered what appears to be a robust relation between a particular cardiac pattern and a class of incentives investigators might call a "discrepant event that is difficult to assimilate." That coherence invites a name, and we have chosen *vigilance*. Recall that when 14-month-olds saw the stimulus in which the most central feature of a person was removed (the head of a woman), or when 20-month-olds saw the three-circled figure with scrambled facial parts, many children showed a stabilization of heart rate. Although the reader may prefer a different term, none of the most popular affect words – fear, interest, or surprise – seems to be the best descriptor. There is no reason to assume that "vigilance" is a less primary affect than interest or surprise. It has not been included as a primary affect because the relevant experiments have not been performed. I suspect that many more coherences remain to be discovered. The fact that the state we call "vigilance to discrepant events" is not currently popular in the vocabulary of either scientists or nonscientists has less to do with its psychological significance than with the fact that it has not been easily detected in the popular sources of evidence that come from changes in the face or molar behavior, but might be.

But biologists did not know that the cell was the primary structure until the power of microscopes was improved, permitting investigators to see them. Before that time, the organ, which was visible to the naked eye, was regarded as the primary structure in living creatures. The basis for the invention of psychological categories in contemporary psychology resembles the foundation for classification in evolutionary biology several centuries ago, when only observable evidence and intuitively reasonable categories were chosen to classify animals. Currently, proteins, enzymes, and paleobiological evidence revealing evolutionary history are used for classification. These data were not available to seventeenth-century naturalists. I do not urge abandoning a priori ideas; only a greater readiness to accommodate to newly discovered relations among incentives, physiological changes, and cognitive processes and to inhibit the easy impulse to assimilate these relations to the popular affect categories. I believe, with Newton, that occasionally investigators should argue from phenomena rather than a priori presumptions.

Issue 3: the measurement of affects

A third occasion for debate centers on the empirical indexes that reflect particular affect states, detected and undetected. This controversy is yet another instance of the ancient problem of the relation of a component to the larger unity in which it participates. Most scholars in the life sciences accept the doctrine that a particular combination of component events creates an emergent synthetic phenomenon different from and not amenable to prediction by examination of each of the individual parts. The mitosis and differentiation of the zygote from the union of male and female gametes is as classic an illustration as any. This principle implies that it is often difficult or impossible to infer the emergent state from any one index that is a participant in that state. First, any single reaction can reflect different emotional states. A rise in heart rate, for example, can accompany both a smile and crying (Emde et al., 1978). On occasion, the same affect state is associated with different indexes. One child may react to the threat of punishment with a rise in heart rate, another with stomach contractions, another with increased muscle tension.

During the first and second years some infants react with a smile to stimuli that are discrepant from a habituated category, others with prolonged looking, still others with a change in heart rate. Many infants do not show all three reactions, but only one of them (Reznick & Kagan, 1983). Are these infants in the same or different emotional states? If we cannot relate the presence (or absence) of the change in face, fixation, or heart rate in this situation to any other variable, theoretically we might ignore the different responses. This is a common strategy in science. All returning honeybees do not perform identical dances for the members of the hive. And if the uniqueness in a dance does not predict anything in the behavior of the other foraging bees, we ignore it, at least for now.

Events are innocent until proven guilty; hence, we should be careful about attributing a meaning to all events. Every mutation that results in a change in a blood protein does not have evolutionary significance. A theory of emotion tries to explain the coherence among incentives, physiological changes, and evaluations. If a change in heart rate or facial expression is not part of a coherence, the investigator can ignore it, at least until someone discovers its relevance.

Further, on occasion, different physiological changes might be used to infer the same emotional state. Consider the following empirical finding as an illustration of the conceptual difficulties associated with making inferences about affect from autonomic data. A group of 3-year-olds, from both working- and middle-class homes, were administered two cognitive tasks while their heart rate was being monitored continuously. In one task, which consisted of nine specially constructed embedded figures, the child was requested to locate a familiar object embedded in an illustration with many confusing lines (Kagan, 1971). In the second task, called memory for locations (Kagan, 1981), the child sat on the mother's lap facing an examiner who hid an attractive toy under one of an increasing number of receptacles (from two to eight receptacles). The receptacles were hidden from view by an opaque screen for a 13-second delay, and then, when the screen was lowered, the child was asked to find the receptacle that covered the toy.

Previous research had shown that children and adults typically show a cardiac deceleration while searching for a stimulus – the required mental set for the embedded figures test – but show a cardiac acceleration during a period when they are trying to remember information – the appropriate mental set during the 13-second delay period in the memory for locations test. And indeed, these were the modal cardiac patterns displayed by these 3-year-olds. But there was considerable variation in the number of trials that contained a deceleration on the embedded figures test, and an acceleration on the memory test, as well as variation in the quality of performance on the memory test. Some children showed frequent *decelerations* on the embedded figures test (more than 60% of the trials) and frequent *accelerations* on the memory test (greater than 40% of the trials), and these children performed better on both tasks than those who showed these two cardiac reactions less frequently. We might regard these more successful children as being in an emotional state psychologists might call *involvement*, *motivation*, or *concern with doing well*. But their heart-rate reactions on the two tests were different. On the embedded figures test the heart rate decelerated 4 to 10 beats per minute while the children scanned the test card searching for the disguised object. On the memory test the children's heart rate increased 4 to 10 beats per minute while they waited for the screen to be lowered. Thus, differential direction of heart-rate change might, depending on conditions, reflect similar motivational states.

Despite these constraints on inference some modern investigators decide that display of any one of the potential indexes of an emotion is sufficient to diagnose the state, and few impose the stiffer criterion that demands the occurrence of more than one index. If a child either stops playing or shows a rise in heart rate following a failure experience, some investigators assume a changed affect state, and typically name it *anxiety*. The problem with this decision is that if the child revealed his anxiety in other ways (became noisy, spoke at a faster rate, or showed stomach contractions), the investigator who did not measure those reactions might conclude that the child was not anxious.

However, both strategies have precedent. If exposure to Anopheles is associated with the malarial parasite in the blood – without any other index – a physician will diagnose the patient as having malaria. However, the same physician would never use the single sign of a high fever to make the same diagnosis. As with disease states, or indeed any classification, the signs of an emotional state differ in centrality, with some being more criterial than others. Thus, behavioral and physiological signs of an affect category will vary in centrality. But unfortunately there is poor agreement on the central signs of the major emotional states. Crying to an unexpected event is a very reliable sign of uncertainty or anxiety; cessation of play and a wary face are slightly less reliable; and an increase in heart rate is the least reliable. The task is empirical. We must determine the relative frequencies of the various physiological and behavioral signs to classes of emotional incentives. These should include, at a minimum: unassimilable discrepancy, present threats to physical integrity, cognitive dissonance, blocking of a goal, threat to the self's conception, failure at a task, loss of an attachment target, the violation of standards (with and without choice), sexual incentives, the belief one has no coping response, the attainment of a goal through effort, the meeting of a standard, sensory delight, witnessing the violation of a standard by another, and the anticipation of threat. When we have charted the sets of physiological and behavioral features that accompany each of these incentives, we can decide on the relative centrality of each. But this must follow a great deal of empirical work; it cannot be decided a priori.

Once again the history of taxonomic scholarship can be instructive. Two major insights that permitted progress were the realization that the many relevant morphological features that defined a species or genus were to be differentially weighted and, second, that the weighting of a particular feature would vary with the genus being classified. These related principles seem relevant to the classification of emotions. If a 1-year-old is placed on the deep side of the visual cliff or watches its care giver leave the room, an observer is likely to see a cardiac acceleration, a facial expression of wariness, and crying. Although the presentation of an unexpected tickle or a piece of cake also produces a reliable cardiac acceleration, facial wariness and crying occur with much lower probability. Thus, although the observer does not ignore the occurrence of the cardiac acceleration to the cliff and to separation from the care giver, he is likely to award it less weight than the cry or wary face. Research on emotional states does not yet have the advantage of sets of weighted qualities.

The complementarity of subjective and objective frames

A serious issue involves the failure to treat the person's subjective report of his or her feeling states as qualitatively different from the observer's descriptions and constructs. Description and explanation in contemporary empirical science adopt an objective frame rather than the subjective frame of the subject studied. The observer uses terms that are presumed to capture the essential qualities of the state or structure of the entity being discussed or to explain the basis for the covariation among observable phenomena. Although some scholars argue that these descriptions should reflect the private experiential states of the person, I am less certain that the scientist's terms must match the constructed experience of the subject. As indicated earlier, from the perspective of a perceiving agent, what Garner (1981) calls the primary epistemology of the subject, the perception of an object is holistic, immediate, and unanalyzed. But the psychologist loyal to an objective epistemology analyzes into separate mechanisms what he knows was unanalyzed by the subject and invents names for processes that may not reflect the subject's construction of his experience.

Consider the phenomenon psychologists call "proactive interference in memory." When we ask a person why he cannot remember a set of three animal terms after he has listened to and successfully recalled two earlier sets, he simply says, "I can't remember them." He does not report experiencing a feeling of *interference*. The psychologist might have said of the same phenomenon that there was elimination, replacement, dampening, or simply forgetting. The connotations of the word "interference," intended to describe the objective data generated by the proactive interference paradigm, do not match the experiences of the subject, and there is no reason why they should.

Parents' perceptions of their children furnish another useful example of the different status of these two frames. Infants and young children differ in their tendency to be fearful, irritable, and active, as well as a host of other qualities. When scientists observe infants and categorize them as fearful, irritable, or labile, based on objective evidence, the categorizations are, at best, in moderate agreement with those of the parents – often they show no agreement at all (Sameroff, Seifer, & Elias, 1982) – and, of course, bear no relation to the infant's evaluations.

I recently listened to recordings of lengthy interviews conducted with 30 mothers of 3-year-olds who came from a broad range of social and economic backgrounds in the Boston metropolitan area. Although the female interviewer asked a specific set of questions in a specified order, many of the questions were open-ended and permitted the mothers to report their feelings and intuitions (e.g., what is your child like now? what would you like her to be at age 10?). More than three-fourths of the mothers repeatedly produced replies that led me to conclude they wanted their children to be "empathic to the distress states of others" and "able to inhibit anxiety to unfamiliar people." However, the actual sentences the mothers used to express these concerns were quite varied.

The concern with empathy appeared in sentences like, "I don't want my child to be mean," "I want her to be a caring person," "I'm pleased with his sensitivity to others' feelings," "I hope he's considerate of other people," "I'm happy he likes to be so loving," "I want her to be careful of how people feel," "I'm proud of her affectionate ways with other people." The concern with controlling anxiety was expressed in words and phrases that reflected the mother's hope that her child would be "bold," "a daredevil," "not intimidated by other children," "not scared to speak her mind," and "confident enough to do what she thought was right."

Because each of these expressions is likely to have some unique connotation for the speaker, is the scientist justified in assuming a single premise shared by all of the statements, namely, a concern with empathy or inhibition of anxiety? These terms are in the objective frame of the investigator. Many mothers who had used one or more of the phrases just noted to describe their child denied that their child was fearful when the interviewer asked them directly, "Is your child fearful?" Further, if the interviewer asked the parent whether she was worried that her child might be fearful, some replied negatively because the term "fearful" did not have the same meaning to the mother that it did for the interrogator.

The use of self-report data to make inferences about a person's emotional state poses a profound problem. The popular solution permits the investigator to invent a concept, like *empathic* or *anxious*, decide on the spoken phrases that belong to the concept, and quantify objectively the subject's statements for instances of the category. If that procedure leads to reliable prediction of theoretically reasonable phenomena, its validity is affirmed. If not, we know nothing. But in no case can the investigator assume he knows the subject's private emotional state. Indeed, when college students were asked to imagine and express nonverbally, during exercise, one of six different emotional states while their heart rate and blood pressure were being monitored, observers' judgments of the subjects' emotional states were in better theoretical accord with the students' physiological changes than with the students' self-reports of their emotions.

"The findings suggested that the observers were seeing relationships that the subjects themselves did not" (Schwartz, 1982, p. 85). Schwartz adds that clinically depressed patients report experiencing more pleasure than observers judge them to be experiencing, while schizophrenic patients report experiencing less pleasure than observers judge them to have.

However, investigators indifferent to this issue ask their subjects what emotion they are feeling and give the reply special priority. I suggest that the replies are of interest and require accommodation but have only slightly greater significance than an eye blink, a smile, or an acceleration of the heart. The words people use to name their feeling states are only a little less disguised as a datum to be used in an objectively framed proposition than a furrowing of the brow. It is common for a 3-year-old who has just committed a mischievous act to run to the mother and say, "I love you, Mummy." It is not obvious that the child is experiencing the emotion we believe *love* refers to when an adult uses the same phrase. Further, it is likely that most psychologists would conclude that the mischievous child was experiencing fear of punishment or guilt, not love. Psychologists should use self-reports of feeling states but must treat them as any other evidence. They always require interpretation (Polivy, 1981).

The attribution of affect states to persons by investigators must always add a statement of the measurement procedures. When we say a child is "involved in a task," we must add, "as indexed by a change in heart rate," "as indexed by a change in performance on a memory task," or "as indexed by the answer to a direct question." These are not equivalent statements. When a nineteenth-century observer made a statement about a child's state, other scientists knew that the source of his statement was the child's overt behavior, for this was the typical method of observation. Today investigators use questionnaires, interviews, projective tests, memory problems, and polygraphic display of autonomic or neural discharge. Even if we ignore the fact that these methods might not evaluate the properties of lability or fear accurately, the scientist makes statements about the degree to which a child possesses these properties and is indifferent to the real possibility that the measurement methods are not equivalent. Most child psychologists believe that the quality of attachment of infant to caretaker is a critical property to assess. But there is disagreement as to the measurement procedures to be used to evaluate this quality. Some use the Ainsworth Strange Situation, others code the person to whom the child goes when it has a choice between caretaker and another person when it is tired, uncertain, or bored. The data produced by these procedures do not always generate similar conclusions.

Statements about the presence of the emotion of *interest* in infants also vary in a serious way with the measurement index used. Duration of fixation time and the facial expression of interest along with the magnitude of cardiac deceleration were coded while infants 2, 4, 6, and 8 months of age were shown an inanimate object, a mannequin, and a woman. These three indexes of *interest* showed the same developmental function to the person; namely, a linear increase with age in each of the three dependent variables. However, to the mannequin, the pattern was somewhat different. The magnitude of cardiac deceleration showed an inverted U relation with a peak at 6 months, but duration of fixation time and the facial expression of "interest" formed a U function with a trough at 4 months. Further, the correlations among the three indexes of interest were only moderate (r = .2 to .5) (Langsdorf et al., 1983). Each measure seemed to reveal a different component of the emotion named interest. Failure to acknowledge the dependence of the meaning of a description of the emotional state of a child on the source of the evidence is a major cause of ambiguity in conclusions about emotions and their development.

Despite these unsolved problems, a popular position, which owes much of its vitality to Izard's (1977) technically elegant procedures, holds that certain facial expressions are the origins of emotional states. (It should be noted that this sequence is not traceable to Darwin, who believed that facial expressions were the products of mental states.) In this view, the spontaneous smile is not an imperfect accompaniment to the emotion of joy: It is the reliable origin of the emotion. It is not possible to judge the validity of these claims at the present time. Because it is not obviously true that every time a smile occurs one can be certain that the same affect state has been experienced, I shall assume that the task of finding indexes for emotional states remains unfinished. One reason I make this claim is the common observation that often no observable change in facial expression occurs to a situation that on other occasions produced a particular facial reaction. (It is possible, of course, that the muscular patterns are subtle and not capable of being perceived by the unaided eye.) All developmental scholars have observed children suddenly stop playing and retreat to their mother following encounter with a stranger or an unexpected event who do not show the changes in facial expression that are presumed to index fear. During the first three years of life one of the most reliable behavioral reactions to an unexpected or threatening event is cessation of play, not a particular arrangement of facial muscles.

For these reasons I favor the implementation of research that attempts to find lawful covariation between incentive events and response classes presumed to reflect similar states. Campos and Stenberg (1981) report that infants are likely to look toward the mother if an unfamiliar person approaches. In the generalized case, infants often look to their care givers when an unexpected and initially unassimilable event occurs. But infants are also likely to stop playing, cease vocalizing, or, on occasion, show a wary face to the same incentives. The reliability of these associations invites the postulation of an emotional state. The thorny issue is to decide what signs or combinations of signs are to be regarded as the valid indexes of an emotional state. The answer lies, of course, with the logical coherence and replicability of the proposed relations. The incentive of maternal departure in an unfamiliar place typically leads to interruption of play in a 1-year-old child. A change in facial expression and crying occur with less regularity. Because these three reactions, which share the inferred dimension of unexpectedness, also occur to phenotypically different incentives, it is justifiable to invent an affect term like *anxiety* that applies to these coherences. But their appeal to the larger community will depend on the intuitions of others: Some claim that the 1-year-old feels sad when the care giver leaves.

The development of affect: the first five years

During the first 3 to 4 months of age, many coherent reaction profiles suggestive of emotional states, but probably involving unevaluated feeling tone, appear in the infant's repertoire. The first is comprised of motor quieting and heart-rate deceleration to the introduction of an unexpected or discrepant event. We might call this combination "surprise to the unexpected." A second set of changes is characterized by increased motor movement, closing of the eyes, heart-rate acceleration, and crying to incentives of pain, cold, and hunger. We might name this combination "distress to physical privation." A third set includes decreased muscle tone and closing of the eyes following feeding, which we might name "relaxation to gratification." A fourth set includes increased motoricity, smiling, and babbling to a moderately familiar event or special class of social interaction, which we might call "excitement to assimilation of the unexpected." During the third month the infant also shows a reaction characterized by attentiveness, namely, smiling to an event that is moderately familiar, especially a face. The incentive is not a particular physical stimulus but is defined in terms of the child's prior experience and, therefore, his expectations. Some might call this emotion "the joy of understanding." One can add many more examples. The point is that the name of the emotion contains a reference to the incentive.

Cognitive evaluations of incentives and internal feelings are probably absent during the first few months, even though the behavioral reactions to certain events are predictable. But because older children do evaluate incentive and feeling, there is a potential danger in attributing to the 3-month-old the same affect state ascribed to the older child, whether the term used is *surprise* or *fear*. It would be wiser to use a different set of affect constructs for the opening four months, when evaluation is likely to be absent or, at the least, diminished. Note that we typically do this when adults are in a state of sleep. Not all psychologists attribute the affect of fear or anxiety to a person having a nightmare, even though the sleeping person's autonomic reactions are similar to those that occur when the adult is awake and behaving as if in a state of fear.

By 4 to 10 months of age new reaction sets have appeared. For example, 8-month-olds react to some discrepant events with a special facial expression, inhibition of play, and, on occasion, crying. This cluster of reactions to discrepant experiences does not occur earlier and implies the appearance of a completely new emotional state, which most would probably call "fear or anxiety to the unfamiliar." It is not necessary to treat this fear as a derivative of the earlier distress to privation or to assume that the distress of the early weeks is a necessary prerequisite for the fear. The fear to discrepant situations becomes possible because of the maturation of new cognitive functions, especially memory and evaluation, not because the 1-month-old cried when he was hungry (Kagan, Kearsley, & Zelazo, 1978).

A second new set of reactions involves resistance and protest to the interruption of a response routine or to the loss of an object of interest, which some might call "anger to frustration." Mandler (1975) awards interruption of a response routine a central place in his essay on emotion because of the detected autonomic changes that typically follow such an event. The principal difference between this emotion and those displayed during the first six months is that fear and anger require relating an incentive event to knowledge; they involve an evaluation of the information. The presentation of a distorted human face elicits attentive interest in a 1-month-old, rarely crying. The same event often elicits both inhibition and crying in 7-month-olds. One way to explain the different reactions to the same incentive is to assume that the older children related the incentive to their schemata.

Similarly, the response of motor protest to loss of a toy requires recognition of its absence. The 1-month-old who drops a toy or has it removed by an adult does not display this behavior. Unlike the incentives for interest in the 1-week-old, typically movement or contrast, the incentives for 4- to 12-month-old children are more often discrepant events. This fact has implications for emotional states, because discrepant events provoke an attempt at assimilation. These three new affects – anxiety to discrepancy, anger to frustration, and surprise to the unexpected – cannot appear until the cognitive ability to relate incentive events to schemata has matured.

The role of the resolution of uncertainty and the problems associated with the labeling of emotion are illustrated in the infant's processing of pictures that inevitably become more familiar as the child matures. The attentiveness, motor behavior, and facial expressions of infants 8, 14, and 20 months of age were videotaped during an experiment in which the children looked at a series of different pictures representing one of four categories: women, infants, dogs, and butterflies. Three behaviors coded were: excited vocalizations, motor excitement (pointing to the screen, leaning toward the stimulus, or banging both arms rhythmically), and smiling.

Most of the 8-month-olds showed maximal display of these three behaviors to the pictures of infants, which are transformations of their schemata for adults, and minimal display of these responses to the butterflies, which should have been unfamiliar to them. By contrast, the 20-month-olds, who should have acquired easy familiarity with adults and infants but only a beginning familiarity with animals, showed maximal display of these responses to dogs. Additionally, smiling decreased with age to women but increased to dogs and to butterflies. This pattern of results implies that moderately discrepant events on the threshold of assimilation have the greatest power to provoke an affect of excitement to assimilable discrepancy. The pictures of women were easily assimilated by the 20-month-olds; hence, the smile did not occur. The schematic representations of dogs and butterflies had become articulated enough so that these two-dimensional representations engaged them but required mental effort for assimilation. Hence, the smile.

Some investigators may be tempted to call a child *happy* when she smiles, but the conditions that produced the smile in this setting invite a descriptive term like *comprehending* or *understanding*, not *happy*. Is it likely that the smile that accompanies the receipt of a cookie or new toy reflects the same state that accompanies assimilating a picture of a butterfly to one's knowledge?

It is not possible to list all the many new coherences that emerge during the second year. Two of the prominent reactions include an initial protest, followed by inhibition and apathy, to the prolonged absence of an attachment object – emotions that are popularly called *depression* or *sadness* to loss of a familiar object. Now children must retrieve schemata of the past, not just relate an event in the field to their schema. Consider the reaction that follows prolonged absence of a caretaker. The 2-year-old must be able to recall the caretaker's former presence, relate that idea to the current situation, and, additionally, hold that information in consciousness so that it is not lost after a few seconds. These phenomena cannot occur without major maturational advances in cognitive function, as well as attachment to the caretaker. There is also increased concern over and interest in events that violate standards, as revealed in smiling to the completion of a task and crying and seeking proximity to a caretaker following anticipated task failure (Kagan, 1981).

During the second year children show a set of reactions that might be called "anxiety to possible task failure." In one experimental setting, the child is playing happily on the floor when an adult comes to the child and asks to join in the play. The adult then acts out some brief behaviors that are on the threshold of the child's sphere of mastery, such as picking up some dolls and a plate and pretending to make dinner or taking three toy animals for a walk. After completing these acts, the adult says "Now it's your turn to play" and returns to her seat. Beginning around 18 months and peaking around the second birthday, children show extreme degrees of upset and distress after the adult returns to the couch. They fret, cry, cling to their mothers, stop playing, protest, or may insist on going home. This reaction occurs in Cambridge children, children growing up in huts on islands in the Fiji chain, as well as those who have recently arrived in northern California from their homes in Vietnam (Kagan, 1981). What name shall we give to this coherence, which does not occur during the first year?

The potential to become concerned with the sight of a broken cup or dirt on a blouse, which occurs in the second year, requires the child to recall that the event violates a standard and to infer that someone produced that violation. Similarly, the smile that follows the successful completion of a task in which one invested effort requires the recognition that ego has met a goal generated earlier. During the second and third years the incentives for affects are more often generated internally, rather than externally. The injection that led to extreme distress in a 1-week-old might produce a quite different affect in a 6-year-old, even though pain was present on both occasions. It might produce pride because the child had planned to be stoic and met that standard.

Because the affective experiences of the first two years seem so canalized, it is useful to ask about the advantages of the emotions of the first two years. From an evolutionary perspective, one possible function of the reactions to discrepant events is to protect the child from physical harm. Inhibition of action to the unfamiliar keeps the child from approaching the unfamiliar event, and the child's crying is likely to bring a protective adult.

The incentives for anger toward another include interruption of a goal-directed sequence, frustration of a motive, or seizure of objects children regard as their own. Because it is not obvious that anger protects children from harm, why do they react with vigor of voice and body to the interruption of a goal-directed action or loss of property? One possibility is that this reaction and its accompanying responses serve to establish a resistant, rather than an acquiescent, response to the intrusion of others. If anger successfully produces retreat on the part of the intruder, it will become part of the child's repertoire. With time, the child will react to interruptions and seizures with angry protests. Consider a 2-year-old who never reacted with anger to any intrusion. The child would lose objects he was holding and cease goal-directed actions when interrupted. If interventions were frequent, the child would eventually become passive to domination and intrusion. Many zoologists and comparative psychologists suggest that an animal's position in a dominance hierarchy has profound implications for its adaptation, especially its reproductive success.

The excitement provoked by interactions with adults (surprise, physical contact, and talking) prolongs the behavior of the adult who produced the excitement originally, leading to longer bouts of interaction. One possible function of the affect, therefore, is to facilitate mutual interaction and mutual bonding of child and adult.

The function of sadness to loss of an attachment object is less obvious. Why should a 2-year-old child react to the prolonged loss of a target of attachment with signs of depression or apathy? One possible purpose is to keep the child close to familiar people. Children approaching the third to fourth birthday are physically and psychologically able to leave the family group, at least temporarily. They can wander from the home, although it is still dangerous for them to do so. The extreme fear of the unusual, which keeps 1-year-olds close to their parents, is less potent, and the new affect of *sadness* to loss may have a similar function by provoking the child to return to family members when this emotion is felt. The child chooses to stay close to the family to avoid the unpleasant feelings that accompany separation from them for a prolonged period.

The function of an emotional reaction to the violation of an adult standard seems obvious. To be accepted by the social group, children must inhibit those behaviors negatively sanctioned by the group, typically destruction, aggression, and lack of cleanliness. If the affects called shame and guilt are classed as undesirable (in part because the accompanying ideas are linked to evaluations that the child is bad), the child will avoid initiating prohibited behaviors. It may have been necessary in human evolution to promote the early development of functions that would inhibit aggression. In most parts of the world for most of our history, mothers gave birth to the next offspring about three years after the birth of the last child. A 3-year-old has both the strength to inflict injury on a younger sibling and, more important, the ability to retain hostile thoughts long after the emotion of anger has subsided. Aggressive behavior toward a younger sibling that can be the product of the jealousy of a 3-year-old must be held in check. It would be adaptive, therefore, if 3-year-olds appreciated that aggression was wrong. The importance of a strong inhibition on aggression to younger children is seen in a rare event in which a 30-month-old killed his 22-month-old regular playmate by pounding the victim's head on the floor and striking his skull with a heavy glass vase. The fact that this is a freak phenomenon indicates that most children have learned to appreciate that such actions are improper by their second or third birthday. These emotions do not appear until the child is mature enough to anticipate the actions of others or, in the case of guilt, to choose whether he should initiate an action sequence that violates a standard.

The appearance of guilt is delayed because the cognitive bases for the emotion need time to mature. The cognitive talent in question is the ability to recognize that one has a choice. A 2-year-old is not capable of recognizing that he could have behaved in a way different from the one he chose. But the 4-year-old has this ability and so experiences the emotion we call guilt.

There seems to be a complementary relation between the emotions of the first year and those of the second and third years. The earlier emotional states, and their accompanying behaviors, offset the child's impotence and protect the child against harm and victimization. The emotions of the next two years, especially those following a violation of standards, restrain the child. The protest to intrusion characteristic of the first year is balanced by the shame of the second, keeping the child distant from both the Scylla of impotence and the Charybdis of destructive arrogance. Nature intended the child to be neither too humble nor too aggressive, just civilized.

The development of affect during childhood

The affects that usually appear during the fifth and sixth years have as their immediate incentive an evaluation of the self's properties in comparison with others − a function less prominent during the first three years of life. The products of that evaluation lead to emotional reactions to which we give names like insecurity, inferiority, humility, pride, and confidence.

The other as referent

Accustomed to assuming that all effects must be the result of an external force actively imposed on an agent, we are reluctant to award psychological potency to the simple presence of another person in the psychological consciousness of an agent, even though the other directs no actions toward the agent. In dominance hierarchies among animals, a more dominant animal will influence the behavior of a less dominant one, even if the two never have a dispute.

Humans select particular others as referents in evaluating their own qualities, typically siblings and peers of similar age, sex, and background. The success and failures of the referent can profoundly alter the mood and aspirations of the agent. A boy with an older, very successful brother may ignore his own real successes and conclude he is inadequate simply because of the competence of the older sibling. The symbolic evaluation of the self's internal private qualities with another, which is likely to be unique in humans, is a profound basis for mood and behavior. Animals respond to physical signals from another; humans react to imagined qualities and that process creates the important incentives for both emotion and action.

American children of 6 or 7 years possess standards for abilities, attractiveness, honesty, bravery, dominance, popularity, and a host of other qualities and are able to rank themselves and their friends on these qualities with remarkable consensus. As a result, the child's concept of self is influenced by private evaluation of the degree to which ego possesses those characteristics relative to others. The crucial new cognitive competence is the ability to evaluate the degree to which the child possesses a particular property in comparison with another. In the language of Piagetian operations, the child can seriate the self with others on a psychological quality.

The child takes another person – peer, sibling, or parent – as a standard. If the evaluation of the self's quality is seriously deviant from the standard (the standard is the quality possessed by the other), an emotion is generated. It will be recalled that when the 2-year-old's behavior deviated from a standard, a distress reaction occurred. For the 7-year-old, the incentive is not a specific action of self that deviates from an internal standard but rather a quality or property of the self that deviates from that same quality in another person. In the popular essays on mental health, the resulting affects are feelings of inferiority, superiority, pride, or humility. The key element is recognition that a property of the self deviates from a standard defined by another.

The ability to compare the events occurring to self and another is also the basis for the emotions we call jealousy and envy. The incentive is the belief that another (whom ego takes as referent) is the recipient of experiences ego desires and to which ego feels entitled. The other's presence is a threat to ego's evaluation of self, even though the other has not acted intentionally to produce that state – the other's presence is a sufficient incentive. The specific other that the child takes as a standard is of course an important issue. The older the referent used for comparison, the more likely the child will evaluate the self as deficient. What determines the referent chosen?

Two-year-olds automatically detect similarities between or among objects (balls, animals, foods). This disposition remains potent throughout life. As the concept of self becomes more articulated, the child automatically compares specific qualities of self with those of other people. In grouping objects, the 2-year-old uses both physical and functional similarities (e.g., round and edible objects). In addition to using physical and functional dimensions in detecting similarities among people, the child also uses membership in a common category like sex, ethnic group, and family. In this mental comparison, the presence of distinctive properties not shared by everyone is an important determinant in the choice of referent. The child is disposed to choose those who share properties that are unusual or infrequent and, therefore, distinctive.

There must be variation on a dimension if it is to function as an incentive for categorization. When persons are the entities grouped, the relevant dimensions are not those shared by all people – arms, eyes, or the ability to talk – but those that distinguish one from another. When people are asked to describe themselves, they usually name distinctive dimensions first (McGuire & Padawer-Singer, 1976). For example, when asked to "tell me about yourself," very few sixth-graders named their gender; many more, however, listed activities (like recreations or daily routines) that would differentiate them from members of their family and relationships that differentiated them from their peers (siblings or pets) or their beliefs. More important, 7% of the children who were born in the United States spontaneously mentioned their birthplace as a distinctive attribute, whereas 44% of the foreign-born children mentioned their place of birth.

If three animals and nine fruits comprise an array, children are most likely to set aside the three animals, not the nine fruits. But if the array contained three fruits and nine animals, children would set the fruits aside. In comparing the self with others, children are disposed to select properties that are less, rather than more, frequent and to regard those who show that property as belonging to a common category. This means that physical properties – red hair, skin color, freckles, or a physical handicap – are potent dimensions for the child's categorization. Gender is a dimension of categorization because half the people a child meets are of a different sex. Hence, girls group themselves with girls, and boys with boys. As early as 2 years of age children are aware of some psychological dimensions that define the sexes, including modal actions, control of fear, and adult vocation (Kuhn, Nash, & Brucken, 1978). Family will be a dimension of importance because the family's last name is a rare property, and certain behaviors typically occur only within the home. Crying, boisterousness, yelling, aggression, and extreme hilarity occur in the home, rarely outside. Children recognize that they behave in this manner, and so regard themselves as more similar to family members than to nonfamily members. When they learn that biological properties are also shared with family members, children are persuaded of membership in a common category.

The belief that one is similar in a significant way to persons in one's family has two important consequences. First, the child is disposed to regard members of the family as primary referents in evaluating self. Second, once the child treats the self and the other as belonging to a common category, it is likely that the child will share vicariously in the affects of those persons who belong to the category.

Because the child is likely to take a member of the family as a referent for comparison, it follows that the greater the differences in particular qualities between the child and the other, the more likely the child will deviate from the standard. Thus, a child with only one older sibling of the same sex will perceive greater deviance between his properties and those of the older sibling than will a third born with both older and younger siblings. The more siblings available for comparison, the more likely the child will take a sibling as primary referent and the less likely the ego will perceive dramatic differences in psychological properties and the emotion that accompanies recognition of serious deviation from a standard of competence, beauty, or power.

Outside the family, attendance at the same school or residence in a common neighborhood can be a basis for similarity. A 7-year-old boy is more likely to compare self with the boys in his classroom than with all the boys he knows or has heard about. One corollary of this assumption is that the smaller the effective peer group available for comparison, the more likely a particular child will evaluate the self as positive on a given psychological property, because there will be fewer children with more outstanding qualities. The child who has a large peer group is likely to compare self with many more children who possess the desired attribute in excess of the self. As a result, the child will regard self as further from the desirable standard and experience distress.

The advantages of some of the emotions that characterize the older child are not obvious because the development of feelings of confidence (or lack of confidence) depends upon the peer group to which the child is exposed. Perhaps these emotions, like the human chin, which was a consequence of the development of the jaw and teeth, were unintended consequences of the cognitive ability to seriate the self with others. On the other hand, it is possible that when all human groups were small in number, the number of referent peers of the same or similar age was rarely more than a half dozen. A typical 7-year-old in a hunter-gatherer group probably had only three or four other children 5 to 9 years old for comparison. Under these conditions, the child would be likely to evaluate the self as coming close to meeting the standard for desirable properties and to generate more positive feelings about the self. By creating large cities, civilized man created a condition in which each child was exposed to many hundreds of youngsters of similar sex and age, leading many to conclude that they deviated from a desirable standard in a serious way. The feeling of inadequacy that results from these conditions may be a culturally invented phenomenon that does not seem to be adaptive.

As adolescence approaches, a new incentive with both cognitive and physiological components appears. Although the physical changes that accompany puberty are interpreted as signs of a change in role, the changes in sexual feelings, which are due in part to hormonal secretions, play an influential role in the emotion we call sexual excitement. One function of this affect is obvious: it facilitates reproduction of the species. But even for this vital feeling state the detection of deviation from standards is relevant. Adolescents are aware of their ability to meet the local standards of sexual attraction and success. In most species the males are in a dominance hierarchy based on their ability to physically dominate others; the less dominant males defer to the more dominant ones in gaining access to females. The analog in humans is the adolescent's evaluation of his or her ability to attract a partner and to maintain a romantic relationship. This principle holds for both sexes. Males and females evaluate their sexual competence and initiate or withdraw from participation in accord with their private evaluation of the degree to which they deviate from the standard of appropriate sexual characteristics.

A final pair of affects that emerges during adolescence and early adulthood also waits upon a cognitive advance. Piaget's description of the stage of formal operations implies that the adolescent becomes capable of examining beliefs, in sets, for logical consistency. On detecting inconsistency, the adolescent automatically tries to rearrange or alter them to attain coherence both among beliefs and between beliefs and behavior. Failure to do so results in a special feeling state we might call dissonance, which is not identical with guilt (which follows recognition that one's voluntary actions deviate from a standard).

The 12-year-old has acquired a new cognitive competence: the disposition to examine the logic and consistency of existing beliefs. The emergence of this competence, which may be dependent upon biological changes in the central nervous system, is catalyzed by experiences that confront the adolescent with phenomena and attitudes that are not easily interpreted with existing ideology. These intrusions nudge preadolescents to begin analytic reexaminations of their knowledge. Of special relevance for this discussion is the fact that the adolescent is disposed to examine beliefs in sets and to search for inconsistencies among them and between the beliefs and related actions. This inclination depends partly on cognitive abilities, because critical examination of the logic of a set of related beliefs requires the capacity to consider multiple rules simultaneously. Thus, the 14-year-old broods about the inconsistency of the following three propositions: (1) God loves man; (2) the world contains many unhappy people; (3) if God loved man, he would not make so many people unhappy.

The adolescent is troubled by the incompatibility that is immediately sensed when these statements are examined together, and has at least four choices. The adolescent can deny the second premise, that man is ever unhappy, but this is unlikely, for its factual basis is overwhelming. Adolescents can deny that God loves man; this is avoided, for love of man is one of the definitional qualities of God. The youngster can assume that such unhappiness serves an ulterior purpose God has for man; this possibility is sometimes chosen. Finally, adolescents can deny the hypothesis of God.

The last alternative, which has become the popular form of resolution for many in Western society, has profound consequences. It is a denial of a belief that has been regarded as true for many years, and therefore invites the implication that if this statement is not tenable, all other beliefs held at the moment are also in jeopardy. Suddenly, what was regarded as permanently valid has become tentative. A 14-year-old girl, asked how her present beliefs differed from those she held several years earlier, replied, "I had a whole philosophy of how the world worked. I was very religious, and I believed that there was unity and harmony, and everything had its proper place. I used to imagine rocks in the right places on the right beaches. It was all very neat, and God ordained it all, and I made up my own religion, but now it seems absolutely ridiculous."

Consider another inconsistency many adolescents try to resolve.

1. Parents are omnipotent and omniscient.
2. My parent has lost a job, or failed to understand me, or behaved irrationally – or any other liability the reader cares to select.
3. If my parents were omniscient, they would not be tainted with failure and vulnerability.

The statements are examined together and the inconsistency noted. As with the first example, the adolescent can deny the truth of the second premise, but it demands too severe a straining of objectivity and is not usually implemented. The adolescent can invent a statement about parental motivation and excuse the show of incompetence on the basis of willingness rather than capacity. This alternative is infrequently chosen because its acceptance elicits another troubling notion; it implies that parents do not care about the emotional consequences of their apathy for the vitality of the family. Hence, the child is tempted to deny the original hypothesis of parental omniscience. As with the denial of God, the fall of this belief weakens all the others.

A third set of propositions placed under analytic scrutiny involves sexuality:

1. Sexual activity – self-administered or heterosexually experienced – is bad.

2. Sexuality provides pleasure.
3. If sex is pleasant, it should not be bad.

We shall forgo the obvious analysis of these propositions and simply note that again the most likely conclusion is that the first assumption is not tenable. Increased masturbation at puberty forces the child to deal with a private violation of a strong social prohibition. However, the consistent sensory pleasure cannot be denied, and this silent violation has to be rationalized. As that rationalization is accomplished, the child is tempted to question a great many other standards and thus begins to examine all prohibitions with the same skepticism.

Each culture presents its children with a different set of beliefs to examine. In our society standards surrounding family, religion, sexuality, drugs, and school are among the major ideological dragons to be tamed. Partial support for these ideas comes from interviews suggesting that American adolescents begin to wonder about the legitimacy of their belief systems, whereas earlier, inconsistent propositions were not examined as a structure. Sometimes this analysis leaves the adolescent temporarily without a commitment to any belief. The author asked a 15-year-old about the beliefs she was most certain of: "None really. I just take in things and analyze them. Maybe it will change my opinion and maybe it won't. It depends, but I'm not really stuck to anything."

A second cognitive competence that is part of formal operations is the ability to know one has exhausted all the solution possibilities to a problem. When a 16-year-old girl is faced with a problem, like rejection by a romantic partner or failure in school, she assesses all the potential coping reactions to the problem and believes she knows when she has exhausted every reasonable solution. This state is accompanied by an affect some might call helplessness (Seligman, 1975); others call it depression. This state can be simulated in animals, for if a dog is allowed to behave in a way that permits it to avoid electric shock and subsequently is prevented from using that response, the animal struggles initially but eventually stops struggling, and becomes passive. If the opportunity to escape occurs later, the animal does not avail himself of the opportunity but remains inactive.

Adults who believe there is nothing they can do to avoid a future tragedy (death from cancer or sorcery), often become inactive and stop eating; some die in hopelessness. This emotional state requires, as a prior condition, the conviction that no coping solution is possible. Five-year-olds are not capable of this affect state because they are not cognitively mature enough to review all solutions and conclude there is nothing they can do. Although it is difficult to see why this emotion would be adaptive, one can argue that it would be adaptive for fatally ill older persons to die quickly and not burden a kin group morally obliged to provide support. The support drains effort and energy from the younger members of the group who are still engaged in reproduction and the care of children.

Summary

This brief tour of the affects that appear from infancy through adolescence has emphasized three principles. The most important is that one class of emotional states is the result of detected and evaluated changes in feeling tone, that is, cognitive processes acting on a perception of altered feelings in specific contexts. Developmental changes in these emotional states are due, in part, to the maturation of new cognitive functions and new knowledge. (Emotional phenomena that do not involve evaluated changes in detected feeling tone may be less dependent on cognitive developments.) Emotional states that involve evaluation of an incentive and perceived changes in feeling tone form a unity that cannot be decomposed without losing the phenomenon. A molecule of insulin has a certain structure; if one of its critical atoms is removed, it loses its biological potency. We can talk or write about the cognitive and visceral elements separately, but the phenomenon is the coherence of these events.

Second, although some emotions seem to have advantages, in the evolutionary sense, it is not obvious that changes in feeling state had to accompany the cognitive functions that evolved with phylogeny. One can imagine our species evolving so that concrete and formal operations matured without any accompanying changes in emotional state. The fact that affects did evolve implies, but does not prove, that they were useful. Because feelings can dominate consciousness in a way that thoughts cannot, one can argue, after the fact, that the perceptual commandingness of feelings keeps the person's mind focused on the desires and events of the moment and directs the person to find ways to maintain the pleasant feelings and eliminate the unpleasant ones.

It is also possible, as many Chinese philosophers but a small number of Western scholars have argued, that affects form the bases for whatever moral standards are universal. Many of the virtues celebrated help to control unpleasant affects. For example, the capacity for empathy with the plight of another lies at the root of ethical demands for justice and the control of aggression. The potential to experience the state of uncertainty following detection of inconsistent beliefs or puzzling events forms a basis for the virtues of wisdom and self-understanding. The ease with which anxiety is generated by anticipation of physical harm in time of war or social rejection when honest leadership is needed invites adherence to standards for courage and loyalty to personal conviction. The unpleasant feelings of exhaustion and ennui can be avoided by loyalty to a standard of temperance, and worry over possible loss of wealth or reputation is muted by adopting a prudent attitude. If humans did not possess the competence for these emotional states, moral standards might be even more diverse and relativistic than they appear to be in this era of ideological tolerance for ethical pluralism.

A third theme is that emotional states can be altered by the acquisition of information. When an infant who is avoiding the deep side of the visual cliff sees her mother smile, her facial expression of wariness changes, and she crosses the deep side (Klinnert et al., 1983). When a child angry at a peer because of an insult later learns that the insult was not intended, the affect of anger is likely to vanish. Similarly, an adolescent's anxiety over a supposed illness vanishes when the medical report is positive. Some emotions are difficult to alter because no information will alleviate the emotional state. Guilt resulting from the belief that one has caused the death of a parent is one example. Affects vary, therefore, with respect to their vulnerability to new information. Some resist new evidence and remain potent. With growth, fear and anxiety become easier to alter because the child can gain information more readily; guilt is more difficult to alleviate because the child cannot change the fact that he acted in a particular way.

The fact that emotions can be altered by knowledge is in accord with the argument that one large class of emotions is dependent upon cognition. During the first years of life, affects are generated most often by external events; by 7 years of age, ideas have become more important. As a result, emotions are easier to alter in younger than in older children. Younger children's emotions are labile because of their responsiveness to changes in external situations, not because young children have a labile physiology. We distinguish, therefore, between acute emotions provoked by specific events and chronic moods based on persistent beliefs. The adult is characterized by fewer changes in acute emotions and more stable moods because feeling states have become more dependent on long-standing belief systems and less responsive to minor perturbations in the environment.

Finally, I have urged that psychologists should question the utility of some popular emotional terms and search for new coherences among related events. This suggestion resembles Cuvier's plea to his fellow taxonomists at the end of the eighteenth century to search for coherences among observable features in defining species.

I have not presented this essay on division that it may serve as the beginnings of the determination of the name of species; an artificial system would be easier for this, and this is only proper. My aim has been to make known more exactly the nature and true relationships of the *animaux à sang blanc* (invertebrates), by reducing to general principles what is known of their structure and general properties (Mayr, 1982, p. 184).

References

Averill, J. R. On the paucity of positive emotions. In K. R. Blankstein, P. Pliner, & J. Polivy (Eds.), *Assessment and modification of emotional behavior*, pp. 7–45. New York: Plenum, 1980.

Berlin, B., Breedlove, D. E., & Raven, P. H. General principles of classification and nomenclature in folk biology. *American Anthropologist*, 1973, *75*, 214–242.

Briggs, J. L. *Never in anger*. Cambridge, Mass.: Harvard University Press, 1970.

Campos, J. J., & Stenberg, C. R. Perception, appraisal, and emotion. In M. Lamb & L. Sherrod (Eds.), *Infant social cognition*, pp. 273–314. Hillsdale, N.J.: Erlbaum, 1981.

Darwin, C. *The expression of emotions in man and animals*. Chicago: Phoenix, University of Chicago Press, 1965.

Doi, T. *The anatomy of dependence*. Tokyo: Kadansha, 1973.

Emde, R. N., Campos, J., Reich, J., & Gaensbauer, T. J. Infant smiling at five and nine months: Analysis of heart rate and movement. *Infant Behavior and Development*, 1978, *1*, 26–35.

Garcia Coll, C. *Psychophysiological correlates of a tendency toward inhibition in infants*. Unpublished doctoral dissertation, Harvard University, 1981.

Garner, W. R. The analysis of unanalyzed perceptions. In M. Kubovy & J. R. Pomerantz (Eds.), *Perceptual organization*, pp. 119–139. Hillsdale, N.J.: Erlbaum, 1981.

Izard, C. E. *Human emotions*. New York: Plenum, 1977.

James, W. *Principles of psychology*, 2 vols., ed. F. Burkhardt. Cambridge, Mass.: Harvard University Press, 1981.

Kagan, J. *Change and continuity in infancy*. New York: Wiley, 1971.

Kagan, J. On emotion and its development: A working paper. In M. Lewis & L. A. Rosenblum (Eds.), *The development of affect*, pp. 11–42. New York: Plenum, 1978.

Kagan, J. *The second year*. Cambridge, Mass.: Harvard University Press, 1981.

Kagan, J., Kearsley, R., & Zelazo, P. *Infancy: Its place in human development*. Cambridge, Mass.: Harvard University Press, 1978.

Klinnert, M. D., Campos, J., Sorce, J. F., Emde, R. N., & Svejda, M. J. Social referencing: Emotional expressions as behavior regulators. In R. Plutchik & H. Kellerman (Eds.), *Emotions in early development*. New York: Academic Press, 1983.

Kuhn, D., Nash, S. C., & Brucken, L. Sex role concepts of two- and three-year-olds. *Child Development*, 1978, *49*, 445–451.

Langsdorf, P., Izard, C. E., Rayias, M., & Hembree, E. A. Interest expression, visual fixation and heart rate changes in two- to eight-month-old infants. *Developmental Psychology*, 1983, *19*, 375–386.

Lutz, C. The domain of emotion words on Ifaluk. *American Ethnologist*, 1982, *9*, 113–128.

Lyons, W. *Emotion*. Cambridge: Cambridge University Press, 1980.

Mandler, G. *Mind and emotion*. New York: Wiley, 1975.

Mayr, E. *The growth of biological thought*. Cambridge, Mass.: Harvard University Press, 1982.

McGuire, W. J., & Padawer-Singer, A. Trait salience in a spontaneous self-concept. *Journal of Personality and Social Psychology*, 1976, *33*, 743–754.

Newman, P. L. Wildman behavior in a New Guinea Highlands community. *American Anthropologist*, 1960, *66*, 1–19.

Obrist, P. A., Light, K. C., & Hastrup, J. L. Emotion and the cardiovascular system: A critical perspective. In C. E. Izard (Ed.), *Measuring emotions in infants and children*, pp. 299–316. Cambridge: Cambridge University Press, 1982.

Polivy, J. On the induction of emotion in the laboratory. *Journal of Personality and Social Psychology*, 1981, *41*, 803–817.

Reznick, J. S. *The development of perceptual and lexical categories in the infant*. Unpublished doctoral dissertation, University of Colorado, 1982.

Reznick, J. S., & Kagan, J. Category detection in infancy. In L. Lipsitt (Ed.), *Advances in infant development* (Vol. 2). Norwood, N.J.: Ablex, 1983.

Rorty, A. O. (Ed.). *Explaining emotions*. Berkeley: University of California Press, 1980.

Rorty, R. *Philosophy and the mirror of nature*. Princeton, N.J.: Princeton University Press, 1979.

Sameroff, A. J., Seifer, R., & Elias, P. K. Sociocultural variability in infant temperament ratings. *Child Development*, 1982, *53*, 164–173.

Schwartz, G. E. Psychophysiological patterning of emotion revisited: A systems perspective. In C. E. Izard (Ed.), *Measuring emotions in infants and children*, pp. 67–93. Cambridge: Cambridge University Press, 1982.

Seligman, M. E. P. *Helplessness*. San Francisco: Freeman, 1975.

Shields, S. A., & Stern, R. M. Emotion: The perception of bodily change. In P. Pliner, K. R. Blankstein, & I. M. Speigel (Eds.), *Perception of emotion in self and others*, pp. 85–106. New York: Plenum, 1979.

Tanji, J., & Evarts, E. V. Anticipatory activity of motor cortex neurons in relation to direction of an intended movement. *Journal of Neurophysiology*, 1976, *39*, 1062–1068.

3   Affect and cognition: the hard interface

R. B. Zajonc and Hazel Markus

In contemporary psychology, cognitive and affective processes are treated within largely separate and distinct conceptual frameworks, and, with few exceptions (e.g., Lang, 1979; Mandler, 1975), scientific publications in one area of research do not cite those in the other. Yet both domains of research investigate processes that interact with one another constantly and vigorously. Even though most theories of emotion assume as necessary the extensive participation of cognitive functions (Lazarus, 1966; Mandler, 1975; Schachter & Singer, 1962), the precise nature of this participation has been seldom explicitly analyzed. And it is equally remarkable that, even though cognitive content is rarely processed without the participation of affect (Piaget, 1981), cognitive theories have no conceptual elements that reflect the contribution of affective factors (Zajonc, 1980). This conceptual isolation of affect and cognition is likely to persist unless we come to understand which elements of these two processes make contact with each other and how the influence of one process over the other is actually effected.

The interface of affect and cognition presents a considerable theoretical and experimental challenge because it is not clear just *how* and *where* the affect-cognition interface should best be studied. Both affect and cognition are complex and manifold processes sharing many subsystems of the organism (e.g., neural, visceral, muscular, glandular, mental) and deriving from a variety of common external and internal sources (e.g., biological states, sensory input, and subjective experiences). Traditionally, however, it has been thought that the contact between affect and cognition takes place primarily or even exclusively at the level of internal mental representations. Implicitly, research and theory have commonly held that for affect to influence information processing, some form of the affective representation (say, the subjective experience of emotion) must make contact with a cognitive representation of the information being processed. Thus, the interaction of affective and cognitive elements is analyzed with a focus on the associative structures that represent both types of elements (Bower, 1981; Isen et al., 1978).

This chapter was prepared as part of a research program supported by the National Science Foundation, Grant BS-8117977.

73

In contrast, it is the premise of this chapter that associative structures are not the only form of representation, and that affect and cognition are in fact represented in multiple ways. This is most obvious with respect to affect. Feelings, emotions, and moods do result in specific sets of mental representations, but they are most readily identified by responses of the motor and visceral systems such as clenched fists, red faces, bulging veins, slumped postures, silly grins, pounding hearts, and queasy stomachs. The motor system is extensively engaged in affective processes, and it is reasonable that affect is at least partially represented by these somatic responses. Cognition, like affect, may also be represented in a variety of the organism's activities. For example, when observers are first exposed to a novel object they do more than just orient their sensory apparatus so as to explore the various attributes and parts of the stimulus. They open their mouths, move their hands over their lips, and shift their weight from one foot to the other. The function of the motor system during nonperceptual tasks such as thinking, recalling, or imaging is even more striking. People engaged in an arithmetic problem often gnash their teeth, bite their pencils, scratch their heads, furrow their brows, or lick their lips. Why? Why do people who are angry squint their eyes and tense their shoulders? Why do people who are thinking hard bite their lips and tap their feet? Are these actions just epiphenomena that accompany the core processes of feeling and thinking or might they themselves be integral parts of these processes? Perhaps both affect and cognition avail themselves of the motor system for representational purposes to a significant degree. In this chapter we will focus on this possibility and examine the motor system as a critical point of contact between affect and cognition. Our analysis is carried out in the expectation that the motor aspects of the affect-cognition interface can provide a rich database revealing affective and cognitive phenomena that can be directly observed, measured, and manipulated.

Representation of affect

In the present context, we need not mean anything more by a "representation" than some event *within* the organism that *stands for* a particular referent, be it an external stimulus (concrete, verbal, or abstract) or an internal stimulus, such as proprioceptive experience or kinesthetic feedback. A representation, like a symbol, is "anything that denotes or refers to anything else" (Kolers & Smythe, 1979), and in the case of affect, the "something else" is some element, feature, or manifestation of affect. In representation of affect, as in language or in cognition generally, there need not be a one-to-one correspondence between a particular representation and its referent. The words *chair* and *table* stand for a variety of objects and meanings. Their meanings in the sentence "The chair may not be moved to the table" can be understood by knowing what information preceded and followed it, and they have quite different meanings than in the sentence "The chair may not move to table a motion." Nor is it required that there be an isomorphism between the representation and its referent, because the representation of affect need not be an analog or a map of its referent. Again, this is so also in language where, except for onomatopoeia, there is no analog correspondence between words and their referents. And the same is true of cognitive representations, such as propositions, categories, and cognitive structures.

Representation of affect according to theories of emotion

There are two broad, partly overlapping classes of recent theories of emotion, and both would lead to similar conclusions about the nature of affective representations. One class – the cognitive theories of emotion – invokes cognition as a necessary factor (e.g., Lazarus, 1966; Mandler, 1975; Schachter & Singer, 1962). The motor system and expressive movements do not figure as significant elements in the cognitive theories of emotion. These elements are central in another class of theories: the somatic theories of emotion. This class of theories also considers cognitive processes to be involved in the generation of emotion, but in these theories the somatic processes play a more prominent role (e.g., Ekman & Friesen, 1975; Izard, 1977; Leventhal, 1980; Tomkins, 1962, 1963). These two classes of theories have generally different orientations and different purposes. The cognitive theories of emotion seek mainly to explicate the subjective manifestations of emotion: They are concerned with the emotional *experience* and with the phenomenology of emotion. The somatic theories of emotion, on the other hand, attempt mainly to describe the *expression* of emotion and to explicate the *perception* of emotional expressions. They are concerned with the universalities of expression of emotion, and they seek to identify the significant parameters of emotional expression so that the various forms of emotion can be identified and classified. Also, they attempt to specify those stimulus properties of emotional expression that allow one person to understand the emotion of another.

The cognitive theories of emotion assume that representation of affect is "imposed" by the individual. According to the Schachter–Singer position, individuals may construe representations of their emotions by combining perceptions of their internal states with those of external events. Thus, subjects who were injected with adrenaline were friendly in a friendly environment and hostile in a hostile environment. Persons' perceptions of their own behavior, too, may help them construct representations of their affective states, according to Bem's (1965) self-perception theory. And in the somatic theories of emotion, the representation of affect derives principally from kinesthetic and proprioceptive feedback that is generated by emotional arousal. In all theories of emotion, therefore, "representation of affect" is rather abstract, and it is inferred by observing behavior and its antecedent conditions. It is invariably understood to be an abstract associative structure, erected from images, propositions, categories, or prototypes that stand for the external events that generated emotional arousal and for the internal states that correspond to that arousal. Its proof of existence rests entirely on inferences made from variations in behavior and their relationships to input. But we have no direct access to these representations and cannot observe them.

In both the cognitive and the somatic theories of emotion the motor and somatic processes are also important elements in the generation of emotion. Nevertheless, in contemporary theories of emotion they are not considered *in themselves* as having significant representational and mnestic functions. Theories of emotion consider instead the kinesthetic *feedback* from muscular acts as the basis for the representation of affect. And in order for this feedback to become representational, the kinesthetic and proprioceptive information must be encoded and processed by the individual in very much the same way as any other information that comes through the senses. This conception of affective representation is true even of motor theories of emotion such as that of Bull (1951), and in fact is true of all theories of emotion. In Izard's (1971, 1977) theory of emotion, it is the proprioceptive and kinesthetic feedback that is the basis for a direct representation of affect as "feeling," and it is feeling – the subjectively experienced emotion – that forms its cognitive representation.

Hard representation of affect

There is another simpler route for affective representations than that mediated by subjective states that, in turn, are generated by kinesthetic and proprioceptive feedback. The motor movement can *in itself – without kinesthetic feedback and without a transformation of that feedback into cognition* – serve representational functions. Thus, the afferent reactions that are elicited by the organism's own motor behavior and not by the external stimulation – what von Holst (1954) called *reafference* – need not be integral parts of motor representations. When a dog withdraws a foreleg in response to a bell signaling an incipient shock, it is utterly reasonable to regard the leg flexion as a "representation" of the bell-shock configuration in itself, independently of its proprioceptive and kinesthetic feedback and certainly without an awareness of this feedback. On some future presentation of the bell, the "memory" of the bell-shock association will be *represented* by low amplitude motor activity in the same muscles of the foreleg that were involved in the flexion. Recall that according to the classic terminology, once conditioned, the response pattern becomes a "signaling system," a concept that is virtually synonymous with "representation." It is important to note that we actually consider the leg flexion *itself* as the representation of the affective episode. An "internal image" of the flexion, another form of a cognition about it, or the neural events that produced the leg flexion can function as representations as well. Similarly, information about the commands controlling the effector system (Festinger & Canon, 1965) need not be part of the representational function of the motor system. But just because they can function in this manner is no reason to suppose that the representational capacity is exclusively theirs.

To be sure, the leg flexion is not the type of representation that has been commonly conceptualized in such terms as "proposition," "image," "category," and "cognitive structure." But except for the fact that leg flexion is observable, its representational function is formally indistinguishable from representations given by associative structures, propositions, images, or scripts. It has all the critical representational properties. It has a fixed referent; it is symbolic in that it can substitute for that referent; it can be combined and interact with other representations; it can become a part of a larger "knowledge" or skill structure; and it can be retained, lost, suppressed, or retrieved. We shall call the representations provided by the motor system *hard* representations mainly to distinguish them from the more abstract, verbal, propositional, analog, or iconic forms of representations, which we will call *soft* representations.

It is obvious that some aspects and features of the motor processes in emotion must, in fact, be representational. Expressions of emotion have distinct meanings, readily grasped even by members of different linguistic and cultural communities (Ekman, 1971). These meanings, therefore, must be readily apprehended by individuals who produce these expressions. Theoretically, therefore, the representational and mnestic functions of the motor system in emotion are simply a matter of acknowledging the obvious. To avoid any misunderstanding, let us clearly acknowledge that all theories of emotion regard motor processes as having some *indirect* representational capacity. However, these theories endow the motor system with representational capacities only through cognitive mediation. That is, the motor output is thought to be important in emotional representation, but only when the organism perceives and thereby obtains a soft representation of that motor output. With this view, motor output serves as a representation of affect only to the extent that the organism perceives it or registers its proprioceptive or kinesthetic feedback. In contrast, we are proposing that the motor responses in themselves – without a cognitive mediation – can serve representational and mnestic functions. The retention of these responses is a form of memory as valid as any other.

Needless to say, motor responses must have neural antecedents. And it may be asked, therefore, whether the neural events that activate a given motor response that acquires representational function may themselves be representational. These neural events, and others that are antecedents of soft representations, play a role in cognition and affect that is not easily established, given the current state of knowledge. The representational function of neural events that underlie soft and hard representations is problematic. We can only speculate. For any afferent or efferent act there is a corresponding neural activity. However, there is a great deal of other simultaneous adjacent neural activity that has little to do with the figural afferent and efferent neural events. If the neural activity that is the correlate of particular information processing or affective event under examination is embedded in a noisy background, its representational usefulness would be limited. At times, however, neural events are more distinctive, whereas sensorimotor activity is diffuse and has no distinctive features that would be useful for representational purposes. Such states occur in dreams, for example. Under these conditions, neural processes may play a more significant representational and mnestic function.

From one point of view, however, it would seem that motor output cannot serve representational functions independently because, according to such views as the close-loop theory (Adams, 1971) or the schema theory (Schmidt, 1975), stable motor patterns are themselves controlled by cognitive programs. These theories require kinesthetic feedback to monitor the execution of the motor program or schema, because it is through such feedback that each successive subroutine is instantiated. Thus, if all recurring motor processes are *themselves* under the control of cognitive programs, their representational functions would be entirely redundant, superfluous, and not independent of the cognitive system. The earlier and the more recent studies on deafferentation, however, show that there is muscular "knowledge" *without kinesthetic feedback*. Taub (1980) severed the afferent fibers from both forelimbs of a monkey, and he blinded the animal to eliminate visual feedback. Yet even then the monkey could still perform previously acquired responses, with rather complex instrumental behavior patterns, "[running] off without requiring the support of sensory feedback of any kind" (p. 378). Thus, if muscular patterns, such as climbing and reaching, that entail extensive contact with particular features of the environment and hence an integration with other sensory input need not be guided by kinesthetic or visual feedback, then motor patterns serving representational functions need such feedback even less, because these patterns are for the most part self-contained and seldom involve any features of the environment.

Other systems, too, such as the autonomic, glandular, or the visceral, can serve representational and mnestic functions in emotion. They, too, are hard representations of emotions. Thus, for example, Bull (1951) observed two distinct reactions when she hypnotized subjects to experience disgust: One was muscular in the form of an aversion to, or turning away from, the imagined source of stimulation, and the second was visceral in the form of nausea, as if the person was about to vomit. The gastrointestinal activity could well constitute a partial representation of disgust. But it must be only a partial representation in this case, because the muscular revulsion pattern is necessary to discriminate disgust from other states, such as seasickness. And recent work by Walker and Sandman (1981) suggests in a more subtle way that the cardiovascular system, too, has representational capacities. These workers found systematic lateralization differences in evoked potentials elicited by visual stimuli during different cardiac events. Thus, potentials to a flash of light recorded from the right hemisphere were quite different when obtained during rapid heart rate and high carotid pulse pressure than when heart rate and pressure were low. No such differences were obtained from the potentials recorded from the left hemisphere. On the basis of these results, Walker and Sandman suggest that "afferent impulses from the cardiovascular system modulate the context with which the brain receives and processes information." These results can be taken to mean that the muscles of the heart have representational capacities for emotion. Thus, we shall assume for the present purposes that the somatic manifestations of emotion, and in particular *the motor manifestations*, have representational and mnestic capacity. The scream, the laugh, the shedding of tears, the rapid withdrawal of a burned finger, are, *in themselves*, all representations of the affective states.

Figure 3.1 illustrates diagrammatically affective representations. Because it is unnecessary to our illustration, we omit neural activity underlying emotion that was to be found in the thalamus according to earlier theories (Bard & Rioch, 1937; Cannon, 1929) and in the limbic system according to more recent views (MacLean, 1958; Pribram, 1981). We assume that an emotional state can be brought about by biological, sensory, or cognitive events. Thus, the injection of heroin produces temporary euphoria, the perception of a looming hawk elicits fright in the quail, and the memory of her husband's death elicits the widow's grief. Whether any of these events can actually generate the basic emotional state with its autonomic, visceral, and muscular correlates depends on a number of gating processes, including attention, ambient mood, the presence of competing emotional arousal that interferes with the elicitation of the new emotion, and competing muscular engagement. One cannot be roused from a depression into euphoria without some doing.

The generation of emotion is associated with three components. One is the *arousal* of autonomic and visceral activity. The second is the *expression* of emotion, which is mainly its motor manifestation. These two forms of discharge – the internal arousal processes and the manifest expression – constitute the basis of the *hard representation* of emotion. The third component is the *experience*[1] of emotion, which is the basis of its *soft representation*. The soft representation requires the mediation of the cognitive system. Thus, the soft representations of emotions are like any other abstract associative structures: They are in propositional or analog form, but in the case of affect, they derive from a transformation of sensory or kinesthetic input. In the present context, the experience of emotion is simply the cognition of having one. In the extreme case, only arousal is a necessary consequence of the generation of emotion. Neither experience nor expression need be part of the emotion process. The latter can be voluntarily suppressed – a skill taught to a high degree of proficiency in the English public school – or simulated even by poor

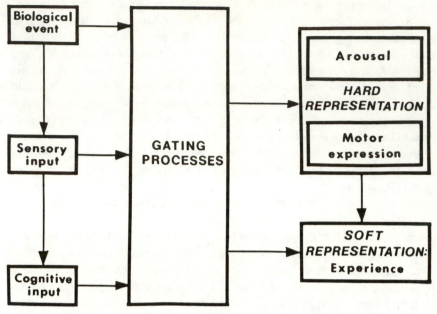

Figure 3.1. The representation of affect.

actors. And with regard to experience, the cognitions involved are sometimes not accessible to awareness, as in repressed guilt, for example.

In current research, the influence of affect on cognition is examined at the level of soft representation, because it is at this level that the critical causal contact whereby affect can influence cognition is thought to occur. How does fear or sadness, for example, influence cognition according to these views? These emotional states have as their consequences proprioceptive and kinesthetic stimulation. This stimulation, although internal, is perceived by the individual just as external stimuli are perceived. The soft representations (associative structures) that derive from the proprioceptive and kinesthetic feedback can thus interact with the associative structures representing the exposed stimuli (Bower, 1981; Isen et al., 1978), implicating processes such as spreading activation (Collins & Loftus, 1975).

Thus when the affect-cognition interaction is viewed entirely at the soft representational level, we do not really analyze how emotion proper influences cognition but only how one component of emotion influences cognition. We analyze instead how the *subjective (soft) representation of emotion* influences cognition, which is not altogether the same thing, because the problem reduces itself to the influence of one associative structure on another.

The role of hard representations in cognition

If we are to consider that cognition involves both soft and hard representations, their nature must be examined and specified. While the participation of motor processes is universally accepted as an integral part of emotion, their role in cognition is considerably more controversial. There have been, of course, several sporadic attempts to elevate the role of the motor system in the processing of information (see M. O. Smith, 1969, for a concise history). However, following the severe critique of the motor theory of speech perception (e.g., Neisser, 1967), there has been a marked hesitation in thinking of the motor system as having anything significant to contribute to higher mental processes. We attempt in this section to rehabilitate the representational and mnestic role of motor processes, for we fear that psychology may have abandoned the problem prematurely.

As noted earlier, affect and cognition share several subsystems of the organism. A given activity of the organism – muscular, visceral, glandular, or cardiovascular – may readily represent a cognitive element, an affective element, or both simultaneously. *In themselves*, hard representations of affect and of cognition are not always distinguishable from each other. Data about the occasion and the origin of the given motor action (or bodily function) must be consulted when it cannot be determined on the basis of the topography of a motor action alone whether it represents a cognitive element, an affective element, or a mixture of both. But this is true of all behavior – its meaning cannot always be fully grasped without knowledge of its antecedents. The marathon runner may look down at his feet because he is depressed over the outcome of the race or because his shoe is untied. In many cases, however, the parameters of the motor processes that represent pure information content can be distinguished from those that represent affect. These parameters have been identified fairly precisely in speech (e.g., Monrad-Krohn, 1963; Scherer, Koivumaki, & Rosenthal, 1972), although even in speech they are not *uniquely* identifiable: the parameters that represent affect in one language (e.g., rising pitch in English) may represent meaning in another (Chinese).

The software and hardware of cognition: extending the computer model

It is clear from the above that the conceptualization of the affect-cognition interface depends mainly on the role we are willing to assign to the motor processes in representational and mnestic functions of cognition. The tendency today is to regard motor processes that occur in association with information processing as secondary and derivative. For example, in the controversy about whether cognitive representations are in the form of propositions (Pylyshyn,

1981) or images (Kosslyn, 1981), no mention was made at all of the possibility that they may have significant motor correlates. Nor is the possible role of motor representation listed by Norman (1980) among the most pressing issues that cognitive science must confront. The reluctance to consider somatic involvement in information processing is not accidental. The analysis of hard components of cognition is virtually incompatible with the type of computer model of information processing prevalent in contemporary psychology – a model that ignores some very important functions of the computer in drawing the analogy. The contents of the mind, according to this model, are regarded in terms analogous to computer memory, similar to patterns of electromagnetic charges on a tape or disk. For some reason, the computer model of information processing, however, came to ignore the multitude of electronic and mechanical events in the machine that produced the electromagnetic deposits. It focuses our conception of memory on the *product* of information processing; it makes us think of the software and ignore the hardware, so to speak. Yet human memory may be more akin to the *process* whereby electromagnetic charges are deposited on a tape than to the resulting patterns of these charges – the end product of this process.[2] The computer model prompts us to conceive of memory as a static store (short term or long term), with retrieval questions reducing themselves to the matter of computerlike search strategies (e.g., direct access vs. location). This form of memory "retains stimuli," their copies, traces, or analogs. In this form of memory, the individual's responses in themselves are not retained nor are they significant components of the representation. It is only recently in computer simulation that a concern with responses and with the dynamic aspects of memory again becomes evident (Schank & Abelson, 1977; Simon, 1979).

Remembering stimuli and remembering responses

Except for a few sporadic publications (e.g., Lang, 1978), the current view of memory is that we remember stimuli not responses. It is the consequence of the language of the information-processing approach that the organism's memory functions are now viewed in terms of storing information. This view, of course, is a departure from the traditional stimulus-response approach in which the response figured as a much more significant conceptual element. Lang (1978) is a clear exception, for in his work responses contribute quite considerably to all sorts of retrieval processes. This secondary role of the individual's responses promoted by the current views of memory is well illustrated in research on articulation effects. The logic of past research, because it considered motor involvement to be secondary and ancillary, focused on the advantage that was gained in cognitive activity through the addition of a motor process. The subject's responses themselves did not figure in the representational and mnestic process. The advantage was considered *as accruing to the stimulus process*. Thus, for example, Murray (1965, 1966, 1967) compared the learning of letter lists by subjects who just looked at them, whispered them, or said them aloud. Loud reading resulted in best recall. Similar findings to those of Murray are reported by Wong and Blevings (1966). Other studies show that seeing one stimulus while saying another often reduces recall by more than one-half (Levy, 1971; Muensterberg, 1890; Murray, 1967; T. L. Smith, 1896; W. G. Smith, 1895). These studies form the basis for the inquiry, largely unresolved, into the role of the encoding and retrieval of acoustical (stimulus) and articulatory (response) properties of the material (Conrad, 1964; Hintzman, 1965, 1967; Levy, 1971; Levy & Murdock, 1968; Wickelgren, 1969). It is of some interest in the present context, therefore, that these authors stress the stimulus features as critical factors in encoding and retrieval even in the case of articulation. The enhancement of recall by articulation is interpreted by invoking kinesthetic feedback that adds to the *enrichment of the stimulus* (Hintzman, 1967; Murray, 1965; Wong & Blevings, 1966). Thus, in the study of articulation effects, motor responses are viewed as serving an intermediary function: They only provide an opportunity for kinesthetic feedback, and it is the kinesthetic feedback that is actually encoded and retained. The articulatory responses *in themselves* are regarded as having no mnestic value. But it is clear that these findings could be very well interpreted by assuming that articulation provides for a more extensive participation of motor processes since more intense and more extensive muscular action is involved in reading a word aloud than in reading it silently or in whispering it. Thus, these motor responses are able to provide a clearer and more stable representation: They are *motor representations of cognition* in very much the same way as flailing arms or thrashing legs are *affective representations of rage*.

Cognitive hardware

Have we discarded the motor elements of cognitive processes prematurely? There is, of course, an enormous motor involvement during mental activity (Baddeley, Eldridge, & Lewis, 1981; Bills, 1937; Block, 1936; Courts, 1939; Jacobson, 1929; Sokolov, 1972). The clearest examples are to be found in attending and orienting. The active organism plays an especially important role in Gibson's theory (1966). People looking at a street scene or at a painting engage a complex set of orienting acts that expose them to different features of the stimulus. The head tilts at a proper angle, the lenses accommodate for the proper distance, and the eyes roam over the various parts of the stimulus. It is entirely possible that the orienting and attending responses have partial representational and mnestic functions. This possibility is strongly suggested by the studies of Held and his associates (e.g., Held & Hein, 1963) in which people or cats were exposed to a given environment either by being allowed to move about on their own or by being transported. In all cases, passive

visual experience alone, without the participation of the individual's own
locomotor system, produced very inefficient spatial behavior. Even more dramatic results are reported by Dru, Walker, and Walker (1975) for rats with
striate lesions. Only rats that were allowed actively to explore their environment recovered their visual functions. The rats remained functionally blind,
however, when their experience involved only a passive exposure to the
stimuli.[3]

Observers are anything but passive when they are exposed to stimuli. If it
is a photograph, for example, they might smile if it is a photograph of a smiling
face or frown if it is angry. It is quite easy to understand why it is that perceivers
roam their eyes over the photograph or accommodate for the proper distance.
But why do they open their mouths? And why do they smile? And what traces
do these reactions leave?

The function of muscular activity present during cognitive tasks is quite
puzzling and not well understood. Why do people scratch their heads and rub
their chins when they try to remember something? Why does chess-playing
require such an enormous *physical* effort?[4] What is "going on in the mind"
that requires muscular output? The arithmetical prodigy Truman Henry Safford
is said to have engaged in rich and peculiar motor activity in the course of his
rapid calculations.[5] " 'What number is that which, being divided by the product
of its digits, the quotient is 3; and if 18 be added, the digits will be inverted?'
He flew out of his chair, whirled around, rolled up his eyes and said in about
a minute, 24. 'Multiply in your head 365,365,365,365,365, by 365,365,365,
365,365,365.' He flew around the room like a top, pulled his pantaloons over
the top of his boots, bit his hand, rolled his eyes in their sockets, sometimes
smiling and talking, and then seeming to be in agony, until, in not more than
one minute, said he, 133,491,850,208,566,925,016,658,299,941,583,225!"
(Scripture, 1891). When asked to suppress subvocalization, people find doing
mental arithmetic impossible (Fryer, 1941) and reading comprehension suffers
similarly (Baddeley, Eldridge, & Lewis, 1981).

The violinist Itzhak Perlman, in trying to play a difficult note, raises his
eyebrows (if it is a high note) and keeps them raised until the note has been
played. His face and body perform a rich program of varied movements. Why,
again? With few exceptions (Piaget, 1954), it is generally believed that these
motions are secondary and ancillary. But suppose that a good part of musical
memory is in fact lodged in these peculiar movements. Suppose that they are
significant. Looking at performing musicians, one is impressed with the possibility that they are engaged in a sort of matching process. It seems as if they
had "*in* their eyebrows" or "*in* their tongue" a muscular representation of the
ideal tone that they wish to produce. They seem to accommodate their hands,
they adjust their bows over the strings of the instrument, and modulate finger
pressure over the board seeking to attain the closest match between the output
and that ideal.

Thus, the issue that must be resolved is whether these movements are *generally* helpful (e.g., they rid the musician of excess energy or express emotion) or whether some of them, or some of their parameters, constitute essential and integral parts of the representation in memory of the music and its finer qualities. It is interesting in this respect that the raising of the eyebrows to high notes occurs *before* the note is actually played. And nobody raises eyebrows to a descending pitch. If the motor system is involved in learning a piece of music, it might also be implicated in learning a poem, in proving a theorem, in encoding a street scene, or in trying to recall a face of an old acquaintance Surely, a person who tries to "mimic" a particular tree or even such an abstract stimulus as a number will register these items more efficiently and will remember them better than a person who remains passive.

Perhaps the head scratching and chin rubbing of people who are trying to solve a difficult problem or to remember something is in some way functional. It is certainly unlikely that these movements are "superstitious," since they occur with such an enormous uniformity in diverse cultures. And there is certainly no possibility that the scratching of the head will "release lost ideas." But it is possible that scratching one's head is a "resetting" action that modifies the individual's ambient muscular "attitude," changes motility, and discontinues a pattern of muscular processes that may have been interfering with a particular muscular pattern that *is* the memory that we seek.

It is an obvious fact that mental processes are accompanied by overt and quasi-overt muscular activity. The overt activity is readily seen by any observer and the quasi-overt activity is revealed by electromyographic (EMG) studies (e.g., Cacioppo & Petty, 1981, 1981a; Jacobson, 1929; Lang, 1978; McGuigan, 1978; Schwartz et al., 1978; Sokolov, 1972). On the assumption that "the arms and fingers of the deaf are the locus of their oral, written and gestural speech," Max (1937) recorded EMG responses from the flexores digitorum of deaf and hearing subjects. Of the deaf subjects, 84% showed significant responses compared with only 31% of hearing subjects. Moreover, the average amplitudes for the two populations were 3.41 and 0.8 microvolts, respectively. The assumption here is that some of this muscular activity has significant representational and mnestic functions.

It is not difficult thus to demonstrate that muscular involvement can be advantageous in the encoding and retrieval of information. However, not all movement that occurs during thinking, recalling, or imaging is significant for affective or cognitive analysis. And in some cases it will be quite difficult to separate the representational motor movements from motor movements that have no such function. It also will be difficult to establish for those movements that are in fact representational just what information they carry. But if we find conditions under which motor output can be demonstrated as significant in the acquisition and retrieval of information, a useful terrain for the study of the affect-cognition interface will have been found.

Empirical research on the hard affect-cognition interface: some possibilities

The proposal to implicate hard representations in the study of the affect-cognition interface and thereby to gain greater knowledge about both processes is based mainly on the *potential* heuristic value of our approach. There is very little evidence at this time to support it directly, and judging by the past record of motor theories of perception and thought, this version will have a rough going as well. The most serious problem to overcome is that motor processes serve many masters. And because motor processes serve so many different functions of the organism, it will be certainly quite difficult to identify those processes that are significant for a particular act of information processing. Yet the multiple functions of the motor system are a fact of nature that the psychologist must accept. Motion, too, occurs in nature in terribly contaminated form, and the physicist had, therefore, to create experimental paradigms such as the vacuum or the inclined plane to observe it in its purified form. No one can predict the trajectory of a boulder tumbling down the side of a mountain. To examine the role of the motor system, it is necessary to discover or to create situations in which motor responses serve primarily representational and mnestic functions. To begin with we have chosen the domains of face recognition, mood, attitudes, and emotional disturbance. Although a diverse set of problem areas, they are alike in their potential for suggesting paradigms that will be useful in designing investigations of hard representations.

Motor reproducibility of visual input and recognition memory

In the initial phase of our research we have chosen to examine the role of hard representations in the affect-cognition interface with respect to the perception and remembering of faces. Face perception seems to involve an extensive participation of affective processes. But it is particularly significant for our purposes because the subject's motor responses that are implicated in face recognition are probably *mainly* representational rather than otherwise instrumental.

It is useful in formulating the face recognition problem to make a distinction between two types of sensory input, a distinction that is highly correlated with sensory channels. Some sensory systems are what we may call *quasi-reproducible* and others are *nonreproducible*. Within some sensory systems, the organism can immediately produce the same or nearly the same physical stimulus energy that reached the sensorium. For other sensory systems, reroducibility is not possible without elaborate external support. Thus, for example, when one *hears* a dog bark one can imitate it fairly well as one heard it and thus *hear* the same stimulus once again. But when one *sees* a dog bark one cannot produce a visual facsimile quite so readily. All sorts of auditory input can be reproduced with some degree of accuracy – a feature that is much less true of the visual input and one that is profoundly involved in speech perception. Thus, we can approximate the sound of an automobile but not its sight. One could argue that we can actually produce visual images. But visual images have no radiant energy that impinges on the visual receptors. Nor can we reproduce odors, tastes, or temperatures.

There is one exception to the superiority of the auditory over the visual channel. This important exception is the visual perception of the human body and its parts, a crucial factor in the perception and recognition of some emotions (e.g., Ekman & Oster, 1979; Izard, 1971; Tomkins, 1980). People can imitate gestures and postures and view and feel their own imitations. The face and its expressions, like other parts of the body, can be partially reproduced by the organism. And it would appear that in the perception of persons such a partial reproduction may in fact be going on. While there is no formal evidence, some preliminary observations in our laboratory indicate that perceivers do not necessarily mimic others' facial expressions to the full extent, but they do produce patterns of low amplitude muscle potentials that often correspond to the face that is seen. Sometimes these muscle potentials can only be revealed through EMG recordings. And, of course, people do not produce the visual stimulus of the perceived face and of its expressions that they themselves can see. But they do produce a fair analog which is readily translated into a visual image. Thus, changes in subjects' own expressions upon viewing photographs of faces (and certainly of actual faces) may play a significant role in encoding and retrieval, a fact that provides us with an opportunity for studying hard representations of affect and cognition. As in language learning and in many motor skills, production may turn out to be the key to efficient acquisition and retrieval (Liberman et al., 1967; Meyer & Gordon, in press).

A series of experiments carried out recently in our laboratory (Pietromonaco, Zajonc, & Bargh, 1981; Zajonc, Pietromonaco, & Bargh, 1982) illustrates how the role of hard representations can be explored in the study of the affect-cognition interface. In one of these experiments, photographs of faces were shown during the study period and subjects were tested for recognition memory in a subsequent session during which the original slides interspersed among an equal number of distractor items were presented for old-new judgments. During the study period, different tasks were assigned to subjects in different groups. Of interest here are three groups. In one group the subjects were required to imitate the person in the photograph. Several points of focus were stressed. Specifically, the subjects were instructed to reproduce the direction of the person's gaze, the expression of the mouth and of the eyes, and the orientation of the head and shoulders. Another group viewed the slides while chewing bubble gum. In this group, we expected that the chewing would engage motor responses that would interfere with those that the subjects might have otherwise used in encoding the faces. The third group of subjects also chewed gum, but in addition they had to make judgments about, but not imitate, the same features that the first group was asked to imitate. Thus, they had to decide whether the person in the photograph looked up or down, in what direction the head was turned, whether it was a smiling or a frowning face, and so on. All groups had an equal amount of time for studying the photographs.

The best performance was obtained by subjects who imitated the exposed faces (73% correct). The worst performance was that of the subjects chewing bubble gum (59% correct). The subjects who had to make judgments of the individual features but were prevented from using their facial musculature for representational purposes showed intermediate performance (70% correct).

It is perhaps in the ability to reproduce and mimic people's faces that an answer to the superior recognition memory for faces (Goldstein & Chance, 1970) may be found. Perhaps upside-down faces are so much harder to recognize than other upside-down objects (Ellis & Shepherd, 1975; Hochberg, 1968; Phillips & Rawles, 1979; Yin, 1969) precisely because one is denied the opportunity of mimicking them. It is interesting that people seem incapable of "mentally rotating" a face and then mimicking it. Even with training, the retention of upside-down faces is enormously difficult. It is a possibility that such mental rotation also involves a motor process, and that this process, involving the muscles of the face, perhaps around the eyes, interferes with muscular movements generating the representation of the face.

Our results indicate that motor processes are significant in encoding material, such as the human face, that has distinct affective elements and that cannot be processed without the participation of some, however minimal, affective reactions. It is, of course, not clear whether these results illustrate the role of hard representations of affect alone (i.e., the subject's emotional reaction to the photograph, such as attraction, empathy, or dislike), or just descriptive information (i.e., the shape of the face or direction of gaze), or in fact both. And it is up to future research to distinguish the features of the motor responses that serve as hard *affective* representations from those that serve as hard *cognitive* representations. Thus far, it is clear, however, that the musculature of the face serves a useful representational function.

Mood-dependent information processing and motor cues

Recent studies on the antecedents and determinants of mood suggest that it also may be a useful domain for the exploration of hard representations in the affect–cognition interface. In recent experiments (Bower, 1981; Isen et al., 1978), mood is translated into a node in memory, as any other information would be translated. Mood effects are treated as a special case of state dependent learning (Ho, Richard, & Chute, 1978), with mood providing cues that become associated with the test items to be acquired and retained. Other studies, however, have revealed that mood is an ambient emotional state that has some distinct motor and visceral correlates. A person who is depressed has a different muscle tonus and motility than a person who feels utter delight (Whatmore & Kohli, 1968). It has been found, for example, that psychomotor speed is substantially decreased under a depressive state (Natale, 1977a, 1977b; Velten 1968) and that posture shows distinct changes (Bull, 1951). Subjects given the Velten mood induction procedure (Natale & Bolan, 1980; Velten, 1968) tend to hang their heads down and contract their corrugator muscles, a motor pattern that Darwin thought to be the paradigmatic expression of grief.

When stimuli that have an emotional content impinge on the individual, the muscular activity deriving from *their* affect must somehow interact with the muscular ambient state deriving from the subject's mood (Schwartz, Davidson, & Goleman, 1978). Miller (1926), for example, reports that reactions to electric shocks are markedly reduced when subjects are very relaxed. Both the speed and amplitude of their responses were found to be lowered by muscular relaxation, and the subjects indicated that the shocks felt less intense than under the normal state of motor readiness. Mood-dependent learning effects, therefore, can be interpreted in terms of the hard affect-cognition interface.

There is now also considerable evidence that the voluntary induction of a motor reaction that is normally associated with a particular emotion, say anger, results in significant cognitive consequences (Colby, Lanzetta, & Kleck, 1977; Duncan & Laird, 1977; Laird, 1974; Laird & Crosby, 1974; Laird et al., 1982; McArthur, Solomon, & Jaffe, 1980; Rhodewalt & Comer, 1979). As one subject in Laird's (1974) experiment said, "When my jaw was clenched and my brows down, I tried not to be angry but it just fit the position. I'm not in an angry mood, but I found my thoughts wandering to things that made me angry" (p. 480).

Why should interference and facilitation be associated with incongruence and congruence of muscular states? Take an agitated and excited individual whose muscles are active and tense. The person receives the word *CALM*, which he or she must encode. If some portion of the muscle pattern associated with the motor representation of *CALM* calls for relaxed muscles, there will be a direct *physical* conflict, as in Miller's (1926) research. Muscles cannot be both tense and relaxed. Washburn (1926) was quite explicit about this point. She wrote that the "normal attitude of a healthy individual is an attitude of cheerfulness. Now, an attitude of cheerfulness is an actual movement system involving certain innervations, and while it is maintained it will inhibit all incompatible innervations" (p. 224). Thus, a person in the attitude of cheerfulness may be temporarily incapable of generating the hard representations that may normally accompany a depressing thought, just as "he cannot pronounce t and g at the same time: the movements involved are incompatible" (p. 225). Note, in this respect, that the meaning of conflict and of limited capacity is quite clear when viewed at the level of hard representations. The same cannot be said for conflict viewed at the level of soft representations, however. It appears that mood-dependent effects in particular and most state-dependent effects in general can be viewed as involving a conflict between ambient muscular state and hard representations of information items that the individual is asked to encode or retrieve. Thus, the hard representation of a given item is simply not the same physical configuration when the overall muscle tonus is changed. The individuals will be handicapped in their attempts, under the given ambient muscle tonus, to recall items that were acquired under another muscular state because the identical muscular representations cannot be faithfully reproduced. The role of muscle tonus in mood-dependent learning can be experimentally examined by varying the subjects' motility independently of their subjective representations of the mood-state dependency that had been suggested to them under hypnosis. In this way we would discover the independent contribution to mood-dependent effects of both the hard and the soft representations.

Motor representations of attitudes

Research on attitudes comprises another broad domain that can be fruitfully reexamined for the role of the motor system and hard representations. Typically, as is the case with mood effects, most attitude effects are assumed to result from an interplay of soft representations. The affective component of attitudes has usually been conceptualized as a mental component and is most often indicated by a mark on a rating scale. Social psychologists who have been the most prolific contributors to the attitude literature have been almost solely concerned with mental attitudes and have accorded little, if any, attention to the importance of the muscular or motor system in the determination and expression of attitudes.

This neglect of motor factors is particularly notable in light of the early history of the attitude concept, which reveals a strong and important emphasis on the motor component (cf. Fleming, 1967). Darwin (1872/1904), for example, defined attitude as an overt physical posture and used the term to mean motor expression. Sherrington (1906) also emphasized the motor component of attitudes and stressed that an attitude was the ordinary posture of the organism – "the steady tonic response" (p. 302).

Even the idea of a mental attitude derives from the concept of motor attitude and results from conceptualizing the mind as "assuming a stable posture, bracing itself in a determinate stance to receive the incoming signals so that the answer will be a resultant of posture and stimulus" (Fleming, 1967, p. 302). Washburn (1926) tried to reconcile the mental and motor aspects of attitudes and went so far as to suggest that all thought was accompanied by motor impulses. Every stimulus, even remembering a stimulus in the form of an image, "conduced to a slight actual performance of some movement" (p. 48). Equally radical are the views of Jousse (1925, 1974) and Wallon (1970). Subsequent work has focused almost exclusively on the mental nature of attitudes and has largely ignored the possible contribution or involvement of the motor system.

A reconsideration of the involvement of the motor system could provide some additional and more comprehensive explanations of existing attitudinal effects and could suggest as well a set of mechanisms that would allow a more complete exploration of the affective nature of attitudes. Many recent approaches to attitudes have been criticized as being excessively "cold" and for failing to uncover significant data about the emotional nature, function, or consequences of attitudes. This, in part, may be due to the emphasis on soft representations of attitudes. It is entirely possible that attention to the hard representations of attitudes could reveal their affective aspect more precisely. For example, it is more than likely that approach and avoidance tendencies are associated with distinct skeletal and muscular "attitudes" toward the target (Bull, 1951). Galton observed these "attitudes" in social interaction, saying that "when two persons have an 'inclination' to one another, they visibly incline or slope together when sitting side by side or at a dinner table, and they throw the stress of their weights on the near legs of their chairs. It does not require much ingenuity to arrange a pressure gauge with an index and dial to indicate changes in stress" (quoted in Pearson, 1924, p. 270). The popular literature on "body language" may not be far off the mark in this respect, and clear motor differences in the face and other parts of the body are revealed in approach and avoidance reactions to tastes and odors, for example. Nodding and shaking one's head are nearly universal gestures indicating agreement and disagreement, gestures that have very powerful semantic content. It is quite difficult and awkward to say "you are absolutely right!" while shaking one's head or to say "that is absolutely wrong!" while nodding. Osgood (1962) assigned a particular role to the kinesthetic system in processing meaning. Wells and Petty (1980) had subjects make these movements, ostensibly to test the quality of the headphones through which the subjects heard editorial statements. Subsequent measures of agreement with these statements indicated definite effects associated with head movement. These motor "attitudes" of approach and avoidance are clearly identifiable in many animal species.

More specifically, it should be possible to conceptualize particular attitudinal effects, such as the mere exposure phenomenon in terms of affective motor preferences. Previous research on exposure indicates that when a stimulus object is presented on repeated occasions, the subjects' attitudes to that stimulus object will eventually become more positive. There are consistent findings in the literature showing that preference for objects increases with the logarithm of their frequency (Harrison, 1977; Matlin & Stang, 1978). Experiments of Kunst-Wilson and Zajonc (1980), Matlin (1971), Moreland and Zajonc (1977, 1979), and Wilson (1979) all show that this effect need not be mediated by the subjective feelings of familiarity that are generated by stimuli with which the subject had repeatedly been confronted. Even when the subject cannot

discriminate objectively old from objectively new stimuli, a clear preference
for the old stimuli is obtained.

We do not know whether preference has a particular type of motor representation, but it is reasonable to assume that it has *some* type of motor representation. The first exposure of a stimulus generates an orienting pattern
with its particular response topography and autonomic and visceral correlates.
The body is tense and the limbs are poised for exploration, potential flight,
or attack. Repeated exposures produce gradual habituation and the body relaxes
and the autonomic arousal decreases. Galvanic skin response (GSR) measures
to Turkish-like words were found to decrease with successive presentations
(Zajonc, 1968). Thus, in making liking judgments of the stimuli that had been
exposed, the subject makes use of the hard representations of his or her affective
state that the stimuli elicit. In future studies, it should be possible to manipulate
the involvement of the motor system during the exposure sequence as well as
during the test sequence, much as was done in our face recognition studies,
and thus investigate the contribution of the hard representations in the course
of acquisition of positive affect for the exposed stimuli.

It was noted in a previous study (Zajonc, 1980) that attempts to change
attitudes by means of persuasive communication are singularly unsuccessful,
largely because persuasive communication does not reach the affective basis
of the attitude. In the light of the present formulation, we can now specify
why this is so. If motor responses are salient and significant in the affective
system, then to change affective reactions from positive to negative one must
also, and perhaps above all, change the motor aspects of these reactions.
Attitudes, because they contain strong affective elements, must also contain
motor components (although these motor components may be primarily of low
amplitudes). Given that the motor system is less amenable to change by means
of verbal control than the abstract representational system, we should not be
surprised that persuasive communications are unsuccessful in changing attitudes.
The significance of the motor system in attitude change must have been appreciated in the practice of brainwashing because the method involves a massive
assault on the body. The victim is very often starved, drugged, tortured, and
emotionally agitated (Lifton, 1956). All these practices may result in a condition
that makes it difficult to retrieve old thoughts and feelings and at the same
time makes the motor system more receptive to new representational input.

Obsessional and hysterical syndromes and tics

The role of the motor system has been given considerable thought in psychoanalysis and may provide yet another area for the exploration of the role of
hard representations in the affect-cognition interface. The obsessional personality, for example, is characterized by meager expression of emotion and
little awareness of affective arousal. These individuals seem to keep emotions

away, although they seem to be aware of the stimulus world around them that can bring about emotional reactions. The hysterical syndrome is just the opposite. The hysteric is overexpressive, exploding frequently with long and powerful motor outbursts. It is, therefore, interesting that the musculature and motility of these two types of pathologies is strikingly different. The obsessional personality is tense, holding his or her muscles under gripping control, lest an emotion be generated. The hysteric's muscle tonus and motility are either totally relaxed or in wild action.

The symptom of the psychogenic tic is paradigmatic for the interplay of hard and soft representations. The tic is thought to reveal the independence of the emotional motor impulses from the organized ego. In tics, the whole action of which the movement forms a part, has been repressed and the repressed motor impulses return against the will of the ego (Fenichel, 1945). In the present language, the hard representations of some affective content thus appear to become separated from their soft representations and gain autonomy. According to psychoanalytic theory, the repressed tendencies whose *motor* intentions return in a tic are highly emotional. Most commonly repressed are instinctual temptations or punishments for warded-off impulses. "In tics, a movement that was once the concomitant sign of an affect (sexual excitement, rage, anxiety, grief, triumph, embarrassment) has become an equivalent of this affect, and appears instead of the warded-off affect" (Fenichel, 1945, p. 318). The tic may occur in several ways, all of which suggest disturbances in the links between the soft and the hard representations of a particular event or situation. For example, the tic may represent part of the original affective disposition whose real significance became inaccessible to awareness. The affective stimulus may have thus received hard representation when it originally occurred, but its soft representation was either never formed, distorted, or repressed. Thus, a facial tic was determined in one case to constitute an arrested act of crying because the patient had been trained never to show emotions (Fenichel, 1945, p. 319). It occurred whenever something came up that might have provoked crying. In another patient, the facial tic apparently constituted a suppressed act of laughter at the patient's own father.

Two other motor phenomena – stuttering and slips of the tongue – are also considered to result from disturbances in the expression of a particular affect. Stuttering is said to reveal a conflict between the expressions of two affects. The individual wishes to say something, and yet he does not wish to do so. According to the psychoanalytic view, stuttering arises when speaking itself acquires threatening significance or when the content of speech has a threatening meaning. Very often individuals begin to stutter when they wish to prove a point or when they are in the presence of an authority figure. Under these circumstances, a tic may arise from the blocking of hostility toward the authority figure. The latent expression of hostility – say an impulse to spit, to growl, or to bite – is incompatible with the motor responses required for the speech production and stuttering occurs as a result. A slip of the tongue can be viewed in similar terms. Something disturbs the individual's hard representation of a particular stimulus. With a slip of the tongue, as opposed to stuttering, however, it is thought to be possible to explore the relationship between the actual utterance and the intended utterance. Thus, the underlying motive or emotion that interfered with the originally intended expression can perhaps be established.

Conclusion

Clearly, this chapter raises more questions than it answers. But many of the questions raised are empirical problems that have answers, some of which are now being obtained in our laboratory and elsewhere. And our approach allows us to formulate these questions quite readily and rather precisely. If the motor system indeed provides the organism with representational and mnestic functions, we should be able to specify them, measure them, observe them, interfere with them, or facilitate them. We could thus verify how they work and what contributions they make to cognitive and affective processes and to their interaction. Knowing these answers, our attempts to understand the nature of soft representations would be on a firmer ground. It is always better to start solving a system of equations after some of the unknowns have been eliminated.

It is not necessary for our purposes to deny or even to question the existence of soft representations, be they propositions (e.g., Pylyshyn, 1981) or analogs (Kosslyn, 1981). In fact, there must surely be a number of parallel representational systems of all kinds to allow for such a fabulous achievement as the acquisition of language by the child. It is, nevertheless, useful to discuss some of the presumed weaknesses of hard representations.

The realities of hard and soft representations

It is certainly the case that no research has ever demonstrated a strict one-to-one correspondence between neuromuscular activity and a particular image or a particular mental memory. There are some casual observations such as, for example, when we ask someone to describe a spiral and see the person make an overt hard representation with his or her hand or when a person describes a particularly vile taste by reproducing the original facial expression. For the most part, however, no firm assertions can be made about the nature of this correspondence. But neither have images and associative structures been accessible to independent observation, manipulation, and verification. No research has thus far been able to generate information about the nature of soft representations and there are doubts whether this information can ever be obtained (Anderson, 1978). There are doubts, furthermore, about whether soft representations of the form that is commonly postulated exist at all (Kolers & Smythe, 1979). Certainly, thus far, they are not available to inspection. At best, it is possible to demonstrate a correspondence between some conditions of input and some parameters of output that are consistent with some of our theories about certain types of soft representations. For example, some forms of categorization (a cognitive activity) during input have been shown to influence retrieval in a systematic way, suggesting an organization that corresponds to these categories (Mandler, 1967). But this research has no *direct* evidence that anything internal – that is, soft – has actually happened in the course, or as a result, of the sorting or categorizing of the items. The findings suggest that *something soft* may have happened, but no one can be sure that it has and what it was. The entire effect could have resulted from the placement of one pile of cards farther to the right than another – a condition that involved distinct muscular patterns.

Motor responses are too diffuse to serve representational functions

A criticism can perhaps be made that although the motor system might provide adequate representations of certain gross affective states, such as moods, for example, it is too diffuse to provide sufficient specificity to reflect faithfully the fine distinctions that are sometimes generated by the cognitive system. However, this limitation of the motor system must surely be illusory. The motor system is capable of extreme specificity. How else could we learn to *speak* a language? Because linguistic productions are readily understandable, even with a variety of subtle nuances, and because modern computer technology has nearly achieved speech recognition and speech identification, there can be hardly any question of motor specificity in language production. And if such specificity exists in language production, why does it not exist in other forms of motor output as well? The dancer, the gymnast, the skater, the sculptor, the diamond cutter, all require an enormous precision of motor output.

The motor system lacks sufficient variability

One criticism frequently voiced against the possible representational and mnestic function of the motor system is that it is simply too constrained and too limited to represent the enormous wealth of the stuff of the mind. There are two answers to this criticism. The first answer is that the motor system is virtually unlimited in its capacity to represent information, both content and affect. Consider the piano with its 88 keys. How many different melodies and each in how many different ways can be played with these 88 keys (disregarding the pedals that add another enormity of variations)? Now, the body has more than 200 bones and many more muscles. Let us just take a subset of these muscles, say 100, because all of them cannot function simultaneously (since when one contracts, its opposite must expand). Given 100 muscles, there are

2^{100} different patterns possible for the *simultaneous* excitation of all the units. If we allow each muscle to be extended or contracted more than once, such that the motor process is allowed to be sequential (like a piece of music) rather than simultaneous, an infinite number of motor representations are possible. And the fact that these muscles may also vary in the amplitude of response, from a fraction of 1 microvolt to a massive contraction, expands the range of variations even more. The facial muscles can literally encode some 6,000 to 7,000 appearance changes (Izard, 1971).

The second answer to the question is that we have no way of knowing the capacity of the soft representational system and no basis for estimating it. Hence, we cannot compare hard and soft representations in this respect.

The same motor response seems to represent different objects or events

The answer to this criticism, which is similar to the criticism regarding the narrow variability of the hard process, is that this need not be so and seldom is so. One needs only to look at the brain activity in the various areas of the motor and premotor system and to make the obvious observation that it is easier to account for the responsiveness to differences than to similarities, because from one fraction of a second to the next the pattern of activity changes radically.

Curarized organisms are able to acquire information

That curarized animals are able to acquire information is often argued as a criticism of the motor theory of perception and thought. Two answers apply to this criticism. First, suppose that the curare evidence is absolutely incontrovertible. Thus, we would conclude that the organism can get along without the participation of the motor system in representing reality. But this would only mean that the motor system is unnecessary. It would not mean that it is insignificant. It could still be possible for the motor system to act as an accessory in representational and mnestic processes.

The second answer is a criticism of the curare studies themselves. Curare does not affect smooth muscles, and such organs as the heart and the lung retain their functions. Thus, if the only muscles available for representational and mnestic functions are the smooth ones, then it will be those, under these circumstances, that will process information presented to the organism. Moreover, curare experiments seldom if ever go "all the way" for fear of damaging the animal. Thus, it is possible that some low voltage potentials might still be detected in the muscles that are involved in the hard representation.

Many of the points raised in this chapter are, of course, not new. It is today taken more or less for granted that affect and cognition are represented in a multitude of ways. Izard (1971) postulates central representations, Lang (1978) implicates both the stimulus and response in representational functions, and Leventhal (1980) speaks of innate, acquired (conditioned) and transformed (propositional) representations. It was our primary purpose, however, to draw attention to a neglected realm of representation of affect and cognition and point to an arena where they could be examined as one influences the other. In doing so we have exaggerated the distinction between what we call "soft" and "hard" representations, and we did so deliberately.

Much of the opposition to the early concept of motor representations was brought about by the extreme position assumed by proponents of motor theories (e.g., Watson, 1914). The early statements of motor theory of thought made the muscular system a *necessary* and central condition for the cognitive process. Some recent positions are also equally categorical (e.g., Jousse, 1974; Wallon, 1970), and they are equally vulnerable to ready criticism. There is nothing in the relevant evidence or in the structure of cognitive theories to suggest that motor representations or indeed representations of any particular kind (subjective, propositional, iconic, somatic, visceral, or neurophysiological) are in themselves *necessary* for cognition or for affect. It is more likely that there are a multitude of representational forms, partially independent and partially redundant, not one of which is absolutely necessary and each one of which is sufficient for some types of cognitive processes.

The proposal to rehabilitate some of the older ideas about the role of motor processes in cognition and affect (Jacobson, 1929), on the grounds that these processes are easy to observe, measure, and manipulate, must surely seem like looking for lost coins under a lamppost. And we admit that this is in part true. But a large number of coins – some of them quite valuable – were lost, and many must have rolled under the light.

Notes

1 The term *experience of emotion* has been equated on occasion with the term *feeling* (e.g., Freud, 1948), and thus it was meant to include other correlates such as arousal. For our purposes, we retain the term *experience* exclusively to refer to cognitive (and perceptual) processes of emotion. Experience of emotion reflects primarily the subjective aspect of emotion. Experience, thus, should not be equated with "registration" because one can "experience" an emotion falsely, that is, without the antecedent arousal and expressive correlates.

2 The computer model is misleading to some extent in the case of the "hardware–software" distinction. In the computer the software and the hardware are perfectly correlated. There is no more in the one realm than in the other. And there is perfect access to both. This, however, is not the case in human information processing. Soft representations may be redundant with hard representations, but they are not fully redundant, and access to either is not yet possible in most instances.

3 Note that the role of motor activity in Gibson's (1966) perceptual theory emphasizes especially the orienting function. The active organism is viewed as better able to gain access to stimulus information than is an inactive organism. In our approach, however, the emphasis is on the role of motor responses as representational and mnestic devices, not as instrumentalities of orientation.

4 Note that an intense emotional reaction can be also physically exhausting. Recall your most recent domestic fight.
5 We are grateful to Geoffrey Fong for drawing our attention to this article.

References

Adams, J. A. A close-loop theory of motor learning. *Journal of Motor Behavior*, 1971, *3*, 111–150, 411–418.

Anderson, J. R. Arguments concerning representations for mental imagery. *Psychological Review*, 1978, *85*, 249–277.

Baddeley, A., Eldridge, M., & Lewis, V. The role of subvocalisation in reading. *Quarterly Journal of Experimental Psychology*, 1981, *33A*, 439–454.

Bard, P., & Rioch, D. A study of four cats deprived of neocortex and additional portions of the forebrain. *Johns Hopkins Hospital Bulletin*, 1937, *60*, 73–147.

Bem, D. J. An experimental analysis of self-persuasion. *Journal of Experimental Social Psychology*, 1965, *1*, 199–218.

Bills, A. G. Facilitation and inhibition of mental work. *Psychological Bulletin*, 1937, *34*, 286–309.

Block, H. The influence of muscular exertion upon mental performance. *Archives of Psychology*, 1936, *No. 202*, 49.

Bower, G. H. Mood and memory. *American Psychologist*, 1981, *36*, 129–148.

Bull, N. The attitude theory of emotion. *Nervous and Mental Disease Monographs*, 1951, *81*.

Cacioppo, J. T., & Petty, R. E. Electromyograms as measures of extent and affectivity of information processing. *American Psychologist*, 1981, *36*, 441–456. (a)

Cannon, W. B. *Bodily changes in pain, hunger, fear and rage*. New York: Appleton, 1929.

Colby, C. Z., Lanzetta, J. T., & Kleck, R. E. Effects of the expression of pain on autonomic and pain tolerance responses to subject-controlled pain. *Psychophysiology*, 1977, *14*, 537–540.

Collins, A. M., & Loftus, E. F. A spreading-activation theory of semantic processing. *Psychological Review*, 1975, *82*, 407–428.

Conrad, R. Acoustic confusions in immediate memorising. *British Journal of Psychology*, 1964, *55*, 75–84.

Courts, F. A. Relations between experimentally induced muscular tension and memorization. *Journal of Experimental Psychology*, 1939, *25*, 235–256.

Darwin, C. *The expression of emotions in man and animals*. London: Murray, 1904. (Originally published, 1872.)

Dru, D., Walker, J. P., & Walker, J. B. Self-produced locomotion restores visual capacity after striate lesions. *Science*, 1975, *187*, 265–267.

Duncan, J. W., & Laird, J. D. Cross-modality consistencies in individual differences in self-attribution. *Journal of Personality*, 1977, *45*, 191–206.

Ekman, P. Universal and cultural differences in facial expression of emotion. In J. K. Cole (Ed.), *Nebraska symposium on motivation*, vol. 19. Lincoln: University of Nebraska Press, 1971.

Ekman, P., & Friesen, W. V. *Unmasking the face*. Englewood Cliffs, N.J.: Prentice-Hall, 1975.

Ekman, P., & Oster, H. Facial expression of emotion. In M. R. Rosenzweig & L. W. Porter (Eds.), *Annual Review of Psychology*, 1979, *30*, 527–554.

Ellis, H. D., & Shepherd, J. W. Recognition of upright and inverted faces in the left and right visual fields. *Cortex*, 1975, *11*, 3–7.

Fenichel, O. *The psychoanalytic theory of neurosis*. New York: Norton, 1945.

Festinger, L., & Canon, L. K. Information about spatial location based on knowledge about efference. *Psychological Review*, 1965, *72*, 373–384.

Fleming, D. Attitude: The history of a concept. In D. Fleming & B. Bailyn (Eds.), *Perspectives in American history* (Vol. 1). Cambridge, Mass.: Charles Warren Center in American History, Harvard University, 1967.

Freud, S. The unconscious. In *Collected Papers* (Vol. 4). London: Hogarth Press, 1948.

Fryer, D. H. Articulation in automatic mental work. *American Journal of Psychology*, 1941, *54*, 504–517.

Gibson, J. J. *The senses considered as perceptual systems*. Boston: Houghton Mifflin, 1966.

Goldstein, A., & Chance, J. E. Visual recognition memory for complex configurations. *Perception and Psychophysics*, 1970, *9*, 237–241.

Harrison, A. A. Mere exposure. In L. Berkowitz (Ed.), *Advances in experimental social psychology* (Vol. 10). New York: Academic Press, 1977.

Held, R., & Hein, A. Movement-produced stimulation in the development of visually guided behavior. *Journal of Comparative and Physiological Psychology*, 1963, *56*, 872–876.

Hintzman, D. L. Classification and aural coding in short-term memory. *Psychonomic Science*, 1965, *3*, 161–162.

Hintzman, D. L. Articulatory coding in short-term memory. *Journal of Verbal Learning and Verbal Behavior*, 1967, *6*, 312–316.

Ho, B. T., Richard, D. W., & Chute, D. L. *Drug discrimination and state dependent learning*. New York: Academic Press, 1978.

Hochberg, J. In the mind's eye. In R. Haber (Ed.), *Contemporary theory and research in visual perception*, pp. 309–331. New York: Holt, Rinehart and Winston, 1968.

Isen, A. M., Shalker, T. E., Clark, M., & Karp, L. Affect, accessibility of material in memory and behavior: A cognitive loop? *Journal of Personality and Social Psychology*, 1978, *36*, 1–12.

Izard, C. E. *The face of emotion*. New York: Appleton-Century-Crofts, 1971.

Izard, C. E. *Human emotions*. New York: Plenum, 1977.

Jacobson, E. *Progressive relaxation*. Chicago: University of Chicago Press, 1929.

Jousse, M. Études de psychologie linguistique: Le style oral rythmique et mnémotechnique chez verbo-moteurs. *Archives de Philosophie*, 1925, *2* (4), 429–676.

Jousse, M. *L'anthropologie du geste*. Paris: Gallimard, 1974.

Kolers, P. A., & Smythe, W. E. Images, symbols, and skills. *Canadian Journal of Psychology*, 1979, *33*, 158–184.

Kosslyn, S. M. The medium and the message in mental imagery: A theory. *Psychological Review*, 1981, *88*, 46–66.

Kunst-Wilson, W. R., & Zajonc, R. B. Affective discrimination of stimuli that cannot be recognized. *Science*, 1980, *207*, 557–558.

Laird, J. D. Self-attribution of emotion: The effects of expressive behavior on the quality of emotional experience. *Journal of Personality and Social Psychology*, 1974, *29*, 475–486.

Laird, J. D., & Crosby, M. Individual differences in the effects of engaging self-attribution of emotion. In H. London & R. Nisbett (Eds.), *Thinking and feeling: The cognitive alteration of feeling states*. Chicago: Aldine, 1974.

Laird, J. D., Wagener, J. J., Halal, M., & Szegda, M. Remembering what you feel: Effects of emotion on memory. *Journal of Personality and Social Psychology*, 1982, *42*, 646–657.

Lang, P. J. Emotional imagery: Theory and experiment on instructed somatovisceral control. In N. Birbaumer & H. D. Kimmel (Eds.), *Biofeedback and self-regulation*. Hillsdale, N.J.: Erlbaum, 1978.

Lang, P. J. Language, image and emotion. In P. Pliner, K. R. Plankstein, & I. M. Speigel (Eds.), *Perception of emotion in self and others* (Vol. 5). New York: Plenum, 1979.

Lazarus, R. S. *Psychological stress and the coping process*. New York: McGraw-Hill, 1966.

Leventhal, H. Toward a comprehensive theory of emotion. In L. Berkowitz (Ed.), *Advances in Experimental Social Psychology*, 1980, *13*, 139–207.

Levy, B. A. Role of articulation in auditory and visual short-term memory. *Journal of Verbal Learning and Verbal Behavior*, 1971, *10*, 123–132.

Levy, B. A., & Murdock, B. B. The effects of delayed auditory feedback and intralist similarity in short-term memory. *Journal of Verbal Learning and Verbal Behavior*, 1968, *7*, 887–894.

Liberman, A. M., Cooper, F. S., Shankweiler, D., & Studdert-Kennedy, M. Perception of the speech code. *Psychological Review*, 1967, *74*, 431–459.

Lifton, R. J. "Thought reform" of Western civilians in Chinese Communist prisons. *Psychiatry*, 1956, *19*, 173–195.

MacLean, P. D. Contrasting functions of limbic and neocortical systems of the brain and their relevance to psychophysiological aspects of medicine. *American Journal of Medicine*, 1958, *25*, 611–626.

Mandler, G. Organization and memory. In K. W. Spence & J. A. Spence (Eds.), *The psychology of learning and motivation* (Vol. 1). New York: Academic Press, 1967.

Mandler, G. *Mind and emotion*. New York: Wiley, 1975.

Matlin, M. W. Response competition, recognition, and affect. *Journal of Personality and Social Psychology*, 1971, *19*, 295–300.

Matlin, M. W., & Stang, D. J. *The Pollyanna principle: Selectivity in language, memory, and thought*. Cambridge, Mass.: Schenkman, 1978.

Max, L. W. Experimental study of the motor theory of consciousness: IV. Action-current responses in the deaf during awakening, kinaesthetic imagery and abstract thinking. *Journal of Comparative Psychology*, 1937, *21*, 301–344.

McArthur, L. Z., Solomon, M. R., & Jaffe, R. H. Weight and sex differences in emotional responsiveness to proprioceptive and pictorial stimuli. *Journal of Personality and Social Psychology*, 1980, *39*, 308–319.

McGuigan, F. J. Imagery and thinking: Covert functioning of the motor system. In G. E. Schwartz & D. Shapiro (Eds.), *Consciousness and self-regulation* (vol. 2). New York: Plenum, 1978.

Meyer, D. E., & Gordon, P. G. Dependencies between rapid speech perception and production: Evidence for a shared sensory-motor timing mechanism. In H. Bowma & D. Bouhuis (Eds.), *Attention and performance X*, (in press).

Miller, M. Changes in the response to electric shock produced by varying muscular conditions. *Journal of Experimental Psychology*, 1926, *9*, 26–44.

Monrad-Krohn, G. H. The third element of speech: Prosody and its disorders. In L. Halpern (Ed.), *Problems of dynamic neurology*, pp. 107–117. Jerusalem: Hebrew University Press, 1963.

Moreland, R. L., & Zajonc, R. B. Is stimulus recognition a necessary condition for the occurrence of exposure effects? *Journal of Personality and Social Psychology*, 1977, *35*, 191–199.

Moreland, R. L., & Zajonc, R. B. Exposure effects may not depend on stimulus recognition. *Journal of Personality and Social Psychology*, 1979, *37*, 1085–1089.

Muensterberg, H. Die Association successiver Vorstellungen. *Zeitschrift für Psychologie*, 1890, *1*, 99–107.

Murray, D. J. Vocalization-at-presentation and immediate recall, with varying presentation rates. *Quarterly Journal of Experimental Psychology*, 1965, *17*, 47–56.

Murray, D. J. Vocalization-at-presentation and immediate recall, with varying recall methods. *Quarterly Journal of Experimental Psychology*, 1966, *18*, 9–18.

Murray, D. J. The role of speech responses in short-term memory. *Canadian Journal of Psychology*, 1967, *21*, 263–276.

Natale, M. Effects of induced elation-depression on speech in the initial interview. *Journal of Consulting and Clinical Psychology*, 1977, *45*, 45–52.(a)

Natale, M. Induction of mood states and their effect on gaze behaviors. *Journal of Consulting and Clinical Psychology*, 1977, *45*, 960. (b)

Natale, M., & Bolan, R. The effect of Velten's mood-induction procedure for depression on hand movement and head-down posture. *Motivation and Emotion*, 1980, *4*, 323–333.

Neisser, U. *Cognitive psychology*. New York: Appleton-Century-Crofts, 1967.

Norman, D. A. Twelve issues for cognitive science. In D. A. Norman (Ed.), *Perspectives on cognitive science: Talks from the LaJolla Conference*. Hillsdale, N.J.: Erlbaum, 1980.

Osgood, C. E. Studies in the generality of affective meaning systems. *American Psychologist*, 1962, *17*, 10–28.

Pearson, K. *The life and labours of Francis Galton*. Cambridge: Cambridge University Press, 1924.

Phillips, R. J., & Rawles, R. E. Recognition of upright and inverted faces: A correlational study. *Perception*, 1979, *8*, 557–583.

Piaget, J. *The construction of reality in the child*. New York: Basic Books, 1954.

Piaget, J. *Intelligence and affectivity: Their relationship during child development*. Palo Alto, Calif.: Annual Reviews, 1981.

Pietromonaco, P., Zajonc, R. B., & Bargh, J. *The role of motor cues in recognition memory for faces*. Paper presented at the Annual Convention of the American Psychological Association, Los Angeles, 1981.

Pribram, K. H. Emotions. In S. B. Filskov & T. J. Boll (Eds.), *Handbook of clinical neuropsychology*. New York: Wiley, 1981.

Pylyshyn, Z. W. The imagery debate: Analogue media versus tacit knowledge. *Psychological Review*, *88*, 16–45.

Rhodewalt, F., & Comer, R. Induced-compliance attitude change: Once more with feeling. *Journal of Experimental Social Psychology*, 1979, *15*, 35–47.

Schachter, S., & Singer, J. Cognitive, social, and physiological determinants of emotional state. *Psychological Review*, 1962, *65*, 379–399.

Schank, R. C., & Abelson, R. P. *Scripts, plans, goals, and understanding*. Hillsdale, N.J.: Erlbaum, 1977.

Scherer, K. R., Koivumaki, J., & Rosenthal, R. Minimal cues in the vocal communication of affect: Judging emotions from content-masked speech. *Journal of Psycholinguistic Research*, 1972, *1*, 269–285.

Schmidt, R. A. A schema theory of discrete motor skill learning. *Psychological Review*, 1975, *82*, 225–260.

Schwartz, G. E., Davidson, R. J., & Goleman, J. Patterning of cognitive and somatic processes in the self-regulation of anxiety: Effects of meditation versus exercise. *Psychosomatic Medicine*, 1978, *40*, 321–328.

Schwartz, G. E., Fair, P. L., Mandel, M. R., Salt, P., Mieske, M., & Klerman, G. L. Facial electromyography in the assessment of improvement in depression. *Psychosomatic Medicine*, 1978, *40*, 355–360.

Scripture, E. W. Arithmetical prodigies. *American Journal of Psychology*, 1891, *4*, 1–59.

Sherrington, C. C. *The integrative action of the nervous system*. New York: Yale University Press, 1906.

Simon, H. A. Information processing models of cognition. In M. R. Rosenzweig & L. W. Porter (Eds.), *Annual Review of Psychology*, 1979, *30*, 363–396.

Smith, M. O. History of the motor theories of attention. *Journal of General Psychology*, 1969, *80*, 243–257.

Smith, T. L. On muscular memory. *American Journal of Psychology*, 1896, *7*, 453–490.

Smith, W. G. The relation of attention to memory. *Mind*, 1895, *4*, 47–73.

Sokolov, A. N. *Inner speech and thought*. New York: Plenum, 1972.

Taub, E. Somato-sensory deafferentiation research with monkeys: Implications for rehabilitation medicine. In L. P. Ince (Ed.), *Behavioral psychology and rehabilitation medicine: Clinical applications*. Baltimore: Williams & Wilkins, 1980.

Tomkins, S. S. *Affect, imagery, consciousness* (Vol. 1). New York: Springer-Verlag, 1962.

Tomkins, S. S. Affect as amplification: Some modifications in theory. In R. Plutchik & H. Kellerman (Eds.), *Emotion: Theory, research, and experience*. New York: Academic Press, 1980.

Velten, E. A laboratory task for the induction of mood. *Behaviour Research and Therapy*, 1968, *6*, 473–482.

Walker, B. B., & Sandman, C. A. Visual evoked potentials change as heart rate and carotid pressure changed. *Psychophysiology*, 1982, *19*, 520–527.

Wallon, H. *De l'acte à la pensée*. Paris: Flammarion, 1970.

Washburn, M. F. *Movement and mental imagery: Outlines of a motor theory of the complexer mental processes*. Boston: Houghton Mifflin, 1926.

Watson, J. B. *Behavior: An introduction to comparative psychology*. New York: Holt, 1914.

Wells, G. L., & Petty, R. E. The effects of overt head movement on persuasion: Compatibility and incompatibility of responses. *Basic and Applied Social Psychology*, 1980, *1*, 219–230.

Whatmore, G. B., & Kohli, D. Dysponesis: A neurophysiologic factor in functional disorders. *Behavioral Science*, 1968, *13*, 102–104.

Wickelgren, W. A. Auditory and articulatory coding in verbal short-term memory. *Psychological Review*, 1969, *76*, 232–235.

Wilson, W. R. Feeling more than we can know: Exposure effects without learning. *Journal of Personality and Social Psychology*, 1979, *37*, 811–821.

Wong, R., & Blevings, G. Presentation modes and immediate recall in children. *Psychonomic Science*, 1966, *5*, 381–382.

Yin, R. K. Looking at upside-down faces. *Journal of Experimental Psychology*, 1969, *81*, 141–145.

Zajonc, R. B. Attitudinal effects of mere exposure. *Journal of Personality and Social Psychology Monographs*, 1968, *9*(2, Part 2), 1–28.

Zajonc, R. B. Feeling and thinking: Preferences need no inferences. *American Psychologist*, 1980, *35*, 151–175.

Zajonc, R. B., Pietromonaco, P., & Bargh, J. Independence and interaction of affect and cognition. In M. S. Clark & S. T. Fiske (Eds.), *Affect and cognition: The seventeenth annual Carnegie symposium on cognition*. Hillsdale, N.J.: Erlbaum, 1982.

4   Interaction of affect and cognition in empathy

Martin L. Hoffman

Empathy seems like a simple concept – one feels what another person feels –
but the more one learns about it, the more complex it becomes, and the complexity
is precisely in the domain of this volume: processes of interaction between
affect and cognition. Empathy thus affords an ideal vantage point from which
to examine these processes. I will first summarize the most recent formulation
of my theory of empathy development, or, more precisely, development of
empathic distress (Hoffman, 1982b), and then examine in more depth than
previously several aspects of the theory in which interactions between affect
and cognition come into sharp relief. The issues include acquisition of "person
permanence" and the transformation of empathic into sympathetic distress,
the impact of language and "person identity" on the empathic experience,
and the role of causal attribution in the shaping and transformation of empathy.
Finally, I will point up the relevance of the theory for other affects.

Development of empathy

Empathy has been defined in two ways: the cognitive awareness of another
person's internal states (thoughts, feelings, perceptions, intentions), and the
vicarious affective response to another person. Our interest here is in affective
empathy. Most writers define affective empathy in outcome terms, that is, a
match between the observer's and the model's feelings. For reasons that will
be apparent, I conceive of empathy more in terms of the *processes underlying*
the match, that is, the processes responsible for one's having a feeling more
appropriate to another's situation than to one's own situation. In direct affect,
one reacts to events impinging on oneself; in empathy, one reacts affectively
to events impinging on someone else. The complexities of this definition and
its assumptions will be discussed later.

Though empathy is an affective response, it has cognitive as well as affective
components. The interaction of affect and cognition can be seen in the various
modes of empathic arousal as well as in the transformations and developmental
levels of empathic experience.

103

Modes of empathic arousal

There are at least six distinct modes of empathic arousal. They vary in the type of eliciting stimulus (e.g., facial, situational, symbolic, imaginal), the depth of processing involved, and the amount and kind of past experience required. They are presented here roughly in order of their development.

Primary circular reaction. It has long been known that infants cry to the sound of someone else's cry. The first controlled study of this reactive cry was done by Simner (1971), who found it in 2- and 3-day-olds. He also established that the cry was not simply a response to a noxious physical stimulus, because the infants did not cry as much to equally loud and intense nonhuman sounds. There thus appears to be something especially unpleasant about the sound of the human cry. Simner's findings have been replicated in 1-day-olds by Sagi and Hoffman (1976), who report in addition that the subject's cry is not a simple imitative vocal response lacking an affective component. Rather, it is vigorous, intense, and indistinguishable from the spontaneous cry of an infant who is in actual discomfort. We do not know the reason for this reactive cry, although it may be a primary circular reaction: The sound of another's cry evokes a cry response in the infant through an innate releasing mechanism; the infant then cries to the sound of its own cry, and so on.

Whether a primary circular reaction or not, it remains that infants respond to a cue of distress in others by experiencing distress themselves. This reactive cry must therefore be considered as a possible early, rudimentary precursor of empathy, though obviously not a full empathic response. The reactive cry may also actually contribute to the development of empathic distress because the resulting co-occurrence of the distress cue in others and the actual distress in self may lead to an expectation of distress in self when one is exposed to distress cues in others. This leads directly to the next arousal mode.

Classical conditioning. Because this mode requires some perceptual discrimination capability, it is therefore prominent a bit later developmentally than the reactive newborn cry. A type of direct classical empathic conditioning, it results from observing the cues of another's affective experience and experiencing simultaneously the same affect directly. Thus the affective cues from others become conditioned stimuli that evoke the same feelings in the self. Aronfreed and Paskal (1965) demonstrated this kind of empathic conditioning with schoolchildren in the laboratory. It often occurs in real life, too, as when the mother's affective state is transferred to the infant through physical handling. For example, when a mother feels anxiety or tension, her body may stiffen, and the child may also experience distress. Subsequently, the mother's facial and verbal expressions that accompanied her anxiety can serve as conditioned stimuli that evoke distress in the child even in the absence of physical contact.

Furthermore, through stimulus generalization, similar expressions by other persons may evoke distress feelings in the child.[1]

Direct association. This mode was described some time ago by Humphrey (1922). When we observe people experiencing an emotion, their facial expression, voice, posture, or any other cue in the situation that reminds us of past situations associated with our experience of that emotion may evoke the emotion in us. The usual example cited is the boy who sees another child cut himself and cry. The sight of the blood, the sound of the cry, or any cue from the victim or the situation that reminds the boy of his own past experiences of pain may evoke an empathic distress response. This mode does not require the immediate co-occurrence of pain or discomfort in self and distress cues from others. The only requirement is the observer's *past* experiences of pain or discomfort. Any feelings of distress that accompanied those past experiences may then be evoked by distress cues from the victim. It is thus a far more general associative mechanism than classical conditioning, and may provide the basis for a variety of distress experiences with which children, and adults as well, may empathize. The advent of words adds to the variety because the physical properties of a word can become associated with an emotion. Someone says "I'm terrified, I may have cancer" and the sound of the word "cancer" alone may evoke fear in the listener.

Mimicry. A fourth mode of empathic arousal was described more than 70 years ago by Lipps (1906). For Lipps, empathy is an innate, isomorphic response to another person's expression of emotion. There are two steps: The observer automatically imitates the other with slight movements in facial expression and posture ("motor mimicry"). This then creates internal kinesthetic cues in the observer that contribute (through afferent feedback) to the observer's understanding and feeling the same emotion. This conception of empathy has been neglected in the literature, perhaps because it seemed too much like an instinctive explanation. Some recent research (reviewed by Hoffman, 1978), however, suggests its plausibility.

Language-mediated association. The fifth mode, like the third, is based on the association between the victim's distress cues and the observer's past pain or discomfort. The victim's distress cues, however, do not communicate feeling directly but through language. They may be emotional labels ("I'm worried") or descriptions of events ("My child was just taken to the hospital"). Further, the victim need not be present. One might respond empathically to a letter describing what happened to someone or describing how they feel. Because it requires the ability to process information semantically, this mode of arousal is relatively advanced. The semantic processing may put some distance between the observer and the model. It may also reduce the involuntary component, though not totally, because the symbols serve primarily as the medium by which the model's affect is communicated; if one understands how the other feels, one can usually be expected to respond empathically. The role of language as a mediator of empathy will be discussed in depth later.

Role taking. The sixth mode usually involves the cognitive act of imagining oneself in another's place. The pertinent research has been done mainly by Stotland and his associates. In one study (Stotland, 1969), subjects were instructed to imagine how they would feel and what sensations they would have in their hands if they were exposed to the same painful heat treatment that was being applied to another person. These subjects gave more evidence of empathic distress, both physiologically and verbally, than (a) subjects instructed to attend closely to the other person's physical movements and (b) subjects instructed to imagine how the other person felt when he or she was undergoing the treatment. The first finding indicates that imagining oneself in the other's place is more empathy arousing than observing another's movements. The second finding suggests, more specifically, that empathic affect is more likely to be generated when the focus of attention is not on the model's feeling but on the model's situation and on how one would feel in that situation, that is, how one would feel if the stimuli impinging on the model were impinging on oneself. The dominance of cognitive and probably voluntary processes in this mode of arousal is indicated by another of Stotland's (1969) findings, namely, that the palmar sweat response of subjects instructed to imagine themselves in the other's place did not begin to increase until as much as 30 seconds after the experimenter had announced that the painful heat was being applied to the victim – a far longer latency than occurs in the absence of such instruction.

These six modes of empathic arousal do not form a strict stage sequence in the sense of subsequent modes encompassing and replacing the preceding mode. The first mode typically drops out after infancy, owing to controls against crying, even though adults feel sad when they hear a cry and some adults even feel like crying themselves, though they usually control it. The sixth mode, being deliberate, may be relatively infrequent – used perhaps mainly by parents and therapists who believe they can be more effective if they experience some of the feeling experienced by the child or patient. The intermediate four modes, however, enter at different points in development and probably continue to operate throughout life.

Which arousal mode operates in a given situation presumably depends on which cues are salient. If the expressive cues from the victim are salient, then mimicry may be the predominant mode. Conditioning and association are apt to predominate when situational cues are salient. Cues based on pictorial or verbal communication will of course require symbolic association. And, in any of these cases, the possibility exists for additional arousal if the observer gives thought to how he or she would feel in the other's situation. In other words, an arousal mode exists for whatever type of cue about the other's feelings may be present, and multiple cues may increase the level of arousal (although, as noted earlier, the response latency of empathy is increased by the addition of the "role-taking" mode). This is important because it indicates that empathy may be an overdetermined response in humans. Empathy may also be a self-reinforcing response. That is, as already noted in connection with the reactive newborn cry, every time we empathize with someone in distress the resulting co-occurrence of our own distress and distress cues from another person may increase the strength of the connection between the cues of another's distress and our own empathic response, and thus increase the likelihood that future distress in others will be accompanied by empathic distress in ourselves. It should also be noted that most arousal modes require rather shallow levels of cognitive processing (e.g., sensory registration, simple pattern matching, conditioning) and are largely involuntary. With several such arousal modes in the human repertoire, it should perhaps not be surprising that empathy appears to be a universal and largely involuntary response – if one attends to the relevant cues one responds empathically – that had survival value in human evolution (Hoffman, 1981a).

Development of a cognitive sense of others

Before discussing the cognitive component of empathy I should note that cognition did enter into the discussion of empathic affect arousal in several ways. The earliest arousal modes, except for the primary circular reaction, require a level of perceptual discrimination and pattern recognition adequate for mediating between the cues from the model and the affect aroused in the observer. The importance of cognitive mediation is especially apparent when the observer responds to the semantic meaning of cues rather than to their physical attributes. And, the most advanced mode, imagining oneself in the other's place, illustrates the role of cognition in actually generating empathic affect. What I mean by the cognitive component of empathy, however, is something more fundamental and unique to empathy.

Although empathy may be aroused by the predominantly simple mechanisms previously described, the subjective experience of empathy is rather complex. To be sure, the essential feature of empathy is the vicarious feeling in the observer of the feeling directly experienced by the model, (although this definition is too simple, as will become clear later). But mature adults who experience distress on observing someone in distress over the death of a loved one, for example, know that their own distress feeling is due to a stimulus event impinging on someone else. They also have an idea of what the other person is feeling – an idea based on how they would feel in the other's situation, their general knowledge about how people feel in such a situation, or their specific knowledge about that other person. Young children who lack the distinction between self and other may have vicarious affect aroused without these cognitions. In other words, the level of empathy depends on the level of cognition. This suggests that empathy development must correspond at least partly to the development of a cognitive sense of others. Because the cognitive sense of others undergoes dramatic changes developmentally, a conceptual basis for a developmental scheme for empathy is thus provided.

Although extensive work has been done on role taking, there is as yet no formal literature on a broader conception of a cognitive sense of the other. I have worked out such a conception, based on several different bodies of research, which will now be summarized.

Person permanence. Person permanence refers to the awareness of another's existence as a separate physical entity. The young infant apparently lacks this awareness; objects, events, and people are not experienced as distinct from the self. Until about 6 months of age, according to Piaget (1954), infants do not organize the fleeting images making up their world into discrete objects and experience them as separate from their own biologically determined sensations. The main empirical evidence comes from studies of object displacement. When a desired object is hidden behind a screen before the infant's eyes, the infant loses interest in it as though it no longer existed. By 6 months of age the infant removes the screen to get the object, which shows that he or she can internally reproduce the image of an object and use the image as a guide to the object. The infant's sense of the object is limited, however, since it is dependent on the presence of an external cue, the screen. When the experimenter places the object in a container and hides the container behind a screen where the object is removed from the container, the 6- to 18-month-old infant will not seek the object on being shown the empty container. By 18 months, however, the child retrieves an object after a succession of such invisible displacements, indicating that he can then evoke an object's image even when there is nothing in sight to attest to its existence. Piaget sees this as the beginning of object permanence – a stable sense of the separate existence of physical objects even when they are outside the individual's immediate perceptual field. The research since Piaget (e.g., Bell, 1970) suggests that "person" permanence may occur several months earlier, that is, children by the age of 1 year can retain a mental image of a person in the person's absence.

There is evidence that acquiring a sense of the object is a gradual process (e.g., Bell, 1970). At the age of 1 year, the child can hold an image of the mother long enough to find her (Bell, 1970) but perhaps not much longer. It seems likely, too, that the child may regress to the level of global self–other fusion when fatigued or emotionally aroused. In other words, at that early age, the emerging image of the other (and perhaps the emerging image of the self) may be unstable. The child may be only vaguely and momentarily aware of the other person as distinct from the self; and the image of the other, being transitory, may often slip in and out of focus with changes in the infant's state. Only later may person permanence be stable enough for self and other to be sharply differentiated throughout the normal course of daily events.

Perspective taking. The child's sense of the separate existence of persons is for some time highly limited. Although aware of people's existence as physical entities, the child does not yet know that they have internal states of their own, and he or she tends to attribute to others the characteristics that belong to the self. Piaget (1932) thought, based on his famous three-mountain landscape research, that it was not until about 7 or 8 years of age that this egocentrism gave way to the recognition that others have their own perspective. Subsequent research has shown that certain aspects of Piaget's original task (e.g., the size and complexity of the objects displayed, their asymmetrical placement, the requirement of a verbal response) served to mask the role-taking competence of younger subjects. With different tasks, 3- and even 2-year-olds can take the spatial perspective of others. The same is true of cognitive role-taking competence. For decades following Piaget's landmark study of moral judgment, for example, children were thought to be incapable of taking another's intentions into account until 8 or 9 years of age. Recent research that has clarified the ambiguities in Piaget's original stories (e.g., whether the child reaching for the jam really had bad intentions) shows that 4- and 5-year-olds make inferences about intentions and use them in making moral judgments (e.g., Imamoglu, 1975). Children of this age can also take the listener's perspective into account; for example, they use simple, attention-getting language when talking to younger children but not with their peers or adults (Shatz & Gelman, 1973).

There is anecdotal evidence that even younger children are capable of role taking in highly motivating, natural settings. Here are two examples. In the first, which I observed, 20-month-old Marcy wanted a toy that her sister was playing with. When she asked for it, her sister refused vehemently. Marcy paused, as if reflecting on what to do, and then went straight to her sister's rocking horse – a favorite toy that her sister never allowed anyone to touch – climbed on it, and began yelling "Nice horsey! Nice horsey!" keeping her eye on her sister all the time. Her sister put down the toy Marcy wanted and came running angrily, whereupon Marcy immediately climbed down from the horse, ran directly to the toy, and grabbed it.

What are the cognitive processes underlying Marcy's actions? She might have gone through a logical role-taking sequence in which she first realized that to get the toy she had to induce her sister to leave it, then figured out that this could be done by getting her sister concerned about something more important to her than the toy, and finally hit upon the horse. Or, she might have thought about what she would do in her sister's place, reasoned that she would give up the toy only if suitably distracted, assumed her sister would do the same, remembered her sister's feelings about the horse, and used this knowledge to lure her sister away from the toy. It seems likely, in view of her age, that Marcy's thought process was based more on imagery and association than on logical inference. For example, she might have noticed the horse, which triggered an image (or script) derived from past experiences in which she climbed on the horse and her sister came running and pushed her off, and then reasoned that getting on the horse was a way of getting her sister away from the toy. Whatever cognitive processes were involved, it seems clear that Marcy realized her sister would not give up the toy voluntarily, that she had to be lured away from it, and that a way to lure her was to climb on her horse. We may conclude that the rudiments of role-taking competence may be present under certain conditions in children under 2 years of age.

In the second incident, 15-month-old Michael and his friend Paul were fighting over a toy and Paul started to cry. Michael appeared disturbed and let go, but Paul continued to cry. Michael paused, then offered his Teddy bear to Paul. When this proved fruitless, Michael paused again. Paul finally stopped crying when Michael gave him his security blanket, which he had located in an adjoining room. Several aspects of this incident deserve comment. First, it is clear that Michael initially assumed that his own Teddy bear, which often comforted him, would also comfort Paul. Second, Paul's continued crying served as negative feedback that led Michael to consider alternatives. Third, Michael's final, successful act has several possible explanations: (a) He simply imitated what he had observed in the past; this is unlikely, as his parents were certain he had never seen Paul being comforted with a blanket; (b) he may have remembered seeing another child soothed by a blanket, which reminded him of Paul's blanket (more complex than it first appears, since Paul's blanket was out of Michael's perceptual field at the time); (c) he was somehow able to reason by analogy that Paul would be comforted by something he loved in the same way that Michael was comforted by his own Teddy bear. Whatever the correct interpretation, this incident, as well as a strikingly similar one reported by Borke (1971), suggests that children under the age of 18 months can, with the most general kind of feedback, assess the specific needs of another person that differ from their own.

If we may generalize tentatively from these two instances, it would appear that the rudiments of role-taking competence in familiar, highly motivating natural settings may be present in some children by the age 2 years or earlier. Role-taking competence of course improves and becomes increasingly complex with age.

Person identity. The third stage pertains to the view of others as having identities of their own — their own life circumstances and internal states beyond the immediate situation. Ignored in the literature, this concept is most closely approximated by Erikson's (1950) ego identity concept, which pertains to the integration of one's own discrete experiences and changing appearance over time and the formation of a concept of oneself as having different feelings and thoughts in different situations but being the same continuous person. The little research available (see review by Hoffman, 1975) suggests that 6- and 7-year-old children recognize their identity in terms of their names, physical appearance, and behaviors. Their sense of continuity over time, however, remains hazy until 8 or 9 years when more covert and personalized differences in feelings and attitudes begin to contribute to self-recognition, although even then their names and physical characteristics continue as the main anchorage points of identity. It thus appears that children's sense of their own continuing identity may begin to emerge somewhere between 6 and 9 years of age. By early adolescence, this sense should have expanded considerably, and once children observe coherence and continuity in their own lives, despite their different reactions in different situations, they should soon be able to perceive this in others. They can then not only take the other's role and assess their reactions in particular situations but also generalize from these situations and construct a concept of the other's general life experience. In sum, the awareness that others are coordinate with oneself expands to include the notion that they, like oneself, have their own personal identities that go beyond the immediate situation.

To summarize, the research suggests that there are four stages in the development of a cognitive sense of others: (1) for most of the first year, children probably experience a fusion between self and other; (2) by the end of the first year, they attain person permanence and become aware of others as physical entities distinct from the self; (3) by two years of age, they acquire a rudimentary sense of others not only as physically distinct but also as having internal states independent of their own. This is the initial step in role taking, and with further development they become able to discern other people's internal states in increasingly complex situations; (4) by late childhood or early adolescence, they become aware of others as having personal identities and life experiences beyond the immediate situation.

Developmental levels of empathy: affective-cognitive synthesis

As children progress through these four social-cognitive stages, the vicarious affect aroused in the previously described ways is experienced differently. I will now describe four hypothetical levels of empathic feeling that result from this coalescence of vicarious affect and the cognitive sense of the other, as exemplified by the empathic response to someone in distress.

Global empathy. Infants can probably experience empathic distress through one or more of the simpler arousal modes (e.g., conditioning, mimicry) long before they acquire a sense of others as distinct physical entities. It follows through much of the first year that witnessing someone in distress probably results in a global empathic distress response. Distress cues from the dimly perceived victim are confounded with the unpleasant feelings empathically aroused in the infant. Since infants cannot yet differentiate themselves from the other, they must often be unclear as to who is experiencing any distress that they witness and they may at times behave as though what is happening to the other is happening to them. For example, a colleague's 11-month-old daughter who saw another child fall and cry first stared at the victim, looking as though she were about to cry herself, and then put her thumb in her mouth and buried her head in her mother's lap, which is what she does when she is hurt herself. Kaplan (1977) described a similar response in a younger child:

At nine months, Hope had already demonstrated strong (empathic) responses to other children's distress. Characteristically, she did not turn away from these distress scenes though they apparently touched off distress in herself. Hope would stare intently, her eyes welling up with tears if another child fell, hurt themselves or cried. At that time, she was overwhelmed with her emotions. She would end up crying herself and crawling quickly to her mother for comfort.

Zahn-Waxler, Radke-Yarrow, and King (1979) found a similar pattern to be characteristic of 10- to 14-month-old infants. This first level of empathic distress is obviously primitive. We call it empathy, although the child does not really put himself in the other's place and imagine what the other is feeling. (Perhaps it would be more correct to call it a precursor of empathy.) The child's response is, rather, a passive, involuntary one based on the pull of surface cues and requiring the shallowest level of cognitive processing. This simple form of empathic distress is important, however, precisely because it shows that as humans we may involuntarily and forcefully experience others' emotional states rather than the emotional states pertinent and appropriate to our own situation, that is, that we are built in such a way that distress will often be contingent not on our own but on someone else's painful experience.

The transition to the second level occurs when the child approaches person permanence. With the emergence of a sense of the other as physically distinct from the self, it seems reasonable to expect the affective portion of the global empathic distress to be extended to the separate image-of-self and image-of-other that emerge. Early in the process, as already suggested, children are probably only vaguely and momentarily aware of the other person as distinct from the self; and the mental image of the other, being transitory, may often slip in and out of focus. Consequently, children at this intermediate stage probably react to another's distress as though the dimly perceived "self" and the dimly perceived "other" were somehow simultaneously, or alternately, in distress. As an example, consider Billy, whose typical response to his own distress beginning late in the first year was to suck his thumb with one hand and pull his ear with the other. He also tended to do this when he saw someone else in distress, an example of the first level of empathic functioning. Something new happened at 12 months. On seeing a sad look on his father's face, he proceeded to look sad and suck his thumb while pulling on his father's ear!

"Egocentric" empathy. The second level is clearly established when the child is fully aware that the other is a physical entity distinct from the self and thus able for the first time to experience empathic distress while also being aware that another person, and not the self, is the victim. Children at this level, however, cannot yet fully distinguish between their own and the other person's internal states and are apt to confuse the other's internal state with their own, as illustrated by their efforts to help others, which consist chiefly of giving the other person what they themselves find most comforting. Examples are a 13-month-old who responded with a distressed look to an adult who looked sad and then offered the adult a beloved doll; and another child who ran to fetch his own mother to comfort a crying friend, even though the friend's mother was in the same room. In labeling this empathic level, I used quotations because it is not purely *egocentric*: Although the child's attempts to help indicate confusion between what comforts the self and what comforts the other, these same attempts to help, together with the child's facial responses, also indicate that the child is responding with appropriate empathic affect.

Empathy for another's feelings. With the beginning of a role-taking capability, at about 2 to 3 years, children become aware that other people's feelings may sometimes differ from their own, and that other people's perspectives are based on their own needs and interpretation of events. More important, because children now know that the real world and their perceptions of it are not the same thing, and that the feelings of others are independent of their own, they become more responsive to cues about what the other is feeling. By 3 or 4 years of age, children can recognize and respond empathically to happiness or sadness in others in simple situations (e.g., Feshbach & Roe, 1968; Strayer, 1980). And, with the acquisition of language, which enables children for the first time to derive meaning from symbolic cues of affect, not just its facial and other physical expressions, they can begin to empathize with a wide range of emotions, including complex emotions like disappointment and feelings of betrayal. Eventually, they become capable of empathizing with several, sometimes conflicting, emotions at once. Thus, while empathizing with the victim's distress, one may also empathize with the victim's desire not to feel obligated or demeaned or the victim's potential feelings of inadequacy and low self-esteem – hence, the victim's desire *not* to be helped. And, finally, children can be aroused empathically by information pertinent to someone's feelings even in that person's absence. This leads to the fourth empathic level.

Empathy for another's general condition. By late childhood, owing to the emerging conception of self and other as continuous persons with separate histories and identities, one becomes aware that others feel pleasure and pain not only in the situation but also in their larger life experience. Consequently, though one may continue to be empathically aroused by another's immediate distress, one's empathic response may be intensified when one knows that the other's distress is not transitory but chronic. This fourth level, then, consists of empathically aroused affect combined with an image of another's general life condition (e.g., general level of distress or deprivation, opportunities available or denied, future prospects). If this image is the only information available (no immediate distress cues), empathy may result from imagining oneself as having the experiences and feelings associated with that life condition.

As an extension of the fourth level, with the ability to group people into categories, children eventually can be empathically aroused by the plight of an entire group or class of people (e.g., poor, oppressed, outcast, retarded). Because of different backgrounds, one's specific distress experience may differ from theirs. All distress experiences have a common affective core, however, which may allow for a generalized empathic distress capability. The combination of empathic affect and the perceived plight of an unfortunate group may be the most developmentally advanced form of empathic distress.

We can now elaborate on the definition of empathy as an affective response more appropriate to another person's situation than to one's own. When one encounters someone in pain, danger, or discomfort, one is exposed to a network of information about the other's affective state. Depending on one's developmental level, the network may include verbal and nonverbal expressive cues from the other, situational cues, and knowledge one has about the other's general affective experience beyond the immediate situation. These sources of information are assumed to be processed differently: Empathy aroused by nonverbal and situational cues is expected to be mediated by the largely involuntary, cognitively "shallow" processing modes. Empathy aroused by verbal messages from the victim, on the other hand, or by one's knowledge about the victim requires more complex processes such as semantic interpretation and imagining oneself in the victim's place. What may be defined as an empathic response for a very young child may thus involve relatively simple levels of processing of visual or auditory cues in the immediate situation, whereas mature empathizers may, in addition, respond in terms of semantic meanings of stimuli and representations of events beyond the situation.

Empathy is thus defined as to the underlying processes involved and the developmental level of the observer. It is also assumed that there is at least a high degree of similarity, if not an exact match, between the observer's affect and the affect experienced by the model in the immediate situation or in the model's general life experience. For the empathic process to result in such a match requires that the observer and the model process information similarly. This means that empathy may be unlikely when the observer and the model are at different developmental levels, at different levels of sanity, or from different cultures. Empathy might even be possible in these cases, however, if the observer had the "code" for the model's processing. A mature adult, for example, might be able to empathize with a child, an insightful therapist with a psychotic patient, and an anthropologist with someone from another culture. In addition to the code, the observer must also have the particular affect in his or her repertoire. I might not be able to empathize with a masochist's pleasure at being beaten, even if I fully understood the basis of his response.

Just how close must the match be for the response to qualify as empathy? I have argued elsewhere against insisting on a high degree of closeness (Hoffman, 1982a). For present purposes I will only note that when one is reminded by another's situation of a similar event in one's own past, one is apt to feel as the model does because people tend to process events similarly (assuming similar backgrounds and developmental levels, as previously discussed). There will always be an idiosyncratic component, however; for example, one's concerns about one's own child have certain nuances that may differ from the model's concerns about his or her child. This limits the degree of similarity possible but I would still call it an empathic response, despite the idiosyncratic component, if one remains aware that the other is having the direct experience and that one's own response is vicarious, and if one's attention remains focused on the other's feelings rather than one's own.

To summarize, one can empathize with someone who processes information in the same way, or with someone who processes information differently if one has the code for that person's processing and the necessary affective range. And one's vicarious affective response qualifies as empathy, despite its idiosyncratic component, if one's attention is focused on the other and the other's situation rather than on the self.

Cognitive transformation of empathy

Many affect theorists (e.g., Schachter & Singer, 1962) suggest that how a person labels or experiences an affect is heavily influenced by his or her cognitive appraisal of the situation. These writers are explaining how we distinguish among specific affects (e.g., anger, fear, joy) aroused *directly*. Whether or not they are right – see Izard (1971) for another view – a different type of appraisal appears to be so intrinsic to *empathically* aroused affect as to alter the quality of the observer's affective experience. This becomes clear when we take a closer look at the developmental processes mentioned earlier.

Person permanence and transformation of empathic into sympathetic distress

I suggested earlier how a child's cognitive sense of others may combine with his or her vicarious unpleasant affect and produce four developmental levels of empathic distress. The transition from the first to the second of these levels may involve an important qualitative shift in the child's feeling. More specifically, once children are aware of others as distinct from themselves, their own empathic distress, which is a parallel response – a more or less exact replication of the victim's presumed feeling of distress – may be transformed at least in part into a more reciprocal concern for the victim. That is, they may continue to respond in a purely empathic manner – to feel uncomfortable and highly distressed themselves – but they also experience a feeling of compassion for the victim. This feeling of compassion, which I call sympathetic distress, may include a conscious desire to help, because they feel sorry for the victim and not just to relieve their own empathic distress.

It is hard to document this shift but there is evidence, already noted, that children seem to progress developmentally from first responding to someone's distress by seeking comfort for the self and later by trying to help the victim and not the self. And, there appears to be an in-between stage, in which children feel sad and comfort both the victim and the self, that occurs about the time that children become aware of others as distinct from themselves. An example may help make the process clear. Recall Billy, who at 12 months reacted to his father's sad look by looking sad, sucking his thumb, and pulling his father's ear. My interpretation is that with the beginning of self–other differentiation Billy experienced a dual emotion: a feeling of his own distress and the wish to alleviate it (empathic distress) along with a feeling of concern for his father's distress (sympathetic distress). In a similar example, Zahn-Waxler and associates (1979) describe a child whose first positive overture to someone in distress occurred at 12 months when he alternated between gently touching the victim and gently touching himself.

What processes may account for this developmental shift? First, as I suggested earlier, with the acquisition of person permanence the unpleasant affect experienced as part of the child's initial global, undifferentiated "self" may be transferred to the separate "self" and "other" that emerge. Second, it seems reasonable to assume that the experience of any unpleasant affect includes some kind of a motive or wish, not necessarily conscious, that it be terminated. Such a motive is therefore probably included in the unpleasant affect transferred to the "other" (as well as to the "self"). Consequently, the child's empathic distress now includes a wish to terminate distress in the other, the sympathetic distress component, and a more purely "empathic," wish to terminate distress in the self.

As mentioned earlier, the process of self–other differentiation is gradual and there is probably an early period in which the child is only vaguely and momentarily aware of the other as distinct from the self. The emerging "self" and the emerging "other" may thus slip in and out of focus. It follows that the child may often respond to another's distress by feeling as though the dimly perceived "self" and the dimly perceived "other" were somehow simultaneously, or alternately, in distress. The child may thus frequently have the experience of wishing to alleviate or terminate distress in the self in close association with a similar wish regarding distress in the other. As a result of this co-occurrence, the child may subsequently be expected to have a strength-ened connection between distress in others and his or her empathic and sym-pathetic response.

An early period of subjectively overlapping concern such as this, in which the "self" and the "other" are experienced as "sharing" the distress, would seem to provide a basis for the positive attitude toward the emerging "other" indicated in the two examples cited above. The gradual nature of self–other differentiation may therefore be important because it gives the child the ex-perience of simultaneously wishing to terminate the other's distress as well as distress in the self, thus providing a link between the initially quasi-egoistic empathic distress response (*quasi*-egoistic because the self was then a fusion of self and other and there was therefore no actual conflict between a self and an other) and the earliest traces of a true sympathetic distress. If the sense of the other were attained suddenly, the child would lack this experience; and on discovering that the pain belonged to someone else, the child might simply experience a feeling of relief (or even blame the other for his or her own empathic distress). The co-occurrence of distress in the emerging "self" and in the emerging "other" may thus be an important factor not only in the transition between the first two levels of empathic distress but also in the partial transformation of empathic into sympathetic distress.

To summarize, there are two significant aspects of the child's early response to another's distress that may account for the seemingly paradoxical notion that self–other differentiation, which might be expected to create a barrier between persons, and empathic distress, which is partially egoistic, combine to produce the developmental basis for sympathetic distress. These aspects are manifest in the earliest stages of self–other differentiation: (1) the transfer of the unpleasant affect – and the urge to terminate it, associated with the initial global self – to its emerging separate parts ("self" and "other") and (2) the subjective experience of "sharing" distress, which is due to the gradual attainment of a sense of the other and gives the child the experience of wishing the other's distress to end.

Insofar as this transformation does occur, the last three developmental levels previously described may be said to apply to sympathetic as well as empathic distress. I will continue to use the term empathic distress generically, however, to refer to both empathic and sympathetic distress.

Language, semantic processing, and empathic experience

As noted earlier, empathy is often mediated in part by language. To highlight the processes involved, consider situations in which language provides the only cue about another's affective state; for example, one receives a letter describing the other's feelings and the surrounding circumstances. In these situations language might produce an empathic response because of the physical properties of the words used or because the words have become signals of a particular affect (e.g., the way the word *cancer* evokes fear). These cases reduce to a type of conditioning or association and are less interesting here. What is special about language are the cases in which the observer must engage in semantic processing, and the meaning obtained from the message mediates the link between the model's and the observer's affective state. The message may pertain to the model's feeling (I'm worried), the model's situation (My child was just taken to the hospital), or, more commonly, both. In any case, empathic affect may be aroused through at least three distinct types of role-taking processes.

These processes, in all of which cognition is heavily implicated, turned up in a number of interviews I conducted with adults about their empathic responses to someone's distressing experience communicated to them by letter or a third person.

Focus on other. On learning of the other's misfortune, one may (a) simply imagine how the other is feeling, which may result in an empathic affective response. The empathic feeling may be enhanced if one also (b) visualizes the other person's bahavioral response. In using visual imagery, one may picture the other's facial expression, posture, and overt behavior; in using auditory imagery, one may imagine the other expressing his or her feelings verbally, for example, with a sad voice or cry. Depending on how vivid the image is, one may then respond empathically to the image, more or less as though the other was physically present. In this way one may provide oneself with the nonverbal cues that are missing, and then respond to them as though the other person was present.

Focus on self. On learning of the other's misfortune, instead of imagining the other's feelings or actions, one may (a) picture oneself in the model's place and imagine how one would feel, that is, one may imagine that the stimuli impinging on the other are impinging on oneself. If one can do this vividly enough, one may experience some of the same affect experienced by the other. One's affective response may be enhanced considerably if one also (b) is reminded of similar events in one's own past in which one actually experienced the emotion. Because of the associative links, some of the earlier emotions may be evoked in the present. This is especially likely if one employs visual or auditory imagery. Even if one lacks the actual experience, one may be able to imagine how it would feel if one had the experience. This might be possible, for example, if one had previously thought or worried a lot about how one would feel if it did happen.

Combination. On learning of the other's misfortune, one may shift back and forth between these "other-focused" and "self-focused" processes.

Empathic responses that are based primarily on self-focused processes are subject to an interesting vulnerability: The focus on one's own affective experience may take control of one's entire response. The result may be that one becomes lost in one's own egoistic concerns and the image of the other and the other's condition that initiated the process may slip out of focus and fade away. This phenomenon, which I call "egoistic drift," may seem to contradict Stotland's finding, noted earlier, that subjects observing someone being given a painful heat treatment and instructed to imagine how they would feel in that situation show *more* empathy than subjects instructed to imagine how the victim feels. My explanation is that the self-focused condition arouses more intense empathy because it makes a direct connection between the other's affective state and the observer's own need system. This very connection, however, may also make the self-focused condition more vulnerable to "egoistic drift." A testable hypothesis that follows is that the self-focused condition produces more intense, but less stable, empathic affect. Regardless of the explanation, the observer's response, though initially triggered by another's affective state, would not qualify as empathy (we might call it an "aborted" empathic response) unless the observer returned to a focus on the other person.

Empathic responses that are mediated entirely by language are also subject to another, more general type of vulnerability: The observer's affect may not match the model's because of the necessary intervening encoding and decoding processes. Consider the encoding process by the model. Words, which are ways of categorizing experience, are typically more effective at portraying the general rather than specific aspects of feeling; putting a feeling into words transforms it in part into the more general class of which it is an instance. For example, words like sad, afraid, and happy may capture what is general about a feeling, what different experiences of it have in common, but the nuances of how one feels at a particular moment may be lost. The verbal message, in other words, is at best a generalized approximation of the model's feeling. And this generalized approximation is the total input available to the observer.

In the process of decoding, the observer will often relate this input to his or her past experience, as discussed previously. Reversing the model's encoding sequence, the observer goes from the general to the specific, imagining, with varying degrees of vividness, past events in which he or she had the feeling in question, and, consequently, reexperiences the feeling. The observer's feeling may have a lot in common with the model's, owing to the normative, shared meaning of the terms used by the model to describe the feeling, but there will also be an "error" component due to the encoding and decoding. The error component may be reduced if the model is particularly good at putting feelings into words and if the observer is intimately related to the model, knows how the model feels in different situations, and perhaps imagines the model's facial expression and behavior in the situation.

Let us now return to the more usual situation, in which the model is present and able to supply direct expressive cues as well as language. These expressive cues, which are largely nonverbal and usually visual or auditory, may have triggered the observer's empathic response in the first place, with the verbal message adding precision or fine-tuning the observer's empathic affect and understanding of the model's feeling. Alternatively, the message's semantic meaning may have led to the observer's initial empathic response and also directed the observer's attention to the model, which then enabled the model's expressive cues to trigger additional empathic affect. In either case, the empathic process may have been kept "alive" by the expressive cues because they are salient, often vivid, and can hold the observer's attention. As a result, the image of the model remains with the observer rather than fading away, and the observer does not drift into an egoistic state. Thus, although language may be an effective mediator of empathy because it can provide more precise information about the other's internal state, the process of deriving meaning from the other's verbal message and connecting it with relevant events in one's past may weaken the hold of the empathic affect aroused. The presence of the model and of nonverbal expressive cues from the model, while lacking the precision of language, may help keep the observer's attention focused on the model and thus maintain the empathic response.

Nonverbal expressive cues may also help the empathic observer to stay on target in another way. Although it is likely that people's verbal descriptions of their feelings are usually expressed in accord with their actual feelings, discrepancies sometimes occur. When this happens, the other's nonverbal expression may give the observer cues about the other's feeling that contradict the other's words. This is due to the tendency of people to "leak" their feelings through changes in facial expression, posture, or tone of voice.[2] Although these cues are often not precise, they may be sufficiently accurate to reflect the other's true feelings and thus prevent the observer from being misled by the verbal message.

Impact of person identity on empathy

The highest empathic level, as discussed earlier, consists of vicarious affect combined with one's concept or image of the other's affective state and life condition beyond the situation. To highlight the effect of person identity on empathy, consider the case in which only information about the other's life condition is available and immediate cues are absent. How does this information produce empathic affect? Empathic affect may be aroused because one is reminded of an event or a series of events in one's own past that resemble aspects of the other's life condition. Or, one may not relate the other's condition to oneself but focus directly on the other and try to imagine what the other is experiencing and feeling. In other words, the earlier discussion of self- and other-focused processes in regard to the role of language in empathy may also apply here. This should not be surprising since our knowledge about other people's affective states beyond the situation is ordinarily obtained through language – someone gives us background information about the person – although we can also build up such knowledge through direct observations of the person over time.

Usually the information about the other's life condition is not all that is available to the observer. Cues about the other's affective state in the immediate situation are also available. As already noted, the observer is responding to a network of information – expressive cues from the other, immediate situational cues, knowledge of the other's life condition – using perhaps several of the empathic affect arousal modes described earlier. The separate sources of information are ordinarily congruent. They may at times be contradictory, however, as when knowledge about the other's life condition conflicts with the immediate situational or expressive cues. When such conflict or disequilibrium occurs, the situational or expressive cues may lose much of their force for the observer who knows that they only reflect a transitory state. Indeed, the image of the other's life condition may sometimes actually be more compelling than the immediate cues because it signifies that the model's affect in the situation is short-lived and suggests many past and possibly future instances in which the model experiences the opposite affect. The opposite affect may then seem more representative of the model's experience. Imagine a person having a good time playing and laughing who does not know that he or she is mentally retarded or has a terminal illness. A young child may simply respond with an empathic joy, whereas an observer who has attained the fourth empathic level is more likely to imagine the events in store for the person and the feelings probably associated with these events. Such an observer may feel sadness rather than joy, thus matching the other's presumed general rather than immediate feeling state, or a mingling of sadness and joy, or an alternation between sadness and joy. Still another possibility is that the observer may temporarily suspend sadness so as to appear to share the other's joy, as a parent or therapist might do. In any case the mature empathizer must deal with the conflict between the situation and the other's life condition.

In other words, I am hypothesizing that the mental image of the other's general life condition may to some extent override contradictory cues in the present. Responding empathically to this image, then, may involve a certain amount of distancing, responding partly to one's mental image of the other rather than to the stimulus immediately presented by the other. Indeed, once this level of empathy is attained one may never again respond totally in terms of the other's feelings in the situation but always at least partly in terms of one's representation of the other's general condition and type of affective experience beyond the situation. If this is true, then we may expect a certain amount of distancing even when there is congruence between the expressive, situational, and life-condition cues.

Knowledge about the other's life condition may sometimes transform a direct affective response into an empathic one. Consider, for example, the situation in which anger at being harmed by another is diminished when one discovers that the harmful act was provoked by extenuating circumstances. In a recent study (Pazer, Slackman, & Hoffman, 1981), children were asked to state how "mad" they would be if someone acted in a harmful manner toward them (e.g., stole their cat). The experimental subjects were given background information about the culprit (e.g., his own cat had run away and his parents would not get him another one). The subjects in this group who were 8 years or older said they would be less mad than control subjects who were given equally wordy background information that was not extenuating. Empathy data were not collected, but since the extenuating circumstances put the culprit in a sympathetic light, it seems reasonable to assume that empathy was aroused and may have led to the decrease in anger.

Causal attribution and the shaping of empathic affect

Another major cognitive input that shapes empathic affect is causal attribution. The burgeoning research on attribution indicates that people of all ages make causal inferences about events. We may therefore expect a person who encounters someone in distress to make inferences about the cause of the victim's plight. The nature of the inference depends primarily on the cues relevant to causality and the inference may serve as a cognitive input, in addition to those already discussed, that helps determine the observer's affective experience.

The simplest type of situation is that in which one is first empathically aroused, through one or more of the mechanisms described earlier, and then receives information about causality. The question is, how does the resulting causal attribution alter the observer's empathic affect? Consider situations in which the cues indicate that the other person is to blame for his or her own plight. Blaming the other may be incompatible with an empathic response because the other may no longer appear to be a victim. This attribution should therefore operate to neutralize the observer's empathic distress, and the observer may end up feeling indifferent or even derogating the victim. One's empathic response may thus be cut short by the assignment of blame to the victim.

Suppose the cues indicate that a third person is to blame for the other's plight. In that case one's attention may be diverted from the victim to the third person, and one may feel anger toward that person because one sympathizes with the victim or because one empathizes with the victim and thus feels attacked. Or, one's affective response may alternate between empathic distress and anger. It is also possible that one's anger may crowd out one's empathy entirely. If, on the other hand, one discovers that the victim previously did something harmful to the third person, the situation may be transformed into the one in which the observer blames the victim. The observer in this case might even begin to empathize with the third person's anger or with the underlying feelings of hurt that presumably led him or her to engage in the aggressive act. Yet another possibility is that one discovers that the victim has a history of being mistreated in the relationship with the third person, in which case one may assume the victim had a choice (why else would he continue the relationship?) and one may then end up blaming the victim.

What happens when the observer has the necessary information and makes the causal attribution beforehand? If one blamed the victim before witnessing his or her distress, would one respond empathically? Are such prior causal attributional processes powerful enough to prevent empathy? For example, might they alter the direction of one's attention so that one does not attend to the expressive cues from the victim (e.g., does not see the victim's face)? Or would one of the more compelling arousal processes like mimicry and conditioning still operate to produce at least a momentary empathic response? And what about situations involving a third person? Would advance knowledge that a third person caused the victim's distress arouse more anger and less empathy than when this knowledge becomes available only after empathy has been aroused? The answers to these questions are unknown. There is some evidence in Stotland's research (1969) that a set to avoid empathizing (with someone being given a painful heat treatment) does *not* reduce empathic distress. But that was an artificial laboratory situation involving no counterempathic causal attribution. There are some situations in which we might confidently expect causal attribution to interfere with empathy, at least empathy with the victim, for example the situation in which one has prior knowledge that the victim has been the aggressor in the past.

Finally, we may ask what happens in situations in which there are no clear cues as to who if anyone is responsible for the victim's plight. In these cases individual differences in personality may play a role. Some people, for example, may use perceptual or cognitive strategies such as blaming the victim precisely for the purpose of reducing the discomfort of empathic distress. There may also be a general human tendency to attribute the cause of another's action to that person's own dispositions (Jones & Nisbett, 1971) and more specifically to blame others for their own misfortune in order to support one's assumptions about a "just world" (Lerner & Simmons, 1966). If, however, we take seriously the research showing a widespread tendency for people to respond empathically to another's distress (Hoffman, 1981a), we can only assume that a derogatory attitude is not necessarily incompatible with an empathic response.

Furthermore, my respondents indicate that thoughtful observers may not always settle for their initial causal attributions in ambiguous situations; they may consider alternatives. An adult male in my sample saw the driver of an expensive sports car being wheeled in a stretcher to the ambulance. He had not seen the accident, coming on the scene just after it had happened. He reported:

"I first assumed it was probably a rich, smart aleck kid driving while drunk or on dope and I did not feel for him. I then thought, this might be unfair, maybe he was rushing because of some emergency, suppose he was taking someone to the hospital, and then I felt for him. But then I thought, that was no excuse, he should have been more careful even if it was an emergency, and my feeling for him decreased. Then I realized the guy might be dying and I felt bad for him again."

This response nicely illustrates the shifts in causal attribution and feeling that may occur in ambiguous situations, and it also shows how derogating another may actually be compatible with empathizing. It does make it appear, however, that the causal attributions changed first and led to appropriate changes in feeling. But, we may ask, what made the attributions change in the first place? In the course of interviewing the subject, who is known as a generally empathic person, he remembered having an initial empathic distress response that was so intensely aversive that it seemed immediately to trigger derogatory attributions to the victim. These attributions seemed to make the situation more tolerable and gave him time to gain control over his aversive feelings. He could then respond to the stark reality of the victim's condition and again empathize. In this case the derogatory attributions were more a consequence than a cause. The conflict between the highly aversive empathic distress caused by the powerful, continuing reality of the victim's condition, and the observer's motivation to avoid that distress may have led to a series of revised causal attributions.

In other words, this may be an instance of a temporary defense against empathic overarousal (see Hoffman, 1978 for a general discussion of empathic overarousal). If one's initial empathic distress is highly aversive, one may distance oneself from the victim by making a series of causal attributions. These causal attributions, especially the first, may operate to transform some of the observer's empathic distress into derogatory feelings. But quite apart from the content of the attributions, the sheer amount of cognitive work involved in making them may serve to divert one's attention from the reality of the victim's condition. One can handle empathic overarousal by mobilizing one's cognitive resources, and thus gain time and control over one's feelings, so that one can then return to one's initial empathic response, though in a more manageable fashion.

It may be that the analysis of empathic distress outlined earlier, including the four developmental levels and the transformation of empathic into sympathetic distress, may apply only when the other's plight is beyond his or her control, like an illness or accident, and perhaps sometimes when the cause is ambiguous.

Culture may play a role in all of this of course. If the victim belongs to an outcast group, for example, his or her misery may be attributed to false causes or responded to with indifference.

Causal attribution and guilt feeling

Thus far in my analysis, the observer is an innocent bystander. A special case of interest is that in which the cues indicate that the observer is the cause of the other's distress. It seems reasonable to assume that empathic distress occasioned by distress in the other caused by the observer will be transformed by self-blame into a feeling of guilt. That is, the temporal conjunction of empathy for someone in distress and the attribution of one's own responsibility for that distress will produce guilt.[3]

Like empathic distress, guilt has affective and cognitive dimensions. The affective dimension pertains to the painful feeling of dis-esteem for the self, which, in the extreme, promotes a sense of being a worthless person. The cognitive dimension is more complex. It includes an awareness of the harmful effects one's behavior might have on others. One aspect of this awareness is the cognitive sense of others that is also important in empathy. If one does not know that others are separate from oneself, one may be uncertain as to who committed the harmful act – oneself or the victim. Another aspect is the ability to make causal inferences about one's actions, for example, the inference from the fact that one's act preceded a change in another's state, that one's act was the cause of that change in state. Consider also guilt over inaction, which requires that one be aware of something one did not do and the consequences of not doing it; and anticipatory guilt, which requires that one be aware of the potential connection between one's intentions and actions before either of them has occurred. Finally, the cognitive dimension of guilt also includes the awareness that one has choice and control over one's actions, without which there might be no reason to feel guilty.

I have presented a developmental scheme for guilt and a theory of how parental discipline contributes to its development elsewhere (Hoffman, 1982b, 1983). I will now summarize the developmental scheme, highlighting the parallels between guilt and empathic distress.

Relation between guilt and empathic distress

First of all, before becoming aware of others as separate physical entities, children respond to simple expressions of pain by others with empathic distress and also at times with a rudimentary guilt feeling, even though they may lack a keen sense of being the causal agent. Once they know that others are separate entities, they experience empathic distress when observing someone who is

physically hurt, and their empathic distress may be transformed into guilt if
they perceive their own actions as having caused the hurt. Similarly, once
aware that others have internal states, the empathic distress one experiences
in the presence of someone having painful or unhappy feelings may be transformed into guilt if one perceives one's actions as causally related to those
feelings.[4] Finally, once aware of the identity of others beyond the immediate
situation, one's empathic response to their general plight may be transformed
into guilt if one feels responsible for their plight.

Although empathic distress is here viewed as a developmental prerequisite
of guilt, it seems likely that guilt may eventually become largely independent
of its empathic origin. In some situations – for example, those in which the
victim is visibly sad or hurt – guilt may continue to be accompanied by empathic
distress. In other situations, however, the victim and his or her hurt may be
less salient than other things – for example, the actor's own behavior or motivation may be more salient. In these cases, the actor may feel guilt without
empathy. And, in most instances of anticipatory guilt, there may rarely be
empathic arousal except in the unusual case in which one imagines the other's
response to one's planned action especially vividly. In general, then, at some
point in development, the awareness of being the causal agent of another's
misfortune may be enough to trigger guilt feelings without empathy. Thus,
although empathic distress may be a necessary factor in the *development* of
guilt, it may not, subsequently, be an inevitable accompaniment of guilt.

It seems likely, moreover, that once the capacity for guilt is attained, especially
guilt over omission or inaction, guilt may become a part of all subsequent
responses to another's distress, at least in situations in which one might have
helped but did not. From then on, even as an innocent bystander, one may
rarely experience empathic distress without some guilt. The line between empathic distress and guilt thus becomes very fine, and being an innocent bystander
is a matter of degree. To the degree that one realizes that one could have acted
to help but did not, one may never feel totally innocent.

Summary and concluding remarks

The model of empathic arousal presented here differs from many other psychological theories in its stress both on emotion and on the interaction between
affective and cognitive processes within a developmental framework. It may
be useful to point up in general outline the main characteristics of the model.
First, the emotion in question, empathic distress (or guilt), has a cognitive as
well as an affective component. The affective component pertains to the arousal
property of the emotion. Six distinct arousal modes were discussed, ranging
from the simplest kind of involuntary conditioning of empathic affect and
mimicry to a far more cognitively demanding process of imagining oneself in
the other's place. The cognitive component pertains to the shaping and trans-

formation of the affective experience that results from the actor's awareness that the event is happening to someone else – an awareness that progresses through four stages, from a total self–other fusion to awareness of the other first as a separate physical entity, then as having independent internal states, and finally as having a life beyond the immediate situation – and the actor's causal attributions about the event and its impact on the other person. Second, the affective and cognitive components are seen as developing largely through distinctly different processes. Third, the affective and cognitive components are constantly interacting, and furthermore, despite the differences in the processes underlying their development, they tend to be experienced not so much as separate states but as a unity. That is, empathic distress (and guilt) are emotionally charged, or what have been called "hot" cognitions. Fourth, at all four developmental levels the experience of these emotions is assumed to include a motivational disposition, although this dimension has not been highlighted here.

Before concluding, I would like to call attention to the definition of empathy and to the potential relevance of the model to other affects. First, although our definition of empathy focuses on the processes involved, it is consistent with a definition based on a match between the observer's and the other's affect. This is because we assume that the observer and the other are structurally similar (same developmental level and cultural background). They should therefore process the same information in a similar manner. And, since the observer is processing information pertinent to the other's affective state, the observer may be expected to have an affective response more in keeping with the other's situation than the observer's own situation. We may therefore expect a match, though not a perfect match for reasons already stated, between the observer's and the other's affective state.

Second, the theory of empathic distress, its development and transformations, presented here involves various cues, arousal modes, levels of processing, and cognitive developmental stages. It also encompasses numerous interactions between affective and cognitive processes. In the interest of theoretical parsimony I will abstract and summarize the basic concepts of the theory and state them in a more generic form so as to show their possible relevance to other affects.

First, when one encounters another person experiencing an emotion one is exposed to a potential network of information about the other's affective state. The network may include verbal and nonverbal expressive cues from the other and from the other's situation and one's own knowledge of the other's general affective experience beyond the situation. These sources of information are processed differently. (a) Empathy aroused by nonverbal expressive and situational cues is usually mediated by the largely involuntary conditioning and mimicry modes, which require only the "shallowest" levels of information processing: sensory registration and pattern recognition. (b) Empathy aroused by verbal messages from the other and by one's knowledge about the other requires "deeper" levels of processing such as semantic organization and imagining oneself in the other's place; shallower levels may also be involved here too, as when imagining oneself in the other's place triggers empathic affect because of associations with one's actual past experiences.

The various cues, arousal modes, and processing levels thus appear to reduce to two general process patterns that, alone or in combination, may account for most instances of empathic affect arousal; a verbal, cognitive process and a nonverbal, perceptual process. To facilitate further discussion I will refer to them simply as verbal and nonverbal processes, but the entire pattern of cues and types of processing associated with each should be kept in mind. Before proceeding it should be noted that both processes usually work in the same direction, contributing to arousal of the same affect, although contradictions sometimes occur between or within processes (e.g., between verbal messages and expressive cues; between facial cues and tone of voice).

Second, although the two processes generally work in the same direction, the process of verbal mediation of empathic affect is vulnerable in two ways. First, whereas some people can verbalize their feelings with precision, especially to close friends and associates, generally, a loss of specificity is experienced when feelings are encoded into words, and the error is compounded when the observer decodes the words into feelings and adds his or her own nuances. The result inevitably is a certain amount of error in the match between the observer's and the other's affect. Second, when empathy is aroused by putting oneself in the other's place and recalling one's own similar past experiences, one may get caught up in the resulting affective experience, lose track of the other person, and consequently drift from an empathic into an egoistic mode.

Usually there are expressive and situational cues also present. When these are salient, the nonverbal arousal processes may exert a corrective and reinforce the verbally mediated empathic affect. Salient expressive cues may, for example, help keep the observer's attention focused on the model and prevent the drift into an egoistic mode. The added information about the other's affect provided by the nonverbal cues should also help reduce the error in affective match caused by encoding and decoding, and it may alert the observer to discrepancies between the other's verbal messages and actual feelings.

Third, the developmental dimension enters in several ways. The very young child, first of all, is limited to having empathy aroused through simple nonverbal processes and to empathizing without awareness, that is, without knowing that the other and not the self is having the direct affective experience. Second, with the acquisition of language, the child's empathic range is expanded enormously, although by the same token his or her empathic responses become vulnerable in the ways just discussed. Third, the child's empathic experience is shaped in important ways by social-cognitive development. Thus a major transformation occurs when the child first becomes aware of the other as a physical entity distinct from the self, as the affect previously linked to the global self–other is transferred to the separately emerging representations of the self and the other. Further advances occur when the child becomes aware that others have internal states independent of the child's own and, eventually, that they lead affective lives beyond the immediate situation.

The theory may be applicable not only to empathic distress, for which it was initially devised, but also to other empathic affects such as fear and joy. Its relevance to anger is problematic. Because anger is often directed at someone in the form of aggressive behavior, one might empathize with the victim rather than with the angry person, and in that case our previous analysis of empathic distress would apply. One might be expected to empathize with another's anger when one knows that the angry, aggressive person was previously the victim of the current victim's behavior.

The theory also appears to be relevant to direct affect, to at least direct affective responses to the behavior of others. To begin with, any of the previously discussed empathic arousal modes may apply to direct affect. Even mimicry, which may be the quintessential mode of empathic arousal, may provide information about the other's internal states, which may then serve as a stimulus that arouses one's affect. Through mimicry one may become aware of another's anger, which may then elicit fear in oneself (see discussion by Hoffman, 1981b, of affective cues in social cognition). For similar reasons, one's cognitive sense of the other, which is so significant in empathy, should also influence one's direct affective response to others. In the case of direct affect, however, the corresponding sense of oneself may play an analogous, more central role than the sense of the other. One's affective response to pain, for example, is of a different order when one is capable of knowing that it may signify a chronic, possibly terminal illness in oneself.

The extension of the theory to direct affect is limited in one important way. Although the theory may encompass even the earliest arousal of empathic affect, it may have little to say about the earliest arousal of direct affects (e.g., the infant's anger at being constrained, sadness at separation from the mother and joy at reunion, and anxiety at a stranger's approach). Arousal mechanisms are effective in producing empathy because they provide links between the other's affect and one's own direct affective experience. The mechanisms thus rely on direct affective experience, but they cannot explain one's earliest direct affective experience. Mimicry does not fit this mold, but because it requires expressive cues from the other person neither can it explain one's own direct affective experience. Nor are the problems of encoding, decoding, and drifting into an egoistic mode, noted earlier in connection with language-mediated empathy, significant in relation to direct affect, although how one feels may be influenced by labeling one's own affective state. Despite these limitations, the theory may still be useful in gaining perspective on interactions between people past infancy, since it can deal with both the empathic and directly experienced affects aroused and expressed in the course of such interactions.

The limitations do emphasize, however, the obvious fact that in empathizing with another, in sharing another's experience, one nevertheless ordinarily remains oneself. Although empathy may be a major, perhaps *the* major, social bond, it does not allow one to become the other.

Notes

1 Classical conditioning may also account for the reactive newborn cry. Thus, the sound of the infant's cry is associated with his or her own past distress – perhaps at birth. Consequently, the sound of an infant's cry may serve as a conditioned stimulus for his or her own cry response. Because the infant cannot distinguish between the sound of his or her own cry and that of someone else, the sound of another's cry may also serve as a conditioned stimulus for the infant's cry response.

2 Because people are often socialized to mask their true feelings, which is best accomplished through controlling one's facial response (Ekman & Friesen, 1974; Littlepage & Pineault, 1979), changes in facial response may be less revealing in older children and adults.

3 It should be clear that this type of guilt differs from the early conception of guilt as a conditioned anxiety response to anticipated punishment. Nor is it the same as Freudian guilt, which is a remnant of earlier fears of punishment or retaliation that resulted in repression of hostile and other impulses and is triggered by the return of the repressed impulses to consciousness. It is rather a true, interpersonal guilt – the bad feeling one has about oneself because one is aware of actually doing harm to someone. Although aware of the necessity of this type of guilt, neither Freud nor his followers ever succeeded in integrating such a conception into the main body of psychoanalytic theory. This is unfortunate, for those early quasi-pathological conceptions may account for the negative reputation of guilt among psychologists and for the dearth of research on the topic.

4 This analysis is most applicable to those instances in which the victim of the child's act exhibits clear signs of being sad and downcast, hurt, or otherwise distressed. If the victim is angry and retaliates, the child may feel anger or fear rather than empathic distress and guilt.

References

Aronfreed, J., & Paskal, V. *Altruism, empathy, and the conditioning of positive affect.* Unpublished manuscript, University of Pennsylvania, 1965.

Bell, S. M. The development of the concept of the object as related to infant–mother attachment. *Child Development*, 1970, *41*, 291–311.

Borke, H. Interpersonal perception of young children: Ego-centrism or empathy? *Developmental Psychology*, 1971, *5*, 263–269.

Ekman, P., & Friesen, W. V. Detecting deception from the body or face. *Journal of Personality and Social Psychology*, 1974, *29*, 188–198.

Erikson, E. H. *Childhood and society.* New York: Norton, 1950.

Feshbach, N. D., & Roe, K. Empathy in six- and seven-year-olds. *Child Development*, 1968, *39*, 133–145.

Hoffman, M. L. Developmental synthesis of affect and cognition and its implications for altruistic motivation. *Developmental Psychology*, 1975, *11*, 607–622.

Hoffman, M. L. Empathy, its development and prosocial implications. In C. B. Keasey (Ed.), *Nebraska symposium on motivation* (Vol. 25), pp. 169–218. Lincoln: University of Nebraska Press, 1978.

Hoffman, M. L. Is altruism part of human nature? *Journal of Personality and Social Psychology*, 1981, *40*, 121–137. (a)

Hoffman, M. L. Perspectives on the difference between understanding people and understanding things: The role of affect. In J. Flavell & L. Ross (Eds.), *Social cognitive development*, pp. 67–81. Cambridge: Cambridge University Press, 1981. (b)

Hoffman, M. L. Measurement of empathy. In C. Izard (Ed.), *Measurement of emotions in infants and children*, pp. 279–296. Cambridge: Cambridge University Press, 1982. (a)

Hoffman, M. L. Development of prosocial motivation: Empathy and guilt. In N. Eisenberg (Ed.), *The development of prosocial behavior*, pp. 281–313. New York: Academic Press, 1982. (b)

Hoffman, M. L. Affective and cognitive processes in moral internalization. In E. T. Higgins, D. Ruble, & S. W. Hartup (Eds.), *Social cognition and social development: A sociocultural perspective*, pp. 236–274. Cambridge: Cambridge University Press, 1983.

Humphrey, G. The conditioned reflex and the elementary social reaction. *Journal of Abnormal and Social Psychology*, 1922, *17*, 113–119.

Imamoglu, E. O. Children's awareness and usage of intention cues. *Child Development*, 1975, *46*, 39–45.

Izard, C. E. *The face of emotion*. New York: Appleton-Century-Crofts, 1971.

Jones, E. E., & Nisbett, R. E. The actor and the observer: Divergent perceptions of the causes of behavior. In E. E. Jones, D. E. Kanouse, H. H. Kelley, R. E. Nisbett, S. Valins, & B. Weiner (Eds.), *Attribution: Perceiving the causes of behavior*. Morristown, N.J.: General Learning Press, 1971.

Kaplan, L. J. The basic dialogue and the capacity for empathy. In N. Freedman & S. Grand (Eds.), *Communicative structures and psychic structures*. New York: Plenum, 1977.

Lerner, M. J., & Simmons, C. Observer's reaction to the innocent victim: Compassion or rejection? *Journal of Personality and Social Psychology*, 1966, *4*, 203–210.

Lipps, T. Das Wissen von fremden Ichen. *Psychologische Untersuchungen*, 1906, *1*, 694–722.

Littlepage, G. E., & Pineault, M. H. Detection of deceptive factual statements from body and the face. *Personality and Social Psychology Bulletin*, 1979, *5*, 325–328.

Pazer, S., Slackman, E., & Hoffman, M. *Age and sex differences in the effect of information on anger*. Unpublished manuscript, City University of New York, 1981.

Piaget, J. *The moral judgment of the child*. New York: Harcourt Brace and World, 1932.

Sagi, A., & Hoffman, M. L. Empathic distress in newborns. *Developmental Psychology*, 1976, *12*, 175–176.

Schacter, S., & Singer, J. E. Cognitive, social and physiological determinants of emotional state. *Psychological Review*, 1962, *69*, 379–399.

Shatz, M., & Gelman, R. The development of communication skills: Modifications in the speech of young children as a function of listener. *Monographs of the Society for Research in Child Development*, 1973, *38* (5, Serial No. 152).

Simner, M. L. Newborn's response to the cry of another infant. *Developmental Psychology*, 1971, *5*, 136–150.

Stotland, E. Exploratory investigations of empathy. In L. Berkowitz (Ed.), *Advances in experimental social psychology* (Vol. 4). New York: Academic Press, 1969.

Strayer, J. A naturalistic study of empathic behaviors and their relation to affective states and perspective-taking skills in preschoolers. *Child Development*, 1980, *51*, 815–822.

Zahn-Waxler, C., Radke-Yarrow, M., & King, R. A. Childrearing and children's prosocial initiations towards victims of distress. *Child Development*, 1979, *50*, 319–330.

5   Emotion, attention, and temperament

Douglas Derryberry and Mary Klevjord Rothbart

Temperament has been a concern of human thought from earliest times. The ancient Greeks, for example, developed a temperament typology based upon individual differences in the patterning of four bodily humours, while the Chinese viewed temperament in terms of the distribution of intrinsic energy, chi. Within the last several decades, however, issues of temperament have been brought into clearer scientific focus. Evidence from psychology and the neurosciences is now converging to provide the basis for new views of human temperament. We believe that this convergence is beginning to provide an integrative framework for considering the emotional, cognitive, and social aspects of personality.

We have defined temperament as constitutional differences in reactivity and self-regulation, with "constitutional" referring to the relatively enduring biological makeup of the individual, influenced over time by heredity, maturation, and experience (Rothbart & Derryberry, 1981). By reactivity we mean the functional state of the somatic, endocrine, autonomic, and central nervous systems as reflected in the response parameters of threshold, latency, intensity, rise time, and recovery time. By self-regulation we mean higher level processes functioning to modulate (enhance or inhibit) the reactive state of these systems.

Self-regulatory processes are best approached in terms of emotions or affective-motivational processes. Indeed, the construct of temperament has traditionally focused upon individual differences in emotionality. When viewed as regulatory, however, affective-motivational processes can be seen to extend beyond the traditional response-oriented domain of emotion, influencing a variety of perceptual and cognitive processes as well. For example, an emotion such as fear regulates somatic, autonomic, and endocrine response systems, while at the same time modulating sensory channels converging upon these response systems. Thus, the regulatory systems of temperament play a high-level role in coordinating attention and response and influence nearly every aspect of experience and behavior.

We wish to thank Michael Posner, Marjorie Reed, Myron Rothbart, and Prentice Starkey for their comments on an earlier version of this chapter. Our research was supported, in part, by NIMH Grant SRO1 MH 26674-04 and by a grant to the University of Oregon Psychology Department from the IBM Corporation.

132

In the following pages we further consider the regulatory organization of temperament systems. We begin with a discussion of contemporary views of emotion and temperament, emphasizing the role of affective-motivational systems in the guidance of attention. We then attempt to integrate some of these ideas within a hierarchical framework and to discuss the organization of this hierarchy within a developmental perspective. In the final section, we report some of the results of our recent research on adult and infant temperament.

Temperament theories

In considering theories of temperament and emotion, we discuss (a) general arousal models, (b) models based on general reward and punishment systems, and (c) models involving more specific affective-motivational systems. The major issues arising from the discussion include the specificity of arousal and emotional processes, the relationships between arousal, emotional, and cognitive processes, and the role of attention in mediating these relationships. The organization of temperament is then viewed in light of these considerations.

General arousal models

The model of temperament developed by H. J. Eysenck (1967, 1976, 1981) approaches emotion in terms of cortical arousal. Following the "optimal level" formulation of Hebb (1955), Eysenck argues that affective tone is related to cortical arousal through an inverted-U function, that is, hedonic tone reaches its highest levels at moderate levels of arousal and gradually decreases as arousal becomes higher or lower in intensity. Thus, individuals will become motivated to avoid stimulation resulting in either too high or too low a level of cortical arousal and to approach stimulation resulting in more moderate arousal levels.

Eysenck extends these familiar ideas to temperament by suggesting that individuals differ in their basic arousability and therefore in their optimal level of stimulation. More specifically, he suggests that variability in the reactivity of the ascending reticular activating system leads some individuals to have relatively aroused cortices and others to have relatively unaroused cortices. These physiological differences give rise to the primary personality dimension of introversion–extraversion. Introverts are said to possess relatively reactive reticular systems and thus to attain their optimal levels of cortical arousal at relatively low levels of stimulation. As a result of their low optimal arousal levels, introverts are expected to prefer and seek out mild forms of stimulation and to avoid more intense and novel forms of stimulation. In contrast, extraverts are said to possess relatively unreactive reticular systems, to have correspondingly high optimal levels of cortical arousal, and to therefore approach more intense and novel forms of stimulation.

While this central form of arousal is seen to influence the affective quality of experience, Eysenck (1967) proposes that a complementary form of limbic (i.e., autonomic) activation influences the intensity of behavior. Variability in the functioning of the limbic activation system underlies an orthogonal personality dimension referred to as "neuroticism-stability." Individuals with reactive limbic systems (i.e., neurotics) are said to be prone to intense autonomic discharges, while those with less reactive limbic systems (i.e., nonneurotics) are thought to demonstrate autonomic stability. On the basis of their reticular and limbic reactivity, individuals are thus classified into four basic types corresponding to the ancient Greek typology: neurotic extravert (choleric), stable extravert (sanguine), neurotic introvert (melancholic), and stable introvert (phlegmatic). Eysenck's model of temperament has generated considerable research in such areas as psychophysiology, behavior genetics, conditioning, performance, and socialization (for reviews see Eysenck, 1976, 1981; Morris, 1979). Although this research is generally supportive, it is by no means consistent (Gray, 1981).

The optimal level approach to emotion has been questioned on several grounds. Theorists such as Schachter (1975) and Mandler (1975) have questioned the directness of the relationship between arousal and emotion, suggesting instead that cognitive processes are a mediating factor. Mandler (1975), for example, proposes that an interruption of ongoing cognitive activity gives rise to a diffuse autonomic discharge. Feedback from this peripheral arousal is encoded in terms of a single dimension of "intensity" and is then evaluated in relation to ongoing situational and personal cues. Varied emotional states are elicited as a result of this cognitive evaluation. Thus, a state of high arousal can be experienced as either pleasant or unpleasant depending upon such cognitive variables as the construed source, intent, and threat of the stimulation. Whereas the role of cognitive processes is stressed in these approaches, the role of arousal is deemphasized. According to Mandler (1975), autonomic arousal functions primarily to signal the mental organization that something important might be going on. He suggests that a more complex encoding of autonomic feedback might strain the limited capacity processor and interfere with the more important situational evaluation.

Although the theories of Eysenck (1967), Mandler (1975), and Schachter (1975) differ concerning the primacy of arousal or cognition in generating emotion, they are nevertheless similar in several ways. First, all three approaches rely upon general constructs of arousal. This is particularly true of Schachter (1975) and Mandler (1975), who limit arousal to the autonomic nervous system and to only a single dimension within that system. Eysenck (1967) recognizes the important additional role of cortical arousal. The overall level of cortical arousal underlies extraversion, and the overall level of limbic activation underlies neuroticism.

In spite of the parsimony of these approaches, physiological evidence indicates that processes of arousal are not this simple. Indeed, arousal has now been shown to be a multidimensional process at the central (Brodal, 1981), autonomic (Lacey, 1967), endocrine (Mason, 1975), and even cellular (Kandel, 1978) levels of analysis. Within the autonomic nervous system, for example, components such as the respiratory, cardiovascular, and electrodermal subsystems form differential patterns of activity across situations and individuals (Lacey, 1967). Such patterns of arousal also appear likely at the cortical level. In particular, the ascending reticular system is no longer viewed as a unidimensional source of diffuse activation. Instead, the system has been found to consist of multiple, detailed subsystems, including the monoamine (i.e., norepinephrine, serotonin, dopamine) projections from the brainstem, the acetylcholine projections from the basal forebrain, and a variety of projections arising from the nonspecific thalamus (Brodal, 1981; Derryberry, 1983). These ascending systems project in different patterns upon the cortex, demonstrate different time courses, and accomplish different target effects. Rather than activating or arousing the cortex, these projections give rise to more subtle processes of *modulation*, that is, they adjust the target systems' reactivity to incoming signals without necessarily activating them. Some of these modulatory systems, such as the cholinergic mechanisms, are primarily facilitatory, whereas others, such as the monoamines, are primarily inhibitory. Moreover, there appear to be multiple forms of facilitation and inhibition. Within the "inhibitory" monoamines, for example, serotonin accomplishes a greater suppression of evoked than of spontaneous cellular activity. In contrast, norepinephrine preferentially suppresses spontaneous activity and may thus serve to enhance the signal-to-noise ratio. Given the existence of these sensitive and highly articulated subsystems, approaches emphasizing the general nature of arousal must be questioned.

A second similarity between the theories of Eysenck (1967), Schachter (1975), and Mandler (1975) involves the direction of the causal relationship between arousal and emotion. These models suggest that emotion results from arousal, with Eysenck proposing that affective tone arises directly from the level of cortical arousal and Mandler and Schachter suggesting that emotion arises from the evaluation of autonomic arousal relative to the situation. It is also necessary, however, to consider the extent to which both arousal and cognition are influenced by emotion. Emotional processes appear to elicit numerous physiological changes, including detailed adjustments of central (monoamine, cholinergic, etc.), somatic (facial, vocal, etc.), and autonomic (cardiovascular, electrodermal, etc.) subsystems (Foote, Ashton-Jones, & Bloom, 1980; Gallistel, 1980; Schwartz, 1982). For example, the noradrenergic and cholinergic reticular systems demonstrate rapid (within the first 200 msec.) differential activity, depending upon the motivational significance of a stimulus (Foote et al., 1980; Rolls, Burton, & Mora, 1980). At a more behavioral level, the ethologists have long suggested that motivational systems monitor incoming information, detect significant stimulus configurations, and adjust effector (e.g., motor, autonomic) systems accordingly (Gallistel, 1980). When viewed in this light, the causal role of arousal in eliciting emotion is weakened. Arousal may thus be secondary to the functioning of emotional processes.

General emotional systems models

A theory of temperament emphasizing the primacy of general affective-motivational systems rather than arousal has been developed by J. A. Gray (1971, 1973, 1981, 1982). The theory focuses on the relative balance between two limbic-centered emotional systems, both considered to have excitatory influences upon the arousal system (ARAS). The "behavioral inhibition system" consists of the septal-hippocampal system, its monoamine afferents, and the frontal cortex. Upon detection of signals of punishment, nonreward, and novelty, the behavioral inhibition system suppresses ongoing behavioral patterns, activates the cortex, and directs attention toward the relevant stimuli. A complementary system involving the medial forebrain bundle responds to signals of reward and nonpunishment by facilitating approach. Individuals in whom the behavioral inhibition system is relatively more reactive than the approach system are seen in Gray's view as introverted, whereas those with relatively reactive approach systems are seen as extraverted. Individuals in whom both systems are highly reactive correspond to Eysenck's "neurotics."

In essence, Gray has carried out a near 45-degree rotation of Eysenck's extraversion–introversion and neuroticism dimensions, thus attributing causation to the dimensions of "impulsivity" (the approach system) and "anxiety" (the behavioral inhibition system). Within this new framework, Eysenck's dimensions are secondary consequences of the interaction between the two emotional systems, with extraversion–introversion resulting from their relative strengths and neuroticism reflecting their joint strength (Gray, 1981).

Although Gray's emotional systems consist of multiple, distributed components, his theorizing often stresses their unified nature. In his early work, Gray (1971) proposed that emotions such as fear and frustration are functions of the behavioral inhibition system, whereas positive emotions such as hope and relief are functions of the approach system. More recently, Gray (1981, 1982) has suggested that neurotic depression resulting from a functional depletion of norepinephrine may also be related to the behavioral inhibition system. Thus, individuals with reactive behavioral inhibition systems (introverts) may be seen as vulnerable to fear, frustration, and depression, whereas those with reactive approach systems (extraverts) may be susceptible to multiple forms of positive affect.

Another temperament theory relying on relatively general emotional systems has been developed by Zuckerman (1979). Based on his studies of the trait of "sensation seeking," Zuckerman proposes that complementary reward-approach and punishment-avoidance systems influence the extent to which novel and/ or stimulating situations are approached. Like Gray, he suggests that arousal is secondary to the functioning of these general emotional systems. In contrast to Gray, however, he suggests that the punishment system is primarily serotonergic and that the reward system is primarily noradrenergic. In addition, Zuckerman allows for a distinction between three kinds of reward systems involving reinforcement (norepinephrine), incentive (dopamine), and drive-reduction (Opioid peptides) effects. Finally, he extends these neurochemical considerations to include individual differences in such neuroregulatory substances as monoamine oxidase and the gonadal hormones.

Although Gray and Zuckerman emphasize general emotional systems, trends can be seen in their theorizing toward more differentiated systems. Such developments should not be surprising, given recent work in both neurophysiology and psychology. A number of physiologists now suggest the existence of multiple reward and punishment systems (Stein, 1980; Rolls et al., 1980). Intracranial self-stimulation research has led Clavier and Routtenberg (1980) to conclude that reward neurons of the brain comprise multiple systems serving different but related functions. Based on the hypothalamic literature, Panksepp (1981) proposes the existence of discrete circuitry for the emotions of fear, rage, anticipation, and panic. If such affect-specific pathways exist, then traits such as fear, frustration, and depression may not necessarily covary within an individual.

Temperament may thus involve the reactivity of relatively independent affective motivational systems, with individuals demonstrating differential patterning of positive and negative subsystems. Thus multiple emotional systems may converge upon multiple central, autonomic, and somatic regulatory systems, providing for more differentiated and flexible behavior. If such an approach is entertained, then an initial issue is that of specifying the basic affective-motivational systems.

Discrete emotional systems models

The work of Izard (1971, 1972, 1977) has been helpful in this respect. Following Tomkin's (1962) pioneering work on emotion and facial expression, Izard has identified ten fundamental emotions: interest, joy, surprise, distress, anger, fear, shame, disgust, contempt, and guilt. These basic emotions are seen as arising from the functioning of innate, underlying neural systems, possessing characteristic neuromuscular patterns and relating to distinct subjective experiences. As the individual develops, these emotional systems become increasingly intercoordinated, so that patterns of basic emotions may result in such complex emotions as anxiety, depression, love, and hostility. In addition, emotional systems become integrated with cognitive aspects of personality, giving rise to relatively stable affective-cognitive structures such as extraversion, skepticism, and egotism. Instead of emphasizing arousal in the genesis of emotion, Izard stresses the effects of feedback from the facial muscles. Neither does he emphasize processes of cognitive evaluation, pointing out instead that emotional processes influence the selectivity of perception and cognition (Izard, 1977). This is a fundamental point to which we will return.

Another important model involving distinct motivational systems has recently been proposed by Gallistel (1980). Integrating findings across the fields of cognitive psychology, ethology, and neurobiology, Gallistel proposes that motivated behavior is best approached in terms of a lattice-hierarchical organization, that is, a hierarchy in which lower units are subject to shared control by multiple higher-level units. The lowest level units (reflexes, oscillators, and servomechanisms) are coordinated by intermediate level units (e.g., approach and avoidance programs), which are in turn coordinated by higher-level motivational programs (e.g., sex, hunger, fear, rage). Upon activation by converging homeostatic, oscillatory, or releasing influences, the motivational systems send potentiating (threshold lowering) and depotentiating (threshold raising) signals to the nodes below them. This patterned regulation does not in itself activate the lower level nodes but facilitates their functioning, given the appropriate sensory trigger input. Provided that the appropriate potentiating and triggering influences are present, the intermediate level systems are activated and effect a more detailed and selective potentiation–depotentiation of lower level nodes. The course of action is thus increasingly elaborated and refined as signals descend through the hierarchy. Gallistel suggests that motivational signals may also be distributed through cognitive structures such as maps, serving to guide goal-oriented behavior through a given environment. Lastly, he proposes that the action hierarchy is "labile," allowing lower-level motives to assume control over higher-level nodes. Because the order of subordination among motivational systems is not fixed, Gallistel suggests that it is unreasonable to attempt to compile a list of the major motives.

Izard's (1977) and Gallistel's (1980) models are of value in a number of ways. Izard's delineation of specific emotional systems complements and extends the more general approaches emphasizing basic reward and punishment systems. Gallistel (1980) provides the useful construct of hierarchical organization, an approach central to psychological (Piaget, 1952), ethological (Tinbergen, 1951), physiological (Pfaff, 1982), and cybernetic (Kent, 1981) theorizing. Before discussing the hierarchy, we need to consider an equally important idea inherent in Izard's and Gallistel's work, namely, the influence of emotion upon cognition.

Emotion and sensory regulation

Although much psychological theory has stressed the primacy of cognition in controlling "lower-level" emotional processes, it is becoming increasingly clear that cognitive processes do not function in isolation. Instead, these processes take shape within physiological contexts established by ongoing moods and elicited emotional states. Research from both psychology and neuroscience suggests that emotion and cognition interact, with each domain making important contributions to the guidance and organization of the other. In this section, we discuss the role of emotion in guiding attention, and then consider the relationship of such sensory regulation to response regulation within a hierarchical framework.

Psychological perspectives

An initial line of research indicates that emotional reactions may be elicited by stimuli outside focal attention (Dixon, 1981; LeDoux, Wilson, & Gazzaniga, 1979; Zajonc, 1980). For example, Dawson and Schell (1982) have demonstrated that an emotional stimulus (i.e., a shock-related word) elicits an electrodermal response, even when presented to the unattended left ear during a dichotic listening task. Similarly, Dixon (1981) reports a number of electrodermal, cortical, and behavioral responses to emotional words presented at visual intensities below the awareness threshold. These studies suggest that emotional reactions may not depend upon extensive cognitive evaluation but rather may result from a form of parallel, affective encoding.

Moreover, this preconscious affective encoding appears capable of influencing ongoing perceptual and evaluative processes. Relevant in this respect are the many demonstrations of "perceptual defense," a tendency for stimuli of negative emotional tone to have relatively high recognition thresholds (Erdelyi, 1974; Dixon, 1981). For example, Broadbent (1973) was able to show a decreased accuracy in the detection of tachistoscopically presented negative words, and Dixon (1981) reports an increased awareness threshold for a faint light stimulus presented to one eye when negative words are presented subliminally to the other eye. Such effects have been found in a variety of experimental designs, and evidence has accumulated supporting their perceptual (rather than response) nature. Reviewing these findings, Dixon (1981) suggests that affective information may build up in discrete "emogen" processing units. In light of this emotional encoding, central control processes may then enhance or attenuate the buildup of information in parallel "logogen" and "imagen" units.

Another line of research demonstrating emotional influences upon cognition involves the study of mood and memory. For example, G. H. Bower's (1981) studies have shown that subjects construct free associations, TAT (Thematic Apperception Test) stories, interpretations of social behavior, and impressions of persons that are congruent with their ongoing, hypnotically induced moods. Bower suggests that emotional information may be stored as nodes in semantic memory and that mood-related activation of these emotional nodes may lead to a spreading of activation to associated nodes. Such top-down spreading activation lowers the threshold of the associated nodes, thus increasing the likelihood that they will be attended to and retrieved. In other words, cognitive processing may be biased toward stored and incoming information congruent with one's ongoing mood.

Although much remains to be investigated concerning the specificity of these effects, their presence indicates that affect may play a very important role in the regulation of cognitive processes. This role is perhaps best approached within the general construct of attention. Many of the perceptual defense effects are compatible with the idea that an affective encoding of information influences the orienting of attention toward or away from certain relevant channels. Bower's effects are also interpretable within an attentional framework, that is, attention tends to be drawn toward channels enhanced by mood-related spreading activation. Moreover, the biological and adaptive utility of such an arrangement should be underscored. Essential to survival is the allocation of attention to "important" sensory channels, and the emotional significance of a stimulus would seem a primary index of such importance.

Physiological perspectives

The relationship between affect and attention is further demonstrated within a physiological framework. First, consider the processing of visual information in the cortex. Visual input is processed through a sequence of association areas where it undergoes cross-modal integration with other sensory modalities. Even before such integration, however, visual information appears to be directed toward the affect-related circuitry of the limbic system. The inferotemporal visual cortex (a unimodal visual association area) projects to the superior temporal sulcus (where it is combined with auditory information), to the amygdala (a limbic structure involved in the detection of affective significance), to the entorhinal cortex (the cortical gateway to the hippocampus, a limbic structure involved in memory, spatial construction, and the detection of novelty), and to the orbitofrontal cortex (a high-level structure involved in the programming and execution of responses) (Mishkin, 1980; Rolls, 1982). Thus, parallel processing may occur for both affective and more abstract spatiotemporal information. There appear to be several abstract cortical routes along with several affective limbic routes. If affective significance is encoded to some extent apart from its higher-level semantic processing, then a mechanism may be provided through which affective processes can influence subsequent cognitive processing.

Consider next the projections of the affective-motivational circuitry of the limbic system. Limbic structures, including the orbital frontal cortex, hippocampus, amygdala, and hypothalamus, play important roles in regulating the activity of the ascending reticular modulatory systems. In turn, the reticular systems (noradrenergic, serotonergic, cholinergic, etc.) play critical roles in regulating the reactivity of the cortical processing circuits and have traditionally been viewed as mechanisms of attention and consciousness (Adrian, 1954). The limbic systems thus appear to be in an excellent position to control (via the reticular systems) information processing within the cortex. A number of researchers have suggested that activated motivational systems (e.g., aggression, defense) regulate the reticular systems so as to bias sensory processing in the cortex. For example, Siegel and Edinger (1981) suggest that the hypothalamus modulates the cortical patterning mechanism via the reticular formation and in this way controls the passage of sensory information to the motor system. In a more general discussion of motivated behavior, Panksepp (1981) suggests that discrete emotional circuitry of the hypothalamus regulates ascending noradrenergic influences so as to provide an attentional focus for developing response processes. Although the specificity of these limbic-reticular-cortical influences remains to be determined, their anatomical and physiological properties are suggestive of a versatile mechanism for rapidly adjusting and readjusting the state of reactivity of cortical processing systems.

Lastly, consider some recent advances in the physiological investigation of attention. Physiological models of attention currently focus upon a selective enhancement of visual information occurring in the parietal cortex approximately 100 msec following a motivationally relevant stimulus (Wurtz, Goldberg, & Robinson, 1980). Affective-motivational processes are suspected of playing a crucial role in this selective enhancement. For example, Mesulam, Van Hoesen, Pandya, and Geschwind (1977) suggest that projections from a motivational space constructed in the cingulate cortex (a cortical convergence area of direct limbic projections) in terms of present needs and past experiences may be in part responsible for the enhancement effect. Similarly, Bushnell, Goldberg, and Robinson (1981) suggest these limbic projections may establish a state of tonic readiness in the parietal cortex, thereby enhancing the responsivity of motivationally relevant spatial locations. Thus direct cortical projections from the limbic systems may serve to alert central processing mechanisms to the presence of a motivationally relevant stimulus and to direct attention toward that stimulus.

Together with the behavioral studies of Broadbent (1973), Dixon (1981), and others, these physiological considerations suggest that affective-motivational systems are intimately involved in processes of sensory modulation and attention. Within the first several hundred milliseconds of information processing, limbic and reticular projections accomplish a multidimensional tuning of cortical pathways. The resulting pattern of reactivity may serve to bias the flow of information toward consciousness and response mechanisms. States such as fear, anger, and depression may be composed of varied patterns of cortical reactivity, thus bringing different aspects of the world into focus. In simplest terms, emotion influences the way we see and interpret the world.

Processes of sensory modulation are perhaps best viewed in relation to complementary processes of response modulation. As Gallistel (1980) has suggested, affective-motivational systems accomplish a multileveled regulation of motor, autonomic, and endocrine systems. At the same time, this emotional circuitry carries out a general regulation of cortical sensory and association areas, thus controlling the sensory channels relevant to the developing response processes. When viewed in terms of the complementary processes of sensory and response modulation, emotion can be seen to involve a high-level coordination of input and output systems. This coordination is accomplished by multiple neurochemical systems, differing in the spatial distribution, time course, and the nature of their effects (Bloom, 1979).

We feel that this dual view of emotion provides a useful framework for considering individual differences. In particular, it extends the construct of temperament to include not only variability in "behavioral style" but also individuality in experience (Escalona, 1968). Researchers have often emphasized the objective expressions of temperament, as reflected in its overt behavioral (Buss & Plomin, 1975; Thomas & Chess, 1977) and social-communicative (Goldsmith & Campos, 1982) aspects. This is only part of the picture, however, for introspection, psychology, and physiology all suggest that emotional processes influence our subjective perception and cognition. Individuals may thus demonstrate similar patterns of behavior, while their experiences differ in a number of ways. The exploration of these differences promises to be a most interesting and rewarding direction of research.

Hierarchical organization of temperament

An equally valuable perspective arising from the motivational literature is that of the hierarchical organization of behavior. When applied to temperament, this view suggests that affective-motivational systems constitute the highest levels of control over behavior (Gallistel, 1980). These systems may be influenced by relatively direct sensory information (Gray, 1973), by more highly processed semantic information (Mandler, 1975), and by interoceptive information involving homeostatic conditions (Pfaff, 1982). At the same time, however, motivational systems appear capable of modulating this converging sensory information (Mayer & Price, 1982) and thus of indirectly regulating themselves. Such regulation is accomplished via motivational controls over intermediate-level systems involved in sensory and response modulation. The sensory-regulating systems establish the general state of alertness and selectivity while the response-regulating circuits set up the general approach and avoidance orientation of behavior. These general response orientations regulate lower level autonomic, endocrine, and motor components, which in turn regulate more specific behavioral details and so on. Control thus exists at a number of levels and in a number of different forms.

This hierarchical approach suggests that individuals may vary at a number of different levels. For example, persons may differ at the higher levels of motivation, with some being relatively insensitive to signals of potential threat and others showing greater sensitivity to such signals (Gray, 1981). Among the more sensitive individuals, some may be skilled at effectively modulating the threatening sensory signals, while others with less adequate attentional control may be more vulnerable to fear reactions. These vulnerable persons may in turn differ at lower levels, with some showing rapid and prolonged autonomic reactivity and others showing relatively mild autonomic reactions of short duration. It thus seems misleading to limit our view of temperament to a single level, for variability at different levels may result in different patterns of behavior and experience. Views of temperament limited to either the higher (e.g., affective-motivational) or lower (e.g., endocrine) levels tend to overlook these different sources of variability.

In addition to variability across hierarchical levels, temperament also arises from the patterning of reactivity within a given level (Rothbart & Derryberry, 1981). At the lower levels, for example, Lacey (1967) and Mason (1975) have demonstrated individual differences in the reactivity of component autonomic and endocrine subsystems. Thus, some individuals may show greater reactivity through the cardiovascular system, others through the electrodermal system, and others through the gastrointestinal system. At the intermediate levels, individuals appear to differ in the relative balance of reactivity within general modulatory systems utilizing norepinephrine, dopamine, and serotonin. Such differences are central to current theories of depression (Weiss, 1979), schizophrenia (Matthysse, 1977), and hyperkinesis (Porges, 1976). At the highest levels, individuals differ in the patterning of their motivational systems. One of the most basic aspects of emotional processes is their tendency to function concurrently and form discrete blends (Izard, 1977; Schwartz, 1982). Thus, variability in the relative balance of systems involving fear, anger, joy, and so on may lead to a rich variety of basic temperamental patterns. No single response, attentional or emotional process can serve as an adequate measure of temperament, for it arises from complex organizations and interactions of components.

Finally, within a single subsystem, temperament can be approached in terms of the system's reactivity. This property is reflected through response characteristics of threshold, intensity, latency, rise time, and recovery time (Rothbart & Derryberry, 1981). These intensive and temporal characteristics are essential in distinguishing individuals who attain similar peak levels of response but nevertheless differ in how rapidly they reach these levels or in how quickly they return to resting levels. As mentioned earlier, the intensity, rate of increase, and duration of cardiovascular reactivity may greatly influence the behavioral and subjective aspects of a fear reaction. Similarly, the rising and falling characteristic of "reticular" systems may influence the flexibility and ease with which an attentional focus is disengaged and reoriented. Together, and across a number of interacting systems, these overlapping, phasic response parameters may contribute greatly to the quality of motivated behavior.

We thus view temperament in terms of hierarchical, multidimensional, and temporally overlapping regulatory systems. The interaction of these systems gives rise to varied states of reactivity, influencing both the experiential and behavioral aspects of temperament. Although this is a rather complex framework, we feel it provides a useful heuristic for considering the many temperament-related studies now appearing. We also feel that the apparent complexity of central neural and behavioral processes requires a broad and detailed theoretical approach without losing sight of the more general influences that may be operating within and across hierarchical levels.

In the next section, we further elaborate the nature of temperament by approaching it within a developmental perspective. As in a number of areas within psychology, the complexity of temperament at the adult level in many ways demands a developmental approach (Posner & Rothbart, 1981). By viewing the maturation and emergence of temperament systems in the relatively simple, developing organism, their structural and functional organization is most clearly revealed. In particular, a developmental perspective provides a view of initial organization prior to the development of complex regulatory skills and strategies. Thus we are able to view the temperament hierarchy as it gradually develops from the lower to the higher levels. By following the young child through the early years of life, we can view developing interactions between underlying biological systems, the social world, and the emerging conceptual world.

Development of temperament

The newborn infant responds in a relatively automatic way to changes in internal and external environments. Soon, however, the infant begins to assume more control over this initial reactivity. States of sleep and wakefulness become better organized, reflexes are intercoordinated with one another, and intention and anticipation develop. J. Hughlings Jackson (1898) approached this developmental process as one involving increasing regulation of lower-level excitatory circuitry by higher-level inhibitory systems. He proposed that the brain matures in a caudal to rostral manner, with higher levels gradually asserting control over the lower levels. As increasingly higher levels of control are added to the system, an intricate, hierarchically organized system of controls is established, and behavior becomes progressively more precise, flexible, and voluntary.

The affective motivational systems of temperament appear to play high-level roles in this developing hierarchy, serving as command systems for organizing broad patterns of behavior (Panksepp, 1981). Taking into account varying internal and external conditions, these motivational systems coordinate intermediate-level processes involving sensory and response modulation, which in turn coordinate lower-level units involving discrete behavioral and sensory processes. Thus, the motivational state of fear may be potentiated by oscillating hormonal substances and released by certain external or internal stimuli. Once activated, the fear system modulates intermediate level systems involving organized escape and defense behaviors, as well as organized patterns of information intake and rejection. These response and sensory-regulating systems then modulate lower level response units and sensory channels, effectively integrating activated response options and incoming sensory information. Although our knowledge of the fine structure of the hierarchy remains limited (see Gallistel, 1980, for a detailed discussion of the response hierarchy), and although we are undoubtedly underestimating its complexity here, we can at least begin to sketch out some aspects important to temperament and development. These properties include the constitutional and developmental status of the response, response-regulating, sensory, sensory-regulating, and motivational systems.

Response systems

The newborn human functions in the relative absence of higher (cortical) levels of control (Bronson, 1982). Often highly organized reflex patterns of rooting and sucking, stepping, orienting, reaching and grasping may be elicited by appropriate forms of stimulation (T. G. R. Bower, 1982), as well as the Moro, tonic neck, Babinski, and other transient reflexes (Prechtl, 1977). Using the Facial Action Coding System, Oster (1978) has determined that virtually all discrete emotional facial movements may be found in both premature and full-term newborns. In other reflex reactions, the eyes may automatically orient to a peripheral auditory stimulus (Muir & Field, 1979), the eyes and head follow a moving target (Kremenitzer et al., 1979), the heart rate accelerates to a tactile stimulus (Graham & Jackson, 1970), and the arm and hand reach for and grasp a moving object (von Hofsten, 1982). At the same time, powerful endogenous biological cycles modulate this early reactivity (Emde, 1979).

Response-regulating systems

Gradually, higher level systems come to coordinate these initial behavioral units, allowing the possibility of still more complex patterns of behavior. An intriguing example of this coordinative process may be reflected in the gradual "disappearance" of the transient reflexes from the infant's response repertoire. Reflexes such as the Moro and Babinski appear to drop out during the early months of life, as if they have served their adaptive function and are no longer of value. However, these reflexes have been found to reappear following forebrain injury in adults, and their course of recovery following injury parallels their course of disappearance during infancy. Teitelbaum (1977) suggests that their disappearance during infancy reflects the increased inhibitory control through which the forebrain integrates these components into voluntary patterns of behavior. The reflexes may not really disappear from behavior but rather take on new forms as a result of coordinating inhibitory and facilitatory influences.

Another interesting view of this inhibitory maturation is provided by recent pharmacological studies of the developing monoamine systems. These studies suggest that initial excitatory processes (e.g., spontaneous motility, motor activity, locomotion) are gradually counterbalanced by sequentially developing monoamine systems. For example, the spontaneous locomotion of rat pups increases from birth to a maximum in two to three weeks and then gradually decreases to adult levels. Mabry and Campbell (1974) have presented evidence that a serotonin-related inhibition begins to function as early as the fifteenth day of life. Other studies indicate that an acetylcholine-related form of inhibition becomes functional around the twentieth day of life (Anisman, 1975) and that a dopamine-related mechanism may also be involved in inhibiting locomotor activity. According to Pradhan and Pradhan (1980), the inhibitory mechanisms imposing regulatory control might involve functionally distinct acetylcholine, serotonin, dopamine, and amino acid components maturing at different rates. Graham, Strock, and Zeigler (1981) suggest that the onset of cardiac decelerative response between 2 and 3 months of age in the human infant may arise from the maturation of cholinergic pathways descending upon medullary cardio-vascular centers. Finally, Lidov and Molliver (1982) have carefully examined the maturation of ascending norepinephrine and serotonin terminal fields in the rat cortex. The course of serotonergic maturation is delayed relative to norepinephrine and extends through the twenty-first day of life, approximately the time of the appearance of mature slow wave and desynchronized sleep.

Bruner (1974) provides a hierarchical perspective for early skilled action, emphasizing the extent to which exercise promotes the incorporation of constituent elements into more complex patterns of action. Through prolonged practice, constituent subroutines become smoother and more economical (i.e., modularized), thus requiring less attention for their regulation. As they become more automatic, the constituent subroutines can then be incorporated into higher order, longer sequence acts, without disrupting those acts through their attentional demands. Particularly interesting is Bruner's suggestion that activated intention directs and sustains these organizational efforts. Gallistel (1980) also suggests that signals descending from the motivational levels provide the sustained organization to keep infants practicing. With maturation and exercise, intermediate levels of organization are refined, and behavior becomes more coordinated, economical, and flexible.

The present account does little justice to the complex and multilevel processes involved in response coordination. For now, we only wish to suggest that coordination at intermediate levels of the hierarchy serves to organize the basic approach and avoidance responses through which the child interacts with the environment. These programs integrate the eyes, hands, arms, legs, voice, and autonomic systems into more coordinated acts, such as touching, grasping, reaching, crawling, walking, withdrawing, avoiding, and escaping. Variability in the flexibility and maturational status of these coordinative systems will influence the functioning of the motivational systems in a number of ways. For example, the goal-oriented infant who cannot yet coordinate a grasping approach may be susceptible to increasing frustration, whereas the avoidant infant who is unable to escape a threatening situation may be vulnerable to increasing fear. Thus, higher-level motivational systems may be partially operative prior to the maturation of the intermediate level systems. Before considering these motivational systems, we first need to examine developing sensory and sensory-regulating capacities, for these are central to functioning at all levels of the hierarchy.

Sensory systems

Bronson (1982) has recently provided a hierarchical analysis of central neural maturation emphasizing the extent to which subcortical processes tend to dominate during the neonatal period. Subcortical sensory systems may allow for relatively simple analyses of stimulus motion, intensity, and contour density, but more complex pattern analyses and representational capacities await the progressive maturation of the primary sensory and association areas of the cortex. It is interesting to note that the processing areas of the cortex may demonstrate some degree of hierarchical organization within themselves. Primary receiving areas project to unimodal association areas where information within each modality undergoes further processing. The unimodal association areas then project upon polymodal association areas where information from two or more modalities is combined. The polymodal association areas in turn project upon the supramodal parietal cortex where information from all modalities is then integrated (Mesulam et al., 1977). Although we know little of the maturational events occurring in these cortical regions, such a hierarchical structuring of processing areas is extremely interesting from a developmental point of view.

In terms of behavior, however, we are concerned with the quality of information these processing areas can provide to developing response and motivational systems. The newborn is seen as being responsive to a relatively limited and immediate sensory world, with motivational processes correspondingly constrained. As the resolving power and representational capacity of the cortex matures, these behavioral systems come to respond to increasingly refined patterns of stimulation and to "match" incoming information with stored patterns and models. The outcome of this matching may give rise to emotional states such as surprise (Charlesworth, 1969), humor (Pien & Rothbart, 1980), and wariness (Bronson & Pankey, 1977). In addition, maturing representational capacities provide the basis for emotional states related to anticipated consequences. For example, joy may be elicited at the sight of the approaching care giver, and fear or distress may arise from anticipating the care giver's departure. Developing sensory and cognitive capacities thus open up new lines of communication to concurrently developing response and motivational systems.

Sensory-regulating systems

These lines of communication are not necessarily direct, however, for the infant is also rapidly acquiring skill in regulating the flow of sensory information. Here we refer to attentional processes that allow the infant to control and coordinate the flow of information toward the response systems. During the early months of life, the central attentional mechanism may not always be well coordinated with peripheral components of orienting (Posner & Rothbart, 1981). Within several months, however, the central, oculomotor, and cardiac (deceleration) components of the orienting reaction function in a more coordinated fashion. Moreover, orienting and defensive patterns become organized in relation to developing higher-level motivational systems, such as those involving pleasurable and distressful interactions. These higher levels of coordination allow for increasingly flexible use of attentional mechanisms, which in turn can contribute to the coordination of eyes, hands, and other response systems.

Increasing flexibility and organization of attentional behavior can be seen across the period of infancy. During the early months, orienting appears to be primarily involuntary, more or less controlled by the properties of exogenous stimulation and endogenous scanning patterns (Haith, 1980). Thus, young infants often demonstrate the phenomenon of "obligatory attention," appearing to be "caught" by a compelling visual stimulus (Stechler & Latz, 1966). When we present 3-month-old infants with a checkerboard pattern, for example, they often appear to have difficulty shifting their visual attention away from the stimulus. Even though they may be showing signs of increasing facial and vocal distress, and even though their heads may turn away from the stimulus, their eyes remain fixed upon the target. With increasing development, however, infants become better able to shift their eyes away from the unpleasant stimulus. In addition, they become better able to shift their visual attention to more pleasant aspects of the situation, such as the mother's face. This capacity to orient selectively to positive and negative aspects of the environment will profoundly affect the responsivity and experience of the infant.

As the child becomes increasingly able to orient attention to semantic memory during later infancy, more flexible and effective modes of regulation become available. If environmental conditions are less than optimal, the child can focus upon a positively toned memory location. In the care giver's absence, distressed children may be able to orient to an image of the absent care giver or verbally anticipate the care giver's return, thereby attaining some degree of comfort and relief. At later ages when children have developed relatively elaborate concepts of the self and other persons (Lamb & Sherrod, 1981), a selective amplification of positively toned channels and attenuation of negatively toned channels may provide an even more effective means of regulating behavior and experience. These attentional strategies become more sophisticated and flexible as development proceeds, providing an increasing capacity to regulate the affective tone of experience. The developing child is thus by no means at the mercy of external or internal input.

Nevertheless, it is important to emphasize the extent of variability in attentional control seen during early development. Although some infants tend to flexibly shift their visual attention away from unpleasant stimuli toward more pleasant ones, other babies appear more vulnerable to obligatory attention. At later ages, children may show related differences in their ability to disengage attention from an unpleasant line of thought, to shift problem-solving behaviors from one approach to another, or to shift their focus between different aspects of an ongoing situation. As school-related tasks demanding a sustained focus of attention become important, students appear to differ in their capacity to resist orienting to distracting peripheral stimulation. Hyperkinesis, for example, may provide an extreme example of the inability to maintain a focus of attention and resist shifting to irrelevant stimuli (Douglas & Peters, 1979).

Less extreme examples of attentional variability may be found in cognitive-style differences such as reflectivity–impulsivity (Zelniker & Jeffrey, 1979), field dependence–independence (Witkin, 1978) and focal attention, field articulation, and leveling–sharpening (Santostefano, 1978). Attentional variability may also be manifested in different coping or defensive styles, such as repression–sensitization (Bell & Byrne, 1978). Individual differences in these and other aspects of attentional control appear to play central roles in the regulation of behavior and experience. To the extent that these capacities are accessed by higher-level motivational programs, their flexibilities and precision should greatly influence the effectiveness of motivated behavior.

Thus far we have discussed some of the lower-level sensory and response processes involved in the development of temperament, as well as some of the intermediate-level processes of sensory and response regulation serving to coordinate them. We now consider the development of the high-level motivational processes serving to organize attentional and response regulation components.

Motivational systems

Several researchers have approached early motivation from a *homeostatic* perspective, viewing fluctuations of cortical arousal as a source of different affective-motivational states (Izard, 1977; Kagan, 1974; Sroufe, 1979). Emphasizing the arousal engendered by the infant's cognitive engagement of the event, Sroufe (1979) suggests that increasing cognitive capacities underlie the differentiation of positive and negative affect. Positive emotions such as pleasure, delight, and laughter are viewed as resulting from fluctuations of arousal around moderate levels, whereas negative emotions such as wariness and rage arise from high levels of unresolved arousal. Thus, engagement of an incongruent event may elicit an increase in arousal as the infant attempts to assimilate the event. If the discrepancy is successfully resolved and tension is reduced, smiling may result, but if the event remains unassimilated and the tension remains high, wariness and distress may occur.

Researchers have also emphasized the *releasing* aspects of stimulation. Izard (1977) points out that innate motivational systems may be selectively sensitive to certain inputs or environmental conditions. Similarly, an ethological perspective suggests that a smiling face may elicit pleasure, a looming stimulus fear, and separation from the care giver distress. Perhaps more important, however, is the direct access to developing motivational systems provided by the infant's increasing anticipatory capacities. As representational capacity develops, the infant becomes able to rapidly anticipate the consequences of a given perceptual environment, thus providing immediate cues to motivational systems. For example, joy may be elicited by the sound of the care giver entering the room, fear by the sight of the pediatrician, and frustration by parental behaviors signaling bedtime (Bronson & Pankey, 1977; Izard, 1977; Sroufe, 1979). Motivational systems are thus freed from the immediate present context and come under conditional control of events ranging across broad time frames.

Other researchers emphasize the *oscillatory* nature of early emotional processes. Emde (1979), for example, stresses that emotional activity is ongoing and fluctuates not only in relation to external events but also to endogenous biological rhythms such as sleep–wake cycles, basic rest activity cycles, and hormonal cycles. He suggests that a variety of endogenous neurochemical processes may modulate the reactivity of developing affective-motivational systems. Thresholds for emotions such as pleasure, fear, and frustration may thus vary as a function of the oscillatory influences converging upon them, with base rates and ranges regulated accordingly. Along with variability in reactivity of the cortex and affective-motivational systems, individual differences in the characteristics of these oscillating influences will contribute greatly to temperament.

It seems likely that each of the above factors (homeostatic, releasing, and oscillatory) plays an important role in the development of motivated behavior and temperament. When we consider the endogenous oscillatory components, we can also appreciate the extent to which motivated behavior may be "spontaneously" released. In a study of fear, surprise, and happiness, Hiatt, Campos, and Emde (1979) found that their 10- to 12-month-old control infants (i.e., those not placed in emotion-eliciting situations) demonstrated a variety of emotional responses. Gallistel (1980) provides an interesting discussion of such spontaneous forms of behavior, suggesting that motivational systems may become progressively potentiated as a function of time, thus becoming activated by nearly any form of stimulation. The play behavior of children seems particularly well suited for such an analysis, as do mood-related aspects of temperament.

Sroufe (1979) has suggested that basic emotional systems involving pleasure-joy, wariness-fear, and rage-anger undergo differentiation as a function of cognitive development. The wariness-fear system, for example, has its roots in early distress arising from obligatory attention, emerges later as wariness in response to incongruity, and still later in more distinct forms such as conditioned fear, anxiety, and shame. In contrast, Izard and Buechler (1979) propose that the basic emotional systems mature independently and gradually become integrated with one another and with developing cognitive processes. This integrative process gives rise to more complex emotions such as sadness, anxiety, love, and hostility.

A hierarchical approach incorporates both differentiation and integration concepts. A basic principle of hierarchical organization is that higher level controls serve to integrate preexisting lower level processes (Satinoff, 1982). By providing an enhanced coordination of existing behaviors, such integration allows for more differentiated and flexible response patterns. For example, early states of interest promote an increasing coordination of attentional and behavioral approach responses. With repeated application across a range of situations, these coordinations culminate in a repertoire of information intake and manipulation strategies. Early states of distress, on the other hand, appear to involve an increasing coordination of components related to attentional and behavioral avoidance. At first, infants have difficulty disengaging their visual attention from an unpleasant stimulus, but gradually they become better able to deflect the impact of the distressing situation (Tennes et al., 1972). Through both maturation and experience, a set of distinct information rejection and behavioral avoidance procedures is built up.

Later developing emotions involve more sophisticated integrations of these lower level components, combining them in new and more complex patterns. The state of wariness, for example, appears to involve a simultaneous coordination of both approach and avoidance components at both the behavioral and attentional levels. When faced with a novel or exciting stimulus, the child's behavior alternates between reaching toward and withdrawing from the object, coupled with visual fixations toward and away from it (Pien & Rothbart, 1980). States of joy and pleasure also demonstrate complex coordinations of approach and avoidance components. When engaged in social interactions, infants' expressions of positive affect appear to be intricately coordinated with visual fixations toward and away from the partner (Stern, 1974). As a result of these higher level integrations, more specific approach–avoidance procedures are added to the behavioral repertoire. These existing elements may in turn be accessed by subsequently maturing motivational systems such as those related to dependency, sadness, defiance, shame, and pride.

A hierarchical approach thus suggests that higher levels of coordination allow for more specific, differentiated motivational states. Socialization plays a central role in this process, encouraging the development of impulse control, delay of gratification, and resistance to temptation (Aronfreed, 1968). Tasks devised by parents and teachers and games devised by children themselves provide training in increased control over attentional and behavioral reactivity (Reed, Pien, & Rothbart, 1982). The verbal system often appears to be incorporated into the child's self-regulation, supporting and complementing the attentional and behavioral components (Ziven, 1979). Although higher levels of control lead to less diffuse reactivity, the lower levels remain functional and may emerge as dominant (e.g., in temper tantrums). Nevertheless, there is an increasing refinement of attentional and behavioral coordination, culminating in the states of intellectual, aesthetic, and spiritual motivation of adulthood.

In addition to interacting with one another, the systems of temperament also influence the social world. Such influences are evident at each level of the hierarchy. At the motivational level, an impulsive approach-oriented child may continue to seek novel and intense forms of stimulation, thus entering into a relationship with care givers based on excitement. The wary, avoiding child, on the other hand, may develop a more selective, controlled interaction with the world and may require gentler engagement and perhaps more comforting from the care givers. At the intermediate levels, two children may have equally reactive "fear" systems, but differences in attentional flexibility may influence the extent to which they are able to attenuate developing fear reactions through sensory regulation. Flexible children may require less intervention on the part of care givers, may view the care givers as "supplementary" means of support, and may be viewed by the care givers as relatively independent. In contrast, the less flexible child may often require intervention, may come to view the parents as necessary sources of security, and may be viewed by them as relatively vulnerable and dependent. Finally, at the lower levels, two children may be similar in terms of fear motivation and attentional flexibility but may nevertheless differ in their autonomic, endocrine, or somatic reactivity. Parameters such as rise time and recovery time of these systems may influence the outcome of self-regulatory processes, as well as the amount of intervention required from the care giver (Rothbart & Derryberry, 1981). Again, such differences are likely to influence the child's and the care giver's view of themselves and of one another. Later social relationships involving the school years, adolescence, and adulthood may be similarly affected by temperament variables.

A temperament perspective involves far more than thinking about variability in the reactivity of affective-motivational systems. It also involves considering individual differences in processes of sensory and response organization, as well as variability in the processes being coordinated. Component elements at each level of this gradually developing hierarchy may differ across individuals, thus giving rise to the remarkable variability seen in behavior. This individuality may be seen to function within varying social environments to influence the nature and quality of social interactions. In brief, temperament characteristics influence the child's experience, behavior, and subsequent development. As higher level motivational systems mature during later childhood, established behavioral and attentional strategies may undergo considerable reorganization. At the adult level we expect the motivational, sensory-modulatory, and response-modulatory components of behavior to be extremely complex.

Research perspectives

Researchers working at many different levels within many different disciplines can contribute to our understanding of temperament. Particularly relevant are domains such as personality, developmental and cognitive psychology, behavior genetics, neurogenetics, psychophysiology, neurophysiology, and neuroendocrinology. At this stage our own research remains basically exploratory in attempting to ascertain the general relationships or patterns existing within and between the levels of temperament. In particular, we have been concerned with the degree of specificity of emotional and arousal systems and with the basic relationships between emotional, arousal, and self-regulatory processes.

Adult temperament research

In an initial study of adult temperament, a 300-item questionnaire was administered to a group of 231 University of Oregon undergraduates. The questionnaire consisted of eight scales assessing different forms of arousal or reactivity, seven scales measuring different forms of emotion, and four scales assessing different forms of self-regulation. Definitions and sample items from these scales are provided in Table 5.1. In developing scales, the construct of reactivity was first decomposed into central, autonomic, and somatic forms. Central reactivity was then assessed in scales measuring sensitivity to external

Table 5.1. *Definitions of temperament scales and sample items*

Temperament scales	Definitions	Sample items
External sensitivity	The amount of detection or perceptual awareness of slight, low-intensity stimulation arising from the external environment	I often notice small changes in the temperature as I enter a room.
Internal sensitivity	The amount of detection or perceptual awareness of slight, low-intensity stimulation arising from within the body	I'm rarely aware of the sensations in my stomach.
Cognitive reactivity	The amount of general cognitive activity in which the person engages, including daydreaming, problem solving, anticipatory cognition, and the ease with which visual imagery or verbal processes are elicited by stimulation	A continuous flow of thoughts and images runs through my head.
Autonomic reactivity	The amount of cardiovascular, electrodermal, gastrointestinal, and respiratory activity elicited under exciting or arousing conditions	My palms usually sweat during an important event.
Motor tension	The amount of tension experienced in various muscle groups throughout the body	My shoulder muscles are usually loose and relaxed.
Motor activation	The extent to which the motor system becomes activated in the form of stereotypical, nondirected actions	I often tap and drum with my hands or feet while reading, writing, or watching TV.
Rising reactivity	The rate at which general arousal rises from its normal to its peak level of intensity	I often find myself becoming suddenly excited about something.
Falling reactivity	The rate at which general arousal decreases from its peak to its normal levels of intensity	I usually fall asleep at night within ten minutes.
Discomfort	The amount of unpleasant affect resulting from the sensory qualities of stimulation, including irritation, pain, and discomfort resulting from the intensity, rate, or complexity of light, movement, sound, and texture	The feeling of rough clothing against my bare skin rarely bothers me.
Fear	The amount of unpleasant affect related to the anticipation of pain or distress, including uneasiness, worry, and nervousness related to potentially threatening situations	I feel very uncomfortable about having to speak in public.

Table 5.1 *(cont.)*

Temperament scales	Definitions	Sample items
Frustration	The amount of unpleasant affect related to the interruption of ongoing tasks and behavior or to the blocking of a desired goal	I rarely become annoyed when I have to wait in a slow-moving line.
Sadness	The amount of unpleasant affect and lowered mood related to the exposure to suffering, disappointment, and object loss	I seldom become sad when I watch a sad movie.
Low pleasures	The amount of pleasure or enjoyment related to stimuli, activities, or situations involving low stimulus intensity, rate, complexity, novelty, and incongruity	Walking barefoot through cool grass gives me great pleasure.
High pleasures	The amount of pleasure or enjoyment related to stimuli, activities, or situations involving high stimulus intensity, rate, complexity, novelty, and incongruity	I would enjoy parachuting from an airplane.
Relief	The amount of pleasure or enjoyment derived from stimuli or situations involving the attenuation or termination of highly arousing stimulation	I greatly enjoy the relaxed feeling that comes when I no longer have to worry about something.
Attentional focusing	The capacity to intentionally hold the attentional focus on desired channels and thereby resist unintentional shifting to irrelevant or distracting channels	My concentration is easily disrupted if there are people talking in the room around me.
Attentional shifting	The capacity to intentionally shift the attentional focus to desired channels, thereby avoiding unintentional focusing on particular channels	It is usually easy for me to alternate between two different tasks.
Behavioral inhibition	The capacity to suppress positively toned impulses and thereby resist the execution of inappropriate approach tendencies	I can easily resist talking out of turn, even when I'm excited and want to express an idea.
Behavioral activation	The capacity to suppress negatively toned impulses and thereby resist the execution of inappropriate avoidance tendencies	Even when I'm very tired, it is easy for me to get myself out of bed in the morning.

stimulation, sensitivity to internal stimulation, and cognitive reactivity. Somatic reactivity was assessed in scales measuring motor tension and motor activation, and autonomic reactivity in a single scale. Temporal characteristics of reactivity were assessed in scales measuring its rising and falling characteristics. The general construct of emotionality was first decomposed into negative and positive emotionality, and negative emotionality was in turn broken down into scales assessing discomfort, fear, frustration, and sadness. Positive emotionality was decomposed into pleasure from intense stimuli, pleasure from low intensity stimuli, and relief. Self-regulation was decomposed into sensory- and response-modulating components, which were in turn broken down into scales assessing attentional focusing, attentional shifting, behavioral inhibition, and behavioral activation. We were then able to ask the following research questions: (1) to what extent do scales within these general constructs reflect unified reactivity, negative affect, positive affect, and self-regulatory systems, and (2) how are the arousal, affective-motivational, and regulatory systems related to one another?

In selecting the items, we attempted to minimize conceptual overlap between scales, overlap with the conceptual domain of personality, and response and social desirability biases. Thus, items were carefully selected to refer to sensations, feelings, and responses in reaction to selected stimuli. The response format involved a 7-point scale ranging from -3 (extremely untrue of me) to $+3$ (extremely true of me). The consistency and appropriateness of subjects' responses were analyzed in terms of intraclass correlations for 38 pairs of oppositely worded items and of their mean score on an "infrequency" scale. Twenty-four subjects were eliminated from item analyses because of inadequate scores on these two measures.

Item analyses involved the correlation of each item with each scale. Ten percent of the items correlated higher with scales other than their own and were dropped from further analyses. Coefficient alphas were then computed for each scale, and items were deleted to maximize each scale's internal consistency. One scale, Behavioral Activation, was eliminated from further analyses because of an inadequate coefficient alpha (.51). Of the remaining 18 scales, coefficient alphas ranged from .59 to .81, with a median of .70. Finally, test–retest reliabilities were computed for each scale based on a sample of 30 subjects who filled the questionnaire out a second time, two weeks after the first administration. Test–retest reliabilities ranged from .33 to .84, with a median of .74. Scale statistics, coefficient alphas, and test–retest reliabilities are provided for each scale in Table 5.2.

Pearson produce-moment correlations were then computed among the 18 scales. Intercorrelations achieving statistical significance at the .01 level (two-tailed test) are reported in Table 5.3. The intercorrelations among scales are modest in size, but they are generally consistent within and across domains. Thus, scales assessing reactivity are intercorrelated with an average of .34

Table 5.2. *Descriptive statistics, item-scale correlations, and reliabilities of temperament scales*

Scale	Scale Statistics			Item-scale correlations		Reliability	
	N	$\bar{X}$	S	Mean	Range	Alpha	Retest
External sensitivity (ES)	10	1.30	.70	.53	.47–.60	.71	.69
Internal sensitivity (IS)	11	.65	.73	.48	.37–.59	.68	.77
Cognitive reactivity (CR)	10	.84	.69	.42	.38–.58	.59	.60
Autonomic reactivity (AR)	10	.86	.86	.56	.45–.65	.76	.82
Motor tension (MT)	7	−.25	1.14	.68	.60–.75	.81	.77
Motor activation (MA)	8	.06	1.03	.61	.48–.68	.76	.53
Rising reactivity (RR)	8	.58	.96	.60	.34–.72	.75	.33
Falling reactivity (FR)	9	−.02	.95	.58	.45–.66	.74	.73
Discomfort (DS)	10	.47	.78	.47	.35–.58	.61	.60
Fear (FE)	13	.31	.81	.47	.39–.60	.71	.75
Frustration (FN)	11	.82	.78	.49	.36–.57	.69	.75
Sadness (SD)	10	1.10	.73	.49	.39–.61	.64	.73
Low pleasures (LP)	7	1.57	.79	.57	.48–.64	.64	.74
High pleasures (HP)	12	1.08	.82	.49	.40–.61	.70	.89
Relief (RE)	14	1.72	.53	.42	.36–.52	.60	.60
Attentional focusing (AF)	9	−.57	.98	.61	.41–.75	.80	.73
Attentional shifting (AS)	11	.23	.76	.47	.39–.52	.65	.84
Behavioral inhibition (BI)	12	−.13	.84	.45	.38–.60	.70	.82

and those assessing the four negative emotions with an average of .38. When the correlations across these two domains are examined, the reactivity and negative emotionality scales are consistently positively related with an average correlation of .24. The two scales assessing attentional control are positively related to one another ($r = .54$) and are consistently and negatively related to the negative affects (mean $r = -.28$). The measure of attentional shifting is positively related to the measure of high intensity pleasure ($r = .27$). Within the positive emotions, low intensity pleasure and relief are positively related to one another ($r = .44$), but neither is related to the high intensity pleasure scale. Low intensity pleasure and relief are also positively related to the negative affect of sadness (mean $r = .33$) and to the measures of "central reactivity" (i.e., external sensitivity, internal sensitivity, and cognitive reactivity; mean $r = .34$).

This pattern of results is not fully consistent with an optimal level formulation of temperament (e.g., Eysenck, 1967, 1981). Such an approach would predict a negative relationship between the low intensity pleasure and high intensity pleasure scales, as well as a negative relationship between the arousal or reactivity scales and high intensity pleasure. Neither of these predictions is supported. The results are also incongruent with approaches emphasizing unitary

Table 5.3. *Scales within and between constructs correlating beyond the .01 level of significance*

Reactivity

ES,IS	=	.52	(.75)
ES,CR	=	.25	(.39)
ES,AR	=	.27	(.37)
IS,CR	=	.35	(.55)
IS,AR	=	.40	(.56)
IS,MT	=	.48	(.65)
IS,MA	=	.25	(.35)
IS,FR	=	−.26	(−.36)
CR,AR	=	.35	(.52)
CR,MT	=	.28	(.41)
CR,MA	=	.37	(.55)
CR,FR	=	−.32	(−.48)
AR,MT	=	.43	(.55)
AR,MA	=	.29	(.38)
AR,RR	=	.26	(.34)
AR,FR	=	−.37	(−.49)
MT,MA	=	.32	(.41)
MT,FR	=	−.40	(−.52)
MA,FR	=	−.28	(−.37)
RR,FR	=	−.34	(−.46)

Reactivity × negative

DS,IS	=	.36	(.56)
AR,DS	=	.23	(.34)
MT,DS	=	.38	(.54)
FR,DS	=	−.37	(−.55)
AR,FE	=	.29	(.39)
MT,FE	=	.22	(.29)
FR,FE	=	−.25	(−.34)
IS,FN	=	.21	(.31)
AR,FN	=	.24	(.33)
MT,FN	=	.25	(.33)
MA,FN	=	.22	(.30)
RR,FN	=	.24	(.31)
FR,FN	=	−.23	(−.32)
ES,SD	=	.31	(.46)
IS,SD	=	.34	(.52)
IS,CR	=	.33	(.54)
AR,SD	=	.42	(.60)
MT,SD	=	.33	(.46)
MA,SD	=	.23	(.33)
FR,SD	=	−.27	(−.39)

Negative affect

DS,FE	=	.34	(.52)
DS,FN	=	.38	(.59)
DS,SD	=	.30	(.48)
FE,FN	=	.42	(.60)
FE,SD	=	.38	(.56)
FN,SD	=	.39	(.59)

Positive affect

RE,LP	=	.44	(.71)

Self-regulation

AS,AF	=	.54	(.75)
AF,BI	=	.21	(.28)
AS,BI	=	.28	(.42)

Positive × negative

LP,SD	=	.24	(.38)
RE,SD	=	.41	(.66)
HP,DS	=	−.34	(−.52)
HP,FE	=	−.37	(−.52)

Reactivity × positive

ES,LP	=	.42	(.71)
IS,LP	=	.37	(.56)
CR,LP	=	.22	(.36)
ES,RE	=	.41	(.63)
IS,RE	=	.30	(.47)
CR,RE	=	.22	(.37)
AR,RE	=	.27	(.40)

Attention × reactivity

AS,AR	=	−.20	(−.28)
AS,MA	=	−.21	(−.30)
AS,FR	=	.27	(.39)

Attention × negative

AF,FE	=	−.26	(−.35)
AF,FN	=	−.31	(−.41)
AS,DS	=	−.32	(−.51)
AS,FE	=	−.40	(−.59)
AS,FN	=	−.40	(−.60)

Attention × positive

AS,HP	=	.27	(.40)

Note: In parentheses: *r* corrected for attenuation.

reward and punishment systems (e.g., Gray, 1971). Although the negative affects demonstrate consistency among themselves, the positive affects are dissociated in several ways. For example, the low intensity pleasure and relief scales are positively correlated with sadness and "central reactivity," whereas high intensity pleasure relates solely to attentional shifting. Less obvious dissociations are evident among the negative emotions, where only sadness relates to the measures of central reactivity. Together with the modest size of these interrelationships, these dissociations within the domains of arousal, positive affect, and negative affect argue against approaching them as general or unitary systems of temperament.

Nevertheless, the consistency of relationships within and between the arousal and negative affect scales suggests that certain unifying influences are at work. Thus, it might be suggested that an underlying "punishment system" gives rise to multiple expressions of negative affect and arousal. Zuckerman's (1979) model, which allows for a general punishment system and multiple reward systems, fits these results fairly well. However, the emotion of sadness appears to require some special status, for it alone among the negative affects is related to central reactivity and low intensity pleasure. It is of interest that sadness has been viewed as a more complex form of emotion than fear, frustration, and discomfort (Izard, 1977) and that its clinical form (i.e., depression) may reflect a depletion of neuroregulatory systems (Weiss et al., 1979).

Another interpretation suggests that consistency among the negative emotions in part arises from their reliance upon shared central attentional systems. Thus, the consistent negative relationships between the attentional and negative affect scales are congruent with the idea that inadequate attentional control may leave an individual vulnerable to a variety of negative emotions and their associated forms of arousal. Such individuals may have difficulty shifting their attention away from the negative aspects and toward the positive aspects of certain situations. This interpretation is further supported by the positive relationship between high intensity pleasure and attentional shifting; persons capable of flexibly shifting their attention may be able to attenuate the negative and enhance the positive aspects of exciting situations, thus allowing them to approach and enjoy such situations. The lack of a relationship between attention and low intensity pleasure may be due to the lower attentional demands required by these forms of pleasure. In any event, it should be clear that the relationship between attention and affect may also run in the opposite direction. That is, chronic negative affect may disrupt the flexible utilization of attention.

In general, we view this pattern of results as reflecting the functioning of related but relatively independent subsystems. Although the reactivity and negative affect measures are consistently related, the correlations account for only 10% to 15% of the variance on the average. Moreover, when viewed as a whole, the domains of reactivity, negative affect, positive affect, and attention demonstrate a number of interesting dissociations. If these results are viewed in hierarchical terms, it may be argued that covariance within domains arises from similar or shared mechanisms of control at higher and lower levels. As previously suggested, shared attentional and response-regulating components may contribute much to the patterning of higher level emotional processes. It is clear, however, that a more detailed study of emotional-attentional interactions is required, and we are now developing laboratory techniques for this purpose.

Infant temperament research

Another valuable approach to temperament involves its developmental study. Our investigations of infant temperament have utilized parent report, home observation, and laboratory assessments (Rothbart, 1981; Rothbart & Derryberry, 1981). This research has approached motor reactivity in terms of a specific (tendency to startle) and a more general (activity level) measure. Emotional states of fear (distress and latency to approach a novel or intense stimulus), frustration (distress to limitations), and smiling and laughter have also been assessed, along with additional measures of duration of orienting, vocal activity, and soothability.

Using parent report on a sample of 149 infants, we found the measures of fear and frustration to be positively correlated at 3, 6, 9, and 12 months of age. In addition, the startle measure was positively related to the fear measure at all four ages and to the frustration measure at 3, 6, and 9 months. As in the adult study, there seems to be a tendency for the negative emotions to relate to one another and to reactivity (at least as measured through startle). Dissociations are again evident, however. Frustration is positively related to general activity level at 6, 9, and 12 months of age, whereas fear is never related to activity level, and startle relates positively to activity level only at 9 months. Thus, the two measures of motor reactivity (startle and activity level) appear to be relatively independent both in their relationship to one another and in their relationship to the negative emotions. Fear and frustration, although related to one another and to startle, differ in their relation to activity level.

The measure of smiling and laughter was found to be negatively related to fear at all four ages, to frustration at 3 and 12 months, and to startle at 3 months. Smiling and laughter was positively related to vocal activity at all four ages, to duration of orienting at 3 and 9 months, and to soothability at 3 and 6 months of age. This pattern of results is suggestive of a general inverse relationship between positive and negative affect, although the underlying processes are difficult to ascertain. The relationship does not appear to involve motor reactivity, since smiling and laughter after 3 months is relatively independent of startle and activity level.

To examine positive and negative affect in relation to longer lasting tonic states of arousal, a second phase of our research included an assessment of sleep–wake records at 3 and 9 months in a longitudinal sample of 46 infants

(Rothbart & Derryberry, 1982). Analysis of three-month sleep–wake measures indicated a negative relationship between number of sleep–wake transitions and smiling and laughter, activity level, soothability, and duration of orienting. Positive correlations were found between number of transitions and the fear and frustration measures. Thus, there appears to be a general early trend for infants with less stable sleep activity to demonstrate less positive affect and more negative affect. These data are interesting in that stabilization of sleep activity may be related to maturation of the ascending monoamine (e.g., serotonin, norepinephrine) projections (Jouvet, 1975). As mentioned earlier, these systems are considered central to motivational and attentional functions.

Recently we have completed data collection on a detailed laboratory study designed to elicit a range of attentional, emotional, and arousal reactions. Infants were presented with visual, auditory, tactile, and social stimuli varying in intensity and novelty, and their motor, vocal, and cardiovascular reactions were recorded on videotape. We assessed their tendency to startle by presenting them with a rapidly opening parasol, their tendency to smile and laugh by presenting rapidly changing stimuli, including social stimuli, and their frustration tolerance by varying the accessibility of attractive toys. We are measuring reactivity both separately by response channel (motor, vocal, autonomic) and in terms of more integrated emotional responses such as fear, frustration, and pleasure. The videotape record allows us to assess the parameters of reactivity (latency, rise time, peak intensity, and recovery) with some precision.

We are especially interested in assessing the self-regulatory systems of the infant, including attentional regulation (e.g., gaze aversions, looking away, looking at mother) and self-soothing (e.g., sucking fingers, rubbing the body). In particular, we wish to consider the temporal location of these behaviors relative to the rising and falling phases of distress reactions. We assess flexibility of attention by examining infants' orientation to peripheral probe lights while engaged in viewing an attractive, centrally located audiovisual display. We also measure shifts of visual attention as infants play with relatively simple toys and as they alternate their visual fixation between two three-dimensional mask displays.

We feel that the analysis of the patterning of tonic arousal, phasic reactivity, emotionality, and self-regulation across the early years of life can greatly contribute to our understanding of adult temperament. In addition, these energetic and regulatory aspects of the developing personality may have an important influence upon cognitive and social development.

Summary

In this chapter we have attempted to develop a general framework for viewing temperament. In this framework, both homeostatic and nonhomeostatic influences are seen to regulate higher level affective-motivational systems. These systems in turn are seen to operate on two kinds of intermediate level systems: Response regulating systems modulate lower level effector systems, while sensory regulating systems modulate the flow of sensory information toward these output mechanisms. Thus emotion has been viewed as a multilevel process coordinating sensation and response.

When applied to temperament, this framework suggests that individuals may differ at a variety of levels. We have emphasized variability in processes of sensory modulation, for these have often been neglected in both temperament and emotional theory. Individuals who can effectively shift and focus their attention appear less vulnerable to a variety of negative emotional states. At the same time, such individuals appear capable of enjoying potentially negative situations. By selectively enhancing and attenuating sensory and semantic information, attentional processes may be central in regulating experience and behavior.

Beyond these theoretical considerations, however, lie the uniqueness and variability of individual temperaments. This uniqueness is present at birth and unfolds in numerous ways as development proceeds. It influences the child's relationships with the physical world, with the social world, and with the self. It must be appreciated, for we have far too often neglected the organism in favor of the environment.

References

Adrian, E. General discussion. In E. Adrian, J. Bemer, & H. H. Jasper (Eds.), *Brain mechanisms and consciousness*. Springfield, Ill.: Thomas, 1954.

Anisman, H. Time-dependent variations in aversively motivated behaviors: Nonassociative effects of cholinergic and catecholaminergic activity. *Psychological Review*, 1975, *82*, 359–385.

Aronfreed, J. *Conduct and conscience*. New York: Academic Press, 1968.

Bell, P. A., & Byrne, E. Repression-sensitization. In H. London & J. E. Exner, Jr. (Eds.), *Dimensions of personality*. New York: Wiley, 1978.

Bloom, F. E. Chemical integrative processes in the central nervous system. In F. O. Schmitt & F. G. Worden (Eds.), *The neurosciences: Fourth study program*. Cambridge, Mass.: MIT Press, 1979.

Bower, G. H. Mood and memory. *American Psychologist*, 1981, *36*, 129–148.

Bower, T. G. R. *Development in infancy*. San Francisco: Freeman, 1982.

Broadbent, D. E. *In defence of empirical psychology*. London: Methuen, 1973.

Brodal, K. A. *Neurological anatomy*. London: Oxford University Press, 1981.

Bronson, G. W. Structure, status, and characteristics of the nervous system at birth. In P. M. Stratton (Ed.), *The psychobiology of the human newborn*. London: Wiley, 1982.

Bronson, G. W., & Pankey, W. On the distinction between fear and wariness. *Child Development*, 1977, *48*, 1167–1183.

Bruner, J. S. The organization of early skilled action. In M. P. M. Richards (Ed.), *The integration of a child into a social world*. Cambridge: Cambridge University Press, 1974.

Bushnell, M. C., Goldberg, M. E., & Robinson, D. L. Behavioral enhancement of visual responses in monkey cerebral cortex. I. Modulation in posterior parietal cortex related to selective visual attention. *Journal of Neurophysiology*, 1981, *46*, 755–772.

Buss, A. H., & Plomin, R. *A temperament theory of personality*. New York: Wiley, 1975.

Charlesworth, W. The role of surprise in cognitive development. In D. Elkind & J. Flavell (Eds.), *Studies in cognitive development*. London: Oxford University Press, 1969.

Clavier, R. M., & Routtenberg, A. In search of reinforcement pathways: A neuroanatomical odyssey. In A. Routtenberg (Ed.), *Biology of reinforcement: Facets of brain-stimulation reward*. New York: Academic Press, 1980.

Dawson, M. E., & Schell, A. M. Electrodermal responses to attended and nonattended significant stimuli during dichotic listening. *Journal of Experimental Psychology: Human Perception and Performance*, 1982, *8*, 315–324.

Derryberry, D. *The regulation of cortical reactivity: Psychological and physiological models of attention*. Manuscript in preparation, University of Oregon, 1983.

Dixon, N. F. *Preconscious processing*. New York: Wiley, 1981.

Douglas, V. I., & Peters, K. G. Toward a clearer definition of the attentional deficit of hyperactive children. In G. A. Hale & M. Lewis (Eds.), *Attention and cognitive development*. New York: Plenum, 1979.

Emde, R. N. *Levels of meaning for infant emotions: A biosocial view*. Unpublished manuscript, University of Colorado Medical Center, 1979.

Erdelyi, M. A new look at the new look: Perceptual defense and vigilance. *Psychological Review*, 1974, *81*, 1–25.

Escalona, S. K. *The roots of individuality: Normal patterns of development in infancy*. Chicago: Aldine, 1968.

Eysenck, H. J. *The biological basis of personality*. Springfield, Ill.: Thomas, 1967.

Eysenck, H. J. (Ed.). *The measurement of personality*. Baltimore, Md.: University Park Press, 1976.

Eysenck, H. J. (Ed.). *A model for personality*. New York: Springer-Verlag, 1981.

Foote, S. L., Ashton-Jones, G., & Bloom, F. E. Impulse activity of locus coeruleus in awake rats and squirrel monkeys is a function of sensory stimulation and arousal. *Proceedings of the National Academy of Sciences*, 1980, *77*, 3033–3037.

Gallistel, C. R. *The organization of action: A new synthesis*. Hillsdale, N.J.: Erlbaum, 1980.

Goldsmith, H. H., & Campos, J. J. Toward a theory of infant temperament. In R. N. Emde & R. J. Harmon (Eds.), *The development of attachment and affiliative systems*. New York: Plenum, 1982.

Graham, F. K., & Jackson, J. C. Arousal systems and infant heart rate responses. In H. W. Reese & L. P. Lipsett (Eds.), *Advances in child development and behavior* (Vol. 5). New York: Academic Press, 1970.

Graham, F. K., Strock, B. D., & Zeigler, B. L. Excitatory and inhibitory influences on reflex responsiveness. In W. A. Collins (Ed.), *Aspects of the development of competence*. Hillsdale, N.J.: Erlbaum, 1981.

Gray, J. A. *The psychology of fear and stress*. New York: McGraw-Hill, 1971.

Gray, J. A. Causal theories of personality and how to test them. In J. R. Royce (Ed.), *Multivariate analysis and psychological theory*. London: Academic Press, 1973.

Gray, J. A. A critique of Eysenck's theory of personality. In H. J. Eysenck (Ed.), *A model for personality*. New York: Springer-Verlag, 1981.

Gray, J. A. *The neuropsychology of anxiety*. London: Oxford University Press, 1982.

Haith, M. M. *Rules that babies look by*. Hillsdale, N.J.: Erlbaum, 1980.

Hebb, D. O. Drives and the C.N.S. (conceptual nervous system). *Psychological Review*, 1955, *62*, 243–255.

Hiatt, S., Campos, J., and Emde, R. Facial patterning and infant emotional expression: Happiness, surprise, and fear. *Child Development*, 1979, *50*, 1020–1035.

Izard, C. E. *The face of emotion*. New York: Appleton-Century-Crofts, 1971.

Izard, C. E. *Patterns of emotions: A new analysis of anxiety and depression*. New York: Academic Press, 1972.

Izard, C. E. *Human emotions*. New York: Plenum, 1977.

Izard, C. E., & Buechler, S. Emotion expressions and personality integration in infancy. In C. E. Izard (Ed.), *Emotions in personality and psychopathology*. New York: Plenum, 1979.

Jackson, J. H. Relations of different divisions of the central nervous system to one another and to parts of the body. *Lancet*, 1898, *i*, 79–87.

Jouvet, M. Cholinergic mechanisms and sleep. In P. G. Waser (Ed.), *Cholinergic mechanisms*, pp. 455–476. New York: Raven Press, 1975.

Kagan, J. Discrepancy, temperament, and infant distress. In M. Lewis & L. A. Rosenblum (Eds.), *The origins of fear*. New York: Wiley, 1974.

Kandel, E. R. *A cell-biological approach to learning*. Bethesda, Md.: Society for Neuroscience, 1978.

Keele, S. W., Neill, W. T., & deLemos, S. M. Individual differences in attentional flexibility. *Center for Cognitive and Perceptual Research Technical Report* (No. 1). Eugene: University of Oregon, 1978.

Kent, E. W. *The brains of men and machines*. Peterborough, N.H.: McGraw-Hill, 1981.

Kremenitzer, J. P., Vaughan, H. G., Kurtzberg, D., & Dowling, K. Smooth-pursuit eye movements in the newborn infant. *Child Development*, 1979, *50*, 442–448.

Lacey, J. I. Somatic response patterning and stress: Some revisions of activation theory. In M. H. Appley & Trumbull (Eds.), *Psychological stress: Issues in research*. New York: Appleton-Century-Crofts, 1967.

Lamb, M. E., & Sherrod, L. R. *Infant social cognition*. Hillsdale, N.J.: Erlbaum, 1981.

LeDoux, J. E., Wilson, D. H., & Gazzaniga, M. S. Beyond commissurotomy: Clues to consciousness. In M. S. Gazzaniga (Ed.), *Handbook of behavioral neurobiology. 2: Neuropsychology*. New York: Plenum, 1979.

Lidov, H. G. W., & Molliver, M. E. An immunohistochemical study of serotonin neuron development in the rat: Ascending pathways and terminal fields. *Brain Research Bulletin*, 1982, *8*, 349–420.

Mabry, P., & Campbell, B. A. Ontogeny of serotonergic inhibition of behavioral arousal in the rat. *Journal of Comparative and Physiological Psychology*, 1974, *86*, 193–206.

Mandler, G. *Mind and emotion*. New York: Wiley, 1975.

Mason, J. W. Emotion as reflected in patterns of endocrine integration. In L. Levi (Ed.), *Emotions – their parameters and measurement*. New York: Raven Press, 1975.

Matthysse, S. Dopamine and selective attention. In E. Costa & G. L. Gessa (Eds.), *Advances in biochemical psychopharmacology* (Vol. 16). New York: Raven Press, 1977.

Mayer, D. J., & Price, D. D. A physiological and psychological analysis of pain: A potential model for motivation. In D. W. Pfaff (Ed.), *The physiological mechanisms of motivation*. New York: Springer-Verlag, 1982.

Mesulam, M., Van Hoesen, G. W., Pandya, D. N., & Geschwind, N. Limbic and sensory connections of the inferior parietal lobule (area PG) in the rhesus monkey: A study with a new method for horseradish peroxidase histo-chemistry. *Brain Research*, 1977, *136*, 393–414.

Mishkin, M. Two cortical visual systems. *Experimental Brain Research*, 1980, *41*, A17–A18.

Morris, L. *Extraversion and introversion*. New York: Wiley, 1979.

Muir, D., & Field, J. Newborn infants orient to sounds. *Child Development*, 1979, *50*, 431–436.

Oster, H. Facial expression and affect development. In M. Lewis & L. A. Rosenblum (Eds.), *The development of affect*. New York: Plenum, 1978.

Panksepp, J. Hypothalamic integration of behavior: Rewards, punishments, and related psychological processes. In P. J. Morgane & J. Panksepp (Eds.), *Handbook of the hypothalamus*. vol. 3, pt. B: *Behavioral studies of the hypothalamus*. New York: Dekker, 1981.

Pfaff, D. W. (Ed.). *The physiological mechanisms of motivation*. New York: Springer-Verlag, 1982.

Piaget, J. *The origins of intelligence in children*. New York: Norton, 1952.

Pien, D., & Rothbart, M. K. Incongruity humour, play and self-regulation of arousal in young children. In P. E. McGhee & A. J. Chapman (Eds.), *Childrens' humour*. New York: Wiley, 1980.

Porges, S. W. Peripheral and neurochemical parallels of psychopathology: A psychophysiological model relating autonomic imbalance to hyperactivity, psychopathy, and autism. In H. W.

Reese (Ed.), *Advances in child development and behavior*, pp. 35–63. New York: Academic Press, 1976.

Posner, M. I., & Rothbart, M. K. The development of attentional mechanisms. In J. Flowers (Ed.), *Nebraska symposium on motivation*, Vol. 28. Lincoln: University of Nebraska Press, 1981.

Pradhan, S. N., & Pradhan, S. Development of central neurotransmitter systems and ontogeny of behavior. In H. Parvez & S. Parvez (Eds.), *Biogenic amines in development*. New York: Elsevier North-Holland, 1980.

Prechtl, H. F. R. *The neurological examination of the full-term newborn infant*, 2nd ed. London: Spastics International/W. Heinemann, 1977.

Reed, M. A., Pien, D., & Rothbart, M. K. *Development of self-regulation in preschool children*. Unpublished manuscript, University of Oregon, 1982.

Rolls, E. T., Burton, M. J., & Mora, F. Neurophysiological analysis of brain stimulation reward in the monkey. *Brain Research*, 1980, *194*, 339–357.

Rolls, E. T., Caan, A. W., Griffiths, C., Murzi, E., Perret, D. I., Thorpe, S. J., & Wilson, F. A. W. Processing beyond the inferior temporal visual cortex. *Behavioral Brain Research*, 1982, *5*, 114–115.

Rothbart, M. K. Measurement of temperament in infancy. *Child Development*, 1981, *52*, 569–578.

Rothbart, M. K., & Derryberry, D. Development of individual differences in temperament. In M. E. Lamb & A. L. Brown (Eds.), *Advances in developmental psychology* (Vol. 1). Hillsdale, N.J.: Erlbaum, 1981.

Rothbart, M. K., & Derryberry, D. *Sleep-wake transitions and infant temperament*. Paper presented at the meetings of the International Conference on Infant Studies, Austin, Texas, March 1982.

Santostefano, S. *A biodevelopmental approach to clinical child psychology*. New York: Wiley, 1978.

Satinoff, E. Are there similarities between thermoregulation and sexual behavior? In D. W. Pfaff (Ed.), *The physiological mechanisms of motivation*. New York: Springer-Verlag, 1982.

Schachter, S. Cognition and centralist-peripheralist controversies in motivation and emotion. In M. S. Gazzaniga & C. W. Blakemore (Eds.), *Handbook of psychobiology*. New York: Plenum, 1975.

Schwartz, G. E. Psychophysiological patterning and emotion revisited: A systems perspective. In C. E. Izard (Ed.), *Measuring emotions in infants and children*. Cambridge: Cambridge University Press, 1982.

Siegel, A., & Edinger, H. Neural control of aggression and rage behavior. In P. J. Morgane & J. Panksepp (Eds.), *Handbook of the hypothalamus*. vol. 3, pt. B: *Behavioral studies of the hypothalamus*. New York: Dekker, 1981.

Sroufe, L. A. Socioemotional development. In J. Osofsky (Ed.), *Handbook of infant development*. New York: Wiley, 1979.

Stechler, G., & Latz, E. Some observations on attention and arousal in the human infant. *Journal of the American Academy of Child Psychiatry*, 1966, *5*, 517–525.

Stein, L. The chemistry of reward. In A. Routtenberg (Ed.), *Biology of reinforcement: Facets of brain-stimulation reward*. New York: Academic Press, 1980.

Stern, D. Mother and infant at play: The dyadic interaction involving facial, vocal and gaze behaviors. In M. Lewis & L. Rosenblum (Eds.), *The effect of the infant on its caregiver*. New York: Wiley, 1974.

Teitelbaum, P. Levels of integration of the operant. In W. K. Honig & J. E. R. Staddon (Eds.), *Handbook of operant behavior*. Englewood Cliffs, N.J.: Prentice-Hall, 1977.

Tennes, K., Emde, R., Kisley, A., & Metcalf, D. The stimulus barrier in early infancy: An exploration of some formulations of John Benjamin. In R. R. Holt & E. Peterfreund (Eds.), *Psychoanalysis and contemporary science* (Vol. 1). New York: Macmillan, 1972.

Thomas, A., & Chess, S. *Temperament and development*. New York: Brunner/Mazel, 1977.

Tinbergen, N. *The study of instinct*. London: Oxford University Press, 1951.

Tomkins, S. S. *Affect, imagery, consciousness.* Vol. 1: *The positive affects.* New York: Springer-Verlag, 1962.

Von Hofsten, C. Eye-hand coordination in the newborn. *Developmental Psychology*, 1982, *18*, 450–461.

Weiss, J. M., Glazer, H. I., Pohorecky, L. A., Bailey, W. H., & Schneider, L. H. Coping behavior and stress-induced behavioral depression: Studies of the role of brain catecholamines. In R. A. Depue (Ed.), *The psychobiology of the depressive disorders.* New York: Academic Press, 1979.

Witkin, H. A. *Cognitive styles in personal and cultural adaptation.* Worcester, Mass.: Clark University Press, 1978.

Wurtz, R. H., Goldberg, M. E., & Robinson, D. L. Behavioral modulation of visual responses in the monkey: Stimulus selection for attention and movement. *Progress in Psychobiology and Physiological Psychology*, 1980, *9*, 43–84.

Zajonc, R. B. Feeling and thinking: Preferences need no inferences. *American Psychologist*, 1980, *35*, 151–175.

Zelniker, T., & Jeffrey, W. E. Attention and cognitive style in children. In G. A. Hale & M. Lewis (Eds.), *Attention and cognitive development.* New York: Plenum, 1979.

Ziven, G. (Ed.). *The development of self-regulation through private speech.* New York: Wiley, 1979.

Zuckerman, M. *Sensation seeking: Beyond the optimal level of arousal.* Hillsdale, N.J.: Erlbaum, 1979.

6 An attributional approach to emotional development

Bernard Weiner and Sandra Graham

The understanding of this chapter will be facilitated if it is acknowledged at the outset that: (1) we are *social* psychologists; (2) we are *cognitive* social psychologists; and (3) we are cognitive social psychologists whose prime interest is in *attributional processes*. The impact of *social* psychology will be evident in our concentration on emotions that are intrinsic to social motivation, specifically anger, guilt, pity, and pride, rather than, say, disgust, distress, and fear. Adults include these social feelings among their most frequent emotional experiences (Bottenberg, 1975). As *cognitive* social psychologists we have been concerned with how people perceive and interpret their social environment. We will document that cognitions about the personal and social world significantly influence emotional experience and the growth of emotional life. The cognitive process that we believe to be of special importance for the study of emotions involves *attributions about causality*.

Causal attributions

A causal attribution answers a "why" question: "Why doesn't Johnny like me?" "Why did Mary get a poor mark on the spelling quiz?" "Why did I fail to get a hit in the baseball game?" Causal search is not indiscriminantly displayed in all situations, for this would place great cognitive strain on the organism. Rather, search is most evident when an outcome is unexpected (e.g., failure when success was anticipated) and when a desire has not been fulfilled (e.g., there is interpersonal rejection; see Folkes, 1982; Lau & Russell, 1980; Wong & Weiner, 1981). Causal search and explanation may be undertaken to reduce surprise (Pettit, 1981). Thus, a young man might be taken aback when he is rejected for a date by his fiancée. A response to his "why" query – "I must meet a friend" or "I have a terrible headache" produces the explanation needed to account for rejection, thereby reducing surprise. The surprise-reducing function of explanation accounts for causal search given an unexpected outcome. Causal search is also undertaken to aid in subsequent goal attainment. Knowing

The first author of this chapter is supported by a grant from the National Science Foundation. The authors thank Deborah Stipek for her comments on an earlier draft.

why one has failed and undertaking corrective actions might increase later chances for success. The instrumental aspect of explanation accounts for the enhanced attributional search given nonattainment of a goal. Attributional analyses therefore also are functional, and attribution theory falls within the broader study of cognitive functionalism.

As intimated above, causal search is not confined to any single motivational domain. Individuals desire to know, for example, why their team has been defeated (an achievement concern; Lau & Russell, 1980), why they have been refused for a date (an affiliative concern; Folkes, 1982), and why they have lost an election (a power concern; Kingdon, 1967). The number of perceived causes is virtually infinite, although the vast majority of answers to the above questions are selected from a rather circumscribed array. In achievement situations, success and failure typically are ascribed to ability (including both aptitude and learned skills), some aspect of motivation (such as short- or long-term effort expenditure, attention), others (friends, family), physiological factors (e.g., mood, maturity, health), the difficulty or the ease of the task, and luck (see Cooper & Burger, 1980). In an affiliative context, acceptance or rejection of a dating request often is ascribed to prior behaviors (e.g., making a good impression, being too assertive), physical appearance, and the desires or state of the potential date (wanting to go out or having a prior engagement; see Folkes, 1982). And in a political contest, election or defeat tends to be attributed to party identification, the personality characteristics of the candidates, and their stance on issues (Kingdon, 1967).

Because the potential list of causes is considerable within any motivational domain, and because the specific causes differ between domains, the creation of a classification scheme or a taxonomy of causes is essential. This allows the identification of the underlying properties of the causes and the determination of their similarities and differences. Causes that denotatively differ (e.g., intelligence as a cause of achievement success, physical beauty as a cause of affiliative success, and personality as a cause of political success) may be connotatively quite similar (e.g., among other similarities, all refer to relatively enduring personal properties). The discovery of these bases for comparison, which are referred to here as causal dimensions, is an indispensable requirement for the construction of a relatively general attributional theory of emotion and emotional development.

Causal dimensions

Two methods of arriving at new knowledge, dialectic and demonstrative (following Rychlak, 1968), have been used to determine the basic dimensions of causality. The dialectic approach involves a logical grouping of causes (thesis), discovery of an apparent contradiction in reasoning (antithesis), and the emergence of a new dimension of causality to resolve the uncovered inconsistency (synthesis). This logical and introspective examination within the attributional domain began with a differentiation between causes located within the person – intelligence, physical beauty, and personality – and causes located outside the person – as, for example, the difficulty of a task, the prior engagement of a dating partner, or the popularity of one's opponent. The internal–external distinction is primarily associated with Rotter's (1966) discussion of locus of control. However, this causal dimension has been captured with various labels, such as person–environment or disposition–situation, and is evident in contrasts between origin–pawn (deCharms, 1968), intrinsic–extrinsic motivation (Deci, 1975), and freedom–constraint (Brehm, 1966; Steiner, 1970). Within the achievement domain, such causes as aptitude, effort, and health commonly are considered internal, whereas task difficulty, help from others, and luck are perceived to be environmental determinants of an outcome. In the affiliative domain, such causes as physical beauty and "charm" are internal, whereas the availability of the desired dating partner is an external determinant of acceptance or rejection.

A shortcoming of this one-dimensional taxonomy became evident when it was observed that causes classified on the same dimension elicited disparate responses. For example, in achievement-related contexts, expectancies of success are lower when failure is perceived as resulting from a lack of ability than when failure is believed to result from a lack of effort (see, e.g., Weiner, Nierenberg, & Goldstein, 1976). Thus, although ability (aptitude) and effort are considered properties of the person, they nevertheless must differ in one or more respects. Consequently, a second dimension of causality was postulated. Labeled causal stability (see Heider, 1958; Weiner, 1979, 1980a), this dimension differentiates causes on the basis of their relative endurance. For example, aptitude, physical beauty, and personality are perceived as lasting, whereas mood and luck can vary within short periods of time. Because ability is perceived as more enduring than effort, outcomes that are ascribed to ability are more predictive of the future than are outcomes that are ascribed to effort, which accounts for the difference in expectancy shifts produced by these two causal ascriptions.

In a similar manner, a third dimension of causality was proposed when it became evident that some causes identically classified on both the locus and stability dimensions yielded dissimilar reactions (see Litman-Adizes, 1978; Rosenbaum, 1972; Weiner, 1979). For example, greater punishment is elicited by failure attributed to lack of effort than by failure ascribed to ill health, although both causes may be conceived as internal and unstable. Thus a third causal property, controllability, was suggested. The concept of control implies that the actor "could have done otherwise" (Hamilton, 1980). Effort is subject to volitional control; individuals are responsible for how hard they try. On the other hand, inherited characteristics such as aptitude or, in most cases, the onset of an illness cannot be controlled. Within the achievement domain, effort is the most evident example of a controllable cause, although so-called traits such as patience or frustration tolerance also often are perceived by others as controllable. Note, then, that ability (aptitude) and effort differ on two dimensions of causality. Although both causes are internal, aptitude is stable and uncontrollable, whereas effort is unstable and controllable. Disparities in punishment given failure resulting from temporary illness versus that resulting from lack of effort, both internal and unstable causes, are ascribable only to their difference on the controllability dimension.

At present, three dimensions of causality have been identified: locus, stability, and controllability. In most instances, such causes as intelligence, physical beauty, and charisma are perceived as internal, stable, and uncontrollable. Thus a fundamental similarity exists between three denotatively different causes that often are invoked to explain positive and negative outcomes in the three motivational domains of achievement, affiliation, and power.

A number of experimental (demonstrative) studies have been undertaken to discover the dimensions of causality (see review in Weiner, 1982). The empirical data demonstrate a high degree of convergence between the dialectic and the empirical procedures, and it certainly appears that locus, stability, and controllability are among the dimensions of causality. These dimensions both reveal the meaning of a cause and represent the manner in which the causal world is organized.

A working definition

Because of our particular concern with the influence of cognitions (attributions) on emotions, it is first necessary to differentiate "cold" cognitions from "hot" emotions. We believe that any given property of an emotion might also describe a thought. But if all the presumed characteristics of an emotion are in evidence, then an emotional state can be inferred with reasonable certainty. First among these properties is that emotions have a positive or a negative experiential quality of a certain magnitude (e.g., contrast the positive aspects of pride, which one wants "more of," with the negative aspects of guilt, which one wants "less of"). An emotional experience may be accompanied by certain facial expressions and bodily postures, such as the expansive posture associated with pride. In addition, affects frequently give rise to particular behaviors; for example, one strikes out to "eliminate" the object of anger, or helps those who elicit pity. Furthermore, and most germane to this chapter, emotions quite often follow particular thoughts. Thus, gratitude seems to presuppose the attribution of a positive outcome to the volitional help of others. However, an emotion may not follow a thought to which it is typically linked and may not give rise to an associated behavior. For example, one might be helped by others yet not experience gratitude. Or, one might experience gratitude, yet not engage in a positive social response. In a similar manner, given an emotion, the linked thought need not have been the antecedent, and a given behavior may be elicited by any of a number of emotions. For example, one might experience guilt without engaging in an act for which one is personally responsible, and helping others can be instigated by either gratitude or pity.

The position we espouse regarding the relation between cognition and emotion can best be compared, perhaps, to hypotheses regarding the relation between frustration and aggression. Although it is now accepted that frustration may not elicit aggression and that aggression is elicited by factors other than frustration, frustration and aggression nevertheless frequently are linked.

Thus far, the role of physiological factors has been absent from this syndrome or cluster definition of emotion. It is suggested that the social emotions examined here, such as gratitude, pity, and pride, will not be associated with a particular pattern of internal activity. It may be that emotions of great intensity or emotions that can be represented across species, such as rage, sexual excitement, and fear, will have physiological correlates or specific internal representation. But this is not very likely for the vast majority of emotions experienced in everyday life.

Causal ascriptions and emotions

The questions addressed in this chapter regarding the development of relations between causal thinking and feeling were an outgrowth of a series of investigations with adult subjects conducted by Weiner, Russell, and Lerman (1978, 1979). These studies, which documented the causal determinants of feelings, also laid the foundation for a systematic mapping of what kinds of attributional thoughts among adults are linked with what kinds of feelings. Further, the studies examined positive as well as negative emotions, in contrast to the typical psychological focus on the negative emotions of fear and anxiety.

In the guiding study of the relation between causal ascriptions and feelings (Weiner et al., 1978), approximately 250 potential affective reactions to success and failure were identified, as well as the dominant causal attributions for achievement performance, such as ability, long-term effort, luck, and other people. Then a cause for success or failure was given within a brief story, the success- or failure-related affects that had been identified were listed, and the participants merely indicated the intensity of the affective reactions they thought would be experienced in this situation. Responses were made on simple rating scales. A typical scenario was:

Francis studied intensely for a test he took. It was very important for Francis to record a high score on this exam. He received an extremely high score on the test. He felt he received this high score because he studied so intensely, [or, because of his ability in the subject; because he was lucky in which questions were selected; etc.]. How do you think that Francis felt upon receiving this score? (p. 10)

To overcome the weaknesses of a simulational and respondent procedure, a follow-up investigation was undertaken (Weiner et al., 1979) in which par-

Table 6.1. *Some relations between causal attributions and feelings*

	Outcome	
Attribution	Success	Failure
Ability	Competence	Incompetence
Long-term effort	Relaxation	Guilt
Others	Gratitude	Anger
Luck	Surprise	Surprise

Source: Weiner, Russell, & Lerman, 1978, 1979.

ticipants reported a "critical incident" in their lives when they actually succeeded or failed on an exam for a particular reason, such as help from others or lack of effort. They then recounted three affects that were experienced.

Both investigations yielded similar, systematic findings. First, there was a set of outcome-dependent, attribution-independent affects representing broad positive or negative reactions to success and failure regardless of the "why" of the outcome (also see Epstein, 1979). Given success, feelings such as happiness were reported regardless of disparate attributional conditions. One is likely to feel happy when receiving an "A" on an exam whether that high grade is due to ability, help from others, or an easy test. In a similar manner, given failure, feelings such as upset and frustration were expressed in all the attributional conditions. These outcome-dependent affects for both success and failure were rated as the most intensely experienced emotions.

In addition, certain emotions were related to particular attributions. Table 6.1 includes four dominant causal attributions (ability, long-term effort, others, and luck) and the specific emotions they elicited following success and failure. The success linkages included ability/competence and confidence, long-term effort/relaxation, others/gratitude, and luck/surprise. For failure, the attribution-affect associations included ability/incompetence, effort/guilt, others/anger, and luck/surprise. Thus, if we succeed because of help from others, we are likely to feel grateful, whereas failure resulting from hindrance from others tends to give rise to anger. Note that the same emotion (surprise) accompanies both the positive and the negative outcomes given a luck attribution. It must be remembered, however, that success produces the affective constellation of surprise plus the outcome-dependent affect of happy, whereas failure produces surprise plus frustration.

Finally, causal dimensions also play an essential role in affective life. Internal attributions for success – ability, effort, and personality – more often produced pride and other esteem-related affects than did external attributions for success.

Among adults, the affects associated with self-esteem and self-worth are elicited when the cause of the outcome is attributed to the self.

The locus of causality is not the only causal dimension that has direct influence on affective life. Causal stability, or the perceived duration of a cause, also influences affective reactions. Affects such as depression, apathy, and resignation primarily were described when the attributions for failure were internal and stable, such as lack of ability or a personality deficit. It appears that only attributions conveying that events will not get better in the future beget feelings of hopelessness and surrender. Later in this chapter it will be documented that the third property of causes, controllability, also is directly linked with emotional reactions. Just as causal attributions are united with specific affective states, the dimensions of causality also are connected with particular feelings.

In sum, the studies suggest that emotions in achievement-related contexts are a function of outcomes, specific causal ascriptions, and the properties of these perceived ascriptions (Weiner et al., 1978, 1979). The latter linkages revealed unique mappings between causal thoughts and both positive and negative feelings.

The following discussion, which focuses on emotional development, considers, in turn, outcome-linked, ascription-linked, and dimension-linked affects. The attributional approach to the study of affective development promoted here is guided by the belief that causal thoughts precede or change the experience and understanding of emotions such as pride, pity, guilt, and anger. Hence, developmental differences in the experience and understanding of these emotions are due to age-related changes in the linkages between causal ascriptions and affective experiences.[1] Following the discussion of emotional development and the presentation of evidence supporting the attributional position, some persisting problems with this approach are examined. A few general issues and concepts in the field of emotion are then considered, including the thought-affect sequence, arousal, and the study of content versus process. This discussion will reveal that the attributional perspective advocated here is part of a broader belief system concerning how emotions might be productively studied.

Outcome-dependent emotions

It has long been suspected that emotional development proceeds from a state of general excitement to one of more specific feelings. For example, Bridges (1930) stated:

The genetic theory of emotions is thus that excitement, the undifferentiated emotion present at birth, becomes differentiated and associated with certain situations and certain motor responses to form the separate emotions of later life. This process of differentiation and integration takes place gradually, so that at different age levels different emotions are distinguishable. (p. 517)

This intuitively appealing point of view has not been documented with supporting empirical evidence. Neither has the process by which more specific emotions evolve from the earlier undifferentiated states been well articulated (see Sroufe, 1979). Our research suggests that happy and sad represent less cognitively mediated (undifferentiated) reactions to positive and negative outcomes than do, for example, pride and gratitude, which are determined by the assignment of causal responsibility (Weiner et al., 1978, 1979). One might therefore provide some support for the position of Bridges by finding a developmental shift in the reactions to success and failure, with younger children showing a greater tendency to display or infer outcome-linked emotions and older children exhibiting or supposing more complex reactions that include attribution-linked emotions.

To test this hypothesis, the following investigation was conducted by Weiner, Kun, and Benesh-Weiner (1980). The subjects, almost 200 children, mean ages 6.4 and 10.4 years, and 200 adults, were presented a story such as:

Peter did not know how to spell any of the words on the list. When it was his turn, he guessed at the spelling word and spelled it right. Peter knew that the reason he did well was because of good luck. How do you think he felt? (p. 114)

In the condition of immediate concern here, this scenario was followed by five affects: (a) sure of himself; (b) proud; (c) thankful; (d) surprised; and (e) happy. Additional stories portrayed causal attributions for success to ability, effort, and other persons. Thus, the response alternatives included an emotion known to be linked to each attribution (ability/sure of himself, short-term effort/proud, others/thankful, and luck/surprised), as well as the outcome-dependent affect of happy. The same attributions were given for failure, with the attribution-linked emotional alternatives of hopeless, ashamed, angry, and surprised, and the outcome-dependent emotion of sad.

Figure 6.1 shows the percentage choice of the "undifferentiated" or outcome-dependent affects of happy and sad across the three age groups. It is quite clear that the use of outcome-linked emotions decreases with increasing age (and, therefore, the use of attribution-linked emotions increases).

These findings have been replicated by Thompson and Paris (1981), who conducted a more complete investigation that included moral as well as achievement themes and free- as well as forced-choice responses. These authors found, for example, that when success was due to help from others or to high effort, young children were more likely to report feelings of happiness, whereas the older participants tended to infer, respectively, gratitude and pride. Again, therefore, there was greater differentiation among the affective inferences with increasing age, and different attributional cues produced different reported feelings.

Speculations about emotional development

As so little is known about emotions and emotional development, particularly from the cognitive perspective, it seems appropriate at this point in time, and

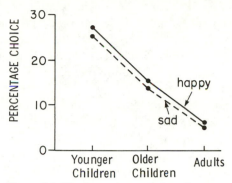

Figure 6.1. Mean percentage choice of outcome-dependent affects (happy and sad) as a function of developmental level. (From Weiner, Kun, & Benesh-Weiner, 1980, p. 118.)

within the context of a review chapter, to offer some speculations that might prove heuristic for future research. We think that outcome-dependent affects, in addition to their reported high intensity, may be of relatively short duration. This is suggested because they are less directly connected with the structure of thought; that is, like other dynamic psychological concepts (e.g., drive), they may have relatively rapid onset and offset. On the other hand, the dimension-linked affects may have great longevity and thus be quite important in life adjustment. For example, feelings related to self-esteem and hopelessness play important roles in depression and coping with stress.

If these thoughts have any truth, and if the responses to the scenarios reported in Weiner and his colleagues (1980) and Thompson and Paris (1981) mirror actual affective experiences, then one might anticipate that children will exhibit great intensity in their emotional responses and that their emotional life will be quite labile or fluctuating. This certainly is in accord with general beliefs about children. In addition, the emotional lives of young children should not be very rich, in the sense that qualitative distinctions between, say, pride and gratitude, manifested by adults given situations that elicit disparate attributions, will be less in evidence among children. Their reasoning about causes is less complex and specific causes may not yet be linked with specific affects. Perhaps, then, cognitive growth both provides a richness to affective life and at the same time dampens the intensity of any single emotional experience. It is sometimes said that the romantic hates the intellectual!

Attribution-dependent emotions

Table 6.1 revealed some of the relations between causal ascriptions and emotions among adults, such as lack of effort/guilt or help from others/gratitude. As already warned, however, it must be remembered that given a causal ascription, the linked emotion does not necessarily follow. For example, one may not put forth effort, yet will be free from guilt. Or one may ascribe success to another, yet not experience gratitude. In addition, one may feel guilty when success is due to luck and when failure is due to lack of ability. But the thought-affect relations shown in Table 6.1 are believed to be quite prevalent in our culture (and perhaps across many cultures).

We have begun to examine the development of relations between specific causal ascriptions and emotional reactions. As thoughts are believed either to determine or to change emotional experience, the attributional perspective advanced here suggests that developmental changes in children's understanding of specific attributions should influence their affective life. In addition, there should be developmental changes in the understanding of attribution-affect linkages that play an important role in social understanding.

In this section we report on research that concerns the understanding of attribution-affect linkages. This research examines inferences made about the inferences of others, or what might be called meta-attributions. In the particular investigation under consideration (Weiner, Graham, Stern, & Lawson, 1982, Experiment 1), the following scenario was described to children and young adults:

A student failed a test and the teacher [became angry, felt pity, etc.]. Why did the teacher think that the student failed? (p. 280)

Note that the subjects are asked to infer what the teacher is inferring. In this manner, it is possible to learn about their understanding of the associations between affects and cognitions. The underlying assumption is that these inferences also would follow if the individual actually was failing and the stated affects were in fact communicated (see Graham, 1982).

Among the affects manipulated were anger, guilt, pity, and surprise (Weiner et al., 1982). The attributional inferences included as possible responses were low ability, insufficient effort, bad luck, and teacher/task ("the teacher made the task too difficult"). The participants indicated on simple rating scales how much each cause was perceived as determining the failure of the student.

In Figure 6.2 the attributional ratings, which are plotted as a function of the affects presented and the age of the subjects, reveal that each affect is associated with a particular causal attribution. Given the expression of anger, the implication is that the student has not tried sufficiently hard. Anger often is an "ought" emotion, indicating a moral evaluation (see Epstein, 1979). Pity, on the other hand, is most expressed when lack of ability is perceived as the cause. In addition, guilt is linked with teacher blame, and surprise is associated with lack of effort in these data.

These relations generally hold among college students and 11- and 9-year-olds (Figure 6.2). The only developmental change concerns the linkage between pity and ability, an association that was clearly in evidence only among the

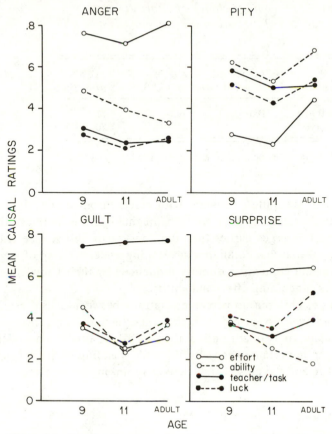

Figure 6.2. Causal ratings as a function of age, plotted within each affect. (From Weiner, Graham, Stern, & Lawson, 1982.)

adult subjects. For the younger age groups, pity was not distinctly linked with any particular emotion (although it was disassociated from effort ascriptions).

In a follow-up investigation (Weiner et al., 1982, Experiment 2), the union between pity and lack of ability, as well as between anger and lack of effort, was examined among even younger children. The participants in this investigation ranged in age from 5 to 9 years old. For these children, only the anger and pity reactions were described and it was possible to select ability or effort as the causal ascription of the teacher. The causal alternative selected, as a function of the communicated affect and the age of the subjects, reveals that both the anger/effort and the pity/ability associations increase with age, with the anger/effort relation the stronger of the two linkages (Table 6.2). Among all subjects, the anger/effort union was significantly greater than chance, whereas this was true only among the 9-year-olds given the pity/ability linkage.

Table 6.2. *Percentage choice of effort given the anger cue and ability given the pity cue, as a function of age*

Linkage	Age 9 (N = 36)	Age 7 (N = 37)	Age 5 (N = 30)
Anger/effort	100	89	77
Pity/ability	72	62	50

Source: Weiner, Graham, Stern, & Lawson, 1982.

These findings are quite consistent with research on the development of attributional understanding. It is well documented in the literature that the concept of effort emerges earlier than the concept of ability (see Nicholls, 1978). It is suggested that children's developing understanding of anger and pity in achievement contexts is directly influenced by their knowledge about causal thoughts concerning effort and ability.

To summarize, children do perceive relations between causal ascriptions and affects, and even 5-year-olds perceive anger/lack of effort linkages. It is anticipated that the study of attribution-affect or affect-attribution associations could provide an important avenue for the understanding of the development of emotional life and the close bonds between thinking and feeling.

Dimension-linked affects

Pity, anger, and guilt

As the data just reported indicate, there are associations between pity and anger and respective inferences about low ability and lack of effort. In addition, among adults, given causal attributions to low ability and lack of effort, the respective affects of pity and anger tend to be elicited. For example, when asked to lend class notes to someone who skipped class to go to the beach (a manifestation of lack of effort), a dominant reaction of the potential help giver is anger (Weiner, 1980b). On the other hand, a request to borrow class notes because of eye problems (a limitation on ability) typically elicits pity and sympathy (Weiner, 1980b). Furthermore, anger gave rise to withdrawal and lack of aid in this situation, whereas sympathy resulted in approach and help giving. In sum, there are associations between lack of effort/anger/no help and between low ability/sympathy/help (also see Weiner, 1980c, for a replication of these findings in nonacademic settings).

Causal dimensions play an important role in these relations. Going to the beach is perceived as subject to volitional control; the individual in need of aid is held personally responsible. A controllable cause for a state of need tends to produce anger. On the other hand, physical disabilities are perceived as uncontrollable. The individual is not held personally accountable for being in a state of need, and more positive social emotions such as sympathy are aroused. In sum, the perceived controllability of the cause mediates between specific attributions, such as lack of ability and low effort, and the affective reactions of pity and anger. In addition, beliefs about controllability, by eliciting disparate affective reactions, influence the behavioral responses of approach and withdrawal (see Brophy & Rohrkemper, 1981; Weiner, 1980b, 1980c).

In a series of studies concerning life events that bear upon the relations between the causal dimension of controllability and affective responses (Graham, Doubleday, & Guarino, in press; Weiner, Graham, & Chandler, 1982), children and adults were asked to report incidents in their lives when they felt pity, anger, or guilt. The participants also rated the controllability of the cause of the event that was recounted.

Among the adults, nearly 90% of the situations that elicited pity were perceived as uncontrollable. This affective reaction frequently accompanied the perception of a physically disabled person or a person who had lost a loved one. On the other hand, guilt and anger were experienced on perceiving an event as subject to volitional control. Guilt was frequently reported when one lied or cheated, whereas anger was experienced when someone else lied or intentionally engaged in a harmful act toward the subject. Note, then, that whether pity or anger is directed toward another depends, in part, on the perceived controllability of the cause of the event. Furthermore, given a controllable cause, the reaction of guilt or anger depends on the locus (self versus other) of the cause.

The data for three groups of children relating these affects to perceived controllability also indicate that pity (communicated with the phrase "feels sorry for") is aroused given uncontrollable causes (Figure 6.3). The situations eliciting pity most often involved accidental injuries, physical disability, or the death or prolonged absence of a loved one. Two representative situations reported by 6-year-olds were: (a) "I felt sorry for my friend when he got hurt; he was helping to build something when a big stack of wood fell on him"; and (b) "I felt sorry for my grandmother when my grandfather died because she felt so lonely and looked so sad." Hence, children of this age do understand pity, although it was reported earlier that they do not exhibit low ability/pity linkages (Weiner et al., 1982). As 6-year-olds and older children apparently have the same concept of pity (perceiving its causal antecedent as an uncontrollable, negative event), it follows that younger children must have a different conception of ability than do adults, perhaps perceiving ability as subject to more change and control (see Weisz, 1980, 1981).

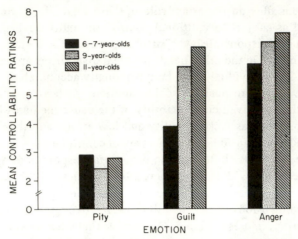

Figure 6.3. Mean controllability ratings for the causes of pity, guilt, and anger as a function of developmental level. (From Graham, Doubleday, & Guarino, in press.)

Given anger, the causes of the eliciting event were perceived as controllable by children in all age groups. Children typically reported feeling angry toward another following incidents of social rejection or humiliation, physical aggression, or intentional goal frustration.

Only in the case of guilt was a developmental trend displayed, with the situations perceived as increasingly controllable across the age groups. All children reported feeling guilty for a generalized class of behavior that can be described as wrongdoing. However, what distinguished the youngest from the older age groups was the unintentional nature of the causes in the accounts given by the 6- and 7-year olds. These children typically experienced guilt for accidental outcomes or after forgetting to carry out a prescribed rule of behavior, such as: (a) "When my brother and I had boxing gloves and I hit him too hard . . . Sometimes I don't know my own strength"; and (b) "When I did the ceremony wrong at my grandfather's funeral . . . I forgot how to do it." In contrast, older children most often reported feeling guilty for intentional wrongdoing or deliberate harm to others: (a) "When I didn't turn in my homework because I was too lazy to do it"; and (b) "When the new girl failed the initiation test into the neighborhood club because we asked questions we knew she couldn't answer."

This pattern of responses suggests that the elicitation of guilt in young children may be more dependent on outcome than on the perceived controllability of the cause of the outcome. There is certainly support for this interpretation in the moral development literature. Moral judgments of preoperational children often are based more on objective outcome information than on intentionality, particularly when accidental or well-intentioned acts have negative consequences (see Karniol, 1978). In addition, the study by Thompson and Paris (1981) found that second graders' inferences about guilt in others were just as likely to be based on outcome as on attributions for the cause of that event.

In sum, it is evident that there are linkages between children's experiences of pity, anger, and guilt and their thoughts about perceived controllability. For all age groups studied, the interpretation of a negative outcome as controllable or uncontrollable by another frequently determined whether children felt pity or anger toward that individual. The developmental trend for guilt suggests that this emotion may be cognitively less complex in younger children because of its closer link to outcome than to perceived controllability.

Pride

The emotions of pity, anger, and guilt were examined in association with the causal dimension of controllability. We now turn to esteem-related affects, particularly pride, and their union with the causal dimension of locus.

As previously indicated, experiments with adults (Folkes, 1982; Weiner et al., 1978, 1979) have documented that pride and positive self-esteem are experienced as a consequence of attributing a positive outcome to the self and negative self-esteem results when a negative outcome is self-attributed, regardless of whether the perceived cause is controllable (e.g., effort) or uncontrollable (e.g., aptitude). Among adults, therefore, pride and personal esteem are self-reflective emotions. To paraphrase Kant, we all can enjoy a good meal, but only the cook can experience pride.

A number of developmental studies have manipulated locus of causality and then assessed affective reactions (e.g., Nicholls, 1975; Ruble, Parsons, & Ross, 1976). For example, Ruble and her colleagues (1976) manipulated causal attributions by providing false normative information concerning the performance of others. Affective reactions to an achievement performance were then examined by having the children indicate their feelings by adjusting the mouth on the face of a clown. Whereas there were no differences as a function of the attributional manipulation for 6-year-olds, children 8 years of age and older adjusted the mouth so that it smiled more given self-ascription for success. We interpret this affective indicator as reflecting, in part, pride in accomplishment, although other data are not available to lend support to this inference.

Rapacz and Kun (1979) more directly examined the development of pride. They asked: "What kinds of things make you feel proud?" Virtually all the replies concerned achievement goals. The kindergarten and adult subjects emphasized personal accomplishments, while the third and sixth graders focused more on competitive success, or doing better than others. Only adults mentioned self-reflection among the antecedents of pride ("thinking about my good points"). But these investigators also did not systematically attempt to relate pride to the locus dimension of causality.

Table 6.3. *Percentage of pride causes classified as internal, intermediate, and external, as a function of age*

Locus	Age 6 (N = 35)	Age 9 (N = 37)	Age 11 (N = 37)
Internal	48	76	82
Intermediate	26	11	16
External	26	ι3	2

In our studies to examine the development of locus/pride relations, children between the ages of 6 and 12 were asked to recall an incident in which they experienced pride. The causes of the reported events were classified as internal (e.g., "I felt proud that I passed the test of swimming around the pool because I kept trying and believing I could do it"), external (e.g., "I felt proud when my uncle got married and had a baby"), or intermediate (e.g., "We beat another basketball team that was really good; I tried hard but everyone else did too so I really didn't do all of it"). The classification of the causes of pride as a function of the age of the subjects (Table 6.3) indicates a growing association between internal causality and feelings of pride with increasing development, although this relationship is evident even among 6-year-olds.

In sum, a number of investigations suggest a developing linkage between positive outcomes attributed to the self and pride. In the data reported by Graham and her associates (in press), pride-eliciting situations were much less differentiated by locus among the youngest subjects, as these children reported experiencing pride even when the cause of the emotion was external. Similarly, in the investigation reported by Ruble and her colleagues (1976), the attribution of success by the youngest participants to themselves and to an easy task produced the same positive affect. Perhaps, then, young children's experiences of pride resemble the joy or happiness felt when positive outcomes occur. As children develop and exercise their capacities to reflect on their own accomplishments, the elicitation of pride becomes more dependent on internal perceptions of causality.

The development of causal dimensions

Three causal dimensions have been identified with some certainty: locus, stability, and controllability. One might speculate that locus will be the first of these dimensions to emerge, as many developmental theorists postulate that infants learn early in life to distinguish the me from the not-me, or what has been called the ego or self from others in the social environment. If this is the case, then attributionally mediated experiences of pride may emerge surprisingly early. Another important aspect of development is the ability to understand and predict the future, which involves the concept of causal stability and seems to require greater cognitive capacities (including seriation) than does the locus dimension. Feelings of optimism, pessimism, and related affective states, such as certain forms of depression and helplessness, might not be experienced before the development of the stability dimension. Finally, the perception of controllability at times relates to principles of justice and "ought," as well as to the concept of intention. These are considered cognitive antecedents of the experience of guilt. Hence, in relation to this aspect of controllability, the affect of guilt may develop later than the affects associated with locus and stability. Such emotions as pity and anger, which could be associated with aspects of controllability unrelated to moral concerns, may follow a different developmental sequence.

Pride, guilt, and achievement strivings

Investigators in the achievement domain typically view shame (which they appear to use synonymously with guilt) and pride as polar opposite reactions to success and failure. They postulate that achievement strivings are determined by a conflict between the anticipation of pride and the anticipation of shame (e.g., see Atkinson, 1964). Yet it has been documented here that the reactions of pride and guilt among adults and older children are partially mediated by different causal perceptions: Pride is associated with locus, and guilt is linked with controllability as well as locus. Consequently, pride and guilt may be qualitatively distinct emotional states rather than the extremes of a continuum. Furthermore, if locus emerges before controllability, as has been suggested here, then attributionally mediated feelings of pride should develop before causally mediated guilt reactions. This creates complexities in the construction of a theory of achievement strivings, as the affective consequences associated with success and failure are not directly comparable.

At this point in time, the sequential development of the dimensions of causality and the relationship of this cognitive growth to affective development and motivated behavior are unknown. We think these are fruitful topics to consider.

Some vexing problems

To facilitate the presentation of the research in the preceding sections, we (cleverly) bypassed a number of extremely complex problems. We turn to these difficulties now, not to offer solutions but to assure readers that we are aware of some of the problems and to invite them to aid in their resolution.

*Are certain emotions experienced before the development of
linked causal attributions?*

This problem has been evident at a number of places in the preceding discussion.
For example, it has been noted that children report feeling guilty for accidental
events. This intimates that guilt can be experienced without linkage to the
concept of controllability or intentionality. What develops, then, is the union
between controllability and guilt. Is the experience of guilt therefore qualitatively
different in children and adults because it has different antecedents? In a
similar manner, young children report feeling pride for an externally caused
event. Can a child also experience pride in initial acts of motor coordination,
that is, before having a clearly defined concept of self? If so, what is developing
is the cognitive linkage between causal attributions and an already-experienced
or developed emotion. But is outcome-related pride the "same" pride felt by
older children and adults or is it qualitative y distinct? Furthermore, are the
younger children really experiencing pride, or is the affect an outcome-linked
experience of happiness or perhaps joy, which often is considered a more
fundamental emotion (Izard, 1977)? Finally, anger and even pity have been
reported in very young children, well before they are likely to have developed
a concept of controllability (see Hoffman, 1978; Izard, 1977).

In contrast to the emotions discussed here, there are often instances in which
causal thoughts appear to be necessary precursors of an emotional experience.
For example, one might contend that gratitude cannot be experienced before
the development of the ability to attribute positive outcomes to help from
others.

A number of difficult issues have been raised in the preceding paragraphs.
For now, it appears most reasonable to contend that at times causal thinking
precedes emotional reactions and at other times attributional beliefs alter the
conditions under which an already-experienced emotion will be elicited.

Are we studying affects or thoughts about affects?

The research findings reviewed here are entirely dependent on the verbal reports
of the participants. Our subjects describe what they might feel if . . . , what
someone else thought or felt when . . . , what happened when they felt or
thought . . . , and so on. Are the research participants merely conforming to
scripts, that is, telling us what they think ought to go with what? Furthermore,
is the study of thoughts about feelings, or reports about prior experiences, a
legitimate approach to the study of emotions? In addition, we have not examined
emotions during their state of activation, with either verbal report, behavioral,
or other techniques.

There are no definitive answers or rebuttals to these questions and criticisms.
It is evident that there are no unambiguous indicators of, for example, pride

in accomplishment and that includes the behavioral, physiological, or verbal correlates of that experience. The systematic nature of our findings, and the integration of the concepts into a viable theory of motivation, lead us to think (and feel) that we are beginning to understand some selected aspects of affective life. But it is evident, and perhaps too trite to admit, that more definitive proof awaits the development and use of other research methodologies.

Where do the linkages come from?

Among virtually all the adults in our samples, many attribution-affect linkages discussed in this chapter are unequivocal. For example, the sight of the blind or the handicapped (uncontrollable states) elicits sympathy; attributing success to oneself (internal attribution) gives rise to pride; and intentional harm or volitional help from others (controllable acts) gives rise to anger and gratitude, respectively. One question that comes to mind, given such intuitively reasonable and pervasive findings, is: "What accounts for these linkages?" Again a comparison with the frustration/aggression hypothesis is instructive, for clear relations exist between these variables even though their source is not understood.

Principles from social learning, such as reward for the socially accepted reaction and imitation of models, surely will explain some of the connections. But perhaps genetic and evolutionary principles also play some role. For example, the display of heightened positive affect by a child on taking his or her first steps seems to indicate some innate union between mastery and positive affect. Whether this can be interpreted as a built-in union between locus of causality and pride is moot, for it is not evident that such a young child can attribute an outcome to the self and even less evident that the emotion is properly labeled "pride." But the possibility that this linkage exists among young children should not merely be dismissed. In addition, one might speculate that there are innate determinants of the relations between uncontrollability, pity, and help giving (see Trivers, 1971). These unions might have survival value, for the young and unable would then be more likely to be aided by caretakers.

General issues in the study of emotion

The research reviewed in this chapter was not undertaken to resolve basic issues in the study of emotion. Nonetheless, the empirical findings are pertinent to a number of contemporary issues in this field. The following discussion is in part based on these data but also greatly reflects our theoretical biases. Any criticisms are communicated in a spirit of inquiry and mutual facilitation. It was once confessed that "it takes great frustration tolerance and, perhaps, a bent toward self-destruction, to pursue the study of experiential states" (Weiner et al., 1980, p. 112). Hence, we commiserate with others working in this area;

faultfinding must be considered within the broader context of admiration. We also suggest that nontenured investigators not initiate emotion research.

The sequence issue

It has been contended that affect often precedes cognition in a variety of psychological phenomena (Zajonc, 1980). The experimental paradigms employed by Zajonc to support this position are so disparate from the ones reported here that direct comparisons are not possible. Concerning the postulated affect-cognition sequence from an attributional framework, it is entirely possible that in some instances feelings antedate causal thoughts. For example, in certain situations anger might be a conditioned reaction that serves as a cue to attribute personal failure to another. As emotional cues can be used to infer the thoughts of others, it is not unreasonable to presume that these cues can also be used to infer our own thoughts. These thoughts may then, in turn, have further affective significance.

Although an affect-cognition sequence is a logical possibility, we believe it to be of secondary importance. There are a number of reasons for not considering this order as fundamental. First, the empirical evidence clearly documents that specific thoughts give rise to particular emotions. Furthermore, affects are changeable by altering thoughts. Anger, for example, will readily dissipate when it is discovered that the faulted other is innocent of wrongdoing. In addition, an affect-thought order does not account for why particular affects, such as anger or pity, are experienced. This is expressly the case when the situational contexts of these disparate reactions are identical. For example, one individual may react to a drunk with anger, whereas another in the same setting feels pity. These disparate reactions are presumed here to be a product of disparate attributional interpretations.

Arousal

The concept of arousal is perhaps most conspicuous in this chapter by its absence. This neglect is somewhat in opposition to the prevailing importance given to arousal in the conceptual analyses of emotion (see Mandler, 1975; Schachter & Singer, 1962), although the alleged functions of arousal are now under question (Marshall & Zimbardo, 1979; Maslach, 1979; Reisenzein, in press). At present, the experimental evidence does not allow one to determine whether arousal precedes, accompanies, or follows cognition and emotional expression, or if all or none of these might describe any specific situation. Feeling gratitude because of an ascription of success to volitional help from others, or feeling pride when reflecting about a self-ascription for success, does not appear to require either a state of arousal that accompanies the affect or arousal that the individual must interpret prior to an emotional experience.

The concept of arousal seems to be entirely superfluous to the attributional analysis outlined here.

As just intimated, there is little evidence to support the position that arousal is necessary for emotional experience or that arousal is a needed concept in the field of emotion (see, e.g., Reisenzein, in press; Valins, 1966). In the area of motivation, the concept of arousal (drive) has been abandoned by even most of the animal psychologists (e.g., Bolles, 1975). We believe that issues in the field of emotion are not clarified with an arousal or drive concept. A nondirective drive concept, in addition to not being able to account for the quality or direction of emotional experience, falls prey to all the issues that caused the drive concept to be discarded in the study of motivation.

For the affects considered in the preceding pages, the antecedent conditions are particular causal cognitions to which the emotions are linked. The implied underlying general process is that cognitions are sufficient determinants of affect.

Process versus content

When psychologists study emotion, they most often are concerned with the emotional process. The search for the emotional process is understandable, as the research psychologist typically is interested in laws that transcend any particular emotional experience. But one wonders about the implicit assumption that there is *an* emotional process. This seems unlikely, given the possibility of conditioned emotions, emotions following logically from particular cognitions, emotions instigated by hormonal conditions, and so forth.

The question of specific emotions and their meaning often is left to philosophers. The differentiation of, for example, gratitude from joy from pride usually is not thought of as an empirical issue. On the other hand, the research presented here is concerned with the nature and meaning of specific feelings, or the content of emotions. Meaning, it has been suggested, is determined by the antecedent conditions and the properties of thought. Furthermore, meaning was ascertained or analyzed by making use of subjects' reports. Mandler (1975) has contended that phenomenological analysis will not lead to an understanding of emotion. That may be correct if he is addressing the emotional process, for most processes, such as learning or perception, are not well understood by those who experience these processes and the processes themselves typically are not capable of verbalization or available to conscious experience. But if one wishes to study the content of emotions, or emotional life, and the meaning of emotions, then one must turn to those who experience these feelings. As the research in this chapter has demonstrated, phenomenological analyses do aid in the understanding and the explanation of emotion.

For the naïve person, the study of emotion should provide insights about envy, jealousy, love, hate, pride, guilt, and so forth, as opposed to knowledge about physiological substratum, muscle movements, or other processes or mechanisms. This is not to imply that psychologists should or must be guided by the person on the street or that these other areas of study are not of great importance. Rather, we think that there should be greater attention paid to the social emotions as they are experienced in everyday life.

Summary

In this chapter we have attempted to map the emergence of some prevalent human emotions, including pride, pity, anger, and guilt, and these emotions have been related to antecedent thoughts called causal attributions. More specifically, it has been documented that:

1. The use of outcome-dependent affects, such as happy and sad, to describe achievement-related emotional reactions decreases developmentally, whereas the use of attribution-mediated emotions, such as pride and gratitude, increases. This suggests an increasing differentiation in emotional life, with affects more determined by the diverse situational cues that promote different causal ascriptions.
2. There are unions between specific affects, such as anger and pity, and inferences about their eliciting causal ascriptions, such as effort and ability. The strengths of these linkages grow with cognitive maturity, with the union between anger/lack of effort occurring prior to a union between pity/low ability.
3. The emotions of anger and pity are associated with the concept of controllability even among 6-year-olds. The association between guilt and controllability shows a more gradual development.
4. Although the linkage between self-ascription for success and feelings of pride is exhibited by 6-year-olds, there is evidence that the linkage develops further with maturation.
5. Young children report feelings of pride and guilt that are not linked with, respectively, internal and controllable causal ascriptions. Among older children and adults, the conditions that elicit these affects are more uniquely tied to particular perceptions of causality.

In discussing the relations between attributions and affect, some underlying beliefs about the study of emotions and emotional development were first implicitly, and later explicitly, communicated. We think there should be a systematic study of common human emotions, partly guided by the phenomenological method and directed by the belief that cognitions are sufficient antecedents of feeling states.

Notes

1 It is well known that Piaget has commented very little on the development of emotions. However, according to Mischel (1971), Piaget's position is close to the one advocated here, that is, "affective life is . . . transformed on the basis of intellectual transformations" (p. 318).

References

Atkinson, J. W. *An introduction to motivation*. Princeton, N.J.: Van Nostand, 1964.

Bolles, R. C. *Theory of motivation* (2nd ed.). New York: Harper & Row, 1975.

Bottenberg, E. H. Phenomenological and operational characterization of factor-analytically derived dimensions of emotion. *Psychological Reports*, 1975, *37*, 1253–1254.

Brehm, J. W. (Ed.). *A theory of psychological reactance*. New York: Academic Press, 1966.

Bridges, K. M. B. A genetic theory of emotions. *Journal of Genetic Psychology*, 1930, *37*, 514–527.

Brophy, J. E., & Rohrkemper, M. M. The influence of problem ownership on teachers' perceptions of and strategies for coping with problem students. *Journal of Educational Psychology*, 1981, *73*, 295–311.

Cooper, H. M., & Burger, J. M. How teachers explain students' academic performance. *American Educational Research Journal*, 1980, *17*, 95–109.

deCharms, R. *Personal causation*. New York: Academic Press, 1968.

Deci, E. L. *Intrinsic motivation*. New York: Plenum, 1975.

Epstein, S. The ecological study of emotions in humans. In P. Pliner, K. R. Blankstein, & I. M. Speigel (Eds.), *Perception of emotion in self and others*. New York: Plenum, 1979.

Folkes, V. S. Communicating the causes of social rejection. *Journal of Experimental Social Psychology*, 1982, *18*, 235–252.

Graham, S. *Communicated sympathy and anger as determinants of self-perception and performance*. Unpublished doctoral dissertation, University of California, Los Angeles, 1982.

Graham, S., Doubleday, C., & Guarino, P. A. The development of relations between perceived controllability and the emotions of pity, anger, and guilt. *Child Development*, in press.

Hamilton, V. L. Intuitive psychologist or intuitive lawyer? Alternative models of the attribution process. *Journal of Personality and Social Psychology*, 1980, *39*, 767–772.

Heider, F. *The psychology of interpersonal relations*. New York: Wiley, 1958.

Hoffman, M. L. Toward a theory of empathic arousal and development. In M. Lewis & L. A. Rosenblum (Eds.), *The development of affect*. New York: Plenum, 1978.

Izard, C. E. *Human emotions*. New York: Plenum, 1977.

Karniol, R. Children's use of intention cues in evaluating behavior. *Psychological Bulletin*, 1978, *85*, 76–85.

Kelley, H. H. Attribution theory in social psychology. In D. Levine (Ed.), *Nebraska symposium on motivation* (Vol. 15). Lincoln: University of Nebraska Press, 1967.

Kingdon, J. W. Politicians' beliefs about voters. *American Political Science Review*, 1967, *61*, 137–145.

Lau, R. R., & Russell, D. Attributions in the sports pages: A field test of some current hypotheses in attribution research. *Journal of Personality and Social Psychology*, 1980, *39*, 29–38.

Litman-Adizes, T. *An attributional model of depression*. Unpublished doctoral dissertation, University of California, Los Angeles, 1978.

Mandler, G. *Mind and emotion*. New York: Wiley, 1975.

Marshall, G. D., & Zimbardo, P. G. Affective consequences of inadequately explained physiological arousal. *Journal of Personality and Social Psychology*, 1979, *37*, 970–988.

Maslach, C. Negative emotional biasing and unexplained arousal. *Journal of Personality and Social Psychology*, 1979, *37*, 953–969.

Mischel, T. Piaget: Cognitive conflict and the motivation of thought. In T. Mischel (Ed.), *Cognitive development and epistemology*. New York: Academic Press, 1971.

Nicholls, J. G. Causal attributions and other achievement-related cognitions: Effects of task outcome, attainment value, and sex. *Journal of Personality and Social Psychology*, 1975, *31*, 379–389.

Nicholls, J. G. The development of the concepts of effort and ability, perception of academic attainment, and the understanding that difficult tasks require more ability. *Child Development*, 1978, *49*, 800–814.

Pettit, P. On actions and explanations. In C. Antaki (Ed.), *The psychology of ordinary explanations*. London: Academic Press, 1981.

Rapacz, J., & Kun, A. *Development of the semantics of emotions: A causal network approach*. Unpublished manuscript, University of California, Santa Barbara, 1979.

Reisenzein, R. The Schachter theory of emotion: Two decades later. *Psychological Bulletin* (in press).

Rosenbaum, R. M. *A dimensional analysis of the perceived causes of success and failure*. Unpublished doctoral dissertation, University of California, Los Angeles, 1972.

Rotter, J. B. Generalized expectancies for internal versus external control of reinforcement. *Psychological Monographs*, 1966, *80* (1, Whole No. 609).

Ruble, D. N., Parsons, J. F., & Ross, J. Self-evaluative responses of children in an achievement setting. *Child Development*, 1976, *47*, 990–997.

Rychlak, J. F. *A philosophy of science for personality theory*. Boston: Houghton Mifflin, 1968.

Schachter, S., & Singer, J. E. Cognitive, social, and physiological determinants of emotional state. *Psychological Review*, 1962, *69*, 379–399.

Steiner, I. D. Perceived freedom. In L. Berkowitz (Ed.), *Advances in experimental social psychology* (Vol. 5). New York: Academic Press, 1970.

Sroufe, L. A. Socioemotional development. In J. Osofsky (Ed.), *Handbook of infant development*. New York: Wiley, 1979.

Thompson, R. A., & Paris, S. G. *Children's inferences about the emotions of others*. Unpublished manuscript, University of Michigan, 1981.

Trivers, R. L. The evolution of reciprocal altruism. *Quarterly Review of Biology*, 1971, *46*, 35–57.

Valins, S. Cognitive effects of false heart-rate feedback. *Journal of Personality and Social Psychology*, 1966, *4*, 400–408.

Weiner, B. A theory of motivation for some classroom experiences. *Journal of Educational Psychology, 1979, 71*, 3–25.

Weiner, B. *Human motivation*. New York: Holt, Rinehart and Winston, 1980. (a)

Weiner, B. May I borrow your class notes? An attributional analysis of judgments of help giving in an achievement-related context. *Journal of Educational Psychology*, 1980, *72*, 676–681. (b)

Weiner, B. A cognitive (attribution) – emotion – action model of motivated behavior: An analysis of judgments of help-giving. *Journal of Personality and Social Psychology*, 1980, *39*, 186–200. (c)

Weiner, B. The emotional consequences of causal attributions. In M. S. Clark & S. T. Fiske (Eds.), *Affect and cognition: The 17th annual Carnegie symposium on cognition*. Hillsdale, N.J.: Erlbaum, 1982.

Weiner, B., Graham, S., & Chandler, C. An attributional analysis of pity, anger and guilt. *Personality and Social Psychology Bulletin*, 1982, *8*, 226–232.

Weiner, B., Graham, S., Stern, P., & Lawson, M. E. Using affective cues to infer causal thoughts. *Developmental Psychology*, 1982, *18*, 278–286.

Weiner, B., Kun, A., & Benesh-Weiner, M. The development of mastery, emotions, and morality from an attributional perspective. In W. A. Collins (Ed.), *Minnesota symposia on child psychology* (Vol. 13). Hillsdale, N.J.: Erlbaum, 1980.

Weiner, B., Nierenberg, R., & Goldstein, M. Social learning (locus of control) versus attributional (causal stability) interpretations of expectancy of success. *Journal of Personality*, 1976, *44*, 52–68.

Weiner, B., Russell, D., & Lerman, D. Affective consequences of causal ascriptions. In J. H. Harvey, W. J. Ickes, & R. F. Kidd (Eds.), *New directions in attribution research* (Vol. 2). Hillsdale, N.J.: Erlbaum, 1978.

Weiner, B., Russell, D., & Lerman, D. The cognition-emotion process in achievement-related contexts. *Journal of Personality and Social Psychology*, 1979, *37*, 1211–1220.

Weisz, J. R. Developmental change in perceived control: Recognizing noncontingency in the laboratory and perceiving it in the world. *Developmental Psychology*, 1980, *16*, 385–390.

Weisz, J. R. Illusory contingency in children at the State Fair. *Developmental Psychology*, 1981, *17*, 481–489.

Wong, P. T. P., & Weiner, B. When people ask why questions and the heuristics of attributional search. *Journal of Personality and Social Psychology*, 1981, *40*, 650–663.

Zajonc, R. B. Feeling and thinking: Preferences need no inferences. *American Psychologist*, 1980, *35*, 151–175.

7 Cognition in emotion: concept and action

Peter J. Lang

Definitions

This chapter is a conjecture on the cognitive events that determine the generation and memory storage of affective response dispositions, events on which ultimately depend, we presume, emotional expression and change. The two words that most require definition in both the title and this opening statement are cognition and emotion. In the present discussion, cognition is defined as the symbolic (or conceptual) processing of information that is required for the central representation and organized expression of a response. This definition of cognition is not restricted to conscious thought (i.e., events described by introspective reports), nor does it hold that cognition is identical with natural language processing. That is to say, I am not presuming that the mind (by which I mean the aggregate of information processing that modulates behavior) is necessarily structured like, or has a fundamental logic wholly consistent with, anyone's phenomenology. The model of cognition on which this discussion is based presumes the brain to be a thinking machine, functionally analogous to a computer, which can accept input from the environment, store it, compare it with other information previously stored in its own memory, change it according to its own internal logic, and use it in the process of modulating its own output systems. Thus, the chapter can be described as an effort to adapt the contemporary cognitive psychology of information processing to the task of analyzing emotional responding. It is an attempt to describe emotional software, or the brain's program for an emotional response. We propose to speculate about the data structure of such a program, indicate when and how the program might be run, and finally to think about how such a program might be changed.

For the present purposes, affect, or an emotion, is defined as a broad response disposition that may include measurable language behavior, organized overt acts, and a physiological support system for these events (somatic and visceral). In several previous papers (Lang, 1964, 1968, 1978; Lang, Rice, & Sternbach, 1972) I have argued that a scientific concept of affect depends on analysis of

The research on which this chapter is based was supported in part by grants from the National Institute of Mental Health, MH-3880, MH-10993.

the broad behavioral database that has come to define emotion in our culture. Emotions cannot be embraced by attending to only one channel of affective expression, such as verbal report. Emotions are also known through overt behavioral acts (facial and postural expressions, avoidance, or performance deficits) and by an expressive visceral and somatic physiology. This three-system approach is commended not in the interests of an obsessive redundancy but because researchers have repeatedly observed that these different response systems (verbal report of feeling, overt acts, expressive physiology) appear to function independently in affect and that correlations between systems, while positive, seldom account for more than a fraction of the total variance in an experiment (e.g., Lacey, 1967; Lang, 1964; Leitenberg et al., 1971). Subjective reports of anger or fear, for example, show very imperfect concordance with supposed behavioral or physiological indices of these affective states and rarely find validation as concepts except as patterns of mean values in group data (see Ax, 1953; Schachter, 1957). Furthermore, systems appear to be modified by therapeutic intervention at different rates and amplitudes of change (Hodgson & Rachman, 1974). Thus, investigators studying the effects of imipramine on phobia find that the dramatic reduction that often occurs in inpatients' demands on nursing staff (for sleep medication, attention, and support, etc.) is often not accompanied by any reduction in the patients' subjective reports of distress (Klein, 1981). Similarly, we are all familiar with the sometimes perplexing outcome of dynamic therapies, in which felt anxiety is much reduced but there is no appreciable change in the behavioral symptoms that originally prompted treatment.

Such findings are troubling because they seem to question the existence of coherent emotional states that are consistent within individuals and subsist across individuals and species. Furthermore, traditional phenomenological concepts of affect have not provided testable theory that survives the confusion of this database. Although the notion of unconscious emotion offers a comforting post hoc explanation of why, for example, avoidance behavior might persist in the absence of acknowledged fear, the hypothesis of a second, hidden phenomenology has shown little predictive validity. By this observation, I do not mean to condemn the empirical study of human subjectivity; patterns of verbally reported affect may well offer a clue to the organization of emotional response. Furthermore, we will not take the position that emotion is not a category of behavior appropriate for scientific study. Although discordance is ubiquitous, there is an equally large body of research (which we have considered elsewhere, Lang, 1971) that shows frequent and quite remarkable behavioral coherence in emotion and seems to support the hypothesis of centrally organized affective states. However, the nature of the organization is not now obvious, and we are well advised to proceed slowly, seeking a parsimonious explanation of the empirical data rather than a broad leap at the ready-made suppositions of human experience.

The dimensions of affect

A serious consideration of reliability of measurement and shared variance of self-description across subjects has consistently reduced the dictionary list of reported affects (fear, anger, surprise, disgust, and the like) to two or sometimes three stable dimensions (see Bush, 1973; Davitz, 1969; Osgood, Suci, & Tannenbaum, 1957; Mehrabian & Russell, 1974). Most typically these are: (1) affective valence, (2) arousal, and (3) control or dominance.

Valence. Almost all investigators find that valence accounts for a majority of variance in affective reports. An emotional response is not neutral but involves a verbal report judgment that can be located along a dimension from maximum pleasure or joy to extreme displeasure, disgust, and repugnance. Reactions in other response systems also may be located in this valence dimension. Thus, an overt action can be characterized as falling somewhere between rapid approach and expeditious avoidance; the peripheral physiology has a dimension extending from a posture of heightened receptivity to environmental stimulation to a rejecting defensive set (Lacey & Lacey, 1970).

Arousal. The dimension of arousal accounts for the second greatest share of variance in descriptions of emotion. Viewed from a three-system perspective, affective reports range along a scale defined at one extreme by excessive anxiety or acute panic and at the other by indifference, apathy, and depersonalization; these reports are in logical synergy with an expressive physiology similarly ranging from gross sympathetic hyperactivity at one end of the dimension to a paradoxical collapse of sympathetic visceral functioning at the other (as in vasovagal fainting); similarly, overt actions may be described between extremes of excessive force or vigor and unusual weakness or softness in behavior.

Control or dominance. Though reported less consistently most researchers also find a third dimension, sometimes called dominance, referring to either a degree of self-control or control over the environment. Along this parameter, subjective reports extend from complaints of compulsions that oversystematize the waking life to a sense of total uncertainty, of being wholly at the mercy of capricious events or impulses; emotional actions vary from being overly controlled, so rigid as to be functionally displastic, to a behavioral confusion of erratic, disorganized acts; the physiology may be similarly described as extending from the highly variable and labile to a response topography without spontaneous fluctuations and with only dampened reactions to environmental stimuli.

   In this chapter we will be interested in the central representation of context-bound response dispositions that can be represented on the the three dimensions of valence, arousal, and control. These labels are meant as descriptors of the broad domain of affective behavior, and we do not invite the reader to presume that they represent substantive theoretical categories in emotion. However, as we noted earlier, these dimensions can be represented in all three responding systems. Furthermore, they seem to have phylogenetic continuity and evolutionary significance. That is, approach and avoidance are fundamental response dispositions for survival (Schneirla, 1959), as is extraordinary energy mobilization in emergency (Cannon, 1936). Of similar relevance is the organization and smooth expression of a behavioral act (Hebb, 1949), particularly when organisms evolve in their complexity. These dimensions also seem appropriate in that they roughly embrace the paths to therapeutic change in pathological emotion. For example, therapists treating fearful or anxious patients may focus directly on the reduction of arousal (through tranquilizing medication or relaxation therapies), or on the modification of negative valence (by evocation of disturbing affects in an ambiance of nurturance and positive support), or on efforts to increase dominance (variously called training in competence, self-efficacy, assertiveness, or self-control).

Affect as action and context

Emotions are considered here to be response dispositions or action sets that can be located along the three dimensions just described. It is also recognized that responses occur in stimulus contexts, which define the function of these behavioral transactions. Thus, stimulus information defines the direction of approach or avoidance and is as pertinent to emotional cognition as is the response code. Indeed, some stimuli, both social (facial expression, sexual postures) and nonsocial (bright colors, spiders, high places), may be hardwired in the brain as part of specific, central sensorimotor programs (e.g., see Lorenz, 1952; Tinbergen, 1951). These so-called prepared (Seligman, 1971) or prepotent stimuli (Gray, 1971; Lang et al., 1972) also occasion special force or vigor in behavior, as well as a base physiology of preparatory arousal. Furthermore, it is clear that a great variety of settings can take on an affective tone through experience or conditioning. Information about stimuli and responses, that is, the meaning of input and output, is also necessarily part of the central data structure of any specific example of emotional expression. Finally, varied learning experiences can lead to the same or similar stimuli prompting more than one motor program. Competing programs disrupt the focus and smoothness of a behavioral act (Hebb, 1949; Mandler, 1975), resulting in inefficient performance and reduced competence.

From this perspective, the terrain of emotion is indeed vast, and in the same sense that every act involves cognitive antecedents, all action could be said to carry an affective tone. To be able to explicate our approach in detail, this presentation will focus mainly on the affective expressions commonly described as fearful, particularly their pathological manifestation in phobia. We will attempt to describe the central information structure of phobia, a stimulus-specific affective state, which has a response topography characterized by negative valence, high arousal, and low dominance/control.

Emotion as information

The present approach is a development of our previous bioinformational analysis of emotional imagery (Lang, 1977, 1979), which we now propose as a more general framework for understanding affective behavior. Emotion is conceived to be an action set, defined by a specific information structure in memory, which, when accessed, is processed as both a conceptual and a motor program. The data structure of an emotion includes three primary categories of information: (1) information about prompting external stimuli and the context in which they occur; (2) information about responding in this context, including expressive verbal behavior, overt acts, and the visceral and somatic events that mediate arousal and action; (3) information that defines the meaning of the stimulus and response data.

In discussing emotional imagery we proposed that emotion information is coded in memory in the form of propositions and that these propositions are organized into an associative network of the general sort first described by Quillian (1966) for semantic knowledge and later adapted to accommodate other types of information (e.g., Anderson & Bower, 1974; Kieras, 1978). The emotion information network is a sort of prototype or schema, which is processed as a unit when a critical number of propositions are accessed. This processing is held to be the cognitive work of emotional expression. Efferent outflow and action are the output events occasioned by the processing of response information (i.e., efferent subroutines) in the network program.

Phobic reactions are characterized by unusually coherent and stable emotion prototypes, which can be accessed readily by a variety of internal and external instigating conditions. For this reason (in addition to the author's clinical interest in fear behavior), phobia is used here as a model of an emotion prototype and as a laboratory illustration. However, other emotional states (e.g., individual conditions of sexual arousal) may be equally focused in content, involving similarly well-organized, readily defined propositional elements of limited number, and might serve equally well as examples.

A phobia prototype

We have suggested elsewhere (Lang, 1977, 1979) that the conceptual network that organizes an emotional response includes two primary information categories, stimulus and response propositions. To this classification we now add a third, meaning propositions, which are construed as analytic and interpretive.

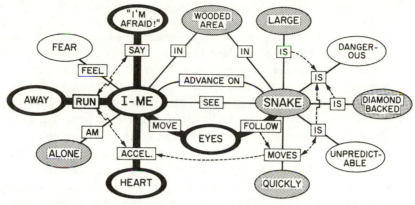

Figure 7.1. A phobia prototype: An associative network of propositionally coded information, presumed to be stored in long-term memory, which is accessed and processed in the expression of a fear response. The development of this propositional notation as a representation of emotional cognitions is described in Lang (1979).

To illustrate with a common focal phobia, the central data structure of the fear response might include the following propositions: (1) *Stimulus propositions* code information critical to the recognition of the frightening animal, including the relevant context of its appearance (e.g., the snake's skin has a diamond pattern; it's moving toward me; no one else is here); (2) *response propositions* describe all the overt and covert responses made in this context, including avoidance, self-referent verbal statements (e.g., God, I'm scared!), and the visceral and somatic responses of physiological arousal (e.g., tachycardia, sweating); (3) *meaning propositions* are interpretive, defining the significance of input and output events, probabilities of stimulus occurrence and consequences of action (e.g., snakes are dangerous and unpredictable; when your heart beats fast you're frightened). An abridged model of a network is presented in Figure 7.1.

The phobia prototype is a conceptual network of propositionally coded information, related by association, which has as functional output a visceral and somatomotor program. The prototype may be activated as a unit by instructional, media, or objective sensory input that contains information matching that in the network. The phobia prototype illustrated in Figure 7.1 could be rendered in descriptive, narrative English as follows: "I am in a wooded area when I see a large snake. It appears to be moving toward me. There's a diamond pattern on its back. This could be a dangerous snake. My eyes jump in my head following a quick, sinuous movement. My heart starts racing. Snakes are unpredictable. 'I'm afraid!' I say it aloud, but nobody is there to hear me. I'm alone and very frightened. I start to run . . ."

Propositions in the network are represented in Figure 7.1 by the oval nodes, containing the concept name, and the labeled, solid black lines that show the links between concepts. In the notation proposed by Kintsch (1974), the lines indicate predicators and the ovals are their arguments (e.g., MOVES, SNAKE, QUICKLY). The dotted lines indicate some of the connections between propositions that could have particularly high probabilities of association. No attempt is made here to indicate all propositions or all possible connections. However, it is suggested that certain propositions are strongly bonded to others and may thus be keys to the broad recruitment of the network, with its action subprograms. For example, (MOVES, SNAKE, QUICKLY) may have a primitive high-probability connection to (ACCELERATE, I, HEART), which in turn unlocks the other fear response propositions, prompting rapid prototype activation.

The network includes three broad classes of information: stimulus, meaning, and response propositions. Stimulus concepts are indicated on the diagram by the shaded ovals, and meaning concepts by the clear ovals. Response propositions are represented by a heavy black connecting line. This is a reminder that such information is doubly coded, that response concepts are represented primitively as motor programs. The view taken here is that the deep structure of the prototype is an action set. Although the prototype can be described in a natural language and processed in part as an independent, exclusively semantic network, these programs are functionally organized to generate efferent output. Thus, the processing of conceptual emotional information always involves some degree of visceral and motor outflow.

An emotion prototype is accessed when a subject attends to information that matches propositions in the network. This matching process is very broadly analogous to the analyzer matching described by Sokolov (1963). However, instead of a mismatch, which prompts orienting, we propose a matching of input information with stored information in the prototype, which activates an associative network. Presently, we assume that a critical number of propositions must be matched for the entire conceptual network to be activated and the associated motor subprogram to be processed. However, certain propositions, or classes of propositions, may be more important than others in accessing an emotion program. Determining the properties of this intranetwork structure is seen as a priority task for future research.

At this point, however, it is sufficient to consider that an emotion prototype may be accessed from memory through a great variety of information input modes and that the instigating information can be from any of the three classes of propositions that determine such conceptual aggregates. Perhaps the most obvious means of evocation involves the exposure of the subject to the actual fear object or context. It is presumed that the fear network is more likely to be accessed by external input when this input includes a critical number of the stimulus propositions that are in the network and when there is no information inconsistent with the prototype. Thus, the sighting of a large snake, which has a diamond pattern on the dorsal surface, by a subject who is alone may be sufficient to initiate the fear prototype. However, the sighting of a 6-inch snake by a subject who is with a crowd of friends may not cause the fear program to be accessed. Alternatively, all stimulus propostions described in the first case might be present along with information that the snake is a battery-operated mechanical toy, which would again not cause the fear prototype to be accessed.

It is not necessary, however, for a fear object to be "real" to access the prototype and run the motor programs. The information in the prototype is conceptual and does not refer to any specific pattern of sensory input. Films, slides, or models may contain enough stimulus propositions to activate the network. Even a verbal description may be sufficient, particularly if the subject is told to process the input as an image. Finally, it is not only stimulus information that can access the prototype. If some of the visceral and somatic response propositions of an emotional prototype are active (perhaps prompted by very different circumstances, such as exercise or drugs; e.g., see Schachter, S., 1964), less stimulus information is required to prompt the total emotional response.

The phobic prototype is held to be relatively easy to activate. The stimulus and meaning information cohere more strongly to the response information and the stimuli are less readily processed independent of the prototype network. The coherence of the network may constitute a definition of severity of phobia. Coherence is defined, in turn, by the number of input propositions required for prototype processing (e.g., the degree to which stimulus information may be degraded and still occasion the efferent outflow of an action set).

Despite phobic prototype hypersensitivity and the high incidence of such fears in the normal population, the majority of phobias are never treated in the clinic. Phobics simply avoid all relevant input information and thus rarely process the fear network. Unless environmental circumstances force confrontation (a snake-phobic geologist is sent to a Central American jungle to evaluate an oil lease), treatment is seldom sought. Thus, the isolation of the network contributes to its stability. If the prototype never moves from the memory into the brain's work space, it is unlikely to undergo modification.

From the perspective presented here, treatment of phobia would involve a breakdown of network coherence and the attachment of the stimulus and meaning information to other response subroutines. Any processing of the prototype through exposure or imagery would facilitate this goal, as the processing context would necessarily add new, possibly inhibitory or incompatible information to the prototype, reducing coherence through this broader association and encouraging a division into smaller subprograms that could be instigated independently by differing environmental circumstances.

Activating an emotional response

To restate our general view briefly, it is held that emotions are represented in memory as specific coherent data structures. The information is stored in propositional form, and these propositions are organized into an associative network called an emotion prototype. An entire network may be activated by a few prompting propositional units. However, probability of prototype access increases with quantity of matching input propositions. Although matching stimulus information provides a powerful prompt, independent instigation of response propositions and meaning propositions can be in many instances the key determinants of access.

The factors that determine emotional activation may be summarized as follows: (1) In general, the more complete and consistent the stimulus information matches the prototype, the more likely it is that the emotion response program will be accessed and run. To state this in terms of output, the probability of an emotional response is reduced with degradation of the input information. Thus, actual exposure to fear objects is more likely to occasion emotional processing than a film, slide show, or verbal description of the same stimulus. (2) Degraded stimulus input is more likely to access the prototype if other propositions in the prototype are independently instigated. For example, watching a film about poisonous snakes at a safari camp in an African jungle (meaning information: Dangerous snakes are nearby) is more likely to prompt fear than watching the same film in a Manhattan apartment. Similarly, watching the film in the New York apartment after unwitting epinepherine intake (response information: a pattern of physiological arousal generally consonant with fear) may increase the probability of an actual fear response (including verbal, behavioral components, and more focused physiology) to the African safari level. (3) The emotion response prototype can be accessed by instructions and/ or description of provocative events in a natural language, as in emotional imagery. However, this is a degraded stimulus input situation relative to exposure and has a lower probability of access. It depends importantly on the subject's ability and inclination to convert semantic input into the deep structural code of the emotion prototype. (4) Because emotions are always about action, prototype activation involves the processing of efferent programs, which, in theory, can be monitored both centrally and at the end organs (muscles or glands).

Emotional imagery: text processing and efferent patterning

It is clear that the evocation of emotional states in human organisms is not dependent on instigation by objective stimuli. Language cues, both as the spontaneous result of internal processing or through external communication, are often the medium of access to the emotional prototype. This occurs formally when descriptions of emotional events are administered to subjects who are under an implicit or explicit instructional set to experience them "as if" they were actually happening. The human response to the novelist's art, an imagery therapist's instructions, the stage hypnotist's commands, or an intimate letter from a close friend all depend on this common underlying process. In these cases the instigation of emotion is essentially a text-processing task. The emotion to be experienced is described by a script and the semantic and lexical structure of the script are critical both to the understanding or comprehension of the semantic content and to the accessing of the relevant emotional prototype from long-term memory storage.

Text-prompted emotional experience is similar to instructionally cued perceptual imagery, as both involve a reprocessing of stimulus information about objects or events that are not objectively present. They both also involve response information processing and the apparent regeneration of related motor programs. Thus, memory images formed during a variety of perceptual tasks have been shown to be accompanied at recall by patterns of efferent activity that are similar to those occurring during the original percept. As early as 1940, Shaw demonstrated that forearm muscle tension levels during imagery recall were proportional in amplitude to the heft of different weights previously employed in a weight-judging task. Several different investigators have found a similar result in visual memory, that is, when a perceptual task requires a stereotyped pattern of ocular scanning, recall trials are accompanied by parallel patterns of eye movement (Brady & Levitt, 1966; Brown, 1968; Deckert, 1964; Jacobson, 1930).

Text-instigated emotional experience has sometimes yielded analogous laboratory findings. In these instances, however, the emphasis is less on a regenerated perceptual physiology and more on a question of demonstrating the affective patterns of physiological arousal. Thus, both Lang, Melamed, and Hart (1970) and Van Egeren, Feather, and Hein (1971) found that passages of descriptive text, hierarchically arranged according to intensity of judged fear content, occasioned in fearful subjects a parallel gradient of visceral arousal, with the greatest heart-rate acceleration and skin conductance responses occurring in reaction to the most frightening text and the smallest responses to the neutral text. A variety of other studies have produced similar results (e.g., Grossberg, 1968; Schwartz, 1971). However, the experimental literature also includes negative findings, instances in which seemingly appropriate instructions and scripts failed to produce a physiologically affective image. For example, Marks and Huson (1973) reported that severely phobic patients showed the expected greater heart-rate acceleration to phobic than to neutral imagery instructions in only three of five experiments conducted at the Maudsley Hospital. Skin conductance fared even more poorly, differentiating these contents in only two of five experiments. Despite this absence of visceral arousal, the patients all reported subjective anxiety or fear during phobic imagery. In point of fact, anxiety reports to frightening or arousing imagery content are relatively easy to obtain; visceral response effects are more rare (e.g., see Weerts &

Lang, 1978). This is particularly troubling in relation to research suggesting that therapeutic imagery may be ineffective unless it includes palpable autonomic activation (Lang et al., 1970; Levin, 1982; Schroeder & Rich, 1976).

Some experimental results

We have recently undertaken a series of experiments designed to explore the circumstances under which the processing of emotional descriptive text does or does not occasion a broad affective response. The previous inconsistent findings are expected by our view insofar as text, compared to fear-object exposure, represents a degraded input. To put this more explicitly: If accessing the fear prototype is facilitated by the number of matching propositional units in the stimulus material, then many previous studies may have failed to elicit responses because the experimental context did not contain enough appropriate information. One obvious difference between our approach and previous imagery theory concerns the role of response information. The classic view of imagery stresses only stimulus information, viewing any efferent activity that may occur as a response to the internal stimulus in the "mind's eye." However, the conception presented here presumes the image to be a network of both stimulus and response information. Thus, the probability of processing the image would be increased if both response and stimulus material were directly instigated, in this case by inclusion in the imagery script. To an extent, probability of prototype access should improve with an increase in the number of any relevant propositions in the input script. However, response propositions also have a special role. While they are coded in the script in a natural language and stored as semantic concepts in the brain, they are also linked to deep structure response propositions that constitute the information base for a motor command system. Thus, processing textual response codes facilitates the access of action programs from memory storage. Activation of the prototype includes innervation (usually at a subovert level) of the designated somatomotor or visceral organ systems. It seems clear that this efferent leakage comes from inhibited motor programs. In fact, such cognitive activity can, under the proper conditions, become dramatically manifest as overt behavior. This occurs routinely in such laboratory tasks as the postural sway test, in which "thinking about" falling produces some sway in the average subject and may prompt actual loss of balance in a susceptible individual (examples abound, from Hull, 1933, to Hilgard, 1965).

It is also clear that the semantic information contained in a script can be processed as "knowledge about" an emotional situation quite independently of any underlying motor subroutines. We presume further that such content comprehension, or processing of the semantic network only, will prompt in many subjects a content-consonant verbal report of subjective distress. In this case, the subject is in effect providing an appraisal of the affective meaning of the script. The extent to which these two modes of processing are independent varies widely among individuals: Some subjects cannot process in the imagery (or subovert action) mode; some subjects cannot not process in the imagery mode; the vast majority of intelligent normals are able to do either, depending on context and instructions.

We have recently developed a brief training program designed to set subjects for imagery processing. Groups are administered imagery scripts and instructed to imagine vividly the events described. Subsequently, they are asked to recall their image and to report to a trainer all the details of the experience they can remember. The trainer then reinforces the subjects specifically for response details (i.e., actions the subject was performing, visceral and somatic responding), priming him or her with instructions to include more such material in subsequent images. In a series of studies, we have contrasted this training procedure with a type of training more oriented to the "mind's eye" view of imagery. In this latter procedure, subjects are reinforced postimagery for only stimulus detail (i.e., the characteristics of the external scene as presented to the receptors). Specifically, we tested the hypothesis that imaging subjects are more likely to generate a psychophysiology of emotion when the prompting text includes response propositions (as well as stimulus information), particularly when subjects have been trained to process response information from text.

The first two experiments were performed by Lang and his associates (1980). Imagery was manipulated by varying the content of the prompting instructions (either stimulus detail or active responding was emphasized in the image script) and by prior imagery training (in which subjects' postimage verbal reports were shaped to emphasize either stimulus or response material). Three thematic contents were examined: neutral, action, and fear scenes. Examples of each script content are presented in Table 7.1. In Experiment 1, a group that received response-oriented imagery training and response scripts was compared to a stimulus-oriented group. The results strongly supported our primary hypothesis. That is, response subjects showed greater physiological activity during imagery than did stimulus-trained subjects. Furthermore, the efferent patterns shown by response subjects generally followed the script content. In Experiment 2, one group again received response training and the other, stimulus training. However, half of each group was later tested on response-structured scripts and the other half on stimulus scripts. Thus, all cells in the interaction between training and script could be examined. Results again supported the primary hypothesis. As in Experiment 1, response-trained subjects tested on response scripts showed substantial, appropriate physiological activity. None of the other groups, which received stimulus training and/or stimulus scripts, showed significant physiological response during imagery. These effects are illustrated in Figure 7.2 for three of the dependent variables studied in Experiment 2.

The physiological patterns obtained in these experiments tended to differ according to type of content, without being wholly concordant with the prop-

Table 7.1. *Experiment 1: Scene contents and sample texts for neutral, stimulus, and response scripts*

Neutral scenes (Trials 1,6)	Action scenes (Trials 2,3,9,10)	Fear scenes (Trials 4,5,7,8)
1. Sitting in the living room	1. Flying a kite	1. Hornet in the car
2. On the sidewalk of a quiet street	2. Playing ping pong	2. Spider on the pillow
	3. Isometric exercises	3. Trapped in a sauna
	4. Studying a difficult text	4. Snake in the water

Imagery scripts

Neutral scene
You are sitting in your living room reading on a Sunday afternoon. Sitting back, relaxed, you look out the window. It is a sunny autumn day. Red and brown leaves drift slowly down from the trees, and several cars and a truck go by in the street. Wind from the cars blows the leaves, which are lying in the street. They scatter onto the pavement and the thick green lawn.

Stimulus
1. You are flying a kite on the beach on a bright summer day. Your red kite shows clearly against the cloudless blue sky and whips quickly up and down in spirals with the wind. The sun glares at you from behind the kite and makes the white sandy beach sparkle with reflection. The long white tail dances from side to side beneath the soaring kite. A strong gust of wind catches the kite, sending it higher and higher into the sky. (Action)

2. You are alone in your car on an interstate highway and you notice an insect on the windshield. It is a large buzzing insect, a yellow jacket that has trapped itself inside your car. The bug has a yellow and black body, and moves back and forth, flying against the windshield trying to get out. It jumps onto the floor and crawls under the seat. It flies around in the back of the car where you can't see what it is doing, and there is no place on the roadside where you can stop so it can escape. (Fear)

Response
1. You breathe deeply as you run along the beach flying a kite. Your eyes trace its path as it whips up and down in spirals with the wind. The sun glares into your eyes from behind the kite, and you tense the muscles in your forehead and around your eyes, squinting to block out the bright sunlight. You follow with your eyes the long white tail, which dances from side to side beneath the soaring kite. (Action)

2. You are alone, driving your car on the interstate highway and you hear the buzzing of an insect on your windshield. Your heart begins to pound as you notice that it is a yellow jacket trapped in your car. You perspire heavily and your eyes dart from the insect to the roadside while you try to watch the bug and look for a place to stop. You tense the muscles of your face and neck as the yellow jacket buzzes to the back of the car where you can't see what it is doing. You breathe in short quick gasps, glancing to the rear to locate the bug. (Fear)

Note: The average number of response propositions per script for action topics was: heart 0.00; respiration .75; muscle 1.75; eye 2.00; sweat 0.00. For fear topics these values were: heart 1.00; respiration 1.00; muscle 1.25; eye 1.25; sweat 0.75. Thus, fear scripts were weighted in favor of heart, respiration, and sweat-gland responses, whereas eye-movement and muscle-tension responses were relatively more frequent in action scripts (Lang et al., 1980).
Source: Lang, P. J., Kozak, M. J., Miller, G. A., Levin, D. N., & McLean, A., Jr. Emotional imagery: Conceptual structure & pattern of somato-visceral response. *Psychophysiology*, 1980, *17*(2), 179–192.

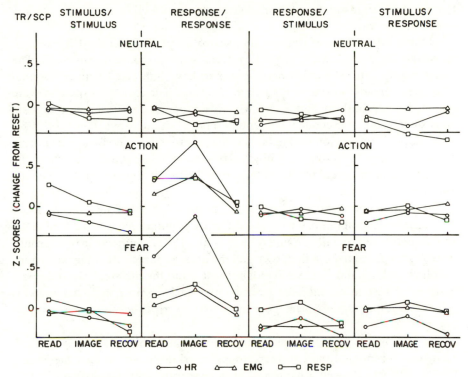

Figure 7.2. Mean change in median heart rate, muscle tension, and respiration cycle length during the presentation of imagery text (read), the imagery period, and an immediately following no-image recovery period. Each measurement period was 30 sec in duration. Experiment 2 results are shown for the four groups separately, during imagery of neutral, action, and fear scenes. The values shown are z-scores, based on the combined data of Experiments 1 and 2. Respiration cycle length change values were multiplied by −1 for plotting. Average heart-rate change for the response-trained/ response-script group during the fear content image period was +7.31 bpm. Muscle tension change was +15.58 volts/min, and respiration cycle length change was −.64 sec (Lang et al., 1980).

ositional structure of the instigating text. Thus, although both fear and action scenes prompted more somatovisceral activity than did the neutral scripts, the pattern of physiological activity differed in these two scene types. Mean muscle potential levels were higher during action images than during fear imagery (the largest response was given to the isometric exercise scene, a context that would reasonably call for considerable muscular effort). On the other hand, heart rate and skin conductance tended to be higher for fear than for action scenes (maximal conductance occurred in response to a public-speaking script). Thus, the results obtained here cannot be attributed to some generalized instruction to be physiologically active, nor are they to be explained by a uni-dimensional concept of arousal. However, they are consistent with the hypothesis that the scripts instigated the processing of an affective prototype already stored in the brain.

In summary, response training and script do partially control the image. However, their influence is shaped by preexisting response dispositions. The image manipulations studied here appear to have interacted with conceptual structures already stored in long-term memory. The largest responses were obtained when both response and stimulus propositions in the scripts were consistent with a precoded perceptual and efferent arousal network, for example, muscle tension during isometric exercise or skin conductance during speech imagery. Training amplified response, increasing the strength of the subject's efferent signal to a level that could be readily measured (Lang et al., 1980).

These phenomena were placed in yet more vivid relief in a recent study conducted in our laboratory with two different populations of fearful subjects: snake phobic and socially anxious (Lang et al., 1983). Subjects in both groups were first exposed to both their own and the other group's actual fear situations (public speaking and a snake-avoidance test), and the different physiological patterns of response generated by these two tasks were noted. All subjects were also administered an imagery task, using scripts based on the two fear contents.

The pattern of means for the physiological responses observed during exposure readily differentiated the two fear groups. During the snake test, the snake-phobic subjects showed a pattern of high heart rate and verbal report of fear arousal significantly different from the low heart rates and low arousal reported by socially anxious subjects. As expected, socially anxious subjects reported greater arousal during the speech task. Curiously, however, the groups did not differ in heart rate during public speaking. Apparently, the task requirements of this performance, in terms of cardiovascular demand, are so great as to obscure any additional load prompted by a differential affective tone.

The group patterns of heart rate and arousal report means observed during imagery of speech and snake contexts paralleled those found at exposure. However, amplitude of physiological response during imagery was low and variance within the sample large, resulting in insignificant statistical tests. Therefore, two new populations of fearful subjects were selected according to the same criteria previously employed, and the experiment was performed again. This time half of each fear group was stimulus trained and half response trained before the administration of fear imagery test scenes. The heart-rate change during imagery found in both experiments is presented in Figure 7.3.

It is readily apparent that subjects respond more to fear material when response trained. As noted previously, the effects on heart rate of stimulus training are little different from those found without training. More pertinent to the present argument, it can be seen that snake phobics responded strongly to the snake scenes; however, even following response training, the reaction of socially

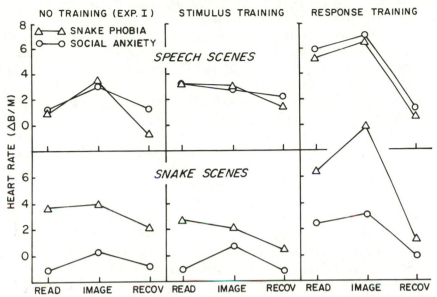

Figure 7.3. Average heart-rate change over read, imagery, and recovery periods for both snake and speech scenes. Data are presented for both no training (Experiment 1) and the comparison of training procedures (Experiment 2). See Lang et al. (1983).

anxious subjects to this material is negligible. On the other hand, both fear groups show cardiac acceleration to the speech scenes after response training. These are exactly the same effects found at exposure. The cardiovascular demands of the speech task itself are apparently so marked as to obscure a specifically affective response in this system. However, the difference between groups is placed in vivid relief when subjects image themselves seated, passively observing a live snake.

It is important to note again that the effect of response training was not to impose a physiology on subjects. Despite having received the same training and response material as the snake phobics, socially anxious subjects did not show an affective physiology to the snake scene. Again, the effect of response information is only to facilitate the access of perceptual-motor programs that are already present in memory.

From a three-system perspective (Lang, 1978), it is also pertinent that response training occasioned greater concordance between ratings of arousal and visceral activation than was found for other subjects. That is, all groups reported arousal during fear and action scenes, and these verbal reports varied significantly with fear diagnosis. However, as already noted, this was accompanied by modest and nonsignificant visceral responses in the stimulus and untrained groups. It is our assumption that a substantial number of subjects processed only the semantic network of the script, with its natural language propositions.

Subjects' reports of arousal were appropriate to the emotional meaning of this information but did not reflect processing of the deep structure with its somatic and visceral programs. The response-training method, which encouraged subjects to attend to somatic and visceral information, probably had two effects: It both increased the probability that efferent programs would be accessed and increased the subject's discrimination of images that actually involved physiological processing. Thus, with response training, physiological arousal and verbal report varied in parallel over scene contents. Furthermore, the relationship between arousal reports and heart-rate response was basically the same as that found in exposure. These data are concordant with the view that imagery instructions and exposure can access the same phobia prototype. That is, different input media access a common data structure from memory.

It is our hypothesis that response training, by setting the subject to process response information, facilitates image mode retrieval and access of the deep structure emotional prototype. However, we further hypothesize that some subjects can perform in this manner spontaneously, with no more help than the instruction to process text in the image mode. Furthermore, if we are correct in assuming a structural similarity between perceptual imagery and emotional imagery, then subjects who profess to have particularly vivid imagery should show a more appropriate physiological response to simple imagery instruction and to the training manipulation (Miller et al., 1983).

In an experimental test of this view, two groups of subjects, good imagers and poor imagers, were selected on the basis of extreme response to the Questionnaire on Mental Imagery (QMI), originally created by Betts (1909) and more recently revised by Sheehan (1967). All subjects were first administered a psychophysiological imagery assessment procedure similar to that used in previous experiments. Subsequently, half of each imagery group was given stimulus training and half response training. All subjects were then reassessed for imagery response.

The results of this experiment did not show a difference between imagery groups before training. The physiological response of these normal subjects to standard emotional scenes was modest at the initial assessment. However, following response training, the good imagers showed a dramatic increase in text concordant reactivity, which the poor imagers failed to match. Results for standard scenes, for both heart rate and skin conductance are presented in Figure 7.4.

The reason good imagery subjects did not, in the above experiment, show a better pretraining response than poor imagers may lie in the fact that the scripted material employed did not match strong, coherent prototypes in these normal subjects. Support for this interpretation is provided by subsequent research with subjects preselected for high fear. Results indicating a greater exposure-concordant physiological response for good imagers than for poor

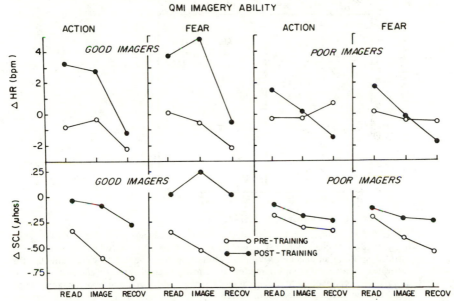

Figure 7.4. Average heart-rate and skin-conductance response during the presentation of the imagery text (read), the imagery period, and during the immediately following no-image recovery period. Each measurement period was 30 sec in duration. Average data for action and fear scenes are presented for both high and low imagery subjects (Betts's questionnaire), before and after response training. See Miller et al. (1981).

imagers has been observed among both volunteer phobics (Levin, 1982) and phobic patients treated at a Fear Clinic (Levin, Cook, & Lang, 1982). In both of these latter experiments the phobics had received no special imagery training before the administration of test imagery. Nevertheless, Levin and his associates (1982) found greater response by good imagers to personal anxiety scenes and a tendency for good imaging patients to begin their response to standard fear scenes earlier than poor imagers. Levin (1982) observed significantly greater initial heart-rate and skin-conductance responses in QMI-defined high-imagery phobic subjects responding to phobia-relevant text than for phobics classified as poor imagers on the QMI responding to the same material (Figure 7.5). Levin's good imager subjects also showed significant habituation of heart rate over fear imagery trials, whereas low QMI subjects were initially nonreactive and showed little change.

The experiments just described exploring text structure and the image mode of text processing, have been a productive beginning. The findings are consistent with the hypothesis that emotional processing can be instigated through the response information included in an imagery script. We have developed a method (response training) that enhances the normal subject's ability to process

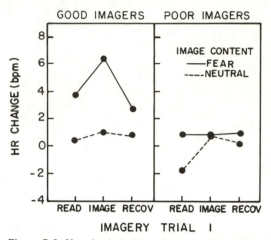

Figure 7.5. Untrained phobic volunteers: Heart-rate change scores of good and poor imagers (Betts's questionnaire) responding to both an affectively neutral script and a script describing an encounter with the phobic object. These data were collected for separate experimental groups immediately following actual exposure and thus represent an imaginal recollection of an actual experience. Both good and poor imager groups responded with marked heart-rate increase to the just preceding objective exposure. See Levin (1982).

text in the imagery mode. The use of this methodology leads subjects to generate, during text-prompted imagery, a subovert efferent pattern that is consistent with the specific arousal pattern shown at actual exposure to the referenced objects or contexts. We have traced a link between perceptual imagery and emotional imagery and shown that response-trained, questionnaire-selected "good" perceptual imagers are more likely to generate a physiology of affect from text than are similarly trained "poor" imagers. Furthermore, among subjects who are presumed to have a more coherent fear prototype (i.e., phobics), this difference between good and poor imagers appears even without supplementary training.

In future studies we plan a more systematic exploration of the propositional structure of emotion-generating text, as it interacts with the learning and retrieval activities of the brain. Bower's (1981) recent work suggests that emotional processing may, through spread of association, broadly influence the content of long-term memory. We intend to evaluate the organization of the prototype network through studies of recall, in which the associative strength of text-based propositions are assessed after subjects process the material in either the imagery or text-comprehension modes. We expect to relate these results to the physiological analyses reported in the present experimental series. It is our view that response propositions (as evidenced by relevant efferent activity) are the primary mediators of affective influence on memory process.

Accessing the prototype: media and emotional change

It is a current working hypothesis that the accessing of an emotion prototype from long-term storage, with its associated motor programs, is facilitated by the quantity of matching propositions at input. In the research just described, we have attempted to prompt such emotional processing by priming the response side of the network. However, a parallel line of research has also been under way in which the amount of stimulus information has been manipulated, as this predicts differences in both the imagery and the exposure physiology of emotion.

With such factors as imagery ability or familiarity of material being equal, it is held that the probability of emotional processing will increase with the quantity of matching stimulus information. Thus, for example, actual exposure to a feared object is more likely to access the prototype than a filmed presentation, which in turn would be a better prompt than a written text. The hypothesis depends, of course, on the absence of serious mismatch, which might result in the access of different, competing material from memory. Furthermore, it will be obvious to the reader that we are entering here the realm of functional aesthetics and that the associative strength of specific stimulus propositions and the organization of the input, as well as the quantity of information, may be of importance. Thus, an artist might well create a poem that would be a surer path to an affective response than a Hollywood extravaganza on the same theme. Our effort here is to describe media differences in terms of their average quantity of information. We are for now skirting the formidable aesthetic problems, as well as the obvious fact that different media require the application of different transformation formulas before either raw stimulus material or semantic representations can be converted into the conceptual information of the prototype (e.g., text in a natural language must be comprehended in terms of the objects and events to which the semantic code refers).

McLean (1981) recently completed an experiment in our laboratory that examined the verbal report and physiological responses of untrained subjects to an imagery script, compared with their response to an elaborate dramatic presentation of the same affective content. The dramatic presentations or playlets took place in a realistic setting, employed trained actors, and engaged the subjects as participant observers. Two contents were studied: The first scenario (fear) involved a live snake that was being ineptly restrained by the actor-handler who described it as poisonous, while the subject watched from a position only a few feet away. The second playlet (anger) cast an actor as a teaching assistant who berated the subject for his lack of intelligence and poor performance on an examination. Both dramatic presentations had great veri-similitude. However, subjects were clearly informed that the events were not "real": for example, the snake was not poisonous, and the actor was only "saying" the subject was stupid for the purposes of the experiment. Thus,

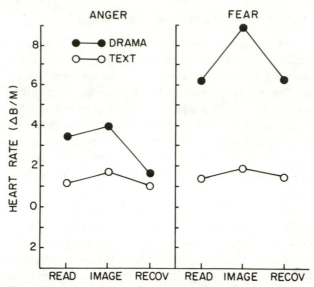

Figure 7.6. Average heart-rate changes observed during text and playlet (drama) prompted imagery. A script was read to the subject during the read period for the text condition; a playlet was presented during the read period in the drama condition. Descriptive fear-inducing (an encounter with a poisonous snake) and anger-inducing (receiving unjust verbal abuse) contents were examined. See McLean (1981).

some of the meaning propositions in the situation were discordant with the presumed emotional prototypes. However, the stimulus information was rendered faithfully in all its physical parmeters, and both the subjects watching the playlets and those hearing the text description were told to imagine the contexts vividly "as if " they were real.

The results of these interventions are presented in Figure 7.6. It is clear that the playlets generated heart-rate change in untrained subjects that was significantly greater than that shown by text-prompted imagery. The modest responses of these subjects to imagery scripts were similar to those observed in previous research by untrained normal subjects. The response to the playlets (with their enriched stimulus information) was comparable in amplitude of physiological response to that previously obtained from response-trained subjects reacting to text (e.g., see Figure 7.3). Furthermore, as with response training and scripted response material, the effect of the playlet on the physiological affective response was enhanced among questionnaire-selected "good" imagers. A comparison of differences between good and poor imagers in response to the playlets is presented in Figure 7.7. It will be noted that the response of females differs from that of males, according to content. Male good imagers responded more to both playlets than did their poor imaging peers. However, good imaging females, while showing a dramatically larger response to the

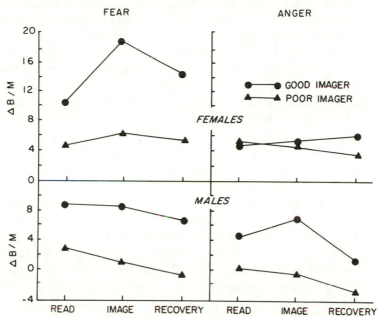

Figure 7.7. Average heart-rate responses of good and poor imagery subjects (Betts's questionnaire) during imagery occasioned by fear- and anger-inducing dramatic presentations. Responses of the two sexes are separately indicated. See McLean (1981).

fear scene, did not differ at all from poor imaging females when they visualized being criticized for poor performance. This reduced response to so-called anger stimuli is consistent with sex differences in affect noted by Frodi, Macaulay, & Thome (1977).

If quantity of matching propositions is the key to prototype access, it is expected that response training would have the same enhancing effect on efferent responding regardless of the input medium. Kozak (1982) recently explored this hypothesis, administering both stimulus and response training to subjects and examining the effects of these procedures on different stimulus materials. Subjects were both administered scripted text and exposed to some of the actual physical stimuli presumed to be part of the stimulus structure of a relevant fear prototype (e.g., for speech anxiety, a view of an audience). For both the physically presented stimuli and the text, response training prompted the enhanced physiological fear pattern predicted; stimulus training occasioned a significantly smaller physiological response to the objective stimulus, as it did to the scripted rendering of the same material, and as it has in our previous comparisons of the effects of training method on emotion-instigating text (Lang et al., 1980).

Two other experiments merit mention in the present context. Both are concerned with emotional change and its relationship to imagery processing. In an earlier study (Lang et al., 1970) it was shown that phobic patients treated by systematic desensitization profited from the therapy to the extent that verbal report of fear during therapy imagery was concordant with a physiology of fear arousal. Recently, Levin (1982) undertook an exploration of the mechanism of this effect. Snake-phobic subjects were exposed repeatedly to a live snake in a habituation paradigm. Between exposure trials, subjects imaged either the snake or a neutral scene (imagery was text prompted). On the basis of QMI scores, subjects were divided into good imager and poor imager groups. The results for good imagers indicated marked habituation of cardiac rate to repeated, objective exposure trials when phobic imagery intervened between these exposure trials; good imagers showed significantly less habituation when the intervening imagery was neutral in content. As noted earlier, the good imagers also showed a significantly greater initial heart-rate response to the intervening phobic imagery than to neutral imagery. Furthermore, the phobic-imagery response of the good imagers (unlike their response to neutral content) habituated with repeated presentations of the scene. None of these same effects were obtained for poor imagers. That is, while poor imagers showed a marked heart-rate response with snake exposure, habituation was not hastened by intervening phobic imagery. Furthermore, again unlike good imagers, the poor imaging group showed no difference in physiological response between neutral and fear imagery.

These results suggest that text-generated imagery processing accesses the same emotion prototype for good imagers as does actual exposure. Furthermore, the prototype's modification over imagery trials transfers directly to the exposure situation. This prompts the hypothesis that for therapies other than those involving direct exposure, effectiveness may depend on the subject's previous ability to generate affect from linguistic representations (instructions to imagine, recall, or discuss emotional content) initiated in the therapeutic interaction. The results of a clinical series (Levin, Cook, & Lang, 1982), conducted in parallel with our laboratory work, provide some support for this view. Among a population of anxious and phobic patients, it was shown that clients who generated appropriate physiological patterning to imagery instructions at an initial diagnostic session were significantly more likely to successfully complete treatment than those who failed to show a palpable initial response. Furthermore, the successful subjects were significantly more likely to be high on the imagery questionnaire than were the subjects who failed to successfully complete the course of treatment.

The psychophysiology of emotion

We began this discourse with a working definition of cognition in emotion, that is, the processing of symbolic information that is required for the central representation in memory and the organized expression of an affective response.

We were at some pains to indicate that this definition contained no implied identity with experienced thought or feeling. That is not to say that subjects might not in any given instance report out in a natural language conceptual information that was part of the cognitive processing in emotion. However, our stance vis-à-vis such data is similar to the view we would take of a teletype report from a computer directing the activities of a factory assembly line. That is, the program might include an output routine that commented on the symbolic manipulations required for the task. However, such a report is not required to be made, or, if present, is not required to be accurate, complete, or even relevant, given that the commentary of the terminal is seldom intrinsic to the information processing required to move the line. The relevance of such reports from either animate or inanimate thinking machinery is determined by independent validating criteria. Thus, our research suggests that verbal report of arousal following an imagined emotional experience could be, depending on the context, an appraisal of the meaning of the content (e.g., "If that happened to me, I'd be frightened") or, alternatively, it could be a pertinent comment on the emotional processing that preceded the report. It is obvious that our method of deciding between these possibilities depends on data obtained from bioelectric recording of the somatic muscles and the viscera. This emphasis is not an arbitrary reification of physiology. It is a dependence founded on paradigmatic requirements of measurement and on a specific theoretical view of emotional expression. The methodological requirement is dictated by problems that stem from the interaction of measurement and observation. Let's assume for a moment that verbal report is a wholly valid comment on internal processing: If the manifest task is emotional expression, its assessment is inevitably confounded when we require that the emoting organism also function as observer of its own expression. Furthermore, if we ask that these tasks be accomplished serially (emotion first; then observation) rather than in parallel, we introduce a delay and confront possible distortions in memory storage and readout. Physiological recording provides a real-time analysis of emotional processing that does not require the subject to perform the confounding second task of observer. From our perspective, it is the most practical method currently available for assessing cognition in emotion.[1]

The theoretical reasons for the use of bioelectric recording lie in our conception of emotion as an action set, a behavioral disposition, and our view that even the subovert processing of response information generates efferent outflow. The practical significance of this approach is highlighted by the therapy studies just considered, in which the psychophysiological link between reality and image appears to be critical to treatment effectiveness. There is, of course, a persisting debate among students of the psychology of emotion concerning the role of physiological responses in affective expression. The two traditional views are: first, that there are emotional states, specific organizations of physiology and behavior, which are isomorphic with and consistent within the various traditional categories of emotional experience; second, that the physiology of emotion is an undifferentiated state of autonomic and somatomotor arousal and that the specific emotion, or the presence of any emotion at all, is determined by interpretive cognitions that arise in response to a felt evaluative need. The approach taken here is not clearly assignable to either side of the debate: The information-processing view blunts the major arguments of this controversy by wholly redefining the terrain of study.

Emotional states

It is our view that activation of an emotion prototype always prompts efferent outflow, whether or not overt behavior is occasioned. The efferent activity is the output of motor subroutines that are linked to the deep structure of response information. The emotion itself is an action set. It is distinguished from other behavior mainly by cultural convention, in that it is behavior with an obvious valence, conveying unusual intensity or arousal, and may be seen as confused or displastic in its expression. Emotions are always about doing something, and setting, meaning, and pattern of action are all coded in the same associative network. Thus, some patterns of emotional expression (visceral and somatic) may be expected to persist across a variety of contexts of evocation. That is, even under conditions of inhibited overt response (e.g., when we are moved by a fearful dramatic presentation or a sexual allusion prompts an unfulfillable fantasy), activity in the somatic and visceral organs cast a shadow of the coded act. We would argue further that specific prototypes and their associated responses are characteristic of certain classes of stimuli and subjects, that is, that both type of emotion context (situational stereotypy) and type of subject (individual stereotypy) may be represented in specific physiological action patterns.[2]

These comments are not meant to imply a belief in physiological patterns that are indices of traditional categories of emotion. However, there are specific task physiologies (i.e., particular organizations of biological events that are the support system of the behavioral acts occasioned by specific stimulus contexts). Situations said to be provocative of a particular emotion may be situations that prompt the same actions in most subjects or in some definable subset of the subject population (e.g., helplessness in depressed or avoidance in phobic patients). To pursue a specific example, a verbal attack or abuse leads many persons to report that they are angry. In some it also occasions a physical counterattack. "Throwing a punch" at a false accuser requires the recruitment of many motor units in specific organization, cardiovascular mobilization tuned to those gross muscles (i.e., blood-pressure and heart-rate increase and other components of a beta-adrenergic pattern), and so on. It seems not unreasonable to presume that the blood-pressure increases usually found in verbally abused subjects, who are however socially restrained, represent an efferent outflow from the central processing of a physical-attack-program prototype (albeit with inhibition of its final step). That such a physiological organization (somewhat attenuated) might also be observed in a person antic- ipating abuse that has not yet taken place or that it might be evoked instructionally or at the theater by an aesthetically valid scenario highlights the persisting, substantive character of the internal data structure.

We are not proposing here another homunculoid view of human purpose or motivation. It is not suggested that there are internal emotional states called anger or fear that are invariably consistent with phenomenological report. What we are suggesting is that the cognitive events in emotion involve infor- mation processing and that the output of the processing program is efferent outflow or action. Although some of the information in the program and some of the logical relationships can be read out as verbal report, the fundamental code is not in the natural language. Sperry (1952) noted many years ago that the brain is best understood not as a sophisticated sense organ or self-contem- plative thought machine but as an organ specialized for the control and mod- ulation of overt responding. Visceral activity, which is not part of routinized, vegetative processes, constitutes the biological support for anticipated or ongoing behavior. Furthermore, in suggesting that a particular stimulus context may tend to prompt a particular action set we do not mean to imply that this rela- tionship is invariant across subjects. The confusion caused by this latter as- sumption has been amply demonstrated in research on sex differences in emotion (Frodi et al., 1977). Apparent differences between men and women in phys- iological response to "anger" stimuli have been shown to be secondary to the differential meaning of the context for the two sexes. In brief, situations that generally prompt attack in males (or its premotor physiological pattern) more often occasion avoidance or efforts at positive social mediation in females (with a different support physiology).

Physiological events, as described by John Lacey (1959), are part of an organism's changing transactions with the environment. Thus, traditional emotional labels such as fear do not consistently reference the same behavior patterns. Indeed, the term is used to designate actions and physiology that at one extreme could involve immobility and hyperattention to the external en- vironment and at the other, unaware, unthinking, headlong flight. However, it is also true that the information structures determining these different response patterns often include some common visceral, stimulus, or meaning propositions. Because of these informational commonalities, different action patterns, even if based on very different learning histories, can appear to be manifestations of a common broad class of affects, that is, fear, anger, or whatever.

Meaning and activation

In recent years, the view put forward by Stanley Schachter (1964) has had a powerful grip on our thinking about emotion. Emotions are held to be a combination of some generalized state of physiological arousal, plus those cognitions that constitute its interpretation or attribution. Thus, high heart rate and increased blood pressure combined with the knowledge that one has just run upstairs does not an emotion make. However, this same physiology following on a verbal attack by the town bully (i.e., the attribution of the physiological arousal to the bully's abuse) generates an affective state. It will already be clear to the reader that we hold the physiology (both visceral and somatic) to be organized around specific response agenda and not to be an undifferentiated behavioral propellant. However, one could hardly argue with the thesis that, in addition to the stimulus information itself, the meaning of a stimulus context may be a significant determinant of subsequent behavior. Semantic elaborations of this sort ("Bullys are dangerous"; "he broke George's arm last week"; "he's a karate expert and I'm not over the flu yet") are likely to be part of data structures that represent an affective response disposition.

However, meaning information of this type is certainly not an invariable link in the accessing of an affective response disposition. Zajonc (1980) provides arresting data arguing that affective expression usually precedes, rather than follows, appraising cognition. Furthermore, it is not difficult to find instances in which such information is simply irrelevant to an emotional response. For example, the agoraphobic may "know" that an open field is not really dangerous, yet the prototype is nevertheless activated by sufficient stimulus and/or response information. Similarly, a woman may correctly attribute her irritability to the period of her menstrual cycle but still behave angrily in response to a minimal external stimulus. Dynamic psychological analysis of such situations has generally proposed that concordant meaning information is present but is outside awareness (e.g., that the agoraphobic, despite protestations, really "deep down" believes the field is dangerous). However, it is at the least more parsimonious to assume, in this instance, that meaning information is simply not critical for prototype activation.

Currently there is considerable interest among behavioral therapists, as there has always been for more traditional psychotherapists, in the interpretive information reported in emotion. Cognitive-behavior therapists (e.g., Ellis, 1962; Meichenbaum, 1977) now emphasize stimulus and response information less in emotion and focus more on altering meaning propositions. Patients are persuaded to talk to themselves positively, to reassess their attributive knowledge of emotional stimuli, and to make coping self-referent statements. It is not clear how powerful a strategy this will be for the modification of emotion. The paradigm developed here could certainly be adapted to its study. Imagery scripts could be modified to include or exclude meaning information. Furthermore, a new imagery training regime could be developed to reinforce subjects for imagery description that included more interpretive information. If such content is a key to emotional image processing, vividness, and prototype activation, its effect should be reflected in augmented amplitude and more appropriate patterns of efferent outflow.

Coda: three systems, three dimensions, three propositions

The approach presented here represents an effort at coping, in very small part, with the ubiquity and diversity of emotional expression. The universe of discourse called emotion has been established through cultural and historical convention. Its general categories are defined by centuries of literary chronicles and philosophical thought. It would be both presumptuous and misguided to attempt at this time anything like a comprehensive theory of emotion. To the extent that affective tone seems to be part of any complex response, it would require that we begin with the manufacture of a general theory of behavior, a task for which our young science hardly seems ready. With respect to these broad goals, what was attempted here involved only a sketching out, broad brushed, of what seem to be consensus characteristics of emotional behavior and a gross outline of the database usually invoked by scientists in its description.

We noted at the outset that definitions of emotion have depended, in different theories and different experiments, on three general classes of dependent variables: verbal report, motor acts, an expressive physiology. It was noted that when these behaviors have been measured in a common experimental setting, correlations seldom accounted for more than a fraction of the total variance in the analysis. It was further suggested that this failure of covariation at the level of quantitative analysis created serious problems for theories that view these measures as indices of substantive states of emotion experienced by a subsisting self. What we have suggested here, as an alternative, is that emotional behavior depends on the specific information processed in the context of its measurement. It is held that emotion information is represented centrally in propositional form and organized into associative networks. Stable networks, such as those found in focal phobia, occasion a reliable behavioral output and thus have the status of emotion prototypes. The units of the network fall readily into the three classes of stimulus, response, and meaning propositions. Response propositions are of particular importance because of their link to motor programs, which coordinate overt and covert efferent expression in emotion. The three-system topography of emotion is expected to vary across subject and context, depending on the specific response information in the prototype.

Although we have emphasized the processing of physiological events, we do not mean to imply that an expressive visceral response is expected every time affective language is used. Certain contexts may occasion only the language behavior of emotion, if neither affective visceral nor overt behavior has been included in the determining cognitive network. I am reminded here of a clinical instance: the young student with an identity crisis who complains of anxiety, fears of failure, and an absence of meaning in his or her life. The clinician may search in vain for evidence in this patient of a physiology of distress or for objective evidence of functional behavioral disturbance (e.g., poor grades, absence of social life). That this unidimensional response topography and the multifaceted response of a severe agoraphobic – heart pounding, cowering at home, and screaming his or her distress – are both called anxiety may be more a linguistic analogy than a categorical association at the level of psychological theory. The view of emotion as information processing presented here has no difficulty dealing with this diversity of phenomena. It is also true that it offers no ready-made integrative theory of emotional life. However, at the present stage of our science this may not be a liability. The categories of emotion are perhaps to be discovered in the research that we do, rather than to be imposed by what may be literary and artistic convention. Similarly, we should not be worried if we have no theory of consciousness or the experiencing self. I do not believe that our field presently needs more grand theories in the *Welterklärung* tradition of our discipline. What we do need are better paradigms for the study of emotion and minitheories that handle well their own parochial data sets. Broad integrative theories require the generation of something worth integrating.

With respect to the three general dimensions of behavior (valence, arousal, and control) proposed as the arena of emotion studies, there was no intention to elevate them to any special theoretical status (any more than the three response systems should constitute a holy trinity!). I mean only to suggest that they seem to conveniently embrace the topic in which we are interested and have further virtue as categories that may permit us to map affect across response systems (a task that has proved difficult with the more varied traditional nomenclature of emotion). Nevertheless, they are only a distillate of Western man's verbal report about emotion and represent more what we want to know than a conclusion about what is already known. How does behavior come to have direction and intensity? Why does it become unstuck, sometimes at times of greatest importance? It is our view that the answers to these questions begin with a definition of the action being prepared, expressed, or inhibited in the particular measurement context of interest. We presume this action to have a differentiated response structure. Thus, there is not an arousal physiology; there are arousal physiologies. Similarly, valence is not unidimensional, and problems in behavioral control are as numerous as the thousand ways we can find to stub a toe. The research endeavor presented here is in its infancy. We have made a toddler's step toward reinterpreting some of the brain's homunculoid functions. There is no question that man's emotional life is conveniently described as the output of what Dennett (1978) calls an intentional system (a system with beliefs organized in the service of goals). The goal of a science of emotion, however, is to reexplain the system as an objective mechanism.

It is only as we begin to realize this quest that we will find a true technology of emotion and effective means for applying our science to human needs.

Summary and conclusions

This chapter is a speculation on the cognitive events that determine the central representation and expression of an emotional response. Cognition is defined here as conceptual information processing. We begin with a description of how the information base of an affective response disposition is organized and its form of representation in memory. An effort is then made to indicate some of the conditions under which such a disposition is accessed and processed as efferent output. Emotions are conceived to be action sets that can evolve three different response systems: verbal report, overt motor response, and expressive physiology. It is held that there is no clear demarcation between affective and nonaffective behavior. However, popular consensus defines the terrain of emotion as including responses that vary in valence, arousal, and control or dominance, and it is toward an explanation of these phenomena that the present chapter is oriented. Because of consistency of response and the reliability of stimulus-instigating conditions (as well as the importance of the clinical problem and the convenience of access to the subject population), focal phobia is used here as a primary case illustration of our approach.

This view of emotion is a development of the bio-informational theory of imagery previously described (Lang, 1977, 1979). Affective dispositions are held to be coded in memory in propositional form. Propositions are organized into networks related by association. The units of a network may be divided into three general information classes: stimulus, meaning, and response propositions. Response propositions are double coded, in that their deep structure is linked to the motor command system that generates efferent output. The information network determining a phobic response is closely bonded and richly interconnected. This coherence of information means that the network has a high probability of being activated as a unit, giving it the status of an action or emotion prototype.

A primary method of accessing the prototype is through input of matching stimulus information. The better the match to the prototype (perhaps optimal with presentation of an actual phobic object), the more likely that the emotion response program will be accessed and run. However, matching information other than stimulus propositions also facilitates access. Thus, under conditions of degraded input (e.g., imagery instructions), probability of access is increased by the simultaneous instigation of the response components in the network. Subjects vary in their basic ability to access affective response codes, independent of the relative coherence of an emotion prototype. This ability appears to be similar to that involved in perceptual imagery recall. Thus, good imagers are more likely to generate affect under conditions of degraded input than are poor imagers. Because of the link between response propositions and motor programs, processing of an affective prototype always involves efferent leakage (even if the implied overt action is inhibited). Therefore, the affective event, as it varies between subjects and/or contents, can be monitored in real time through bioelectric recording.

Two lines of research supporting this view are described. The first group of experiments represents an exploration of text-prompted emotional imagery. Subjects were instructed to imagine emotional situations described by propositionally coded scripts. It was determined that the inclusion of response propositions in the text, in conjunction with prior response training in processing this material, resulted in the largest and most concordant affective reactions (verbal report and physiological pattern). Emphasis on stimulus material, including a "mind's eye" oriented imagery training program, did not facilitate the affective imagery response. The same methodology was subsequently used in a study of two distinct types of fearful subjects. Following response training, reliable differences in the two fear groups were observed, consistent with exposure physiology and hypothesized differences in the two fear types. It was also established that questionnaire-defined good imagers, responding to scripted material, generated more appropriate affective responses than did poor imagers, and that these effects were particularly large and spontaneous when the good imagers were also phobics imaging phobic material.

The second research line involved a systematic varying of affective stimulus information. It was found that affective responses were larger when subjects reacted to a dramatic presentation than when they reacted to scripted text. Furthermore, good imagers showed the same superior performance with the dramatic scenes as they did in our previous studies of text based imagery. Good imagers also showed significant differentiation of response, according to the content of the dramatic scene and hypothesized individual differences in the target emotion prototypes (in this case the expected differences were based on sex rather than fear type). Again, comparable to studies of text, response training prior to objective stimulus presentation was significantly more effective than stimulus training in amplifying appropriate affective patterns of response. Finally, the results obtained for both phobic volunteers and clinical patients support the view that prototype access is crucial to therapeutic behavior change.

In conclusion, it is noted that the present view is wholly consistent neither with the traditional conception of specific states of emotion (subsisting patterns of physiology and behavior that are consistent with the phenomenology of fear, anger, joy, etc.), nor with the concept of emotion as a coincidence of unidimensional arousal and affect-appraising cognitions. The information processing view radically redefines theoretical categories in emotion studies. Emotion is held to be a differentiated action set, often context bound, based on a specific information structure in memory. The research problems this view poses for the future include: a further study of prototype structure and organization, and an assessment of the effects of prototype processing on other memory content; further exploration of individual differences in accessing of affective information; study of how quantity and quality of input information (including the significance of the specific transformational rules required by different media) influence ease of access of an emotional prototype; and finally, systematic examination of the processes of prototype consolidation and change, with a practical view to the improvement of methods for the therapeutic modification of aversive emotional states.

Notes

1 From this perspective, the limitations of the method lie in the fact that stimulus and meaning information can be less directly accessed. These conceptual elements must be tested from the input side, and their processing inferred from measurement of perceptual response code, e.g., efferent activity associated with postural orienting or sense organ adjustments (see Levin, 1982). While more direct access through cortical recording could be hoped for, the current state of the art does not promise realization of this goal in the near future.

2 From the perspective of the psychophysiological investigator, the difficulties in assessing non-exposure response code are considerable. He must often sort through three different but coincident physiologies. For example, when a socially anxious person imagines performing in a public-speaking context there is, first, the physiological code of speech presentation (efferent representations of the motor task of speaking and the cognitive demands of generating or reading the required text); for the anxious subject there is a second coded physiology of alertness and preparation for disapproval and to repel attack (usually the target physiology of the emotion researcher); finally, there is a third physiology of the imaginal act itself, i.e., the immediate biological cost of memory retrieval, regeneration of the relevant conceptual network, and its central processing (see Lang et al., 1983).

References

Anderson, J. R., & Bower, G. H. A propositional theory of recognition memory. *Memory and Cognition*, 1974, *2* (3), 406–412.

Ax, A. F. The physiological differentiation between fear and anger in humans. *Psychosomatic Medicine*, 1953, *15*, 433–442.

Betts, G. H. *The distributions and functions of mental imagery*. New York: Columbia University Teachers College, Contributions to Educational Series, No. 26, 1909.

Bower, G. H. Mood and memory. *American Psychologist*, 1981, *36* (2), 129–148.

Brady, J. P., & Levitt, E. E. Hypnotically induced visual hallucinations. *Psychosomatic Medicine*, 1966, *28*, 351–353.

Brown, B. B. Visual recall ability and eye movements. *Psychophysiology*, 1968, *4*, 300–306.

Bush, L. E., II. Individual differences in multi-dimensional scaling of adjectives denoting feelings. *Journal of Personality and Social Psychology*, 1973, *25*, 50–57.

Cannon, W. B. *Bodily changes in pain, hunger, fear, and rage* (2nd ed.). New York: Appleton-Century-Crofts, 1936.

Davitz, J. R. *The language of emotion*. New York: Academic Press, 1969.

Deckert, G. H. Pursuit eye movements in the absence of a moving visual stimulus. *Science*, 1964, *143*, 1192–1193.

Dennett, B. *Brainstorms: Philosophical essays on mind and psychology.* Montgomery, Vt.: Bradford Books, 1978.

Ellis, A. *Reason and emotion in psychotherapy.* New York: Lyle Stuart, 1962.

Ellis, A. Emotional education in the classroom: The living school. *Journal of Clinical Child Psychology*, 1971, *1*, 19–22.

Frodi, A., Macaulay, J., & Thome, P. R. Are women always less aggressive than men? A review of the experimental literature. *Psychological Bulletin*, 1977, *84*, 634–660.

Gray, J. A. *The psychology of fear and stress.* New York: McGraw-Hill, 1971.

Grossberg, J. M., & Wilson, H. K. Physiological changes accompanying the visualization of fearful and neutral situations. *Journal of Personality and Social Psychology*, 1968, *10*, 124–133.

Hebb, D. O. *Organization of behavior.* New York: Wiley, 1949.

Hilgard, E. R. *Hypnotic susceptibility.* New York: Harcourt, Brace, & World, 1965.

Hodgson, R. O., & Rachman, S. J., II. Desynchrony in measures of fear. *Behavior Research and Therapy*, 1974, *12*, 314–326.

Hull, C. L. *Hypnosis and suggestibility: An experimental approach.* New York: Appleton-Century-Crofts, 1933.

Jacobson, E. Electrical measurements of neuromuscular state during mental activities: III. Visual imagination and recollections. *American Journal of Physiology*, 1930, *95* (3), 694–702.

Kieras, D. Beyond pictures and words: Alternate information processing models for imagery effects in verbal memory. *Psychological Bulletin*, 1978, *85*, 532–554.

Kintsch, W. *The representation of meaning in memory.* Hillsdale, N.J.: Erlbaum, 1974.

Klein, D. F. Anxiety reconceptualized. In D. F. Klein & J. Rabkin (Eds.), *Anxiety: New research and changing concepts.* New York: Raven Press, 1981.

Kozak, M. J. *The psychophysiological effects of training on variously elicited imaginings.* Unpublished doctoral dissertation, University of Wisconsin, Madison, 1982.

Lacey, J. I. Psychophysiological approaches to the evaluation of psychotherapeutic process and outcome. In E. A. Rubinstein & M. B. Parloff (Eds.), *Research in psychotherapy* (Vol. 1), pp. 160–208. Washington, D.C.: American Psychological Association, 1959.

Lacey, J. I. Somatic response patterning and stress: Some revisions of activation theory. In M. H. Appley & R. Turnbull (Eds.), *Psychological Stress: Issues in research.* New York: Appleton, 1967.

Lacey, J. I., & Lacey, B. C. Some autonomic-central nervous system interrelationships. In P. Black (Ed.), *Physiological correlates of emotion*, pp. 205–228. New York: Academic Press, 1970.

Lang, P. J. Experimental studies of desensitization psychotherapy. In J. Wolpe (Ed.), *The conditioning therapies.* New York: Holt, Rinehart and Winston, 1964.

Lang, P. J. Fear reduction and fear behavior: Problems in treating a construct. In J. M. Shlien (Ed.), *Research in psychotherapy* (Vol. 3), pp. 90–103. Washington, D.C.: American Psychological Association, 1968.

Lang, P. J. The application of psychophysiological methods to the study of psychotherapy and behavior modification. In A. E. Bergin & S. L. Garfield (Eds.), *Handbook of psychotherapy and behavior change.* New York: Wiley, 1971.

Lang, P. J. Fear imagery: An information processing analysis. *Behavior Therapy*, 1977, *8*, 862–886.

Lang, P. J. Anxiety: Toward a psychophysiological definition. In H. S. Akiskal & W. L. Webb (Eds.), *Psychiatric diagnosis: Exploration of biological predictors*, pp. 365–389. New York: Spectrum, 1978.

Lang, P. J. A bio-informational theory of emotional imagery. *Psychophysiology*, 1979, *16*, 495–512.

Lang, P. J., Kozak, M. J., Miller, G. A., Levin, D. N., & McLean, A., Jr. Emotional imagery: Conceptual structure & pattern of somato-visceral response. *Psychophysiology*, 1980, *17*(2), 179–192.

Lang, P. J., Levin, D. N., Miller, G. A., & Kozak, M. J. Fear behavior, fear imagery, and the psychophysiology of emotion: The problem of affective response integration. *Journal of Abnormal Psychology*, 1983, *92*, 276–306.

Lang, P. J., Melamed, B. G., & Hart, J. D. A psychophysiological analysis of fear modification using an automated desensitization procedure. *Journal of Abnormal Psychology*, 1970, *76*, 220–234.

Lang, P. J., Rice, D. G., & Sternback, R. A. The psychophysiology of emotion. In N. Greenfield & R. A. Sternback (Eds.), *Handbook of Psychophysiology*. New York: Holt, Rinehart and Winston, 1972.

Leitenberg, H., Agras, S., Butz, R., & Wincze, J. Relationship between heart rate and behavioral change during the treatment of phobias. *Journal of Abnormal Psychology*, 1971, *78*, 59–68.

Levin, D. N. *The psychophysiology of fear reduction: Role of response activation during emotional imagery*. Unpublished doctoral dissertation, University of Wisconsin, Madison, 1982.

Levin, D. N., Cook, E. W. III, & Lang, P. J. Fear imagery and fear behavior: Psychophysiological analysis of clients receiving treatment for anxiety disorders. *Psychophysiology*, 1982, *19*, 571–572 (abstract).

Levin, D. N., Miller, G. A., Kozak, M. J., & Lang, P. J. Emotional imagery: Effects of imagery training and phobia classification. Abstract of a paper presented at the annual meeting of the Society for Psychophysiological Research in Washington, Oct. 29–Nov. 1, 1981. Reprinted in *Psychophysiology*, 1982, *19* (3), 333.

Lorenz, K. Z. *King Solomon's ring*. New York: Crowell, 1952.

Mandler, G. *Mind and emotion*. New York: Wiley, 1975.

Marks, I. M., & Huson, J. Physiological aspects of neutral and phobic imagery. *British Journal of Psychiatry*, 1973, *122*, 567–572.

McLean, A., Jr. *Emotional imagery: Stimulus information, imagery ability, and patterns of physiological response*. Unpublished doctoral dissertation, University of Wisconsin-Madison, 1981.

Mehrabian, A., & Russell, J. A. *An approach to environmental psychology*. Cambridge, Mass.: MIT Press, 1974.

Meichenbaum, D. *Cognitive-behavior modification: An integrative approach*. New York: Plenum, 1977.

Miller, G. A., Levin, D. N., Kozak, M. J., Cook, E. W., McLean, A., Carroll, J., & Lang, P. J. Emotional imagery: Individual differences in imagery ability and physiological responses. *Psychophysiology*, 1981, *18*, 196.

Miller, G. A., Levin, D. N., Kozak, M. J., Cook, E. W., III, McLean, A., & Lang, P. J. *Emotional imagery: Effects of individual differences in perceptual imagery on physiological response*. Manuscript submitted for publication, 1983.

Osgood, C. E., Suci, G. J., & Tannenbaum, P. H. *The measurement of meaning*. Urbana: University of Illinois Press, 1957.

Quillian, M. R. Semantic memory. In M. L. Minsky (Ed.). *Semantic information processing*. Cambridge, Mass.: MIT Press, 1966.

Schachter, J. Pain, fear, and anger in hypertensives and normotensives. *Psychosomatic Medicine*, 1957, *19*, 17–28.

Schachter, S. The interaction of cognitive and physiological determinants of emotional state. In L. Berkowitz (Ed.), *Advances in experimental social psychology* (Vol. 1), pp. 48–80. New York: Academic Press, 1964.

Schneirla, T. C. An evolutionary and developmental theory of bi-phasic processes underlying approach and withdrawal. In M. R. Jones (Ed.), *Nebraska symposium on motivation*. Lincoln: University of Nebraska Press, 1959.

Schroeder, H. E., & Rich, A. R. The process of fear reduction through systematic de-sensitization. *Journal of Consulting and Clinical Psychology*, 1976, *44*, 191–199.

Schwartz, G. E. Cardiac responses to self-induced thoughts. *Psychophysiology*, 1971, *8* (4), 462–467.

Seligman, M. E. P. Phobias and preparedness. *Behavior Therapy*, 1971, *2*, 307–321.

Shaw, W. A. The relation of muscular action potentials to imaginal weight lifting. *Archives of Psychology*, 1940, *23*, 380–389.

Sheehan, P. Q. A shortened form of Betts' questionnaire upon mental imagery. *Journal of Clinical Psychology*, 1967, *23*, 386–389.

Sokolov, Y. N. *Perception and the conditioned reflex*. New York: Macmillan, 1963.

Sperry, R. V. Neurology and the mind-brain problem. *American Scientist*, 1952, *40*, 291–312.

Tinbergen, N. *The study of instincts*. New York: Oxford University Press, 1951.

Van Egeren, L. F., Feather, B. W., & Hein, P. L. Desensitization of phobias: Some psychophysiological propositions. *Psychophysiology*, 1971, *8*, 213–228.

Weerts, T. C., & Lang, P. J. The psychophysiology of fear imagery: Differences between focal phobia and social-performance anxiety. *Consulting and Clinical Psychology*, 1978, *46*, 1157–1159.

Zajonc, R. B. Feeling and thinking: Preferences need no inferences. *American Psychologist*, 1980, *35* (2), 151–175.

Part II

Emotion and cognition in early development

8   Toward a new understanding of emotions and their development

Joseph J. Campos and Karen Caplovitz Barrett

The working definition of emotion to be taken here is a functionalist one: It assumes that emotions are not subject to ostensive definition (because emotions are manifested in so many alternative ways), but that they can be identified on the basis of the conjunction of three criteria. One is that, like language, emotions are crucial regulators of social and interpersonal behavior, primarily through their multiple expressive channels. The second criterion is that, like cognition, emotions regulate the flow of information and the selection of response processes or outputs of the organism. And the third is that, unlike either language or cognition, the basic emotions, which we believe include joy, anger, disgust, surprise, sadness, fear, and possibly sexual ardor, affection, and others, regulate behavior through a noncodified, prewired communication process. This process is widely believed to be innate: No social learning appears necessary either for the *reception* of facial and gestural signals (Kenney, Mason, & Hill, 1979; Mendelson, Haith, & Goldman-Rakic, 1982; Sackett, 1966), or for the *production* of such (Boucher & Carlson, 1980; Ekman & Friesen, 1972; Ekman, Sorenson, & Friesen, 1969; Steiner, 1973).

Moreover, given this emphasis upon an unlearned basis for emotionality, the study of emotion during infancy may be particularly useful in substantiating the definition. Research regarding infantile emotionality has therefore profoundly influenced the model we will propose. However, the proposed framework is by no means limited in application to the period of infancy; it is relevant to the study of older children, adolescents, and adults as well.

Shifts in attitudes about human emotions

Emotions: from central constructs to explanatory fictions

Not long ago (until approximately 1972), emotions suffered a not-very-benign neglect by psychologists. The neglect seemed well justified: Emotions appeared

This chapter was written in conjunction with the preparation of a much larger chapter in socioemotional development: M. Haith & J. Campos (Eds.), *Infancy and Developmental Psychobiology*. Vol. 2 of Mussen (Series editor), *Handbook of Child Psychology*. New York: Wiley, in press. Support to the first author for the writing of this chapter was provided by NIMH grant MH-23556; to the second author, by a fellowship from the American Association of University Women. We wish to thank Wanda Mayberry, Donna Bradshaw, and Rosemary Campos for their comments on earlier versions, and Helen Strautman and Denise Hall for their prompt and efficient work in preparing the chapter for publication. Special thanks are due Professor Izard for his patience and support.

unamenable to measurement with any degree of specificity; they seemed to play no causal role in behavioral explanations; they appeared to be irrelevant to the most central aspects of human behavior, especially those originating within experimental psychology; and they were much too closely linked to naive, romanticized, and unscientific language. What progress was made in understanding emotion had been made not by psychologists but by neurophysiologists working with brain structures or with neural transmitters (Grossman, 1967).

This neglect did not always exist. At one time, the *conscious* aspect of emotions, called "affect" or "hedonic tone" by theorists like Wundt (1904), Titchener (1905), or Beebe-Center (1932), constituted one of the three central topics in psychological theory, along with sensation and association. Moreover, in Freud's early theory, affect also played a central explanatory role. Recall that Breuer and Freud's (1895) theory of "strangulated affect" was one of the early explanations of the formation of neurotic symptoms in hysteric patients. So long as introspection and verbal reports were the preferred methods in psychological theory, affect was revealed directly and unequivocally. Some controversies surrounded the construct of affect in the early history of psychology, but the disputes concerned not its reality but the number of dimensions of which affect was constituted. Early behaviorist theorists such as Watson (1930) also felt the need to explain emotion, not as a feeling in consciousness, of course, but rather as overtly observable instrumental behaviors, facial responses, and vocal expressions. Watson postulated the existence in neonates of three basic emotions and described at length their biological adaptive value.

By the late 1920s, however, the theoretical importance of both affect and behavioral expressions of emotions began to be questioned. By that time, the method of introspection had been discredited, and affect thus lost both its theoretical appeal and its method of verification. Freud abandoned his notions linking repressed affect to symptom formation and proposed his well-known instinct or drive theories, in which the experience of affect was the *result* of increases or decreases in drive rather than the *cause* of symptom formation. Furthermore, not long after Watson proposed his theory of three innate emotions, research by Sherman (1927a, 1927b), and later Dennis (1940) led to dissatisfaction with the behavioral and expressive criteria for emotion. Although Watson had proposed that knowing the response, the researcher can predict the stimulus, Sherman argued that emotions can be identified by observers only if one already knows the stimulus circumstances. Sherman's data and arguments implied that emotions were ways of categorizing stimuli: The construct of emotion was unnecessary at best and a fiction at worst (Skinner, 1953).

By 1933, some psychologists were predicting that the term *emotion* would eventually disappear from psychology (Duffy, 1934; Meyer, 1933), a prediction that almost came true in the 1970s. Consider that in 1954, Woodworth and Schlosberg's *Experimental Psychology*, one of the standard reference sources of the time, included 3 chapters devoted to emotion, out of a total of 24. These described difficulties involved in measuring emotion, and proposed a dimensional approach to conceptualizing both psychophysiological reactions and the recognition of emotional expression in others. By 1971, when Kling and Riggs edited the next edition of the same reference work, however, there were *no* chapters devoted to emotion out of a total of 21 in the book. Moreover, there was not even an entry under "emotion" in the index, and only scattered references to related phenomena such as "conditioned emotional response" or "emotionality." Consider also the treatment of emotion in *Carmichael's Manual of Child Psychology* (Mussen, 1970). Although every edition prior to the 1970 version had a chapter on emotion, neither volume of the 1970 version did, and the indexes were equally skimpy on the topic, being limited to 23 entries. As seemed appropriate to phenomena of secondary importance, any topics of significance in the field of emotion were subsumed under other rubrics considered to be more central (e.g., Early Experience, Aggression, Attachment, Cognition).

Of course, there seemed to be noteworthy exceptions to the neglect of emotion, but these exceptions proved to be more apparent than real. Two influential ones deserve special mention. One is Schachter and Singer's (1962; Schachter, 1970) theory of physiological arousal, cognition, and emotion. In that approach, emotion was conceptualized as a composite of autonomic arousal plus cognition (i.e., the labeling by the subject of the reason for the arousal). By explicitly proposing that physiological arousal was the same for all emotions but that the cognitive labeling was not, Schachter and Singer implied that to understand emotion one must really understand cognition. Accordingly, Schachter's work fostered, rather than challenged, the beliefs that emotions had no specificity and were processes of secondary significance. Neither did Schachter and Singer discuss the role emotions played in perception, cognition, or behavior. Indeed, they treated emotion much like researchers treat color vision: They stopped at the level of self-report. For Schachter, then, like for many others, emotions were essentially epiphenomenal.

The second apparent exception took place within developmental psychology. From the 1940s through the 1960s, there was an abundance of studies of social smiling, anaclitic depression, stranger anxiety, separation anxiety, and numerous similar phenomena. However, except for the conceptualizations of theorists like Spitz (1965) and Bowlby (1951), the motivation for conducting such studies was to use emotions to index something else – usually a cognitive process. For instance, Kagan's interest in the emergence of smiling at 6–10 weeks of age was based on his theory that smiling results when sensory input is assimilated, effortfully, to emergent "schemas" (i.e., representations of prior inputs). His interest was in memory, not emotion. Accordingly, he never followed up his important early research with work on how joy may motivate rehearsal of a new memory skill, how it may help consolidate information into memory, or how it may mediate generalization of the skill to new tasks. His interests led him to study how memory changes with age and how it seems to have a maturational substrate (Kagan, 1976). The smile for Kagan and others (e.g., McCall, 1972; Watson, 1972) was thus just a convenient dependent variable, but any other dependent variable could as easily have served the same purpose.

Stranger and separation distress were also of interest at the time primarily because they provided information about cognitive development (Decarie, 1974; Schaffer, 1974). For instance, they were believed to measure discrepancies from schemes (Bronson, 1968), the establishment of a permanent image of the mother (Brossard, 1974), or the formation of unconfirmed hypotheses (Kagan, Kearsley, & Zelazo, 1978). Besides their theoretical promise as measures of cognitive development, stranger and separation distress had the methodological virtue of being indexed by discrete responses like crying or cessation of play – responses that were easily recorded and readily quantified. However, those investigating separation or stranger anxiety, like those studying the smile, only rarely speculated about the possible consequences or functions that these processes played in the social or intellectual life of the infant. (An exception: Emde, Gaensbauer, & Harmon, 1976.) As in Schachter and Singer's work, the emphasis was placed upon understanding "cold" cognition. Thus, although the developmental work was titularly on emotion, it surprisingly had little to do with it.

The shift in the Zeitgeist

This bleak background has been replaced in recent years with a dramatic reevaluation of the importance of emotion, as well as of its consequences. From the field of information processing – long noted for ignoring emotion – important theorists now consider the role of emotion in information processing to be one of the most critical contemporary problems for that field (Norman, 1980). A symposium on cognition-emotion relationships has recently been held at Carnegie-Mellon University (Fiske & Clarke, 1982), the very center of artificial intelligence and computer modeling of cognition. Attempts are now being made to use computers to simulate affective processes. Moreover, important applications of memory and cognitive research, such as studies of eyewitness testimony, have in particular begun to struggle with how emotions affect the registration, storage, and retrieval of information from memory (Goodman & Haith, 1982).

Researchers of social development are increasingly realizing that the study of interaction is predicated upon the study of emotions as goals, regulators, and monitors of dyadic relationships (Cohn & Tronick, 1982; Sroufe, 1979; Stern, 1977). Theorists who once specified "arousal and activation" as the goals of interaction have begun to propose hedonic processes instead to explain dyadic interaction (Brazelton, 1983). Such changes, in turn, have fostered research regarding individual differences in the ability of each dyad member to "read" emotional signals and to "transmit" such signals to the other (Emde, Harmon, & Gaensbauer, 1982; Field, 1982).

In the field of language, there is increasing interest in tracing the roots of symbolic communication to their possible nonverbal origins in human emotional interchanges (Bruner, 1977; Bullowa, 1979; Ziajka, 1981).

In perception, there is growing realization that emotional expressions constitute prototypic "affordances" (Gibson, 1979). Affordances are perceptual invariants that derive their meaning from the action consequences they specify for both the expressor and the perceiver – for example, a smiling person is likely to be approachable and is also likely to respond to the perceiver's overtures. Fascinating questions are being raised about the extent to which the perception of emotion in another generates an empathic, resonant reaction in oneself (Hoffman, 1978; Neisser, 1976).

Psychiatrists and clinical psychologists, who always viewed emotion as somewhat significant, are more frequently conceptualizing phenomena like empathy and moral development in affective, rather than purely cognitive, terms (e.g., Feshbach, 1982; Hoffman, 1978; Radke-Yarrow & Zahn-Waxler, 1982). Furthermore, new and excitingly detailed proposals for reviving the importance of affect in psychoanalytic theory are now being articulated (Emde, 1980a, 1980b).

It is customary to believe that important changes in the *Zeitgeist*, such as those currently taking place, represent merely the swing of the pendulum backward toward an unimaginative rediscovery of the problems and issues of an earlier day. However, this is not the case with the changes taking place today. There is a new and very different perspective on emotions – what Emde (1980a, 1980b) and Sroufe (1979) are calling the "organizational approach" – an approach, based on systems theory, that emphasizes the role of emotions as regulators and determinants of *both* intrapersonal and interpersonal behaviors, as well as stressing the adaptive role of emotions. Current research is thus abandoning the prior tendency to merely measure or index a central neurophysiological or feeling state and is beginning to explore how a subject's feeling state or emotional behavior impacts the perceptions, thoughts, or behaviors of that person or others (Charlesworth, 1982).

A second difference between contemporary emotion theory and that of the turn of the century is the proliferation of technologies of emotion measurement. These methodological advances are crucial to the organizational approach, which emphasizes the many alternative ways in which the same emotional state can be expressed. Among the new technologies of emotion measurement are several extremely sensitive methods of measuring facial movements (e.g., Ekman & Friesen, 1978; Izard, 1979; Schwartz, 1982). There now exists a means of recording electromyographic patterns of *covert* facial movement (e.g., Schwartz et al., 1976), a procedure that has proven extremely useful in documenting the characteristic expressive dampening of depressed patients and that shows promise as a diagnostic tool. There have also been major strides in the measurement of features in the voice that communicate emotional states (e.g., Scherer, 1981, 1982; Williams & Stevens, 1981), as well as how those vocal patterns influence therapeutic and family interaction. Gaze patterns and gestural expressions of emotional states, although not studied as thoroughly as the face or the voice, now are showing specificity of measurement (Exline, 1982; Scherer & Ekman, 1982). Furthermore, there have been important developments in the measurement of hemispheric specialization of emotion using the electroencephalograph (EEG) (Davidson & Fox, 1982; Fox & Davidson, 1983; Tucker, 1981). These advances in the application of EEG measurement may prove to be quite significant clinically in relationship to effects of brain lesions on patients. Perceptual, cognitive, and motoric deficits have previously been studied, but emotional changes all too often have been neglected in cases of brain damage.

A third difference between the new approaches to emotion and early conceptions concerns the types of questions researchers are asking – questions that would have been alien to Wundt (1904), James (1890), Watson (1930), Cannon (1927), and Allport (1924), although definitely not to McDougall (1908). These questions have to do with what produces emotions. Early approaches tended only cursorily to conceptualize how emotions were elicited. Many assumed that discrete stimuli, such as odors, restraint, pain, shock, conditioned stimuli, and so on, were prototypical of all instances of emotion elicitation. Today, by contrast, we are beginning to realize that the elicitation of emotion has less to do with discrete properties of stimulation and more to do with *how the individual relates past, present, and future events to his or her goals and strivings* (Roseman, 1979). This has also led to a major revision of our understanding of how cognition and emotion relate to one another – a revision reflected, albeit inadequately, in the current distinction between "hot" and "cold" cognitions. General intellectual capacities (e.g., object permanence, representational thought, perspective taking), which were once thought to be necessary and sufficient for the elicitation of emotion, are now known to be uncorrelated with the emotional phenomena they were once thought to explain. A special class of cognitions – those that monitor the relationship between events and the organism's goals – now seems to be the key to understanding both the elicitation of emotion and its specific quality.

The failure to consider these goal-relevant cognitions (i.e., what we call "appreciations" and Arnold [1960] and Lazarus [1968] have called "appraisals") has been one of the consistent problems in prior attempts to understand emotion. We use the term *appreciation* to reflect our conviction that high-level cognitions are neither necessary nor sufficient for the elicitation of emotion. For instance, it is well known by clinicians that merely cognizing a problem does not inevitably result in emotional changes. Moreover, in everyday life, we can fully "know" that an event is not dangerous, yet fear can persist in full intensity. The concept of appreciation is designed to take into consideration that *value* has been added to sensation, perception, or cognition, and that the value results from relating input to goal. It is also intended to connote that even stimuli that are believed reflexively to elicit emotional reactions will fail to do so depending upon the organism's goal. For instance, swaddling, contrary to widespread belief, does not invariably soothe a neonate: When the baby is hungry, swaddling is effective in reducing crying, but when the baby is satiated, it is not (Giacoman, 1971).

Because most human goals are socially constructed, most emotional reactions will be intimately linked to evaluations of how one fares in relation to those social goals. But not all goals are socialized. Some are prewired and relate to the survival of the neonate (a point implied by Emde [1982] in discussing the "pre-representational self "). Thus, if neonates possess such prewired goals, the possibility arises that the neonate's emotional life may be much more differentiated than has been believed previously. These theoretical consider-ations, along with very consistent maternal reports that 1- to 3-month-old infants show many more differentiated and contextually appropriate expressions than was ever thought possible (cf. Johnson et al., 1982; Klinnert et al., 1983) have led Izard (1977), Emde (1982), and Campos and his colleagues (1983) separately to propose that *there may be a core of differentiated affective continuity throughout the life-span*. It has led also to the proposition that the *relationships* of events to goals may constitute developmental invariants even though specific goals may change and new cognitive skills arise in the course of development. For example, a sensory event (e.g., impeding babies' movement when they are not hungry), related to a pre-adapted end-state, may induce anger in neonates (Stenberg, 1982); anticipation that an event may impede progress to a concrete goal may produce anger in 8-month-olds; nonverbal prohibitions frustrating an unseen goal of 24-month olds, may result in anger; a verbal remark thwarting progress toward a symbolic goal may inculcate anger in adults or adolescents, and so forth. Similar considerations apply to other fundamental emotions. We will discuss this assertion further in the following proposed framework.

Emotions as organizational constructs

Earlier, we mentioned that the new *Zeitgeist* in emotion theory involves an "organizational approach." In this section, we provide a summary and extension of major aspects of this approach. There are three ways in which emotions are considered to be organizational constructs: (1) Emotion terms permit quick and convenient summary of multiple functional relationships between stimulation and responses; (2) emotions influence both intrapsychic processes and inter-personal interactions; and (3) emotions are inextricably linked to the active and purposeful striving of the organism. We shall briefly expound on each of these uses of the "organizational" term.

Emotion words as constructs

One of the perplexing features of psychological phenomena is that the very same input to the organism can result in multiple outputs, and very different inputs can result in the same output. Strictly operationalist attempts to summarize these complex event–outcome relationships usually end in failure or in ecologically invalid experimentation that constrains unduly the possibilities of action by the organism. The most orthodox use of the concept of emotion as organizational involves the logic of underlying constructs. A construct is, of course, a term that simplifies the multiple functional relationships possible between variables. Constructs are particularly useful in cases when dependent variables are not highly correlated with one another, yet show some factor-analytic or theoretical coherence. They are also useful when very different independent variables are thought, again on a priori or a posteriori grounds, to tap a similar process in the organism. Miller (1959) used this approach to link multiple experimental means of increasing drives in laboratory rats with multiple means of measurement of drive increase.

One of the most important characteristics of emotions, like drives, is that they are manifested in multiple and somewhat independent ways and are elicited by multiple situational and imaginal events. For instance, a single event can elicit at least five different manifestations of an emotion such as anger: a particular facial configuration, a characteristic tone of voice, an abrupt gesture, a hostile reaction, or a specific autonomic pattern such as flushing of the face, dilation of certain arteries, and increases in diastolic blood pressure. It is rare that a given episode of anger results in changes across all the modes of expression, for at least three reasons.

First, individual differences influence the patterning of responses to stressors. The work of Jones (1930, 1950), Buck (1975, 1977), and Eysenck (1967) has demonstrated that subjects who are facially very expressive are often autonomically hyporesponsive, and subjects who are facially unresponsive are autonomically very reactive. Thus, across *sets* of response variables, very consistent event–reaction relationships can be found, but within a single response category, facial or autonomic, considerable variance is found.

Second, some testing contexts constrain the use of vocal, instrumental, or facial expressive reactions. One example of such a testing context influence is when a subject is tested in the company of another rather than alone. Ekman (1972) reported that Japanese subjects masked their negative facial expressions elicited by films when tested in the presence of an interviewer. A different contextual influence has been noted in studies of infants' reactions to strangers, where rather different outcomes are obtained depending upon whether the infant is permitted to move about freely or is constrained from movement (Horner, 1980).

Third, the manner of expression of an emotional construct can change dramatically in the course of development, yet the construct itself retains its significance in explaining behavior. Consider how the measurement of attachment can change in the course of development: Early in life, attachment of the infant to the care giver can be expressed primarily by the differential reinforcing potential of the mother (DeCasper & Fifer, 1980 on neonates); later, it is manifested by differential smiling (Spitz & Wolf, 1946); still later, by differential cardiac reactions to stressors in the presence of the care giver (Campos, 1976); still later by differential patterns of proximity-seeking, contact-maintenance, distance interaction, and so forth (Ainsworth et al., 1978); and during late toddlerhood, by language and gestural communication.

Failure to consider these alternative manifestations of attachment led not long ago to a sterile controversy about the utility of the construct of attachment. Some investigators, blindly equating the construct of attachment with a single index, discovered that 20-month-olds showed much less physical proximity-seeking than did 10-month-olds faced with similar stressors. The investigators then argued that the construct of attachment was useless, because the index of attachment suggested a sharp but counterintuitive decline in attachment between the first and second year of life. However, later research showed the fallacy of equating the construct of attachment with a single index: When attachment was measured by various alternative means, permitting both distal and proximal alternatives to physical closeness (such as smiling and soothing upon the mother's return) to define the nature of the child's attachment to the mother, stable individual differences were reported between the ages of 12 and 18 months (Waters, 1978). As Sroufe and Waters put it:

Infants who did not initiate contact and turned away when being held by mother on reunion, for example, may or may not have exhibited this *behavior* on reunion at 18 months. But they were likely to show some kind of avoidance (turning away, ignoring, gaze aversion, etc.). It is the organization of behavior, the adaptational patterns, the quality of the affective bond that has been shown to be stable, not particular discrete behaviors maintained by contingent maternal responses (1977a, p. 1193).

Not only can emotions be expressed in a multiplicity of ways, they can also be elicited by a plethora of events. For instance, anger can be elicited by prohibitions, insults, physical restraint, removal of desired objects, and numerous other events. Thus, if one has n possible elicitors of an emotional reaction, n possible means of expressing the hypothetical state, there are n^2 possible functional relationships, a state of affairs graphically portrayed in Figure 8.1A. It is here that the use of emotion terms as organizational constructs is useful. As can be seen in Figure 8.1B, the construct of "anger" neatly summarizes the multiple functional relationships possible between eliciting events and response outputs. In that figure, 9 functional relationships are reduced to 3 between input and construct, and 3 between construct and output. As Hinde (1972) points out, the greater the number of eliciting circumstances and the greater the number of response modes, the greater the economy of description provided by the emotion term. Moreover, given the typically low intercorrelations among alternative emotional reactions, there is a potentially

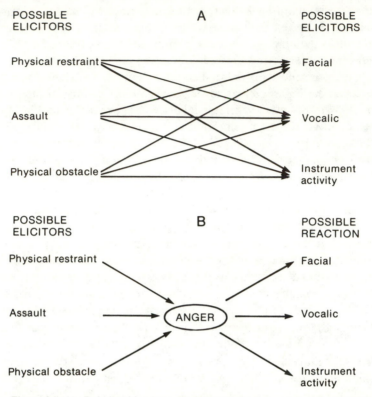

Figure 8.1(A). Relationships between four independent and four dependent variables (adapted from Hinde, 1972, which was based on Miller, 1959). (B) Relationships between four independent variables, one emotional construct, and four dependent variables (adapted from Hinde, 1972, which was based on Miller, 1959).

great increase in explanatory value gained through the use of the construct of anger.

Is there evidence that alternative means of measuring emotion exist? The use of emotion terms as organizational constructs depends upon the existence of several valid means of measuring emotion. Much research is still needed to determine whether facial, vocal, gestural, and instrumental behaviors *are* alternative measures of the same construct. However, results to date are quite promising. We know from the scholarly reviews of Izard (1971), Ekman, Friesen, and Ellsworth (1972), and Ekman (1972) that a once widespread belief that human observers *cannot* identify facial expressions of emotion in the absence of information about stimulus context is categorically wrong. Observers from both Western and non-Western cultures (Ekman, 1972; Izard, 1971), and even preliterate tribes (Ekman & Friesen, 1972; Ekman, Sorensen, & Friesen, 1969) can reliably identify six or seven actor-posed facial expressions (joy, sadness, surprise, anger, disgust, fear, and interest), (although preliterate groups had difficulty distinguishing fear from surprise [cf. Ekman & Friesen, 1972; Ekman, Sorensen, & Friesen, 1969; Heider, 1974]). Boucher & Carlson (1980) recently confirmed the studies with preliterate tribes, including the difficulty in identifying actor-posed fear expressions.

Although there should be some correspondence between actor-posed facial expressions and elicited facial expressions, studies of the latter are scarce. However, recent studies with human infants using a variety of naturalistic elicitors such as heights, vanishing objects, physical restraint, stranger approach, and the injection of medication have generated very good evidence for the theory-predicted facial expression patterning of anger, joy, pain, surprise, disgust, and, to a slight extent, fear (cf. Hiatt, Campos, & Emde, 1979; Izard et al., 1983; Izard et al., 1980; Stenberg & Campos, 1983; Stenberg, Campos, & Emde, 1983). Most of these studies were characterized by very precise scoring of facial movements, careful exclusion of contextual information, and concern to avoid statistical artifact in data analysis.

Much more research is needed to confirm these early findings with human infants, but results to date support the validity of theory-based templates of facial patterns.

The outcomes of studies regarding vocalic emotion are similar to those concerning facial emotion. Judgments of vocal expressions of emotion reveal high levels of agreement regarding which of the six to eight discrete emotions is being expressed (Scherer, 1981). However, in other respects, even more research is needed regarding vocal expression of emotion than regarding facial expression: To date, no studies have been made of preliterate tribes' identification of vocalic emotion, no breakthrough has taken place in identification of the vocal features and patterns specifying emotion, and preciously little research has used real-life situations to elicit emotional expressions in the voice. Nevertheless, despite the use made of artificial verbal content-eliminating devices (e.g., high-frequency filtration, random tape splicing, standard-content paragraph reading), there has been surprisingly high agreement among judges about the nature of the emotion expressed (see Scherer, 1981, 1982). A particularly dramatic study of the power of acoustic patterns to specify emotions has come from Scherer's work using the Moog synthesizer (Scherer & Oshinsky, 1977): By manipulating seven acoustic parameters, Scherer was able to demonstrate statistically significant interjudge agreement for pleasantness, activity, anger, surprise, sadness, and happiness. Scherer's pioneering work on how parameters of *music* can specify affect is likely to spawn much research on the emotion-eliciting capacities of musical passages.

The studies to date on vocal expression of emotion by young human infants (expected to have had minimal socialization) have been few and disappointing. All are seriously flawed in design and data analysis. For instance, Wolff (1969) excited developmentalists with his pronouncement that neonates utter cries specifying hunger, anger, or pain. Later research, however, has failed to confirm Wolff's findings, which were based on a very small sample (Murray, 1979), and which apparently confounded acoustic *intensity* with acoustic patterning in the identification of the three types of cries. Research on vocal emotions using methodologically sound but ecologically valid designs is desperately needed. Since we now have ascertained which facial expression patterns are elicited by certain situations, we can use this information to help anchor inferences regarding the emotion specified by vocal expressions under the same eliciting conditions.

Research on autonomic patterns related to emotions has primarily concerned heart rate. A large number of studies now confirm the early findings that heart rate in infancy slows down in states of nondistressed attentiveness and accelerates in conditions of fear or distress (Campos, 1976; Graham & Jackson, 1970; Provost & Decarie, 1979; Skarin, 1977; Sroufe & Waters, 1977b; Vaughn & Sroufe, 1979). However, no studies have attempted to show that heart-rate acceleration is specific to discrete emotional states, and such a finding seems unlikely. Evidence to date links heart-rate accelerations to states that antedate crying or fussing (Campos & Emde, 1978) or preparation for motor activity (Campos, 1976; Obrist, 1976). Since fussing and motor activity accompany many negative emotions, one would expect heart rate to increase when the infant is in any of these states. Indeed, there is some evidence that in states of intense joy infants show a cardiac acceleration, although one that is much more modest than that shown in states that precede eventual distress (Reich et al., 1978).

Heart-rate levels and variability in response to cognitively engaging stimuli have been related to the temperamental dimension of wariness and inhibition by Kagan and his co-workers (Kagan, 1982; Kagan et al., 1983). Wary infants show high and nonfluctuating heart-rate levels; nonwary infants show low and variable heart rates. Kagan's results are thus consistent with those obtained by other researchers on the relationship between heart-rate reactivity and distress, wariness, or fear; they promise to open anew the study of biological processes that underlie temperamental dimensions in infants and young children. His most recent findings demonstrate a remarkable degree of continuity between 2 and 5 years of age in patterns of wariness in his samples of subjects (Kagan et al., 1983).

Recently, Campos and his associates (1983) have speculated that autonomic reactions are far from "vegetative" (in the sense of having no interaction with the environment), and that certain autonomic reactions (usually the ones with clear social communicative significance) seem prima facie to have emotional specificity. Reactions to sexual ardor are a good example: Penile erection and vaginal lubrication are autonomically mediated reactions very specific to, and strongly communicative of, that state, although in our culture these are physically masked by clothing. Tears are another case in point, usually being expressed in states of sadness or when sadness is blended with other fundamental emotional expressions. Other examples include reddening of the ears in embarrassment, dryness of the mouth in anxiety, flushing of the face in anger, and blanching of the face in fear. Moreover, to the extent that vocalizations show emotional response specificity, and to the extent that respiratory maneuvers support vocalizations, respiration parameters seem likely to show response specificity as well. Most autonomic psychophysiologists have not seriously considered these possibilities when discussing the age-old question regarding whether specific autonomic response patterns are associated with particular emotional states. However, psychophysiologists may be like the proverbial man searching for the key under the lamppost: They have centered their research on the measures for which easy quantification exists (GSR, heart rate, finger pulse volume, etc.), rather than on the measures that, albeit more difficult to quantify, seem more likely to yield the long-sought autonomic response specificity.

Stenberg, Campos, and Emde (1983) and Stenberg and Campos (1983) have studied facial flushing as an index of anger in infancy and obtained promising results; however, because neither study attempted to demonstrate differentiation of anger-eliciting information from nonanger conditions, the specificity of emotional measurement provided by facial flushing has not yet been documented.

Respiration has rarely been studied in human infants, perhaps because it is more difficult to quantify than are many other autonomically mediated responses. However, as noted earlier, because of the very close relationship between respiratory parameters and vocal expressions, and because of the specificity evident to date in studies of vocal expression of emotion, this response parameter deserves further investigation.

Action tendencies have been widely used as indexes of discrete emotional states (see Hiatt, Campos, & Emde, 1979). Avoidance and retreat have been used often to index fear; aggression and attack to index anger; repetition of a successful action to index joy; continuation of looking to index surprise; and slumped posture and prolonged immobility to index sadness.

Alternative methods of measuring feeling states related to discrete emotions have also recently been developed and validated (Kotsch, Gerbing, & Schwartz, 1982).

Taken as a whole, then, the findings to date suggest that emotion as a construct organizes many very different responses and expressive reactions. Researchers, however, face a serious problem in certain applications of this organizational notion. When different infants express the same state in differing ways and with different latencies of reactions, enormous statistical and conceptual problems arise. How does the researcher analyze the obtained response pattern in an intelligent and yet unbiased fashion? If the researcher samples only those behaviors that are predicted to reflect the hypothesized emotion, Type 1 error can easily result. On the other hand, if he or she samples only those behaviors that fall within a time window specified a priori, Type 2 error as well as underestimation of the elicitation of the emotion takes place. This problem may well be one of the most crucial ones in emotion measurement

today, especially given the emphasis on both naturalistic and home observations
of emotional expression.

Emotion as organizer of intrapsychic and interpersonal processes

One of the reasons for the recent generation of interest in human emotions is
that, contrary to once-widespread opinion, emotions clearly influence psychological functions. As we alluded earlier, affect and emotion have long been
treated as epiphenomenal (Kagan, 1978; Ryle, 1950). Moreover, when *not*
considered epiphenomenal, emotions were considered to be *disorganizing*,
that is, disruptions to the smooth execution of cognitive or motoric plans.
However, the new systems view gives every aspect of the organism a role in
total adaptation, leading researchers to look for the possible adaptive functions
for "regulatory" roles of emotions rather than the disorganizing functions. In
systems theory, *regulation* is distinguished from causation insofar as the role
is context-dependent. As we shall soon see, the role of emotions is extremely
context-dependent – a fact that has created difficulties for those proposing
linear models of the influence of affect and emotion. Thus, under some conditions, which unfortunately we have only recently begun to conceptualize,
emotions will play a crucial and adaptive role in human functioning; in other
circumstances, they will play no role at all; and in still others, the role will
range from negligible to disruptive.

Emotion as an organizer of behavior in social settings. The most exciting
contemporary research is taking a contextually dependent view of the way in
which emotions influence social, perceptual, or cognitive processes. Consider
the recent research on affective communication in infancy, including that on
the so-called social referencing phenomenon (Campos & Stenberg, 1981;
Feinman, 1982; Klinnert et al., 1983). In the context of experiencing an uncertain
event, a person tends to seek out and utilize the facial, vocal, and gestural
emotional expressions of others to help disambiguate the uncertainty (Campos
& Stenberg, 1981). A particularly dramatic study with 1-year-old infants using
a modified visual cliff exemplifies the power of this phenomenon of social
referencing, as well as the contextual-dependence of regulation by emotional
communication (Sorce et al., 1981). When an infant attempting to cross to
the mother over a visual cliff is faced with an apparent 4-foot drop-off, she
or he avoids crossing to her. If there is no drop-off at all on a modified deep
side, the baby usually does not even seek affective information, and the information that is received does not influence the tendency to cross to the
mother. However, if the drop-off on the deep side is set at an intermediate
level – somewhat intrinsically fear provoking but not so much that crossing
is impeded entirely – infants characteristically (a) look to the mother and (b)

use the specific *facial* affective information the mother provides to determine whether to cross to her or not. If mothers in the Sorce study posed a fear face, no infant, out of 17 tested, crossed the deep side. On the other hand, if the mother was instructed to pose a joy face, 15 of 19 infants crossed – a highly significant difference. Similar findings were obtained when mothers posed anger or interest faces: Only 11% of infants tested crossed when mother posed anger, whereas 75% crossed when she posed interest. When another group of infants was exposed to the mother's pose of sadness (an emotion contextually inappropriate to crossing or not crossing the deep side of the visual cliff), an intermediate number of infants crossed (33%), and infants showed evidence of extensive vacillation over whether to cross or not.

Subsequent research (Klinnert et al., 1983) has demonstrated that emotional expressions of other adults, and not merely the attachment figure, regulate infants' behavior. When an ambiguous toy moves into a room where baby, mother, and a familiarized female adult are located, the familiarized adult's facial expressions strongly influence the baby's behavior. If the adult poses a joy face, the infant tends to approach and touch the toy significantly more than when the adult poses a fear face even when the mother's expressions are controlled.

Other studies have demonstrated that vocal expressions of emotion (specifically, fear, anger, and joy) significantly influence the reactions to a novel toy of infants as young as 8.5 months (Svejda & Campos, 1982): Infants approach a toy more closely, and resume activity more quickly, following a happy vocalization from the mother than following either an angry or fearful vocalization.

Finally, even the infant's reactions to strangers, long considered to be a biologically prewired phenomenon (Freedman, 1974), can be influenced by the emotional communication between the mother and her infant (Boccia & Campos, 1983). It is now known that the entry and approach of a stranger is an uncertain event for the infant: The infant's checking back-and-forth between the mother and the stranger does *not* seem to be a facial comparison process eventually eliciting a "discrepancy" reaction (Campos & Stenberg, 1981). Rather, it seems to be a deliberate search for emotional information from the mother (Feinman, 1982; Sorce, Emde, & Frank, 1982). If, upon the entrance of a stranger, the mother utters a single abrupt and unfriendly hello and poses a slight frown on her face, 8.5-month-old infants show marked cardiac accelerations to the approach of the stranger and less smiling and more distress than when the mother poses a cheery hello and a smiling face. In the latter condition, the baby's heart rate *decelerates*.

Thus, both social and nonsocial environmental stimuli can acquire very different valences as a result of the process of emotional communication between one person and another. Although the studies to date have concerned infants, the power of emotional expressive communication is not limited to the period of childhood. On the contrary, it is part of everyday interpersonal interaction, influencing everything from friendship to the doctor–patient relationship, as several researchers (e.g., Milmoe et al., 1974) have argued. However, the studies to date also emphasize the importance of context for understanding emotional communication and call for extensive elaboration of what could be called "a theory of context-dependence." Sroufe, Waters, and Matas (1974), for different reasons, have also emphasized the importance of context in understanding the quality and the intensity of emotional reactions.

Emotion as an organizer of cognitive processes. If emotional communication by face, voice, and gesture is such a powerful regulator of behavior in social settings, it is no less an influence on cognitive processing. Emotional communication can mediate learning processes, which are crucial for survival. Infants and toddlers need not learn to avoid dangerous plants, electric outlets, and similar hazards by directly experiencing harmful effects. Nor are verbal communication skills necessary for such learning. Is it not likely that the infant acquires such adaptive habits (and sometimes some maladaptive ones also) by associating specific hazards with the care giver's emotional communications?

Such a learning process may help explain the development of fear of heights in human infants: A wealth of data now demonstrates that infants become wary of heights only *after* the acquisition of crawling (Bertenthal, Campos, & Barrett, 1983; Campos et al., 1978), despite the widespread belief that fear of heights is innate. But precisely how does crawling influence wariness of heights? By providing for increased possibility of falling accidents? That is not likely. Neither our research nor that of Walk (1966) supports such an explanation for the typical subject's reactions. Is it possible that the infant acquires such a fear by associating heights with the mother's emotional reactions to near falls and to precarious situations? Bowlby (1973) has discussed how emotional expressions can mediate fear contagion, as has Bandura (1977). Like Bowlby and Bandura, we propose that emotional communication subserves biologically adaptive learning. If that is so, then it is particularly surprising that no studies on such expression-mediated learning have been attempted with either human infants or toddlers and that only a few studies with monkeys have been attempted (Miller, 1967).

There have been many other recent attempts to relate emotions to the registration, storage, and retrieval of information from memory. These studies differ from the preceding in manipulating feeling states or central affective processes rather than expressions. This new line of research revives, although in methodologically much more sophisticated ways, a theory that has a long but frequently interrupted history. For instance, Bain and Spencer had proposed in the nineteenth century that humans tend to remember pleasant experiences and to forget unpleasant ones, and Freud had proposed in numerous places that one is prone to deny unpleasant perceptions and to repress undesired memories. Rapaport (1961) summarized many of these classic views and presented the findings of several experiments related to the issue of whether the *quality* or the *intensity* of an emotional reaction influences memory.

Recently, these questions have been addressed again in a well-designed series of investigations by Bower (1981) and his associates at Stanford. One of Bower's experiments captures particularly well the importance of emotions as organizational constructs. In that study, subjects were presented with lists of material to be learned while they were in each of four hypnotically induced states: joy, sadness, anger or fear. The subjects were then brought back to the laboratory for a recall test that was conducted while the subjects were in either the same or a different emotional state as the one during initial memorization of the list. Bower's preliminary findings were dramatic: Retention was highest when recall of a list took place in the same emotional state as in acquisition – regardless of what that state was; it was poorest when recall occurred in the emotional state opposite to that in acquisition (e.g., sadness/joy; anger/fear); and it was intermediate when recall took place in the other two emotional states. Bower concluded that hypnotically induced feeling states created "nodes" around which registration of information into memory was organized, which nodes were reinstated when the subject was later in the same affective state but not when he or she was later in a different state.

Bower (1981) also described how emotions influence the cognitive processes of free association, semantic elaboration, interpretation of imaginative stories, and selective learning, as well as certain perceptual effects. The influence of emotion on cognition thus was shown to be powerful and widespread.

Zajonc (1980) has also been influential in restoring interest in how emotions influence both cognitions and perceptions. He has sharply challenged the belief that affect necessarily follows cognition and has presented evidence in support of the notion that affect and cognition show different functional relationships with environmental stimulation presented at the threshold of identification. Beginning with the assumption, established by some of his earlier work, that familiarity with a stimulus leads to preference for it, Zajonc familiarized subjects with some nonsense figures and not others. Then, he presented both familiar and unfamiliar figures at perceptual threshold to these subjects and asked them to rate the figures (whether correctly identified or not) for the degree of their preference for them and for whether or not they had seen them before. His results indicated that subjects showed an affective preference for familiar stimuli even when they could not identify the stimulus as familiar or not (Kunst-Wilson & Zajonc, 1980). From this and other lines of evidence, Zajonc concluded that affect and cognition show separate sources of determination.

Emotions have always been known to influence performance on various tasks, with the intensity of emotional arousal influencing performance in an inverted-U-shaped fashion (the Yerkes-Dodson Law). As usually conceptualized, however, the quality of the discrete emotional state has not been treated as a parameter of the relationship between intensity of arousal and performance. It is conceivable, however, that positive emotions like joy may show inverted-U-shaped functions, which peak at very high levels of arousal, with performance suffering only when joy approaches mania. On the other hand, anger might show inverted-U performance, which peaks at fairly low levels of intensity. This possibility has been recently investigated by Meng and her associates (1983) with 16-month-old infants. The infants were divided into two groups, one of which underwent the stress of two maternal separations and the other of which played intently with a series of puppets. After a brief interval, the subjects were given a problem to solve adapted from one designed by Bruner and Koslowski (1972): The infants rotated a bar away from them in order to bring a toy on the other side of the bar toward them. The results obtained were quite promising: The greater the intensity of happiness in the puppet task, the better the performance up to a certain point, then performance decreased. On the other hand, the greater the intensity of distress elicited by the separation, the poorer the subsequent performance. In short, different functions – one curvilinear and one linear – related emotional intensity and performance for the two hedonically different background conditions.

We know from classic studies, such as those of Easterbrook (1959), that emotion influences perception by constricting the visual field toward the center of vision, and we also know that the social class (and hence the probable value to a child of money) influences the child's report of the apparent size of a coin (Bruner & Postman, 1947). However, most of the classic research has not related perception to discrete emotions. Yet, if discrete emotions are adaptive, one would expect certain perceptual processes to be influenced quite specifically by the nature of the emotion. Does anger, for instance, *raise* pain thresholds as an adaptive preparation for the likelihood of injury following attack? Does fear lower thresholds of sensitivity to sudden stimuli and to certain environmental events that can specify danger? Does the emotion of disgust influence taste and smell thresholds? Investigation of questions such as these deserves careful attention (Erdelyi, 1974).

Emotions as related to the strivings of the individual

If one made a census of studies on emotions, one would find that most investigations fall into three categories: Those on the central nervous system mechanisms of emotion, those on the peripheral autonomic, facial, and skeletal expressions of emotion, and finally, those on how peripheral feedback influences both the central processes and the reports of conscious feeling states. Remarkably few studies are directed at specifying the conditions under which a discrete emotional state is elicited and when the state is not elicited. The studies that have been made of the elicitation of emotion have been inordinately mechanistic, such as the studies on the conditioning of various emotions, usually fear and dependency or affection, and the studies of autonomic reactions to cold, ischemic pain, loud noises, or other physical stressors.

In the 1960s and 1970s many developmental psychologists thought they had abandoned mechanistic interpretations of the elicitation of emotion by postulating the important role that cognitions have in eliciting affect. However, as we shall see, those studies were based on just as mechanistic a conception of the organism, and were just as unsuccessful in explaining emotional elicitation, as were the studies using conditioning and discrete stressors.

Hebb's (1946) theory was the inspiration for most of these explanatory attempts. Initially, the theory attempted to explain fear of unusual or novel events without reference either to maturational factors or to conditioning. It was an attractively simple theory: When stimulation was processed in the central nervous system, it laid down residues in the form of "phase sequences." An input that was sufficiently similar to previous inputs to activate the phase sequences but not similar enough to maintain the correct timing and patterning of neural events in the brain would create neurological disorganization. Such disorganization, in turn, would be expressed peripherally as fear.

This simple theory promised to explain a broad array of emotional reactions besides fear, such as surprise, boredom, interest, laughter, and so on (see McCall & McGhee, 1977, for elaboration of these points). Without past experience with stimuli, according to Hebb's discrepancy theory and its many subsequent revisions (e.g., Bronson, 1968; McCall & McGhee, 1977), new stimuli do not produce disruption: The stimulus is ignored or attended to minimally. If the stimulus is very familiar, it matches the central store too well and does not command attention either – habituation or boredom results (Berlyne, 1960; Sokolov, 1963) and so forth. Although the theory did not attempt to explain sadness, disgust, and anger, it was nevertheless very influential. Unfortunately, the theory was not successful in explaining the elicitation of discrete emotions. It could not account for the extensive time gap between the infant's initial discrimination of mother from stranger (variously placed at 6 to 12 weeks) and the emergence of prevalent overt fear of strangers (which occurs at 7 to 9 months). It also could not account for the fact that some types of discrepant events (e.g., receipt of an unexpected windfall profit) elicited joy, while other discrepant events elicited anger, and still others elicited sadness. Hebb himself, in a later publication (1949), pointed out that under some conditions discrepancy elicited joy, in others anger, in still others puzzlement, and so forth. He left unexplained precisely what converted a discrepancy reaction into a specific emotional state.

We propose that for a discrepant event (or, for that matter, any event) to acquire emotional "meaning" it must be related to the goals of the individual. Thus, an unexpected snowfall will bring joy to someone who wants to ski, fear to someone needing to travel a long distance to another city, anger to someone who needs to shovel a driveway, pride to someone whose theory predicted it, and even guilt, if someone interprets it as the punishment expected from God for a transgression.

A few recent attempts to conceptualize emotion elicitation have noted the central importance of goals. Roseman (1979), for instance, described six factors in all that enter into the elicitation of most discrete emotions. Two we have already mentioned: One is a dimension of "motivational state" – defined as what the organism wants or does not want; the other is the person's "situational state" – the extent to which the goal appears achievable. The simplest emotions – joy, distress, sorrow, and relief – involve a comparison between what a person wants and what he has. According to Roseman, the experience of more complex emotions involves the interplay of other factors related to the comparison between state and goal. For instance, a third factor, "probability," by which Roseman means the subject's estimate of the likelihood that something desirable or undesirable will happen, is related to the elicitation of hope and fear. Hope is the anticipation of joy or relief, whereas fear is the anticipation of sorrow or distress. When a fourth factor, "agency," is added, pride, dislike, and a shamelike state called regret can be predicted. Agency refers to one's attribution of causality for the ongoing situation. A fifth factor, called "legitimacy," involves the perception of the fairness of the actions of others to oneself. It plays a role in elicitation of anger and guilt. Finally, the unexpectedness of an event influences emotion primarily by increasing the intensity of its experience and expression.

Roseman's approach has many difficulties. A major one is its failure to consider the developmental roots of some of the emotions he is attempting to explain. Thus, anger expressions are clearly observable by 4 months of age, but are we to say that the 4-month-old has a sense of "legitimacy"? Two-month-olds express fear to looming stimuli. Are we to say that such a young infant has a well-developed sense of probability? Moreover, the theory in its original form ignores important complexities in the development of certain emotions. Guilt, for instance, may require experience in perceiving the emotional reactions of others in certain situations (Hoffman, 1982), as well as complex capacities to internalize social rules. Roseman's approach does not do full justice to these complexities. Nevertheless, his conceptual framework represents a valuable first step in postulating some of the processes influencing the elicitation of emotion.

A new perspective on emotional development

Postulates

Not only have our views regarding the nature of *emotion* changed, our conceptualization of how emotions *develop* has changed as well. Until recently, it was generally believed that each primary emotion *emerged* at a particular age, much as crawling or sitting up emerge. Now, however, the field is beginning to view emotional development as a much more complex process. We would like to propose five postulates to describe the most important features of emotional development:

1. There is an invariant core of affective continuity across the life-span.
2. The relationship between emotional expression and emotional experience changes with development.
3. Coping responses to emotion change with development.
4. The complexity of emotion changes with development.
5. Receptivity to the emotional expressions of others changes with development.

We will now examine each of these postulates in turn.

There is an invariant core of affective continuity. Although Izard (1977, 1978) and Emde (1982) have also proposed related notions, the idea of an invariant core of affective continuity is unfamiliar. We believe that each basic emotion (e.g., anger, surprise, joy, affection, sexual ardor, fear, or sadness) is best represented as a *family* of closely related emotions. Each family is specified by an invariant relationship between a *type* of goal and a particular *appreciation* of where the person stands relative to attaining that goal. Table 8.1 presents types of goals and appreciations associated with some basic emotion families.

We view each basic emotion as a family because, despite the existence of an invariant *core* emotion, each particular instance of the emotion is likely to differ somewhat from all others. This is especially true when one examines emotion across the life-span. For example, the fear that a 3-month-old seems to express in response to a looming stimulus (cf. Yonas, 1981) is likely to be different from that of an adult upon hearing that all of his/her financial assets are in jeopardy because of a projected change in the stock market. In these two examples, the *level of goal* differs: The threat to the baby is loss of the physical integrity of the self, whereas the threat to the adult is loss of the integrity of the self-concept. Moreover, the level of the *appreciation* differs: The baby faces the quick approach of a concrete object, whereas the adult *thinks* of an impending event's effect on a symbolic, socialized goal. Obviously, maintenance of respect for oneself as a provider for one's family would not be a goal for a child. What is invariant is the type of goal (the maintenance of integrity of the self) and the appreciation (that there is a low probability of achieving a goal unless remedial action is taken).

The relationship between emotional expression and emotional experience changes with development. We believe that during a brief period after birth, the emotional expressions manifested by the infant (e.g., the smile or a fully patterned angry facial expression) may be poorly coordinated with the underlying

Table 8.1. *Generalized schema for predicting elicitation of some basic emotions*

Emotion	Goal	Appreciation	Action tendency	Adaptive function
Joy	Any *significant* objective	Goal is perceived or predicted to be attained	Approach, energizing	Reinforcement of successful strategy; facilitation of rehearsal of new skill; encouragement of response to new challenges; social message to initiate or continue interaction
Anger	Same as above	Perception of, or anticipation of, an obstacle to attainment of goal; perception of obstacle as not easily removable	Elimination (not just removal) of properties of an object that make it an obstacle	Restoration of progress toward a goal; effecting a change in behavior of a social other; in later development, revenge, retaliation
Sadness	Securing or maintaining an engagement with either an animate or an inanimate object	Perception of the goal as unattainable	Disengagement	Conservation of energy; eventual redirection of resources to other pursuits perceived to be more attainable; encouragement of nurturance from others
Fear	Maintenance of integrity of the self, including self-survival and later, self-esteem	Perception that the goal is not likely to be attained, *unless* protective action is taken	Flight, withdrawal	Survival; avoidance of pain; maintenance of self-esteem; alerting others to avoid the situation and/or help one
Interest	Engagement or involvement in a task or event	Perception that information is potentially relevant to *any* goal	Receptor orientation; processing of information	Extraction of information from environment; communication of willingness to enter into a relationship, consider future action

emotional state, probably because of neurological immaturity. Stenberg and Campos (1983), for example, found that, in response to restraint, neonates manifest some nonanger facial components (eye closing and tongue protrusion) along with anger components. It seems possible that the inappropriate components constitute "overflow" or "noise" in the expression. That is, because of neurological immaturity, both contextually inappropriate (e.g., those related to disgust or pain states) and appropriate components are expressed simultaneously. Another example is the rapid eye movement sleep state smile of the neonate. Although it is now clear that this smile is not associated with gas, as had once been believed (cf. Emde & Harmon, 1972), it is not clear what does trigger it. It seems quite possible and even likely that this smile is *not* a reflection of joy, as later smiles will be.

After this early period, expressions are likely to become more closely coordinated with the corresponding emotional state. However, as early as 3 months of age, infants may begin to be exposed to socialization aimed at dissociating expression of emotion from the emotional state (Malatesta & Haviland, 1982). By late childhood and early adulthood, few emotions are expressed completely freely; all may be subject to control in accordance with cultural "display rules," personal display rules, and so on (cf. Ekman, 1980). It is likely that control of expression in turn influences the emotional state of the expressor (cf. Izard, 1971; Laird, 1974). Moreover, it is also possible that minute, covert facial muscle movements corresponding to the "true" emotion continue to promote some experience of that emotion (cf. Schwartz et al., 1976). Still, there is no doubt that overt expression may not resemble underlying emotion.

Coping responses to emotion change with development. Our third postulate concerns an obvious yet neglected feature of emotional development. As a person becomes more competent motorically and cognitively, there arise new capacities for coping with emotions and for short-circuiting elicitation of a particular emotion. Such coping capacities dramatically influence the impact of emotion by (a) changing the phenomenological *experience* of emotion and (b) changing the *regulatory impact* of emotion. For example, when infants acquire the ability to crawl, they can better control interactions with strangers. As mobile individuals, they may ensure that their sensorimotor goals are not thwarted by the actions of strangers. Accordingly, an infant who would otherwise be distressed at interacting with a stranger may not only avoid becoming distressed but may even show pleasure at interacting with the unfamiliar person. Alternatively, if the stranger's actions begin to arouse wariness in the infant, the infant may withdraw and thus prevent the negative emotion from becoming intense. In fact, as Gunnar (Gunnar-Von Gnechten, 1978; Gunnar, 1980) has demonstrated, coping skills may transform negative emotion into pleasurable feelings of efficacy, feelings that should motivate further exploration of novel events.

The complexity of emotion changes with development. One way in which emotions become more complex has been discussed: Expression may not match feeling. Additionally, cognitive development may potentiate the development of a new appreciation of the relevance of events to goals. Whereas a young infant may be able to relate only one aspect of ongoing events to his or her current goals, an older infant may bring to bear multiple aspects of the situation. For example, whereas a young infant may invariably be upset by a loud, novel toy, an older infant may become pleased by the event if adults who are present react with encouraging, positive emotions (Klinnert, 1981). Furthermore, complex emotions, which we believe include shame, guilt, envy, pride, depression, and many others, may become part of the child's emotional life once he or she can appreciate the relevance of many aspects of the situation to socialized goals.

We believe that complex emotions are best conceptualized as patterns (Izard, 1972), or intercoordinations among particular emotions, each of which is relevant to attaining a particular socialized goal. Table 8.2 summarizes the goals and appreciations involved in some complex emotions. The basic emotions involved in each complex state are detectable in the expressions, gestures, and action tendencies of the complex emotions, as well as in the feelings and appreciations involved. Shame, for example, which involves sadness at losing the love or esteem of others, includes a drooping posture, tucked head, and occasional tears. Guilt, moreover, which involves anger at oneself for thwarting one's view of oneself as moral, includes an action tendency of expiation. As Berscheid and Walster (1967), Regan, Williams, and Sparling (1972), and others have demonstrated, inculcation of guilt in a subject increases the likelihood that the subject will engage in altruism, perhaps to reinstate a view of himself or herself as moral. Interestingly, given that guilt seems also to involve a fear of punishment, such a subject is often most altruistic toward persons *other* than the one injured by the guilt-inducing transgression. Perhaps fear of retribution arouses an action tendency to avoid the recipient of the offense.

Receptivity to the emotional expressions of others changes with development. Because emotions are intimately connected with the process of social communication, the study of emotional development is incomplete without an analysis of how receptivity to emotional signals changes with age. The study of the receptive aspects of emotion, however, is among the most neglected topic in the entire field. To date, the most thorough developmental analysis is that of Charlotte Buhler (e.g., Buhler, 1930; Buhler & Hetzer, 1928, cited in Kreutzer & Charlesworth, 1973). She studied infants' responses to a positive face, a negative face, to postive and negative voices, and to threatening and

Table 8.2. *Generalized schema for predicting elicitation of more complex emotions*

Emotion	Goal	Appreciation	Action tendency	Adaptive function
Shame	Maintenance of others' respect and affection; preservation of self-esteem	Perception of loss of another's respect/affection; perception that others have observed one doing something bad	Like those of sadness, anger (at self), and fear	Maintenance of social standards
Guilt	Meeting one's own internalized standards	Anticipation of punishment because one has not lived up to an internalized standard	Like those of fear and anger	Encouragement of moral behavior
Envy	Obtaining a desired object	Perception that an object cannot be had because another has it and one's deficits prevent oneself from attaining the object	Like those of sadness and anger	Motivation of achievement to obtain similar goods
Depression	Having the respect and affection of *both* others and oneself	Perception of lack of love or respect from both others and oneself; perception of lack of possibility of attaining any very significant goal	Like sadness and anger (at self)	Elicitation of affection and nurturance from others

affectionate arm gestures, and reported that by the fifth month of age, some infants were capable of "responding appropriately" to angry facial expressions. By 7 months, the reaction to such expressions was evident in her entire sample.

Buhler (1930) subsequently constructed a developmental scale, suggesting that at 5 months infants responded with the appropriate emotional or behavioral expression to *combinations* of vocal and facial information, at 6 months they responded to vocal emotional information without accompanying facial information, and at 7 months they responded to facial emotional information without vocal accompaniment. At 9 months, infants were expected to respond differently to threatening versus friendly gestural information.

These important findings have been followed up by remarkably few studies, and these have been unpublished (e.g., Kreutzer & Charlesworth, 1973; Klinnert, Sorce, & Emde, 1982). In a recent article, Klinnert and her associates (1983) attempted to integrate what was known about the development of a child's utilization of facial expression information and proposed that such utilization proceeded through several levels.

The first level, predicted to last from birth to about 6 weeks of age, is characterized by minimal attention to internal details of visual gestalts like the face (Hainline, 1978; Haith, Bergman, & Moore, 1977; Maurer & Salapatek, 1976). This characteristic impedes visual access to the areas of the face that specify emotional information; hence, the neonate is not expected to discriminate consistently among facial expressions of emotion, let alone utilize the information for behavior regulation.

The second level, predicted to last from the time that infants reliably begin scanning interior details of the face until about 4 or 5 months, is characterized by the ability to *discriminate* facial expressions that specify emotional states without necessarily appreciating the emotional *meaning* of such expressions. Numerous studies (e.g., Barrera & Maurer, 1981; LaBarbera et al., 1976; Young-Browne, Rosenfeld, & Horowitz, 1977) have shown that 3- and 4-month-olds dishabituate to changes in facial expressions in pictorial displays. However, as has been pointed out repeatedly in the literature on infant perception (e.g., Appel & Campos, 1977; Lamb & Campos, 1982), dishabituation to changes in complex visual displays (e.g., change from a happy to an angry face) may be mediated by a featural, rather than a configurational, discrimination. For instance, Oster and Ewy (cited in Oster, 1981) demonstrated discrimination of smiling from nonsmiling faces only when teeth were visible in the smile, thus raising the possibility that contour density may have mediated the apparent discrimination of happiness from other emotions.

Other studies that at first seemed to imply early appreciation of others' emotions can be explained more parsimoniously. Studies by Tronick (e.g., Cohn & Tronick, 1982; Tronick et al., 1978) have shown that when mothers remain still-faced or depress their level of interaction, 1- to 3-month-olds withdraw and become fussy. These findings, however, are interpretable as effects of maternal noncontingency to infants' responses. They lack the experimental operations necessary to infer that infants appreciate the emotional state of the mother.

The third level involves what we have called "emotional resonance": The infant reacts with a positive or negative expression, depending upon the affective quality specified by the facial configuration. It is during this age period, which Klinnert and her associates (1983) predicted to last from 4 or 5 months to 9 months of age, that infants in both Buhler's (1930) and Kreutzer and Charlesworth's (1973) studies began responding emotionally to others' facial and vocal displays of emotion.

Whereas in the third level, discrete emotional communication may first take place between the infant and another person, in the fourth level, which begins at about 8 to 9 months of age, the communication between infant and another may be extended to include a third event in the environment. During this period, the infant can appreciate the environmental target of the other person's emotional reaction, much as the infant at this age begins to understand the referent of the mother's pointing or gaze behavior (cf. Scaife & Bruner, 1975). Accordingly, during this period, social referencing may begin.

Further changes in the understanding of emotions take place in subsequent years and have been well described by Harter (1979; Harter & Buddin, 1983): At first, children do not seem to understand that an individual can feel two emotions at the same time; later, they understand that a person can feel two emotions, but sequentially; ultimately, at about 10 years of age, children understand that a person can feel two quite opposite emotions simultaneously.

The lack of replicated work in this area makes any proposal regarding emotional development very tentative, and several issues raised by very recent studies need to be addressed. For instance, Field and her colleagues (1982) have reported that 3-day-old infants imitate components of facial expressions of sadness, joy, and surprise. These remarkable findings raise fundamental questions about whether the receptive capacities of neonates are as well developed as their expressive capacities seem to be. However, previous work on neonatal imitation (Meltzoff & Moore, 1977) has failed to replicate (Hayes & Watson, 1981). Will this more recent study of neonatal imitation replicate? Is it possible that, as with certain neonatal reflexes (e.g., Zelazo, 1976), a capacity present at a reflexive level in the neonate submerges only to reappear at a higher level of organization later (T. Bower, 1976)? Is the imitation of facial movements an instance of nothing more than motor mimicry, or is it a surprisingly early manifestation of emotional resonance measurable in expressive responses other than facial ones? These questions not only deserve careful attention but also highlight the dearth of knowledge regarding the origins and developmental course of emotional receptivity.

Conclusion

In this chapter, we have highlighted important changes in the conceptualization of emotion and emotional development. Whereas emotions were once viewed as unimportant outcomes of "cold" cognitive processes, lacking adaptive value at best or constituting maladaptive functioning at worst, now the crucial significance of emotions is becoming apparent. It is now clear that emotions are useful as organizational constructs, lending clarity to the relationship between various aspects of situations and various aspects of an organism's responses to those situations. Emotions function as both intrapersonal regulators, as when they impact cognitive or perceptual processes, and as interpersonal regulators, as when emotional expressions or coping reactions of one person influence the behavior of another. We have presented a model of the development of emotion, including the development of appreciation of *others'* emotional expressions. In this model, we have underscored the importance for emotion elicitation of the organism's *goals*, as well as the organism's appreciation of how events are relevant to those goals. We have stressed that neither "goal" nor "appreciation" imply high-level cognitive processing. Thus, there may be a core of differentiated affective continuity evidenced in the neonate as well as in the adult.

The study of emotion has truly become an exciting and enlightening enterprise. Much remains to be researched: Fascinating questions remain unanswered. The new methodological and theoretical advances offer promise to this reawakening field, as well as hope that emotion will remain a topic of interest to psychology for many generations to come.

References

Ainsworth, M., Blehar, M., Waters, E., & Wall, S. *Patterns of attachment*. Hillsdale, N.J.: Erlbaum, 1978.

Allport, F. *Social psychology*. Boston: Houghton Mifflin, 1924.

Appel, M., & Campos, J. Binocular disparity as a discriminable stimulus parameter for young infants. *Journal of Experimental Child Psychology*, 1977, *23*, 47–56.

Arnold, M. *Emotion and personality*. New York: Columbia University Press, 1960.

Bandura, A. *Social learning theory*. Englewood Cliffs, N.J.: Prentice-Hall, 1977.

Barrera, M., & Maurer, D. The perception of facial expressions by the three-month-old. *Child Development*, 1981, *52*, 203–206.

Beebe-Center, J. *The psychology of pleasantness and unpleasantness*. New York: Van Nostrand, 1932.

Berlyne, D. *Conflict, arousal, and curiosity*. New York: McGraw-Hill, 1960.

Berscheid, E., & Walster, E. When does a harm-doer compensate a victim? *Journal of Personality and Social Psychology*, 1967, *6*, 435–441.

Bertenthal, B., Campos, J., & Barrett, K. Self-produced locomotion: An organizer of emotional, cognitive, and social development in infancy. In R. Emde & R. Harmon (Eds.), *Continuities and discontinuities in development*. New York: Plenum, 1983.

Boccia, M., & Campos, J. *Maternal emotional signalling: Its effect on infants' reactions to strangers.* Paper presented at the meeting of the Society for Research in Child Development, Detroit, April 1983.

Boucher, J., & Carlson, G. Recognition of facial expressions in three cultures. *Journal of Cross-Cultural Psychology*, 1980, *11*, 263–280.

Bower, G. Mood and memory. *American Psychologist*, 1981, *36*, 128–148.

Bower, T. Repetitive processes in child development. *Scientific American*, 1976, *235*, 38–47.

Bowlby, J. *Maternal care and mental health.* Geneva: World Health Organization, 1951.

Bowlby, J. *Attachment and loss* Vol. 2: *Separation.* New York: Basic Books, 1973.

Brazelton, T. Precursors for the development of emotions in early infancy. In R. Plutchik & H. Kellerman (Eds.), *Emotions in early development* Vol. 2: *The emotions.* New York: Academic Press, 1983.

Breuer, J., & Freud, S. Studies in hysteria. *Nervous and Mental Disease Monographs*, 1895, *No. 61*.

Bronson, G. The fear of novelty. *Psychological Bulletin*, 1968, *69*, 350–358.

Brossard, M. The infant's conception of object permanence and his reactions to strangers. In T. Decarie (Ed.), *The infant's reactions to strangers.* New York: International Universities Press, 1974.

Bruner, J. Early social interaction and language acquisition. In H. Schaffer (Ed.), *Studies in mother-infant interaction.* New York: Academic Press, 1977.

Bruner, J., & Koslowski, B. Learning to use a lever. *Child Development*, 1972, *43*, 790–799.

Bruner, J., & Postman, L. Emotional selectivity in perception and reaction. *Journal of Personality*, 1947, *16*, 69–77.

Buck, R. Nonverbal communication of affect in children. *Journal of Personality and Social Psychology*, 1975, *31*, 644–653.

Buck, R. Nonverbal communication of affect in preschool children: Relationships with personality and skin conductance. *Journal of Personality and Social Psychology*, 1977, *35*, 225–236.

Buhler, C. *The first year of life.* New York: John Day, 1930.

Buhler, C., & Hetzer, M., Uber das erste verständnis für ausdrück im ersten lebensjahr. *Zeitschrift für Psychologie*, 1928, *107*, 50–61.

Bullowa, M. *Before speech: The beginning of interpersonal communication.* Cambridge: Cambridge University Press, 1979.

Campos, J. Heart rate: A sensitive tool for the study of emotional development. In L. Lipsitt (Ed.), *Developmental psychobiology: The significance of infancy.* Hillsdale, N.J.: Erlbaum, 1976.

Campos, J., & Emde, R. *Three paradigmatic uses of heart rate in infant research.* Paper presented at the International Conference on Infant Studies, Providence, R.I., 1978.

Campos, J., Barrett, K., Lamb, M., Goldsmith, H., & Stenberg, C. Socioemotional development. In M. Haith & J. Campos (Eds.), *Infancy and developmental psychobiology* (Vol. 2). P. Mussen (General Series Editor), *Handbook of child psychology.* New York: Wiley, 1983.

Campos, J., Hiatt, S., Ramsay, D., Henderson, C., & Svejda, M. The emergence of fear of heights. In M. Lewis & L. Rosenblum (Eds.), *The development of affect.* New York: Plenum, 1978.

Campos, J., & Stenberg, C. Perception, appraisal, and emotion: The onset of social referencing. In M. Lamb & L. Sherrod (Eds.), *Infant social cognition.* Hillsdale, N.J.: Erlbaum, 1981.

Cannon, W. The James-Lange theory of emotions: A critical examination and an alternative theory. *American Journal of Psychology*, 1927, *39*, 106–124.

Charlesworth, W. An ethological approach to research on facial expressions. In C. Izard (Ed.), *Measuring emotions in infants and children.* Cambridge: Cambridge University Press, 1982.

Charlesworth, W., & Kreutzer, M. Facial expressions of infants and children. In P. Ekman (Ed.), *Darwin and facial expression.* New York: Academic Press, 1973.

Cohn, J., & Tronick, E. Communicative rules and the sequential structure of infant behavior during normal and depressed interaction. In E. Tronick (Ed.), *The development of human communication and the joint regulation of behavior*. Baltimore, Md.: University Park Press, 1982.

Davidson, R., & Fox, N. Asymmetrical brain activity discriminates between positive and negative affective stimuli in human infants. *Science*, 1982, *218*, 1235–1237.

Decarie, T. *The infant's reactions to strangers*. New York: International Universities Press, 1974.

DeCasper, A., & Fifer, W. Of human bonding: Newborns prefer their mothers' voices. *Science*, 1980, *208*, 1174–1176.

Dennis, W. Infant reactions to restraint. *Transactions of the New York Academy of Science*, 1940, *2*, 202–217.

Duffy, E. Emotion: An example of the need for reorientation in psychology. *Psychological Review*, 1934, *41*, 184–198.

Easterbrook, J. The effect of emotion on cue utilization and the organization of behavior. *Psychological Review*, 1959, *66*, 183–201.

Ekman, P. Universals and cultural differences in facial expressions of emotion. In J. Cole (Ed.), *Nebraska symposium on motivation* (Vol. 19). Lincoln: University of Nebraska Press, 1972.

Ekman, P. Biological and cultural contributions to body and facial movement in the expression of emotions. In A. Rorty (Ed.), *Explaining emotions*. Berkeley: University of California Press, 1980.

Ekman, P., & Friesen, W. Constants across cultures in the face and emotion. *Journal of Personality and Social Psychology*, 1972, *17*, 124–129.

Ekman, P., & Friesen, W. *Facial action coding system*. Palo Alto, Calif.: Consulting Psychologists Press, 1978.

Ekman, P., Friesen, W., & Ellsworth, P. *Emotion in the human face: Guidelines for research and an integration of findings*. New York: Pergamon Press, 1972.

Ekman, P., Sorenson, E., & Friesen, W. Pancultural elements in the facial expression of emotion. *Science*, 1969, *164*, 86–88.

Emde, R. Toward a psychoanalytic theory of affect. I. The organizational model and its propositions. In S. Greenspan & G. Pollock (Eds.), *The course of life: Psychoanalytic contributions toward understanding personality development*. Washington, D.C.: U.S. Government Printing Office, 1980. (a)

Emde, R. Toward a psychoanalytic theory of affect. II. Emerging models of emotional development in infancy. In S. Greenspan & G. Pollock (Eds.), *The course of life: Psychoanalytic contributions toward understanding personality development*. Washington, D.C.: U.S. Government Printing Office, 1980. (b)

Emde, R. *The pre-representational self and its affective core*. Paper presented at the meeting of the Los Angeles Psychoanalytic Society, February 1982.

Emde, R., Gaensbauer, T., & Harmon, R. Emotional expression in infancy: A biobehavioral study. *Psychological issues*, Vol. 10, No. 37. New York: International Universities Press, 1976.

Emde, R., & Harmon, R. Endogenous and exogenous smiling systems in early infancy. *Journal of the American Academy of Child Psychiatry*, 1972, *11*, 77–100.

Emde, R., Harmon, R., & Gaensbauer, T. Using our emotions: Principles for appraising emotional deviance and intervention. In *Assessing the handicapped infant*. New Brunswick, N.J.: Johnson & Johnson Foundation, 1982.

Erdelyi, M. A new look at the new look: Perceptual defense and vigilance. *Psychological Review*, 1974, *81*, 1–25.

Exline, R. Gaze behavior in infants and children: A tool for the study of emotions? In C. Izard (Ed.), *Measuring emotions in infants and children*. Cambridge: Cambridge University Press, 1982.

Eysenck, H. *The biological basis of personality*. Springfield, Ill.: Thomas, 1967.

Feinman, S. Social referencing in infancy. *Merrill-Palmer Quarterly*, 1982, *28*, 445–470.

Feshbach, N. Sex differences in empathy and social behavior in children. In N. Eisenberg-Berg (Ed.), *The development of prosocial behavior*. New York: Academic Press, 1982.

Field, T. Individual differences in the expressivity of neonates and young infants. In R. Feldman (Ed.), *Development of nonverbal behavior in children*. New York: Jossey-Bass, 1982.

Field, T., Woodson, R., Greenberg, R., & Cohen, D. Discrimination and imitation of facial expressions by neonates. *Science*, 1982, *218*, 179–181.

Fiske, M., & Clarke, S. *Cognition and emotion: The Carnegie-Mellon symposium*. Hillsdale, N.J.: Erlbaum, 1982.

Fox, N., & Davidson, R. *EEG asymmetries in newborn infants in response to tastes differing in affective valence*. Paper presented at the meeting of the Society for Research in Child Development, Detroit, April 1983.

Freedman, D. *Human infancy: An evolutionary perspective*. Hillsdale, N.J.: Erlbaum, 1974.

Giacoman, S. Hunger and motor restraint on arousal and visual attention in the infant. *Child Development*, 1971, *42*, 605–614.

Gibson, J. *The ecological approach to visual perception*. Boston: Houghton Mifflin, 1979.

Goodman, G., & Haith, M. *Eyewitness testimony in children*. Grant application submitted to the Developmental Psychobiology Research Group, University of Colorado Health Sciences Center, 1982.

Graham, F., & Jackson, J. Arousal systems and infant heart rate responses. In H. Reese & L. Lipsitt (Eds.), *Advances in child development and behavior* (Vol. 5). New York: Academic Press, 1970.

Grossman, S. *A textbook of physiological psychology*. New York: Wiley, 1967.

Gunnar, M. Control, warning signals, and distress in infancy. *Developmental Psychology*, 1980, *16*, 281–289.

Gunnar-Von Gnechten, M. Changing a frightening toy into a pleasant toy by allowing the infant to control its actions. *Developmental Psychology*, 1978, *14*, 157–162.

Hainline, L. Developmental changes in visual scanning of face and nonface patterns by infants. *Journal of Experimental Child Psychology*, 1978, *25*, 90–115.

Haith, M., Bergman, T., & Moore, M. Eye contact and face scanning in early infancy. *Science*, 1977, *198*, 853–855.

Harter, S. *Children's understanding of multiple emotions: A cognitive-developmental approach*. Address presented at the Jean Piaget Society, Philadelphia, 1979.

Harter, S., & Buddin, B. *Children's understanding of the simultaneity of two emotions: A developmental sequence*. Paper presented at the meetings of the Society for Research in Child Development, Detroit, April 1983.

Hayes, L., & Watson, J. Neonatal imitation: Fact or artifact? *Developmental Psychology*, 1981, *17*, 655–660.

Hebb, D. On the nature of fear. *Psychological Review*, 1946, *53*, 259–276.

Hebb, D. *The organization of behavior*. New York: Wiley, 1949.

Heider, K. *Affect display rules in the Dani*. Paper presented at the meeting of the American Anthropological Association, New Orleans, 1974.

Hiatt, S., Campos, J., & Emde, R. Facial patterning and infant emotional expression: Happiness, surprise, and fear. *Child Development*, 1979, *50*, 1020–1035.

Hinde, R. Concepts of emotion. In *Physiology, emotion, and psychosomatic illness*, Ciba Foundation Symposium Number 8. Amsterdam: Elsevier, 1972.

Hoffman, M. Toward a theory of empathic arousal and development. In M. Lewis & L. Rosenblum (Eds.), *The development of affect*. New York: Plenum, 1978.

Hoffman, M. The measurement of empathy. In C. Izard (Ed.), *Measuring emotions in infants and children*. Cambridge: Cambridge University Press, 1982.

Horner, T. Two methods of studying stranger reactivity in infants: A review. *Journal of Child Psychology and Psychiatry*, 1980, *21*, 203–219.

Izard, C. *The face of emotion*. New York: Appleton-Century-Crofts, 1971.

Izard, C. *Patterns of emotion*. New York: Academic Press, 1972.

Izard, C. *Human emotions*. New York: Plenum, 1977.

Izard, C. On the ontogenesis of emotions and emotion-cognition relationships in infancy. In M. Lewis & L. Rosenblum (Eds.), *The development of affect*. New York: Plenum, 1978.

Izard, C. *The maximally discriminative facial movement coding system*. Newark, Del.: University of Delaware, 1979.

Izard, C., Hembree, E., Dougherty, L., & Coss, C. Changes in two- to nineteen-month-old infants' facial expressions following acute pain. *Developmental Psychology*, 1983, *19*, 418–426.

Izard, C., Huebner, R., Risser, D., McGinness, G., & Dougherty, L. The young infant's ability to produce discrete emotion expressions. *Developmental Psychology*, 1980, *16*, 132–140.

James, W. *Principles of psychology*. New York: Holt, 1890.

Johnson, W., Emde, R., Pannabecker, B., Stenberg, C., & Davis, M. Maternal perception of infant emotion from birth through 18 months. *Infant Behavior and Development*, 1982, *5*, 313–322.

Jones, H. The galvanic skin reflex as related to overt emotional expression. *Child Development*, 1930, *1*, 106–110.

Jones, H. The study of patterns of emotional expression. In M. Reymert (Ed.), *Feelings and emotions*. New York: McGraw-Hill, 1950.

Kagan, J. *Change and continuity in infancy*. New York: Wiley, 1971.

Kagan, J. Emergent themes in human development. *American Scientist*, 1976, *64*, 186–196.

Kagan, J. On emotion and its development: A working paper. In M. Lewis & L. Rosenblum (Eds.), *The development of affect*. New York: Plenum, 1978.

Kagan, J. Heart rate and heart rate variability as signs of a temperamental dimension in infants. In C. Izard (Ed.), *Measuring emotions in infants and children*. Cambridge: Cambridge University Press, 1982.

Kagan, J., Kearsley, R., & Zelazo, P. *Infancy: Its place in human development*. Cambridge, Mass.: Harvard University Press, 1978.

Kagan, J., Reznick, S., Clarke, C., Snidman, N., & Garcia-Coll, C. Cardiac correlates of behavioral inhibition in the young child. In M. Coles, J. Jennings, & J. Stern (Eds.), *Festschrift for John Lacey*. Stroudsburg, Pa.: Hutchinson Ross, 1983.

Kenney, M., Mason, W., & Hill, S. Effects of age, objects, and visual experience on affective responses of rhesus monkeys to strangers. *Developmental Psychology*, 1979, *15*, 176–184.

Kling, L., & Riggs, E. (Eds.). *Woodworth and Schlosberg's experimental psychology*. (3rd ed.). New York: Holt, Rinehart and Winston, 1971.

Klinnert, M. *The regulation of infant behavior by maternal facial expression*. Unpublished doctoral dissertation, University of Denver, 1981.

Klinnert, M., Campos, J., Sorce, J., Emde, R., & Svejda, M. Emotions as behavior regulators: Social referencing in infancy. In R. Plutchik & H. Kellerman (Eds.), *Emotions in early development*, Vol. 2: *The emotions*. New York: Academic Press, 1983.

Klinnert, M., Emde, R., Butterfield, P., & Campos, J. *Emotional communication from familiarized adults influences infants' behavior*. Paper presented at the meeting of the Society for Research in Child Development, Detroit, April 1983.

Klinnert, M., Sorce, J., & Emde, R. *Differential reactions of one-year-olds to discrete emotional expressions*. Paper presented at the International Conference on Infant Studies, Austin, Texas, March 1982.

Klinnert, M., Sorce, J., Emde, R., Stenberg, C., & Gaensbauer, T. Continuities and change in early affective life: Maternal perceptions of surprise, fear, and anger. In R. Emde & R. Harmon (Eds.), *Continuities and discontinuities in development*. New York: Plenum, 1983.

Kotsch, W., Gerbing, D., & Schwartz, L. The construct validity of the Differential Emotions Scale as adapted for children and adolescents. In C. Izard (Ed.), *Measuring emotions in infants and children*. New York: McGraw-Hill, 1982.

Kreutzer, M., & Charlesworth, W. *Infants' reactions to different expressions of emotions*. Paper presented at the meetings of the Society for Research in Child Development, Philadelphia, March 1973.

Kunst-Wilson, W., & Zajonc, R. Affective discrimination of stimuli that cannot be recognized. *Science*, 1980, *207*, 557–558.

LaBarbera, J., Izard, C., Vietze, P., & Parisi, S. Four- and six-month-old infants' visual responses to joy, anger and neutral expressions. *Child Development*, 1976, *47*, 535–538.

Laird, J. Self-attribution of emotion: The effects of expressive behavior on the quality of emotional experience. *Journal of Personality and Social Psychology*, 1974, *29*, 475–486.

Lamb, M., & Campos, J. *Development in infancy*. New York: Random House, 1982.

Lazarus, R. Emotions and adaptation: Conceptual and empirical relations. In W. Arnold (Ed.), *Nebraska symposium on motivation*. Lincoln: University of Nebraska Press, 1968.

Malatesta, C., & Haviland, J. Learning display rules: The socialization of emotion expression in infancy. *Child Development*, 1982, *53*, 991–1003.

Maurer, D., & Salapatek, P. Developmental changes in the scanning of faces by young infants. *Child Development*, 1976, *47*, 523–527.

McCall, R. Smiling and vocalization in infants as indices of perceptual-cognitive processes. *Merrill-Palmer Quarterly*, 1972, *18*, 341–347.

McCall, R., & McGhee, P. The discrepancy hypothesis of attention and affect in infants. In I. Uzgiris & F. Weizman (Eds.), *The structuring of experience*. New York: Plenum, 1977.

McDougall, W. *An introduction to social psychology*. London: Methuen, 1908.

Meltzoff, A., & Moore, M. Imitation of facial and manual gestures by human neonates. *Science*, 1977, *198*, 75–78.

Mendelson, M., Haith, M., & Goldman-Rakic, P. Face scanning and responsiveness to social cues in infant rhesus monkeys. *Developmental Psychology*, 1982, *18*, 222–228.

Meng, Z., Henderson, C., Campos, J., & Emde, R. *The effects of background emotional elicitation on subsequent problem solving in the toddler*. Unpublished manuscript, University of Denver, 1983.

Meyer, M. That whale among the fishes—the theory of the emotions. *Psychological Review*, 1933, *40*, 292–300.

Miller, N. Liberalization of basic S-R concepts. In S. Koch (Ed.), *Psychology: A study of a science*. New York: McGraw-Hill, 1959.

Miller, R. Experimental approaches to the physiological and behavioral concomitants of affective communication in rhesus monkeys. In S. Altman (Ed.), *Social communication among primates*. Chicago: University of Chicago Press, 1967.

Milmoe, S., Novey, M., Kagan, J., & Rosenthal, R. The mother's voice: Postdictor of aspects of her baby's behavior. In S. Weitz (Ed.), *Nonverbal communication: Readings with commentary*. New York: Oxford University Press, 1974.

Murray, A. Infant crying as an elicitor of parental behavior: An examination of two models. *Psychological Bulletin*, 1979, *86*, 191–215.

Mussen, P. *Carmichael's Manual of Child Psychology*. New York: Wiley, 1970.

Neisser, U. *Cognitive psychology*. New York: Appleton-Century-Crofts, 1967.

Neisser, U. *Cognition and reality*. San Francisco: Freeman, 1976.

Norman, D. Twelve issues for cognitive science. *Cognitive Science*, 1980, *4*, 1–32.

Obrist, P. The cardiovascular-behavioral interaction – as it appears today. *Psychophysiology*, 1976, *13*, 95–107.

Oster, H., & Ewy, R. Discrimination of sad vs. happy faces by 4-month-olds. Cited in H. Oster, "Recognition" of emotional expression in infancy? In M. Lamb & L. Sherrod (Eds.), *Infant social cognition*. Hillsdale, N.J.: Erlbaum, 1981.

Provost, M., & Decarie, T. Heart rate reactivity of 9- and 12-month old infants showing specific emotions in natural settings. *International Journal of Behavioral Development*, 1979, *2*, 109–120.

Radke-Yarrow, M., & Zahn-Waxler, C. Roots, motives, and patterns in children's prosocial behavior. In J. Reykowski, J. Karylowski, D. Bartal., & E. Staub (Eds.), *Origins and maintenance of prosocial behaviors*. New York: Plenum, 1982.

Rapaport, D. *Emotions and memory*. New York: Science Editions, 1961.

Regan, D., Williams, M., & Sparling, S. Voluntary expiation of guilt. *Journal of Personality and Social Psychology*, 1972, *24*, 42–45.

Reich, J., Emde, R., Campos, J., & Gaensbauer, T. Infant smiling at five and nine months: Analysis of heart rate and movement. *Infant Behavior and Development*, 1978, *1*, 26–35.

Roseman, I. *Cognitive aspects of emotion and emotional behavior.* Paper presented at the meetings of the American Psychological Association, New York City, September 1979.

Ryle, G. *The concept of mind.* New York: Barnes & Noble, 1950.

Sackett, G. Monkeys reared in isolation with pictures as visual input: Evidence for an innate releasing mechanism. *Science*, 1966, *154*, 1468–1472.

Scaife, M., & Bruner, J. The capacity for joint visual attention in the infant. *Nature*, 1975, *253*, 265–266.

Schachter, S. *Emotion, obesity, and crime.* New York: Academic Press, 1970.

Schachter, S., & Singer, J. Cognitive, social, and physiological determinants of emotional state. *Psychological Review*, 1962, *69*, 379–399.

Schaffer, H. Cognitive components of the infant's response to strangeness. In M. Lewis & L. Rosenblum (Eds.), *The origins of fear*. New York: Wiley, 1974.

Scherer, K. Speech and emotional states. In J. Darby (Ed.), *Speech evaluation in psychiatry*. New York: Grune & Stratton, 1981.

Scherer, K. The assessment of vocal expression in infants and children. In C. Izard (Ed.), *Measuring emotions in infants and children*. Cambridge: Cambridge University Press, 1982.

Scherer, K., & Ekman, P. *Handbook of methods in nonverbal research*. Cambridge: Cambridge University Press, 1982.

Scherer, K., & Oshinsky, J. Cue utilization in emotion attribution from auditory stimuli. *Motivation and Emotion*, 1977, *1*, 331–346.

Schwartz, G. Psychophysiological patterning and emotion revisited. In C. Izard (Ed.), *Measuring emotions in infants and children*. Cambridge: Cambridge University Press, 1982.

Schwartz, G., Fair, P., Salt, P., Mandel, M., & Klerman, G. Facial muscle patterning to affective imagery in depressed and non-depressed subjects. *Science*, 1976, *192*, 489–491.

Sherman, M. The differentiation of emotional responses in infants: I. Judgments of emotional responses from motion picture views and from actual observations. *Journal of Comparative Psychology*, 1927, *7*, 265–284. (a)

Sherman, M. The differentiation of emotional responses in infants: II. The ability of observers to judge the emotional characteristics of the crying of infants and of the voice of an adult. *Journal of Comparative Psychology*, 1927, *7*, 335–351. (b)

Skarin, K. Cognitive and contextual determinants of stranger fear in six- and eleven-month-old infants. *Child Development*, 1977, *48*, 537–544.

Skinner, B. *Science and human behavior.* Glencoe, Ill.: Free Press, 1953.

Sokolov, Y. *Perception and the conditioned reflex.* New York: Pergamon Press, 1963.

Sorce, J., Emde, R., Campos, J., & Klinnert, M. *Maternal emotional signaling: Its effect on the visual cliff behavior of one-year-olds.* Paper presented at the meeting of the Society for Research in Child Development, Boston, April 1981.

Sorce, J., Emde, R., & Frank, M. Maternal referencing in normal and Down's syndrome infants: A longitudinal study. In R. Emde & R. Harmon (Eds.), *The development of attachment and affiliative systems*. New York: Plenum, 1982.

Spitz, R. *The first year of life.* New York: International Universities Press, 1965.

Spitz, R., & Wolf, K. The smiling response: A contribution to the ontogenesis of social relations. *Genetic Psychology Monographs*, 1946, *34*, 57–125.

Sroufe, L. Socioemotional development. In J. Osofsky (Ed.), *Handbook of infant development*. New York: Wiley, 1979.

Sroufe, L., & Waters, E. Attachment as an organizational construct. *Child Development*, 1977, *48*, 1184–1199. (a)

Sroufe, L., & Waters, E. Heart rate as a convergent measure in clinical and developmental research. *Merrill-Palmer Quarterly*, 1977, *23*, 3–27. (b)

Sroufe, L., Waters, E., & Matas, L. Contextual determinants of infant affective response. In M. Lewis & L. Rosenblum (Eds.), *The origins of fear*. New York: Wiley, 1974.

Steiner, J. The gustofacial response: Observation on normal and anencephalic newborn infants. In J. Bosma (Ed.), *Fourth symposium on oral sensation and perception.* DHEW Publication No. NIH 73-546. Bethesda, Md.: U.S. Department of Health, Education, and Welfare, 1973.

Stenberg, C. *The development of anger facial expressions in infancy.* Unpublished doctoral dissertation, University of Denver, 1982.

Stenberg, C., & Campos, J. The development of the expression of anger in human infants. In M. Lewis & C. Saarni (Eds.), *The socialization of affect.* New York: Plenum, 1983.

Stenberg, C., Campos, J., & Emde, R. The facial expression of anger in seven-month-old infants. *Child Development,* 1983, *54,* 178–184.

Stern, D. *The first relationship: Infant and mother.* Cambridge, Mass.: Harvard University Press, 1977.

Svejda, M., & Campos, J. *The mother's voice as a regulator of the infant's behavior.* Paper presented at the International Conference on Infant Studies, Austin, Texas, 1982.

Titchener, E. *Experimental psychology: A manual of laboratory experiments.* New York: Macmillan, 1905.

Tronick, E., Als, H., Adamson, L., Wise, S., & Brazelton, T. The infant's response to entrapment between contradictory messages in face-to-face interaction. *Journal of the American Academy of Child Psychiatry,* 1978, *17,* 1–13.

Tucker, D. Lateral brain function, emotion and conceptualization. *Psychological Bulletin,* 1981, *89,* 19–46.

Vaughn, B., & Sroufe, L. The temporal relationship between infant heart rate acceleration and crying in an aversive situation. *Child Development,* 1979, *50,* 565–567.

Walk, R. The development of depth perception in animals and human infants. *Monographs of the Society for Research in Child Development,* 1966, *31* (Whole No. 5).

Waters, E. The reliability and stability of individual differences in infant–mother attachment. *Child Development,* 1978, *49,* 483–494.

Watson, J. *Behaviorism.* Chicago: University of Chicago Press, 1930.

Watson, J. Smiling, cooing, and "the game." *Merrill-Palmer Quarterly,* 1972, *18,* 341–347.

Williams, C., & Stevens, K. Vocal correlates of emotional states. In J. Darby (Ed.), *Speech evaluation in psychiatry.* New York: Grune & Stratton, 1981.

Wolff, P. The natural history of crying and other vocalizations in early infancy. In B. Foss (Ed.), *Determinants of infant behavior.* New York: Wiley, 1969.

Woodworth, R., & Schlosberg, H. *Experimental psychology.* New York: Holt, 1954.

Wundt, W. *Principles of physiological psychology.* New York: Macmillan, 1904.

Yonas, A. Infants' responses to optical information for collision. In R. Aslin (Ed.), *Development of perception* (Vol. 2). New York: Academic Press, 1981.

Young-Browne, G., Rosenfeld, H., & Horowitz, F. Infant discrimination of facial expressions. *Child Development,* 1977, *48,* 555–562.

Zajonc, R. Feeling and thinking: Preferences need no inferences. *American Psychologist,* 1980, *35,* 151–175.

Zelazo, P. From reflexive to instrumental behavior. In L. Lipsitt (Ed.), *Developmental psychobiology: The significance of infancy.* Hillsdale, N.J.: Erlbaum, 1976.

Ziajka, A. *Prelinguistic communication in infancy.* New York: Praeger, 1981.

9   The cognitive-emotional fugue

Michael Lewis, Margaret Wolan Sullivan,
and Linda Michalson

Fugue: The theme is first given out by one voice or part, and then, while that pursues its way, it is repeated by another at the interval of a fifth or a fourth, and so on, until all the parts have answered one by one, *continuing their several melodies and interweaving them in one complex and progressive whole, in which the theme is often lost and reappears.* (*Webster's International Dictionary*, 1905)

The relationship between cognition and emotion is a topic of concern to developmental theorists (Kagan, 1974; Lewis & Goldberg, 1969; McCall, 1972; Ulvund, 1980). Although recognizing that a certain level of cognitive development is necessary for the expression of complex emotions (e.g., guilt), many investigators have argued that early in development information processing is associated with emotional responses. For example, the failure to assimilate an event is thought to produce wariness or fear, whereas mastery is likely to result in enjoyment. In this model, emotion is viewed as the consequence of certain cognitive processes.

A second model of the relationship between emotion and cognition is one in which emotional responses are thought to precede cognitive processing. According to this model, emotion is a motive or drive with an action-producing or maintenance function. Such a view stresses the independent nature of emotion and implies that emotions may be events that do not require cognitive processes for their occurrence.

We have chosen the title "The Cognitive-Emotional Fugue" to suggest that a third model may better represent the relationship between cognition and emotion. In this model, emotion and cognition are neither separate nor independent processes. Rather both are elements of a continuous, inseparable stream of behavior, like the parts of a fugue "in which the theme is often lost and reappears." This alternative view, derived from Hofstadter's *Gödel, Escher, Bach* (1980), depicts an interplay of forces or themes without beginning or end. This idea is illustrated in Escher's *Ascending and Descending*. In this painting, as in much of Escher's art, the theme of movement without beginning or end is portrayed. So, too, cognition and emotion can be conceived as continuous and interwoven strands of behavior.

The authors are grateful to the W. T. Grant Foundation for its support of the research and preparation of this chapter.

The first two models are well represented in the literature, as we will show subsequently. After considering some of the issues pertaining to these two models, we will present our alternative model and describe an empirical investigation of the interplay between emotion and cognition in a simple learning task. The two traditional models will be shown to be inadequate, and the third model, the fugue, will be developed more fully.

Models of the relationship between emotion and cognition

Model A: emotion as a consequence of cognition

To understand models in which emotions are viewed as the consequence of cognitive processes, we must first distinguish among the various components of emotion, as the role of cognition in each may be quite different (Lewis & Michalson, 1983). Elsewhere we have postulated that emotion consists of five major components: elicitors, receptors, states, expressions, and experiences (Lewis & Rosenblum, 1978). *Emotional elicitors* refer to situations or stimulus events that trigger an organism's emotional receptors. These stimuli may be internal or external, and the capacity of these elicitors to evoke responses may be innate or learned. *Emotional receptors* are relatively specific loci or pathways in the central nervous system that mediate changes in the physiological and/or cognitive state of the organism. The process through which these receptors attain their emotional function and the types of events that trigger their activity may be genetically encoded or acquired through experience. *Emotional states* are the particular constellations of changes in somatic and/or neuronal activity that accompany the activation of emotional receptors. Emotional states are largely specific, transient, patterned alterations in ongoing levels of physiological activity. *Emotional expressions* are the potentially observable surface features of changes in the face, body, voice, and activity level that accompany emotional states. The constituent elements and their patterning, as well as the regularity with which they are associated with particular emotional states, may be either learned or innate. Finally, *emotional experiences* are individuals' conscious or unconscious perception, interpretation, and evaluation of their own emotional state and expression. This cognitive process is influenced by a range of prior social experiences in which the nature of the eliciting stimuli and the appropriateness of particular expressions have in part been articulated and defined for the individual by others.

The tendency of some investigators to blur the distinctions among these components often prevents a clear understanding of the roles that cognition may play in emotion, particularly at the level of elicitors, expressions, and experiences.

The role of cognition at the level of elicitors. Cognition may elicit an emotion by influencing the effect of an emotional elicitor. For instance, past associations of a stimulus with either a noxious or a pleasant outcome are cognitions that will affect the individual's subsequent emotional response to the stimulus. Watson and Rayner (1920) laid the groundwork for research on conditioned emotional responses by demonstrating that a rat associated with a sudden loud noise could cause fear in a child who once had shown only approach behaviors to the rat. This fear was long-lasting and generalized to other animals and objects.

Alternatively, cognition may play a more direct role in the actual creation of emotion through the interpretation of the elicitor. Theories postulating that emotions arise from certain cognitive activities can be categorized into appraisal and discrepancy theories. Both focus on the quality of the elicitor.

Appraisal theories. Appraisal theories posit that emotion results from the evaluation of a stimulus. According to Arnold (1960, 1970), appraisal is defined as the immediate, automatic evaluation of anything encountered as either "good" (i.e., beneficial to one's well-being) or "bad" (i.e., harmful to one's well-being). This appraisal results in a tendency to approach that which is evaluated as good and to avoid that which is bad. What is judged as neither good nor bad is ignored.

The basis of most appraisals is memory. A new object will evoke a memory of the feelings associated with past experiences with similar objects. Imagination may also play a role in the emotional process to the degree that before people act, they may try to imagine whether the consequences of that action will be beneficial or harmful. Both the appraisal of the conditions and the possibility of action determine the nature of the emotional tendency (e.g., fear or courage). If conscious judgment warrants, the emotional tendency will result in overt action.

In Lazarus's (1966, 1982; Lazarus, Averill, & Optin, 1970) theory, emotions are also thought to originate in particular kinds of cognitive appraisals. Organisms are viewed as constantly appraising and reappraising stimuli with regard to their personal relevance and whether or not the organism can adapt. These appraisals may lead to certain kinds of activities (physiological, cognitive, and behavioral) in an attempt to cope with the appraised situation. Benign appraisals result in an automatic, emotionless adaptation to a situation, reappraisal if additional information warrants, or positive emotional states. Threatening appraisals, on the other hand, lead either to direct action in an attempt to remove the threat or, when no direct action is possible, to reappraisal. Fluctuations in emotion occur as objects and events are reappraised.

Discrepancy theories. In discrepancy theories, emotions are regarded as the product of certain discrepancies or incongruities between external events and internal representations or schemas. Hebb (1946, 1949) first related incongruity to emotion by demonstrating that events highly discrepant from previous experience evoke fear. For example, the detached head of a monkey shown to other monkeys produced extreme fear because of its incongruity.

Berlyne (1960) suggested that unfamiliar or novel events may evoke either fear or pleasure, contingent on the conditions. Pleasure is evoked when a stimulus is novel or curious "to the right degree" (Berlyne, 1970). A lack of information about a stimulus event will generate uncertainty. To reduce the uncertainty, the organism may actively explore and perhaps reappraise the event.

More recently Kagan (1974, 1978) suggested that the organism's first response to a discrepancy or an unexpected change in the physical parameters of a stimulus is a "special state" characterized by an inhibition of motor activity and decreased heart rate. Different outcomes are possible, depending on the cognitive processes that follow. For example, if an event is easily assimilated, boredom is likely to be observed. Events that cannot be assimilated or are assimilated with difficulty may result in fear. A special competence, which emerges between 7 and 9 months of age in Western infants, has been hypothesized to play a major role in the child's emotional reaction to discrepant events. This competence has been described as the "activation of hypotheses" (Kagan, 1974) and as the ability to perform simultaneous comparisons (Schaffer, 1974).

In another version of discrepancy theory, emotion is defined as the consequence of the organism's "need for information" with respect to reaching a goal multiplied by the difference between "necessary information" and "available information" (Siminov, 1970). Information is viewed as the possibility of reaching a goal. As people continually strive to attain the behavioral and physiological state of satisfied needs, the quantity of information vis-à-vis the attainment of this goal determines the emotional response. A lack of information will prevent appropriate organization; in this case, the nervous system is activated in a way to produce negative emotions. Positive emotions, in contrast, result from a surplus of information over and above that which is necessary for the satisfaction of needs.

Lewis and Goldberg (1969) suggested that the initial effect of violation of expectancy (i.e., discrepancy) is to alert the organism. Emotions characterized by approach or withdrawal occur only subsequently. These investigators measured emotion by observing expressions of surprise on the faces of preschool children. Of 14 instances of surprise, 13 occurred in response to a violation of expectancy. Positive emotional behavior (smiling) was observed after the initial surprise response. Apparently the discrepancy served to alert the child, thereby producing an emotional response without hedonic quality.

The specific emotion that follows alerting may depend on the context of the violation as well as the other cognitions of the child at that point. For example, a mother's putting on a mask may be a violation of expectancy for infants and produce alerting. Whether infants laugh or cry depends on the context, their specific cognitions, and their adaptive strategies for dealing with this event. Infants may cry if the mask is put on when the mother is expected to read a bedtime story but laugh when it is put on during play. In both cases infants perceived the discrepancy. However, in one case it produced fear because the infants understood the discrepancy to be unrelated to bedtime and in the other it produced delight because they understood it to be related to play. Thus, the discrepancy produced by the mask has only an alerting effect; other cognitions determine its hedonic tone.

Control over a stimulus event is another factor determining emotional response to a particular situation (Lewis, 1980). For example, when allowed to control the actions of an intrusive toy, infants exhibit significantly fewer distress responses and are more willing to approach and interact with the toy than are infants who have no control over the toy (Gunnar, 1980).

Related to the notion of control is the concept of contingency experience. Similar to Piaget's (1952) notion of circular reactions, contingency experiences may be defined as "if-then" relationships. For example, *if* the infant pulls on a string, *then* a mobile revolves. If specific behavioral responses to contingent outcomes increase with time, the infant is said to have learned the contingency. Continued experience with such stimulation is hypothesized to result in a generalized expectancy that one can act upon and control the environment and a motivation to do so in novel situations (Lewis & Goldberg, 1969). This motivation may manifest itself in increased positive emotion (Watson, 1966, 1972).

Other investigators have also attempted to document changes in emotional behaviors (i.e., smiling, vocalization, and crying) resulting from contingency experience (Sullivan, Rovee-Collier, & Tynes, 1979). Brinker and Lewis (1982) reported increased smiling and vocalizing and decreased crying in young, severely handicapped children in response to learning simple contingencies. DeCasper and Carstens (1981) found that previous experience with contingent stimulation rendered subsequent encounters with noncontingent stimulation "upsetting" to neonates. Initial experience with noncontingent stimulation was not associated with any emotional reaction. Thus, there is some evidence that both positive and negative emotional changes accompany contingency experience or the expectation of control.

The mechanism by which cognition or information processing produces emotion is unknown. One possibility is that the connection is prewired into the organism's nervous system. When activated by certain elicitors, cognition may "release" particular emotional states. The way in which biological necessity controls the activation of emotions is not known, however. Cognitive processing itself might be considered an elicitor of subsequent emotions. From this point of view, the failure to assimilate an event, the acquisition or violation of an expectancy, or even the approach of a stranger may constitute cognitive elicitors of emotional states through their direct action on as yet unspecified receptors.

On the other hand, one could argue that the effect of these cognitive events is a function of their past association with negative or positive outcomes. If this is the case, events may produce emotion because of their associational connections as described previously. Discrepancy theories generally focus on perturbations in the process rather than on the content of thought. The demonstration by Gunnar (1980) and others of the effects of stimulus control on distress responses forces one to consider not only perturbations but their nature as they relate to other factors, including past experience, the content of thought, and subsequent emotional behavior. In these ways – either through learning or prewired connections and interpretive acts – cognitive processes might produce emotion.

The role of cognition at the level of emotional expressions. Emotional expressions have been viewed as the direct consequence of an emotional state (Darwin, 1872/1965; Ekman, Friesen, & Ellsworth, 1972; Izard, 1971, 1977; Tomkins, 1962, 1963) or as the consequence of an emotional state and past socialization experiences (Lewis & Michalson, 1982, 1983). According to the first position, fixed neuromusculature connections exist between internal state changes and facial expressions as well as select postural and vocal behaviors. These natural, biologically determined connections are hypothesized to exist on the basis of the reported universality of facial expressions across vastly different cultures (Ekman, 1973). If, in fact, facial, postural, and vocal expressions are universal and isomorphic with emotional states, the need to postulate a cognitive role in emotional expressions becomes superfluous.

In contrast to more biologically oriented theories, socialization theories assume that expressive behaviors do not necessarily have a one-to-one correspondence with internal states. Upon reflection, even if facial expressions are biologically connected to internal states, the rules governing their appropriate expression are learned through socialization experiences. We know that people often express emotions incongruent with internal emotional states. This circumstance could be due either to knowledge that the expression of a particular emotion is inappropriate in a particular situation (e.g., expressing anger toward one's boss) or to a refusal to acknowledge a particular emotion (e.g., denying anger when insulted). There are many reasons why emotional expressions and emotional states may not be isomorphic, making the postulation of some form of learning necessary.

Lewis & Michalson (1983, in press) have recently outlined a developmental model relating emotional expressions and states. In this model, infants' facial expressions observed in the first months of life are more differentiated than the infants' internal states. Consequently, one cannot assume that expressions and states are automatically connected. For example, even though muscle movements associated with a contempt face have been observed occasionally in very young infants (Izard, 1979), it seems unlikely that the infants have the discrete internal state analogous to the adult state of scorn or disdain, given the cognitive and social requirements associated with this emotion. Another example of a facial expression unrelated to state is the endogenous smile (Emde & Koenig, 1969). Such examples as these suggest that at least in the first months of life facial expressions may be relatively unrelated to internal states. Although the point at which facial expressions correspond to emotional states is difficult to determine, it is reasonable to assume that by the time infants are 6 months of age, emotional states are differentiated sufficiently to be more isomorphic with facial expressions.

The degree of correspondence between expressions and states may vary as a function of the particular emotion, the intensity of the precipitating stimuli, the amount of social reinforcement, and the degree to which children have learned to be aware of and to control their emotional expressions (Brooks-Gunn & Lewis, 1982; Lewis & Michalson, 1982). Some expressions (e.g., smiling) may exhibit considerable synchrony with emotional states in the first few months of life; for other emotions, the synchrony between state and facial expression may evolve more slowly. The correspondence between facial expressions and emotional states is likely to remain high until the socialization experiences of children influence and alter their spontaneous facial displays (Saarni, 1979, 1980, 1982). By 10 months of age, infants appear to be influenced by others to an important degree (Campos & Stenberg, 1982; Feinman & Lewis, 1983). Thus, a greater correspondence between internal emotional states and facial expressions is likely to exist between the ages of 6 and 18 months than either before or after (Lewis & Michalson, in press). These ages appear to be reasonable but conservative boundaries. As such, they are open to empirical study and are likely to be refined with the collection of further data.

The role of cognition at the level of emotional experiences. Cognitive processes may affect emotional experience through (1) the perception of unique physiological changes that occur within one's own body or (2) the cognitive interpretation and evaluation of a general arousal state. The first role of cognition is illustrated in James's (1884, 1890) theory of emotion. For James, the *perception* of the bodily changes as they occur constitutes the emotion. All that is cognitively required on the organism's part is the perception of these internal changes of state. Tomkins (1962, 1963, 1970) also believed that a minimal amount of cognitive processing is involved beyond the perception or registration of bodily (primarily facial) changes. The mental representation of these responses constitutes the experience of the emotion.

Cognition may also affect emotional experience through the interpretation and evaluation of a general arousal state. Indeed, some theorists regard emotion as nothing but "interpretive cognitive action and arousal" (Mandler, 1975, 1980; Royce & Diamond, 1980; Schachter, 1964). Since a general arousal state is common to all emotions, some cognitive interpretation and evaluation of the arousal is necessary to distinguish among emotional experiences. According to Schachter and Singer (1962), this "cognitive context" is provided by external cues. From knowledge of the situation in which the arousal occurs, including the social behavior of other people, the individual creates, as it were, the emotional experience.

In Mandler's (1975, 1980) theory, cognition seems to play a dual role in emotion, first as an elicitor of an emotional state, then as an interpretive-evaluative act. For Mandler, the interruption of an ongoing activity produces a general arousal, which is responsible for the intensity of the emotional experience. The quality of the emotion depends on the accompanying evaluation of the internal state and the environment. Although autonomic reactions only produce emotional experiences in conjunction with cognitive evaluations (which are usually previously acquired or assigned), cognitive evaluations and judgments may occur in the absence of autonomic activity. Thus, one can experience happiness or sadness in the absence of an internal state of happiness or sadness. For example, patients with spinal cord lesions (and thus without physical sensation) report they experience "a cognitive kind of emotion" in the absence of any physiological state (see Buck, 1980). In Mandler's theory, "pure" cognitive activity can generate autonomic activity and produce a "full-blown emotional reaction" through the retrieval of the appropriate context.

Whether emotion involves a specific physiological state or a general state such as arousal, the interpretation of that state may provide emotions with their particular phenomenological quality. For theories in which general arousal constitutes the internal emotional state, specific emotional experiences are facilitated either by the individual's interpretation, knowledge about, and direct observation of the expressions of others in the situation or by knowledge about what emotion is "appropriate" to a particular situation (e.g., we know to feel sad at funerals and not when someone wins a lottery). For theories in which specific physiological changes define different emotions, the interpretation of that state may rely more on specific somatic, visceral, or neural responses. For instance, making a face distinctive to a specific emotion may generate the corresponding emotional experience (Laird, 1974), presumably because the subject has produced a set of unique responses related to that specific emotion.

Although cognitive theories of emotion stress the need to consider the role of appraisal as well as the roles of physiological and situational cues that play a part in emotion, more work is needed in detailing the particular cognitive processes that affect various emotional responses and in specifying their antecedent conditions. There can be no doubt that the perception of the stimulus plus an evaluation of it with respect to its personal significance are contributing factors to emotion.

Model B: emotion as an antecedent of cognition

Theories that view emotion as an antecedent of cognition usually are concerned with whether it is possible to experience an emotion in the absence of thought, or to feel without thinking (Zajonc, 1980). More to the point is the issue of whether emotions can actually *produce* different ways of thinking or different cognitive processes.

At least one theory suggests that thought may be the consequence of certain feeling states. According to developmental theory, the emotions produced by the delay of immediate gratification facilitate the development of more mature thought processes. Cognitive structures are produced by delays through processes labeled "secondary thought" (Freud, 1960) or "elaborated thought" (e.g., Hartmann, 1958; Mischel, 1974). For instance, if individuals cannot eat immediately when they are hungry, they may imagine themselves eating in order to feel good. Imagination is the consequence of an unfulfilled (i.e., negative) emotional state.

The position that emotion precedes cognition has been recently argued by Zajonc (1980). To address this model, we will view emotion as an antecedent of cognition from the perspectives of emotions as motives, as markers, and as instigators.

Emotions as motives. Since Darwin (1872/1965), the notion of emotions as motives to act has appeared in many emotion theories (see Strongman, 1978). Although in the majority of such discussions the general category of action is considered, the arguments easily apply to cognitive activities as well. Theories that regard emotions as motives that impel action can be divided into two classes: (1) those that view emotion as a consequence and thereby a reinforcement of an action pattern and (2) those that view emotion as producing an action pattern based on the evolutionary history of the species.

Central to the hedonic tradition is the belief that people act or think in ways that produce pleasure and avoid pain. The emotional consequences of action or thought are regarded as the primary cause of that action. Action or thought patterns that are likely to result in pleasure or to reduce pain will be taken; action or thought patterns that are likely to lead to pain will not be taken (e.g., consider Festinger's [1957] notion of cognitive dissonance).

This view of emotions as motivating action through the emotional consequences of the action appears reasonable. For example, students may study for examinations because it feels good to pass and it feels bad to fail; children engage in symbolic play to experience the pleasures associated with problem solving. It should be noted that according to this view behavior is motivated by the possibility of its emotional consequence. Even though the emotional experience occurs *after* the action, it is thought that the reinforcement value of this experience serves to produce the same set of behaviors in order to reexperience the particular emotion. So although emotion is initially a consequence of action, the expectation or memory of the emotion may precede and influence subsequent actions.

If one thinks of emotion in this way, then emotions, especially positive and negative feelings, act as reinforcers of particular actions or thoughts. In many cases, these hedonic reinforcers seem to be unlearned. For example, it is unlikely that the good feeling produced by eating when hungry is learned. Rather, eating feels good because of an innate biological connection between food in some part of the digestive tract and relief from hunger. On the other hand, some emotional reinforcers seem, at least at first glance, to be learned. There is no intrinsic reason that it should feel good to get an "A" on a French examination. The issue, however, becomes more complex when one moves from the particular event, such as doing well on a test, to its more general form, such as being competent. It may be the case that being successful in anything (depending on the cultural definition of success) is rewarding, that is, produces a positive state. In this event, the developmental issue pertains only to specifying which particular actions will be associated with positive or negative states.

Emotion may be not only the reinforcing outcome of action, but also its antecedent. This view of emotion is usually associated with biological explanations of emotion. Darwin (1872/1965) argued that the process of evolution applies not only to anatomical structures but to intellectual and expressive behaviors as well. Emotions by their nature are associated with action patterns necessary for survival. For example, the sight of a predator elicits fear in the organism, the action pattern of which is to flee. Or, a baby's cry elicits nurturance in the mother with a concomitant behavioral repertoire of nursing, holding, or retrieving the infant. Viewed in this way, emotion is both a state of the organism and a response basic to survival. Plutchik (1980) enumerated eight adaptive patterns of behavior that may be the functional basis of all emotions: incorporation, rejection, destruction, protection, reproduction, reintegration, orientation, and exploration. The emotions that accompany these basic patterns are acceptance, disgust, anger, fear, joy, sadness, surprise, and expectancy, respectively. Although the specific behaviors associated with these patterns may vary across different species, their survival function is common to all species.

Recently, Zajonc (1980) offered a view similar to the evolutionary position. For Zajonc, some of the behaviors associated with an emotional state may have "hard wire" cognitive representations; that is, they may be independent of cognitive systems and, in fact, may precede perceptual and cognitive operations. Zajonc discusses the primacy of emotion with regard to preferences and attitudes, but his argument is essentially that emotion "accompanies all cognitions, that it arises early in the process of registration and retrieval . . . and it derives from a parallel, separate, and partly independent system in the organism" (p. 154). In short, emotions may be associated with basic adaptive functions and have as their biological consequence a set of dispositions, including thoughts as well as actions.

Emotions as markers. Much attention has been focused on the roles of "hot" versus "cold" cognitions. The general assumption underlying this issue is that many cognitive processes have different levels of efficiency or different outcomes depending on whether these cognitive processes are "marked" or tagged with specific emotional tones (see Zajonc [1980] for a comprehensive review of this topic). Two effects of markers are briefly considered here. First, one might argue that cognitive processes marked with emotion might be more efficient than those not marked. For example, the retrieval of past events from short-term and long-term memory may be facilitated by emotional markers (Norman & Rumelhart, 1975). Information may enter memory not only as a function of the content or sequence of the material but also as a function of the emotional tag. Clearly, the schema of a person in a white coat is more likely to be remembered if it is associated with fear than the same schema not marked with fear.

Second, markers may be associated with the emotional contents of events as they relate to the emotional state of the organism. Bower's (1981) research indicates that emotions may have a powerful influence on cognitive processes, including free recall, fantasies, and social perception. Bower found, for example, that people recalled more events that were affectively congruent with their mood during recall. Here, the view of emotions as markers refers not only to the emotional tag attached to the cognitive event but also to the emotional state of the individual as the individual interacts with the cognitive event.

Emotions as instigators. The third role of emotion in cognition focuses on whether certain feelings can cause people to think in particular ways. One way to approach this issue is to regard thought in the same way that one considers other action patterns as related to specific emotions. Emotions may not only elicit, in some biological fashion, certain action patterns (Plutchik, 1980), but, in fact, emotions may produce specific thinking patterns.

One aspect of this topic concerns the nature or the content of the thought. For instance, imagine that you are told either that your cousin was hit by a car or that your cousin won the lottery. The different emotions produced as a result of the message's content in these two cases are likely to create certain moods that will influence subsequent, although unrelated, thoughts.

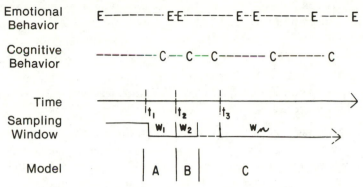

Figure 9.1. Models of cognition, emotion, and the stream of behavior

With the exception of the view of emotions as motives, relatively little empirical work has been carried out with respect to Model B. Model B also lacks the elaborate theoretical underpinnings of Model A. The paucity of theory and information supporting the model of emotions as antecedents of cognition may be the consequence of a Western view of motivation in which human behavior is regarded as the product of a rational mind. The bias inherent in the extensive attention to Model A and relative neglect of Model B in the literature becomes apparent when one considers that many non-Western cultures stress the primacy of feelings over thought. In such cultures Model B may have the greater intuitive appeal.

Model C: the cognitive-emotional fugue

In the preceding sections, two linear models of the relationship between cognition and emotion were considered and some of the issues underlying empirical investigations were reviewed. From this discussion one soon realizes that a simple linear model is insufficient; both cognition and emotion must be viewed as continual processes that are interwoven in highly complex ways. To separate them into arbitrary units serves to produce an artificial temporal and causal sequence. Although linear models have intrinsic appeal to empiricists, the artificial boundaries imposed by such models both restrict one's perspective and are responsible for theories that in their simplicity distort or overlook the continuous interplay between these domains.

For example, consider an alternating sequence of emotion and cognition. The face validity of one's model will depend on the time the stream of behavior is sampled and the width of the sampling window. Figure 9.1 depicts two ongoing streams of behavior, emotional (E) and cognitive (C), as they occur over time. If behavior is sampled between times t_1 and t_2, an observer would see emotion following cognition and find support for Model A. If behavior is sampled between times t_2 and t_3, the observer would discover an emotion preceding a cognition and Model B would be confirmed. If the width of the sampling window is varied (w_n), the sequence of events and the length of the chain of behavior will vary and reflect Model C.

An empirical investigation of the relationship between emotion and learning

In the preceding discussion, we articulated three models of the cognitive-emotional relationship. To explore empirically the relationship between these domains, we chose to observe infants in a simple contingency learning situation in which facial expressions and the learning of an arm-pull response were measured. Before presenting the data, however, each of the three models previously described will be considered as it applies to this particular learning context.

The models and learning

In the experimental task, infants had to learn that a single motor response, an arm pull, resulted in a favorable outcome, the onset of an audiovisual event. Learning was indexed by appropriate changes in arm-pull rate. The hypothesized relationship of emotion to contingency learning, as suggested by each of the three models, is presented in Figure 9.2. For each model a theoretical learning curve is represented by a solid line. In Model A, emotion associated with learning peaks as a consequence of learning the contingency relationship. In Model B, emotion is elevated before the infant actually learns the contingency, possibly as the result of prewired interest and approach mechanisms. Emotion may (1) decline or (2) remain high until the infant ceases to respond. In Model C, emotion occurs both before and after contingency learning. Whereas positive emotional expressions (e.g., smiling and vocalizing) may be the consequence of learning and mastery (i.e., learning feels good!), they also may be a necessary prerequisite for learning (i.e., I cannot learn unless all is well). Positive emotions may occur *not only* at beginning or at end of the learning experience but also during both phases and even throughout the process. Furthermore, emotions other than positive emotions may accompany the learning process. Negative feelings as well, such as stress and frustration, also may accompany increased effort. Does the infant's ability to cope with stress affect learning and at what stage? In Model C the separation of emotion into a number of constituents is essential if the interplay of cognition and emotion are to be considered.

Procedure

The subjects of the study were among 60 infants who participated in a larger study of learning in the first 6 months of life. In this study infants sat in a

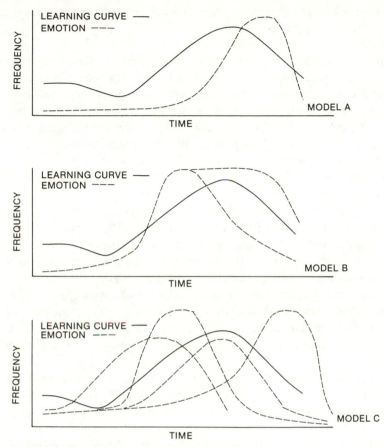

Figure 9.2. Models of the relationship between learning and emotion

contingency apparatus that delivered a 3-sec presentation of an audiovisual stimulus (a color slide of a happy baby and a recording of the *Sesame Street* theme song). Stimulus onset was contingent upon an arm-pull response. Arm-pull responses were automatically recorded by means of a ribbon connected to a Velcro wrist cuff. Deflection of the ribbon activated a microswitch in a lever mounted above the subject. In addition to on-line recording of arm-pull responses, attention, smiling, and vocalizing behaviors were recorded. Facial expressions were videotaped throughout the course of the experimental session. Subjects remained in the session as long as they continued to respond. Two minutes of inactivity or 30 sec of fussy behavior or crying were the criteria for terminating the session.

From the original sample of 60 infants, five 6-month-old infants (three boys and two girls) were selected randomly, the only criterion being that they exhibited classic and well-differentiated learning curves. The temporal param-

eters of each learning curve were identified and each of the curves was segmented
into the following phases:

Baseline: 1 min of nonreinforcement (1).

Initial orientation to stimulus event: the first minute following baseline (2).
This minute is the infant's first encounter with the contingent stimulus.

Contingency awareness: 1 minute prior to response acceleration (3) (that
point where arm-pull responses exceeded and stayed above baseline) as well
as the first minute following this point (4). Although some children's learning
curves showed more rapid acceleration than did others, the point of acceleration
and the minutes prior to and following this point were constant across subjects.

Response asymptote: 1 min prior to the point of highest arm-pull response
(5) as well as the first minute of the highest level (6).

Postasymptote: 1 min prior to decline in arm-pull response (7), first minute
after the sustained decline (8), and last minute of the session (9). Typically,
responses dropped off quite dramatically during this period, although responding
did not invariably return to baseline level. The decline in response may signify
either habituation to the contingency problem or fatigue.

Because individual session lengths and rates of learning varied, the length
of each phase also varied. However, by carefully marking the specific phases
of each curve, one can sample comparable points of the learning curve and
thus compare qualitatively similar moments during the learning experience.

Coding facial behavior. Facial movements were coded from videotapes of the
infants using the Maximally Discriminative Facial Movement Coding System,
referred to as "Max" (Izard, 1979), which was chosen because training manuals
are available and it can be used reliably (Izard & Dougherty, 1982). The coders
completed approximately 46 hours of practice with Max and achieved a reliability
of .85 or greater.

The coder sampled infants' facial behavior from the videotapes in 3-sec
segments based on the predetermined points of the learning curve: (1) 1 min
of baseline, (2) the first 60 sec of the contingency, (3) 60 sec before response
acceleration, (4) 60 sec of initial acceleration, (5) 60 sec before peak response,
(6) first 60 sec after peak response, (7) 60 sec before sustained decline, (8)
first 60 sec of decline, and (9) last 60 sec in the session. A total of 9 min of
facial behavior was coded for each subject.

During the coding, four passes were made through each tape. In the first
three, with the volume off and at slow speed, brow, eye, and mouth regions
of the face were coded. During the fourth pass, with the volume on and at
normal speed, vocalization and fuss/cry were noted. To code facial expressions,
the coder recorded all codable movements in sequence for each 3-sec segment
of behavior. Having coded each component, expressions were determined by
Max formulas. One expression per 3-sec segment was most common, although
two to three facial changes occasionally occurred, particularly during phases

2 and 3. If a facial movement began in one segment and persisted into the following segment, it was coded for the interval in which it first appeared. Duration of appearance changes were not measured. In our experience it appeared that some facial expressions, such as interest, were relatively enduring, whereas others, such an enjoyment (i.e., smiling) were typically brief. The dependent variable then was the number of 3-sec intervals in which a given expression was visible without regard to its duration.

In addition to coding facial expressions, a number of other behaviors of particular interest in a contingency experiment were recorded. Orientation of the head when other than a frontal full face served as an index of inattention to the contingency consequence. Infants might look away from the reinforcing stimulus either by casting their eyes down (which is codable in Max) or by looking to either side (which is not codable). "Looks at hand" is an interesting behavior in the contingency context, as it suggests an awareness of the ribbon and possible perception of the means–end contingency. "Looks at hand" was scored when both the subject's hand with the Velcro bracelet and the subject's eyes were in view and the subject's gaze was oriented toward that hand. Sucking lower lip, thumb, and/or hand were also coded for several reasons. First, their obstruction of the mouth clearly limits judgments of emotion to the rating of only the upper region of the face. It is useful to know the reason that an important emotional cue is missing. Second, sucking and other oral behaviors, although not emotional behaviors per se, may be motivated by stress or boredom (i.e., they may serve pacifying, comforting, or self-stimulation functions). And finally, vocalizing, fussing, and crying were coded.

Results

Figures 9.3, 9.4, and 9.5 present the mean number of expressed emotions as a function of the specific phases of the learning curve. It should be kept in mind that the temporal parameters associated with each phase were different for each subject. Nevertheless, the coding system allowed for the observation of emotional responses by phase across subjects. Since 3-sec intervals across a minute of coding were used, the maximum number of facial expressions per min was 20. However, since more than one facial expression could occur in a 3-sec period, each facial expression could occur a maximum of 20 times per minute. Thus, the total number of different expressions per coded period could (and indeed sometimes did) total more than 20.

The positive emotions of interest, surprise, and enjoyment showed distinct patterns in relation to the learning curve (Figure 9.3). During the base period (1), after the child was placed in this new situation, interest was quite high, whereas surprise and enjoyment were low. At the onset of the reinforcement (2), interest declined markedly and surprise increased slightly; enjoyment remained low. The same patterns continued into the last phase of the orienting

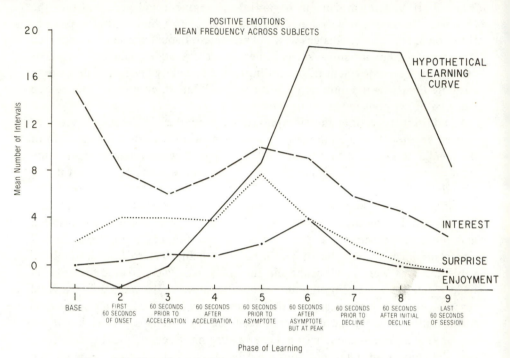

Figure 9.3. The relationship between positive emotions and learning

period (3). The acceleration phase of learning (4, 5) was characterized by an increase in interest and surprise and a slight increase in enjoyment. Enjoyment peaked at asymptote (6), whereas interest and surprise began to decline. All positive emotions declined thereafter. This pattern was observed for 4 out of 5 subjects. The fifth subject showed increased interest and enjoyment but very little surprise.

With regard to expressions of negative emotion, almost none were observed during base (1) (Figure 9.4). Negative expressions were most frequent during the orientation phase (2, 3), with fear reaching its highest level during this period. During the acquisition phase (4, 5), fear declined and remained low thereafter. This pattern held for all five subjects. Sadness showed relatively little change across the learning process, rising only in the postasymptotic period (8, 9). At this point, when interest and other positive expressions declined, sadness reached its highest point. The negative facial expressions appear to be reciprocals of the positive expressions. Four out of five subjects showed this pattern.

Figure 9.5 presents the course of the two self-regulating responses, gaze aversion and oral behavior. These behaviors showed still a different pattern

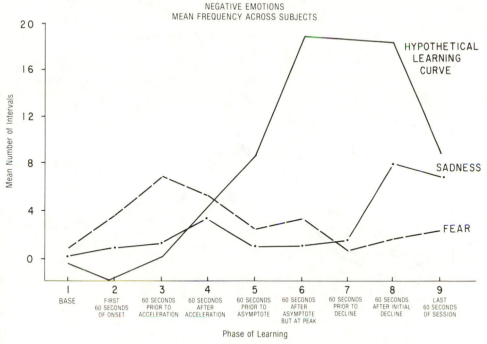

Figure 9.4. The relationship between negative emotions and learning

of occurrence. Relatively few self-regulating responses were observed during the base (1) and orienting (2, 3) phases. Both classes of behavior increased markedly during the acceleration phase (4) and remained high throughout the rest of the session until the last phase (9). Most notably, these behaviors increased at the time when negative expressions declined and positive expressions increased. However, they remained high during the asymptotic and post-asymptotic phases (6, 7, 8, 9), when positive expressions declined. Although more individual variations occurred in these patterns than in others, four of the five subjects showed a decline in self-regulatory behavior in the last minute of the session (9).

Thus far, our discussion has focused on patterns of facial expressions with little attention given to the frequency of their occurrence. Without a doubt, the most frequent expression was interest. This is not surprising, as the task was designed specifically to interest children. The next most frequent responses were surprise expressions and control behaviors. Enjoyment, fear, and sadness were relatively infrequent expressions. In fact, in only one phase corresponding to response asymptote did enjoyment occur more than 20% of the time. Fear and sadness, on the other hand, occurred more than 20% of the time in three

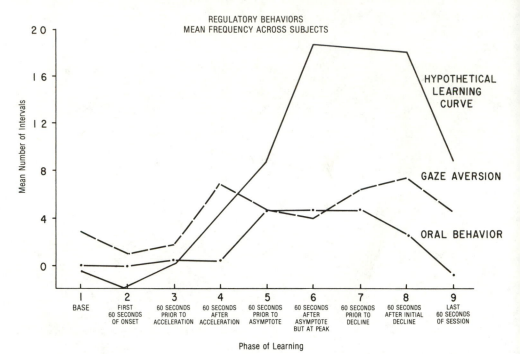

Figure 9.5. The relationship between self-regulatory behaviors and learning

periods (prior to acceleration, during decline, and in the final minute of the session).

Learning and emotional expression

The results of the contingency learning study bear on several issues. First, consider the metaphor of a fugue comprised of two themes, cognition and emotion. The infant is placed in a new situation. The fugue begins. Surprise is present and interest is high. The experiment starts; reinforcement is delivered for an arm-pull response. For the infant, something new is happening; surprise and fear increase, interest decreases. The activity level of the infant also decreases as arm-pulling declines below baseline. This dip in frequency of response may reflect the infant's awareness: "Something is happening. What is going on?" We label this period the orienting phase because of the infant's cessation of activity and increased vigilance and/or wariness. The increase in fear may reflect the infant's lack of information about and lack of control over the new event.

The decline in activity serves to diminish the reinforcement. A response causes reinforcement to recur. During this phase, which is viewed as the end of orientation and the beginning of acceleration, the infant begins to realize the relationship between action and outcome. Fear decreases; interest begins to rise. During the acquisition phase, interest and surprise continue to increase as fear declines. The infant continues to be alert and it now becomes necessary to modulate arousal. Self-regulatory behaviors (gaze aversion and oral activity) appear for this purpose and are observed at relatively high levels.

Learning is achieved by the asymptotic phase, when enjoyment also peaks. Fear remains at a low level and self-regulatory behaviors remain high. Following the solution of the problem, arm-pulling responses decline along with many of the emotional expressions. This decline may reflect a drop in arousal and interest. With the decline in arousal, the infant no longer needs the self-regulatory behaviors that remained high until the beginning of the postasymptotic phase. Cognitive solution brings enjoyment, a decline in arousal, and a decline in self-regulatory behavior.

During the postasymptotic phase, an interesting emotion appears, that of sadness. This expression may be a function of several factors. One strong possibility is that sadness is associated with fatigue or boredom. If this were the case, however, one would also expect to see an increase in self-regulatory responses, particularly oral behavior. This did not occur. Another possibility is that the large increase in sadness reflects "postsolution recoil." Although we do not believe that it reflects the equivalent of adult processes, such an expression may have a parallel in older children who appear unhappy after the successful completion of an activity. Self-reflection suggests that the happiest time is during the solution of a problem rather than after the problem is solved.

If the cognitive-emotional process is viewed in terms of well-defined temporal bouts, each of which has a definitive beginning and an end, then one would expect to observe a decline in all responses at the end of the experiment. That sadness increased at the end of the session, however, suggests that the termination of the experiment may constitute an artificial event imposed by the investigator on the ongoing flow of emotional and cognitive behaviors. One might imagine that the negative emotion of sadness acts as the first note in the next sequence of the cognitive-emotional fugue. From the perspective of opponent-process theory, the appearance of a negative emotion may be precipitated by a preceding positive emotion (Solomon & Corbitt, 1974). For adults the "post-task blues" may be a vital factor in motivating and reorienting the individual to new tasks.

The orienting reflex. One issue raised by the data pertains to the orienting response and learning. It has been argued that in order for learning to take place there must be habituation of the orienting response (Sokolov, 1963). Our data suggest that this is the case. The orienting reaction that occurred at the onset of reinforcement produced a complex set of responses. First, arm-pulling behavior declined as expected, since orienting results in the cessation of activity (Lewis, Goldberg, & Campbell, 1969). In addition, fear responses, perhaps a sign of wariness and/or vigilance, increased during the orienting phase only to decline shortly thereafter. It was following this orienting period that learning seemed to occur. Once the subject's arm-pulling responses returned to baseline, arm-pulling gradually increased. In addition, once fear diminished, interest began to increase. It appears that the habituation of the orienting response consists of a decline in fear, a resumption of activity, and an increase in interest.

It should be noted that this change in emotional behavior accompanying the habituation of orienting had as a concomitant response an increase in self-regulatory behavior. Self-regulation may facilitate the transition to emotions associated with renewed task-oriented activity. For example, for infants to become less fearful and more interested, they may need to regulate their arousal through self-stimulation. Although there are no data to support this view, the control of fear through self-regulation may permit an increase in interest and learning.

The orienting response appears to be comprised of emotional states non-conducive to learning. In this particular study, the cessation of activity was associated with wariness. Not until infants could respond did they learn the association between arm-pulling and outcome. Self-regulation may have reduced this wariness, thereby causing a reduction in the orienting reflex. Once orienting was habituated, behavior resumed. In this sense, orienting is envisioned as an emotional, not cognitive, process.

Individual differences. Individual variations may also influence the tempo and cadence of the fugue. Individual differences may include purely cognitive variables, such as the ability to recognize, store, and retrieve information about the co-occurrence of action and outcome. Of more interest, however, are individual differences related to the emotional components of the fugue. At each stage of learning, individual differences appeared in terms of the amount of emotion expressed, although relatively few individual differences were observed in the type or pattern of emotion expressed.

The variability among subjects was most pronounced in self-regulatory responses. Such individual differences may be related to what has been called "temperament." Part of the child's task in the cognitive-emotional process may be to regulate the level of negative emotion associated with the early phases of learning. This regulation may vary as a function of (1) the amount of negative emotion initially produced and (2) the efficiency of the child's ability to regulate this negative emotion. Both may be associated with the temperament dimensions of excitability and soothability (Thomas et al., 1963). For example, for some infants with difficult temperaments, the intense emotions associated with orienting may be overwhelming and prevent learning. Unable to habituate, these children may become increasingly fretful and ultimately drop out of the learning situation. Alternatively, other infants with difficult temperaments (high excitability, moderate soothability) might take a prolonged period to regulate their orienting response, thereby demonstrating learning only much later. For some of these infants who gain control later, new state variables, such as fatigue, might appear before the learning phase and these infants also might drop out of the learning situation. From another point of view, lethargic children (sometimes considered to have easy temperaments) may not become sufficiently aroused to orient; thus, they may not be able to initiate the learning process. Down's syndrome children may be a case in point. These children typically have low muscle tone, are lethargic, and are often reported to have easy temperaments. Their learning problems may result, in fact, from an inability to become activated.

One would expect that in the study of the cognitive-emotional interface, individual differences in the type of emotion as well as in the amount of emotion expressed would be found. Although the five subjects in the present study were remarkably similar in terms of the types of emotion expressed, there were some idiosyncratic facial appearances, which might be attributed to measurement error. It is not surprising that individual differences exist in the cognitive-emotional interface. Indeed, with age, individual differences in some of the minor themes of the fugue might become even more visible and play a major role in later idiosyncratic behavior. Individual differences are not a problem in the proposed model since, in Hofstadter's (1980) words, "there are standard kinds of things to do but not so standard that one can merely compose a fugue by formula" (p. 9).

Conclusions

The results of this study are particularly relevant to the three models described earlier. First, it is important to distinguish between different emotions and their relationships to cognition. Discussions of global emotional states (i.e., positive or negative) obscure interesting and significant aspects of the dynamic interplay between emotional and cognitive threads of behavior. Second, with regard to the issue of precedence, it seems clear that some emotions occur before what is traditionally viewed as the solution of a problem, or learning, and others come later. The particular emotions observed, rather than causing or resulting from a cognitive process, seem to interface with learning, providing the setting for each learning phase as well as resulting from that learning. The idea of precedence appears too simple in light of the complex relationship between learning and facial expression found in the present study. The data indicated that linear models of the relationship between cognition and emotion are inadequate. The relationship between these domains is complex, continuous, and more finely tuned than depicted by such models. In conceptualizing the relationship between emotion and cognition, neither should be described as causing the other; rather, each continually and progressively chases the other, weaving separate threads of behavior into a single composition, a fugue.

References

Arnold, M. B. *Emotion and personality* (2 vols.). New York: Columbia University Press, 1960.

Arnold, M. B. Brain function in emotion: A phenomenological analysis. In P. Black (Ed.), *Physiological correlates of emotion*. New York: Academic Press, 1970.

Berlyne, D. E. *Conflict, arousal and curiosity*. New York: McGraw-Hill, 1960.

Berlyne, D. E. Children's reasoning and thinking. In P. Mussen (Ed.), *Carmichael's manual of child psychology* (Vol. 1). New York: Wiley, 1970.

Bower, G. H. Mood and memory. *American Psychologist*, 1981, *36*, 129–148.

Brinker, R. P., & Lewis, M. Contingency intervention in infancy. In J. Anderson & J. Cox (Eds.), *Curriculum materials for high risk and handicapped infants*. Chapel Hill, N.C.: Technical Assistance & Development Systems, 1982.

Brooks-Gunn, J., & Lewis, M. Affective exchanges between normal and handicapped infants and their mothers. In T. Field & A. Fogel (Eds.), *Emotion and early interaction*. Hillsdale, N.J.: Erlbaum, 1982.

Buck, R. Nonverbal behavior and the theory of emotion: The facial feedback hypothesis. *Journal of Personality and Social Psychology*, 1980, *38*, 811–824.

Campos, J. J., & Stenberg, C. R. Perception, appraisal, and emotion: The onset of social referencing. In. M. Lamb & L. Sherrod (Eds.), *Infant social cognition: Empirical data and theoretical considerations*. Hillsdale, N.J.: Erlbaum, 1982.

Darwin, C. *The expression of emotions in man and animals*. Chicago: University of Chicago Press, 1965. (Originally published, 1872.)

DeCasper, A. J., & Carstens, A. A. Contingencies of stimulation: Effects on learning and motivation. *Infant Behavior and Development*, 1981, *4*, 19–35.

Ekman, P. Cross-cultural studies of facial expression. In P. Ekman (Ed.), *Darwin and facial expression: A century of research in review*. New York: Academic Press, 1973.

Ekman, P., Friesen, W. V., & Ellsworth, P. *Emotion in the human face*. New York: Pergamon Press, 1972.

Emde, R. N., & Koenig, K. L. Neonatal smiling and rapid eye movement states. *American Academy of Child Psychiatry*, 1969, *8*, 57–67.

Feinman, S., & Lewis, M. Social referencing and second order effects in 10-month-old infants. *Child Development*, 1983, *54*, 878–887.

Festinger, L. *A theory of cognitive dissonance*. Stanford: Stanford University Press, 1957.

Freud, S. *The psychopathology of everyday life* (A. Tyson, trans.) New York: Norton, 1960.

Gunnar, M. R. Control, warning signals, and distress in infancy. *Developmental Psychology*, 1980, *16*, 281–289.

Hartmann, H. *Ego psychology and the problem of adaptation*. New York: International Universities Press, 1958.

Hebb, D. O. On the nature of fear. *Psychological Review*, 1946, *53*, 256–276.

Hebb, D. O. *The organization of behavior*. New York: Wiley, 1949.

Hofstadter, D. *Gödel, Escher, Bach: An eternal golden braid*. New York: Random House, 1980.

Izard, C. E. *The face of emotion*. New York: Appleton-Century-Crofts, 1971.

Izard, C. E. *Human emotions*. New York: Plenum, 1977.

Izard, C. E. *The Maximally Discriminative Facial Movement Coding System* (Max). Newark, Del.: Instructional Resources Center, University of Delaware, 1979.

Izard, C. E., & Dougherty, L. M. Two systems for measuring facial expressions. In C. E. Izard (Ed.), *Measuring emotions in infants and children*. Cambridge: Cambridge University Press, 1982.

James, W. "What is an emotion?" *Mind*, 1884, *9*, 188–205.

James, W. *Principles of psychology*. New York: Holt, 1890.

Kagan, J. Discrepancy, temperament, and infant distress. In M. Lewis & L. Rosenblum (Eds.), *The origins of fear*. New York: Wiley, 1974.

Kagan, J. On emotion and its development: A working paper. In M. Lewis & L. Rosenblum (Eds.), *The development of affect*. New York: Plenum, 1978.

Laird, J. D. Self-attribution of emotion: The effects of expressive behavior on the quality of emotional experience. *Journal of Personality and Social Psychology*, 1974, *29*, 475–486.

Lazarus, R. S. *Psychological stress and the coping process*. New York: McGraw-Hill, 1966.

Lazarus, R. S. Thoughts on the relations between emotion and cognition. *American Psychologist*, 1982, *37*, 1019–1024.

Lazarus, R. S., Averill, J. R., & Optin, E. M., Jr. Towards a cognitive theory of emotion. In M. B. Arnold (Ed.), *Feelings and emotions*. New York: Academic Press, 1970.

Lewis, M. Developmental theories. In I. L. Kutash & L. B. Schlesinger (Eds.), *Handbook on stress and anxiety*. San Francisco: Jossey-Bass, 1980.

Lewis, M., & Goldberg, S. Perceptual-cognitive development in infancy: A generalized expectancy model as a function of mother–infant interaction. *Merrill-Palmer Quarterly*, 1969, *15*, 81–100.

Lewis, M., Goldberg, S., & Campbell, H. A developmental study of information processing in the first three years of life: Response decrement to a redundant signal. *Monographs of the Society for Research in Child Development*, 1969, *34* (9, Serial No. 133).

Lewis, M., & Michalson, L. The socialization of emotions. In T. Field & A. Fogel (Eds.), *Emotion and early interaction*. Hillsdale, N.J.: Erlbaum, 1982.

Lewis, M., & Michalson, L. *Children's emotions and moods: Developmental theory and measurement*. New York: Plenum, 1983.

Lewis, M., & Michalson, L. From emotional state to emotional expression. In D. Magnusson & V. L. Allen (Eds.), *Human development: An interactional perspective*. New York: Academic Press, in press.

Lewis, M., & Rosenblum, L. Introduction: Issues in affect development. In M. Lewis & L. Rosenblum (Eds.), *The development of affect*. New York: Plenum, 1978.

Mandler, G. *Mind and emotion*. New York: Wiley, 1975.

Mandler, G. The generation of emotion: A psychological theory. In R. Plutchik & H. Kellerman (Eds.), *Emotion: Theory, research, and experience*, Vol. 1: *Theories of emotion*. New York: Academic Press, 1980.

McCall, R. B. Smiling and vocalization in infants as indices of perceptual-cognitive processes. *Merrill-Palmer Quarterly*, 1972, *18*, 341–347.

Mischel, W. Processes in delay of gratification. In L. Berkowitz (Ed.), *Advances in experimental social psychology* (Vol. 7). New York: Academic Press, 1974.

Norman, D. A., & Rumelhart, D. F. *Explorations in cognition*. San Francisco: Freeman, 1975.

Piaget, J. *The origin of intelligence in children*. New York: Norton, 1952.

Plutchik, R. A general psychoevolutionary theory of emotion. In R. Plutchik & H. Kellerman (Eds.), *Emotion: Theory, research, and experience*, Vol. 1: *Theories of emotion*. New York: Academic Press, 1980.

Royce, J. R., & Diamond, S. R. A multifactor-system dynamics theory of emotion: Cognitive-affective interaction. *Motivation and Emotion*, 1980, *4*, 263–298.

Saarni, C. Children's understanding of display rules for expressive behavior. *Developmental Psychology*, 1979, *15*, 424–429.

Saarni, C. Observing children's use of display rules: Age and sex differences. Paper presented at the annual meeting of the American Psychological Association, Montreal, September 1980.

Saarni, C. Social and affective functions of nonverbal behavior: Developmental concerns. In R. Feldman (Ed.), *Development of nonverbal behavior*. New York: Springer-Verlag, 1982.

Schachter, S. The interaction of cognitive and physiological determinants of emotional state. In L. Berkowitz (Ed.), *Advances in experimental social psychology* (Vol. 1). New York: Academic Press, 1964.

Schachter, S., & Singer, J. Cognitive, social and physiological determinants of emotional state. *Psychological Review*, 1962, *69*, 378–399.

Schaffer, H. R. Cognitive components of infants' response to strangeness. In M. Lewis & L. Rosenblum (Eds.), *The origins of fear*. New York: Wiley, 1974.

Simonov, P. V. The information theory of emotion. In M. B. Arnold (Ed.), *Feelings and emotions*. New York: Academic Press, 1970.

Sokolov, E. N. *Perception and the conditioned reflex*. New York: Macmillan, 1963.

Solomon, R. L., & Corbitt, J. D. An opponent-process theory of motivation: I. Temporal dynamics of affect. *Psychological Review*, 1974, *81*, 119–146.

Strongman, K. T. *The psychology of emotion*, 2nd ed. New York: Wiley, 1978.

Sullivan, M. W., Rovee-Collier, C. K., & Tynes, D. M. A conditioning analysis of long-term memory in 3-month-old infants. *Child Development*, 1979, *50*, 152–162.

Thomas, A., Chess, S., Birch, H. G., Hertzig, M. E., & Korn, S. *Behavioral individuality in early childhood*. New York: New York University Press, 1963.

Tomkins, S. *Affect, imagery, consciousness*, Vol. 1: *The positive affects*. New York: Springer-Verlag, 1962.

Tomkins, S. *Affect, imagery, consciousness*, Vol. 2: *The negative affects*. New York: Springer-Verlag, 1963.

Tomkins, S. Affect as the primary motivational system. In M. B. Arnold (Ed.), *Feelings and emotions*. New York: Academic Press, 1970.

Ulvund, S. E. Cognition and motivation in early infancy: An interactionistic approach. *Human Development*, 1980, *23*, 17–32.

Watson, J. B., & Rayner, R. Conditioned emotional reactions. *Journal of Experimental Psychology*, 1920, *3*, 1–14.

Watson, J. S. The development of and generalization of "contingency awareness" in early infancy. *Merrill-Palmer Quarterly*, 1966, *12*, 123–125.

Watson, J. S. Smiling, cooing, and "the game." *Merrill-Palmer Quarterly*, 1972, *18*, 323–339.

Zajonc, R. B. Feeling and thinking: Preferences need no inferences. *American Psychologist*, 1980, *35*, 151–175.

10 The role of affect in social competence

*L. Alan Sroufe, Edward Schork, Frosso Motti,
Nancy Lawroski, and Peter LaFreniere*

Observation of free-flowing behavior among preschool-age children makes obvious the vital role of affect in promoting and maintaining interaction and in promoting the emergence of the peer group social structure. Consider this example. Three preschool-age children run down a hill to a richly outfitted playground and begin exploring various toys and physical structures at the edge of a large sand area. Suddenly, one child calls out excitedly, "Hey look! It's a boat," pointing to a large wooden climbing apparatus in the center of the sand area. The structure, made from logs, ropes, and tires and containing ladders and slides, looks nothing like a boat. However, its placement in the middle of the sand inspires the creative imagination of the preschoolers. The others run over, and when the lead child squeals "Come on, let's climb on," all scramble onto the structure. There they play, smiling and laughing, for some time, taking turns at the "wheel" and climbing through the various parts of the "boat." In time, the excitement begins to subside. It is at that point that the first child, again in an expressive voice, calls out: "Oh no, the boat is sinking – we better get into the water!" All scramble into the sand. "Swim!" With great laughter and shouting, the children make their way toward "shore."

In these and countless other observations, we have seen the important role played by affect in both attaining leadership status in the group and promoting and sustaining interaction. The child observed here was, first, excited by the idea of the "boat." Beyond this, she *conveyed* her enthusiasm to the others through voice, body posture, and facial expression. Having a good idea is an important starting point for a positive interaction, but often it is not enough. Pointing to a barrel and stating flatly that "it's a space capsule" seldom engages others, whereas an enthusiastic *"Hey, it's a space capsule"* brings children running. Our main character here attracted the others through her expressed positive affect, and her enthusiasm was contagious.

It is also clear that expressed affect was important in sustaining the fantasy play. When the game slowed, a timely suggestion of a new variation kept the play alive. This was more than simple timing. Without the affect, it is less

This chapter was supported by a grant from the National Science Foundation (NSF/ BNS 8004572) and by a program project grant from the National Institute of Child Health and Human Development (5 POI HO 05027).

289

likely that the others would have been captured by the idea. This child's ability to have fun and to share the fun with others is no doubt one reason she was the sociometric star of her preschool class.

In our view, affect, as the expressive and experiential part of emotion,[1] has a central role in the organization of individual behavior and therefore social interaction (Sroufe, 1979a, 1982). As Zajonc put it: "Affect dominates social interaction, and it is the major currency in which social interaction is transacted" (1980, p. 753). It is not merely a by-product of cognition or the end point of an appraisal process; rather, affect is what cognition serves (Piaget & Inhelder, 1969). The emotions are motivators and organizers of behavior, and the "appraisal process" itself is motivated and directed by emotion (Izard & Buechler, 1980).

Whereas thus far there has been little research on the role of affect in competent functioning, in general, or social competence, in particular, a number of findings are provocative. In reporting on the results of her landmark longitudinal study on the "capacity to cope with the opportunities, challenges and frustrations of the environment," Murphy stated that IQ was less obviously a factor than a child's resources for gratification and "his capacity for zest, pleasure, interest, and enjoyment of activities" (1962, p. 231). Moreover, the capacity for joy and "investment in the environment" were not closely related to IQ, SES, or "physiological variables," though they were related to the capacity for affective expression. Relevant here is the finding of Birns and Golden (1972) that zest in approaching tasks in infancy better predicted later IQ than did infant developmental quotient measures per se.

Rothenberg (1970) reported a correlation between "social sensitivity" and social competence, as assessed through teacher ratings and peer nominations. Social sensitivity was defined as the ability to accurately perceive and comprehend the behavior, feelings, and motives of other individuals.

Izard (1971) cites data on both humans and animals suggestive of a role for affect in social competence. In the one study, teachers' ratings of adjustment correlated with emotional labeling ability. In an experimental animal study, the facial nerves of a group of rhesus monkeys were sectioned, which eliminated the facial expression of emotions. Thus handicapped, these animals were more often involved in aggressive encounters. These data suggest a vital role for affective expressions in regulating the social behavior of the rhesus and, by analogy, human children.

In our previous research at Minnesota we have established a number of empirical relationships relevant to the organizational significance of affect. First, in our longitudinal studies, assessments of competence at each age through the preschool years have had strong affective correlates, for example, attachment and affective sharing (Waters, Wippman, & Sroufe, 1979), toddler problem-solving competence and enthusiasm and positive affect (Matas, Arend, & Sroufe, 1978). Also, our measures of attachment in infancy (defined in terms of affect regulation) and affect expression in the toddler period have strongly predicted competence in the preschool classroom (Arend, Gove, & Sroufe, 1979; Sroufe, 1983; Waters et al., 1979). Finally, prior to the study to be reported here, we had obtained a significant correlation between attention rank (number of looks and glances received in the classroom, a well-validated measure of competence; Vaughn & Waters, 1980) and independent rankings on affective expressiveness (unpublished data).

One other finding is so provocative that it deserves special note. These results were obtained by LaFreniere in an ongoing stdy of the correlates of preschool social structure. Initially, it was found that photograph rankings of children on "physical attractiveness" were significantly correlated with various measures of social competence, including attention rank. However, the "physical attractiveness" rankings were made by persons who knew the children (though not their ranking on the other measures). When persons unfamiliar with the children ranked them on physical attractiveness, using the same photographs, the correlation with attention rank disappeared. One interpretation of these results is that the rankings of the first set of judges were based on "persona"; that is, their experience with what the children projected affectively. Affective expressiveness, interpersonal and otherwise, may turn out to be a much more powerful variable than physical attractiveness per se in regulating social responses.

Conceptual links between social competence and affect

The findings just presented suggest that social competence may be influenced by a range of affective variables, from zestful involvement in activities, to affective expressiveness, to recognition of the emotions of others and oneself. In this section we will present a brief catalogue of the roles that affect may play in promoting social interaction and social competence.

Initiating social exchanges

As suggested in our opening vignette, positive affect plays an inviting role in social interaction. Across cultures, the smile communicates affiliative intent and, as will be discussed later under shared affect, tends to elicit positive responses in others (e.g., Izard, 1977; Sroufe & Waters, 1976; Vine, 1973). It probably also contributes to the development of a positive "set" in the perception of the child by ongoing social partners, increasing their positive feelings toward the child and the likelihood of their making positive future initiations or responses to the child.

The communicative role

Perhaps especially in the case of young children, expressions of affect allow interpretations by others of the meaning of one's socially directed acts as well as the meaning of others' responses to those actions. The meaning of offering or taking objects, so central in the role of early play, must rest heavily on the accompanying affect, and affect expressed by the partner suggests the need to alter or continue a particular behavior. Through affect, the child shows what he or she means by the offer or take, and the other child shows how he or she construes the behavior. This provides valuable information to each child for understanding social interactions, and, in time, a child can both anticipate the other's reaction and fit his or her behavior to the other's intentions and desires.

The regulation of social exchanges

Closely related to the communicative role, the pacing, switching, and termination of exchanges are guided by affect. Activities are commonly sustained through the timely intensification of affective response. The role of positive affect in initiating and guiding social interaction has been most thoroughly documented in the case of care-giver–infant interaction (e.g., Stern, 1974).

Shared affect-contagion

A number of writers have discussed the reciprocal influence of affect on children. Sherman (1975) describes "group glee" and Izard (1977) and Murphy (1962) speak of "contagion."

Feelings expressed can be shared. When these are feelings of satisfaction and delight, interest and zest, sharing them produces contagious responses in the other children and . . . positive feedback to the first child, who is then stimulated to more active responses, new ideas for utilizing the situation and for new goals (Murphy, 1962, p. 242).

Shared affect is the bond that ties children together. Relationships are essentially what people share, and affect is an essential part of what is shared.

Injecting life into the interaction

It would seem likely that the capacity to have fun and to help others have fun (Erikson's "sending power") plays a crucial role in being liked by peers. Such fun is part of what makes interactions among young children rewarding. The zestful child who conveys his or her sense of fun to others is likely to be well liked and sought out. As Greenson puts it: "People who are prone to evoke enthusiasm often become leaders, and it is indeed one of the most valuable characteristics in determining leadership potential" (1977, p. 314).

There are, of course, other aspects of affective-behavioral organization that are vital to social competence. Prominent among these are appropriateness of affect, the ability to express negative affect, and, in general, the ability to modulate affect, for example, excitement without loss of control. Murphy (1962) cites the "capacity to protest, resist and terminate unwanted stimuli" as being of parallel importance to the positive affect correlates of competence. Moreover, attraction of others to exciting activities would not be expected to lead to one's esteem by the group if such activities routinely led to overarousal and, ultimately, disorganized behavior and negative affect. The socially competent child would be expected to express the range of affects clearly and appropriately, to tolerate disappointments well, and to modulate affect in serving the goal of sustained positive interaction.

The social roots of affect modulation and expressiveness

Although the central theme of this chapter concerns the role of affect in emerging social competence, within an integrative developmental perspective there is an equally important role for social experiences in promoting development in the affect domain. Along with others (Ainsworth et al., 1978; Brazelton, Koslowski, & Main, 1974; Stern, 1974), we, in fact, view early sensitive care in terms of the effective modulation of affect. Moreover, we define patterns of attachment in terms of individual differences in the regulation of affect (Sroufe & Waters, 1977). The secure attachment relationship is one in which the infant can use the care giver as a base for affectively engaging the object world and as a ready source of comfort when frightened or distressed. Such security is based on a history of the emotional availability of the care giver and the care giver's dependable responses to the infant's affective signals, positive or negative. From such a relationship history, it is posited, the child enters the preschool social world with confident and positive expectations concerning others and the capacity for both sharing affect and enjoying social exchanges and maintaining organized behavior in the face of considerable arousal. Regulation within the child–care-giver dyad in infancy promotes the capacity for self-regulation in the preschooler (Sander, 1975). Such a child will show a relative absence of anger and hostility, which are pervasive only when the infancy has been characterized by the emotional unavailability or inconsistent responsiveness, of the care giver. In contrast, as a result of their participation in affectively reciprocal interaction, secure children display notable empathic capacity. Documentation for these points is found in numerous papers (e.g., Ainsworth et al., 1978; Arend, Gove, & Sroufe, 1979; Egeland & Sroufe, 1981; Matas et al., 1978; Sroufe, 1983).

In brief, in the research to be described we seek to further document the ties between early relational history and affective control and expression and, especially, the relations between affective variables and social competence in the preschool years. Although the studies to be reported are correlational, the network of relationships is sufficient to imply a clear role for affective variables in promoting social development.

Description of the Minnesota Preschool Project

Despite the intuitively compelling links between affect expression, affect modulation, and social competence, the empirical demonstration of such ties presents complex assessment problems. On both the affective side and the social side we are dealing with broad constructs, which cannot readily be reduced to any single behavior. Moreover, a process is clearly involved, that is, that children find their place in the peer group social structure over time as a consequence of a substantial history of affective exchanges. At the least, one would require assessments of both social competence and affective aspects of interaction based on a considerable period of observation, preferably in a naturalistic setting and preferably across a range of contexts. Understanding the role of affect in a child's ultimate status (and effectiveness) within the peer group probably cannot be addressed in single-session laboratory experiments, however well conceived.

Recently, with funding from the National Science Foundation, we had the opportunity to carry out a detailed, observational study of two consecutive preschool classrooms, one spanning 10 weeks, the other 20 weeks. We were able to observe the children daily in the classroom, in the van, and on the playground, in large and small groups, and in structured and unstructured activities. We were able to observe with great frequency the entire range of affective experience, from unrestrained exuberance through very negative reactions to frustration and disappointment.

The children who participated in our preschool project were part of an ongoing longitudinal study of an urban poverty sample (Egeland & Sroufe, 1981). A large amount of information is available on these children, their care givers, and their life circumstances from before their births to the present time. Included in this data is information on the quality of care received and the early organization of the child's behavior. Prominent aspects of the early child assessments included the regulation of affect in the face of separations from and reunions with, the care giver (Ainsworth's Strange Situation attachment assessments at 12 and 18 months) and affective reactions to progressively more difficult problems at 2 years of age. Thus, we had available affective aspects of early object competence and the roots of social competence as they are manifest within a smoothly functioning care-giver–infant dyad.

Sample characteristics and subject selection

As a representative urban poverty group, the larger sample from which our preschool subjects were selected has certain characteristic features. Many of the mothers were young (mean age of 20 when the child was born), and few had stable partnerships: Two-thirds were unmarried at the time of birth and by the time the children were 18 months old only about one-eighth of the mothers were still living with the child's father. Their lives were highly changeable, in terms of people, residence, and jobs, as well as highly stressful. Nonetheless, the sample contains the entire range of child-care quality and child adaptation. Along with numerous cases of physical abuse, psychological abuse, and neglect (Egeland & Sroufe, 1981), there are also many cases in which both care giver and child functioned quite well.

The primary basis for selecting children to participate in the nursery-school project was stable attachment history. Since Ainsworth attachment assessments are the most widely validated assessment of quality of early adaptation (Ainsworth et al., 1978; Sroufe, 1979, 1983), selection on this basis ensured a wide range of social competence, even given the preponderance of developmental problems in this sample.

All but one of the children in the larger second class (20 weeks) had shown either a pattern of secure attachment (flexible and effective use of the care giver as a support for exploration and a source of reassurance when distressed) at both 12 and 18 months or a pattern of anxious attachment at both ages (either unable to be settled by the care giver when distressed or avoidant of her following a brief separation). There were 12 boys and 12 girls. In the first class, which lasted only 10 weeks, there were 7 children with stable, secure attachments (4 girls), 4 children with mixed histories (2 girls), and 4 children who showed anxious patterns of attachment at both 12 and 18 months (all boys). Again, for our purposes here, the important characteristic of this sample is that a considerable spread in social functioning would be expected. In both classes intellectual potential ranged from low normal to gifted, with the 24-month Bayley Mental Development Index (the measure available at the time) equated across attachment groups.

Description of the preschool program

A salient feature of our preschool program was the ample opportunity allowed for spontaneous social interchange among the children. For transportation reasons, half the children in each class arrived and departed about an hour before their classmates. On arrival, the first group immediately participated in large-motor play outdoors (or at times indoors), which was followed by small-group structured activities. When the second group arrived, the entire class engaged in free play for 50 minutes. Following a snack (and in the first class large-circle time), the "early" children departed, and the "late" children participated in small-group and then outdoor play. This split class format was especially important for the large second class. When all 24 children were present, the free flow of behavior was somewhat constrained. Because the formation of a coherent group structure was impaired, more children opted for individual activity. But even in the large class, outdoor free play was limited to 12 children at a time, so that both behavioral and observational opportunities were maximized.

There was a ratio of at least 1 adult per 6 children. There were 2 full-time teachers, 1 full-time assistant, and 3 part-time assistants. Despite differences in style, classroom rules and procedures were clear and coherent. Because social and emotional development were considered important parts of the pre-school experience, a great amount of spontaneity and free-flowing social interaction was accepted. Nonetheless, aggressive behavior was controlled quite tightly, and there were rules against running in the classroom, jumping off of high places, and throwing objects.

Observation and data-collection procedures

Almost all observation in the classroom was done from a screened booth, elevated and located at the side of the classroom and entered from the outside hallway. Children were informed that observers were present, but they could see only very dimly into the booth, and the observers maintained silence. Children very quickly adapted to this observer presence, certainly within the first week or two of the class. Each day of the first week of class, and then once weekly thereafter, videotapes were made in the classroom. When the children were outdoors, observers flanked the play yard. Observers maintained a strict noninteractive stance, and soon became of little interest to the children who had more important things to do.

Many data-gathering approaches were used, from time sampling to child sampling to event sampling. Measures ranged from the most discrete (frequency counts of interaction) to the most molar (rankings of social competence). Some were based on 10-second periods of observation, and some were based on impressions derived over the entire course of the class.

Assessment of affect

Two procedures were used to assess affect during this project. In the first class a simple, sraightforward measure of affect was used; for the second class, a more complex and comprehensive assessment device was developed. The first procedure involved recording social initiations and responses as positive, negative, or neutral in hedonic tone, based primarily on facial expression and tone of voice.[2] More than 4,000 social interactions involving affiliation, altruism, petitioning, assertiveness, and aggression were coded, using a zone-event sampling technique. (Because of its large size, the classroom was divided into three zones with one observer assigned to each zone.) Observer agreement (number of agreements divided by number of agreements plus number of errors of commission) was consistently greater than 80%. In various analyses, frequencies or proportions of positive and negative affect were used.

In the second class a child-sampling procedure was used. Each child was observed for 5-minute periods over the course of the 20-week session. At the end of the 5-minute period the observer filled out a detailed checklist (Appendix) to record the occurrence of certain events. These codings included affective expression in both interactive and, occasionally, noninteractive contexts, and they included aspects of behavior outside the affective domain (especially impulse control, atypical behavior, and self-management). In addition, qualitative aspects of the child's behavior were included, such as the appropriateness of the affect, the expressiveness, and so forth. Whereas some events also could have been observed using time-sampling procedures, others were amenable only to this technique. For example, certain events required considerable time to unfold. "Using positive affect to sustain an interaction" requires that the interaction be viewed over some time. Similarly, "showing negative affect in response to frustration" requires that the observer witness the frustrating event as well as the consequent negative affect. Although this procedure yields less data in terms of frequency, it yields richer data in terms of process. While the basic data to be reported in this chapter involve composites across various affective items, in-time profiles of each child across affect and impulse control items will be available.

In addition to the attachment classifications at 12 and 18 months, two measures of affect were available from our two-year assessments. The first was enthusiasm in approaching the tool problems (a 7-point scale, see Matas et al., 1978). The second was a clearly identified affect factor from a factor analysis of our current sample (with high loadings on positive affect during free play, enthusiasm and positive affect during the tools, and a high negative loading on negative affect during the tools).

Assessment of social competence

Social competence is best viewed as a construct (e.g., Waters & Sroufe, 1983). One is interested in the child's effectiveness and status in the peer group and, perhaps especially, the child's ability to learn from, and generally draw upon, peer group experiences to further enhance development. From this broad perspective, individual measures are seldom completely adequate. For example, frequency of social interaction is measured easily but would only be imperfectly related to competence. Although, for the most part, frequent social participation would imply more competence than would nonparticipation, even this is not always true. Some children participate frequently but with no skill. And excluding social isolation, frequency of participation within the mid to upper frequencies would carry little information about competence without considering quality of interaction. As a different example, qualitative assessments, such as teacher rankings, are likely to be more robust, but they are subject to halo effects based upon the *teacher's* interactions with the child.

Based on these considerations, we employed a broad-band approach to social competence based on several data sources and a range of procedures. We did obtain data on frequency of social participation. And we used teacher ratings and rankings despite their subjectivity, as based upon their cumulative experiences as highly skilled observers directly involved in the classroom, they are the most integrative measures available. To rule out individual biases, the median rankings of the 3 full-time teachers were used. In addition, we used a measure of sociometric status, determined through a combination of standard nomination procedures (cf. Asher et al., 1979) and forced groupings. Finally, for the first class we had available a time-sampling observation measure of attention rank. In using this measure, which is based on the number of looks and glances received, it is assumed that children learn to look to more competent children for direction, for fun, and simply out of interest. The attention-rank measure has been shown to have an impressive number of competence-related correlates, including teacher rankings, sociometric status, and frequency of being imitated and winning object struggles (Vaughn & Waters, 1980).

Initial empirical relationships: the first preschool class

The first preschool class was considered a pilot sample, because class size was small ($N = 15$) and because our elaborated scheme for coding affect was still being developed. Nonetheless, the small class size offered certain advantages. First, a clear group structure emerged, as reflected by a stable attention structure and strong associations across measures of social competence. In part, this likely reflected more group coherence and, in part, more error-free assessment because of the relative lack of turmoil in the classroom. And, of course, ranking 15 children (as in the teacher judgments and peer sociometric assessment) is simpler than ranking 24 children, as was required in the second class. Nevertheless, despite the small sample size and a rather coarse measure of affect, we expected an association between affect expression and social competence.

Affectively positive social engagement and teacher judgments
of social competence

Relationships between assessments of social competence and affective expression were uniformly strong. We began with the teacher ranking on social competence as the criterion, since it involves the composite observations of three skilled teachers, based across contexts and across time. The correlation between teacher ranking and a combined affective score (the frequency of affectively positive social interaction minus the frequency of negative interaction) was $\rho = .76$ ($p < .001$). A similar relationship was found using the frequency of positive affective interactions alone ($\rho = .70$, $p < .002$). Using negative affect alone did not yield a significant correlation with teacher ranking (or with the other criteria discussed later).

Sociometric status and attention rank data

The association between affectively positive social enounters and teacher judgments of social competence was corroborated by the sociometric status and attention structure data. Children more frequently nominated as liked (and not disliked, a weighted total score) were observed to show more affectively positive social behavior ($\rho = .70$, $p < .002$). (Positive minus negative affect produced similar results; $\rho = .71$, $p < .002$.) Moreover, the children gave more attention to (more frequently looked at) children who were ranked high on positive affective interaction ($\rho = .83$, $p < .001$).

Thus, observer, teacher, and child-based data (with each set obtained by different teams of investigators) converged to suggest that positive affective exchanges are strongly related to social competence. Moreover, these results cannot be reduced simply to social participation. Children high on positive affective engagement, not surprisingly, do tend to be high on social participation ($\rho = .79$, $p < .001$). But social participation does not correlate as strongly as does positive affect with, for example, attention structure ($\rho = .69$, vs. .83), and the relations between affect and social competence held up when proportion values, rather than sheer frequencies, were used. Competent children are not just more frequently involved with other children; they are more positively, affectively involved.

Extending the relationships: Class 2 findings

The Affect Checklist (Appendix) provided a much more differentiated affect assessment. More attention was paid to facial expression, to the timing of the reaction, and, especially, to its place in the ongoing stream of interaction. All of this was promoted by the 5-minute child-sampling procedure. Also, a considerable portion of this data was obtained during large-motor play (outdoors and in the large room allocated to motor activity), during which only 12 children at a time were present. Interaction was promoted in these contexts and observation was somewhat easier than it was during free play in a crowded classroom. Offsetting these advantages, no *coherent* attention structure emerged in this class, and the teachers thus had more difficulty making the social-competence rankings.

Data reduction and reliability

Forty-seven items were coded with sufficient frequency to be included in the final set. (Starred items on the appendix checklist were eliminated.) Two coders independently made 119 observations (52 large motor, 67 free play) evenly distributed across the 24 children. Percent of agreement on the presence or absence of the particular reaction was uniformly high, ranging from 71% to 100%, with agreement above 90% for two-thirds of the items.

With low frequency data, however (or with very high frequency data as existed in some cases), percent agreement resulted in inflated estimates of reliability, which simply were due to base rates. Therefore, a conservative estimate (the phi coefficient) was also computed. These ranged from .23 to 1.00, with a mean of .56. The reliabilities for 3 of the items were in the .20s, with 6 in the .30s, 6 in the .40s, and 32 at .50 or above. The average phi for the large-motor observations alone (the data to be reported) was .58. For individual items, such reliability estimates are quite satisfactory. The disagreements commonly were within category; for example, one coder seeing a display of positive affect as a response to another child, the other seeing it as undirected ("positive affect directed to no one in particular"). It was not the case that one coder saw the behavior as a positive affective response and the other as a negative affective response. Thus, the reliability of "positive affect to no one" was .43, and the reliability for the broader positive affect base line (any positive affect) was .68. Moreover, when items within categories were combined to form mega-items, reliabilities increased appreciably. The use of mega-items is also an important step in reducing the number of statistical tests to be computed (see Table 10.1 for mega-item descriptions).

Antecedents of affective expression and control

Although this chapter focuses on the contemporary affective correlates of social competence, affective assessments from the toddler period are relevant to the construct validity of our current measures. We first correlated the two affect measures available from our two-year assessment (enthusiasm rating and positive-affect factor score) to the principal positive-affect (POSAFF) and negative-affect (NEGAFF) mega-items as defined in Table 10.1. Enthusiasm at age 2 correlated $r = .38$ ($p < .07$) with POSAFF and $-.16$ ($p < .10$) with NEGAFF. The parallel correlations for the two-year positive-affect factor scores were .47 ($p < .03$) and $-.12$ (ns). Such stability over a three-year period is impressive, especially given that these correlations are not corrected for attenuation.

Because our assessments of attachment at 12 and 18 months are viewed as assessments of affect regulation, it is of interest that attachment quality predicted preschool affect expression and control. As noted earlier in this chapter (Sroufe, 1983), children who had been classified as secure in their attachments were

Table 10.1. *Definition of mega-items (large motor data)*

Mega-item	Definitions
POSAFF	Positive initiation, positive response, positive affect directed to no one in particular, very positive affect (exuberance), ongoing high enjoyment, pride in accomplishment, very positive expressive face when communicating with others
NEGAFF	Negative initiation, negative response, very negative expressive face when communicating with others, depressed facial expression, very negative affect (anger, crying), whines
POSADJ	POSAFF + engrossed, independent involvement in activity, tolerates well, successful leadership, interpersonal awareness, empathy, helps child (unsolicited), approach
NEGADJ	NEGAFF + negative response to other's positive/neutral overture, pleasure in other's distress, no response to other's overture, tension bursts, vacant (emotionally absent), listless, wandering (no involvement), diffuse (cannot focus attention on one activity), response to frustration or emotional arousal is: very angry, withdraws, disorganized (not goal directed), mannerisms (stereotypes), no social interaction continuously for 3 min, unprovoked aggression, hazing-teasing, inept leadership, pouty-sullen, hits objects
TOTADJ	POSADJ-NEGADJ

significantly higher on composite positive affect, and especially lower on negative affect, in the preschool setting than were children who had been classed as anxiously attached. These data currently are being analyzed in detail.[3] Again, such predictions attest to the validity of the data based on the Preschool Affect Checklist.

We found also that the attachment assessments (Sroufe, 1983) and the two-year affect measures related to measures of social competence in the preschool. Two-year affect-factor scores correlated significantly with both teacher ranking of social competence ($\rho = .80$, $p < .002$) and sociometric status ($\rho = .60$, $p < .03$), but the two-year enthusiasm rating did not yield significant results.

Contemporaneous relationships between affect expression and control and social competence

The central finding in the Class 1 data was the strong relationship between affectively positive social interaction and the teacher rankings, the most compelling single index of social competence. This finding was replicated in the Class 2 results by the relationship between the large-motor-play mega-item POSAFF and teacher rankings ($\rho = -.50$, $p < .006$). The relationship between POSAFF and sociometric status was not significant ($\rho = .21$, $p < .17$). In contrast, these relationships were reversed for the negative-affect mega-item (NEGAFF). Here, the relationship with teacher ranking of social competence

Table 10.2. *Correlations of affect mega-items (large-motor data) with teacher competence judgment and sociometric status* (*Class 2*)

Mega-item	Social competence	Sociometric status
POSAFF	.50	.21
NEGAFF	−.25	−.56
POSADJ	.54	.25
NEGADJ	−.52	−.69
TOTADJ	.67	.74

fell short of significance ($\rho = -.25$, $p < .12$), whereas the relationship with sociometric status was highly significant ($\rho = -.56$, $p < .002$).

These findings may be elaborated and extended by a further compositing of mega-items (see "positive adjustment," "negative adjustment," and "total adjustment" in Table 10.1). "Positive adjustment" (POSADJ) included the positive-affect mega-item, plus characteristics such as engrossment in activities, tolerating frustration well, and social awareness. The correlation of POSADJ with teacher rankings of social competence was .54 ($p < .004$), whereas the correlation between POSADJ and sociometric status was still short of significance ($\rho = .25$, $p < .12$, see Table 10.2). On the other hand, "negative adjustment" (NEGADJ), which includes all negative affect, frustration behavior, aggression, acting out, and atypical behavior, was strongly correlated with sociometric status ($\rho = -.69$, $p < .001$) and also with teacher ranking on social competence ($\rho = -.52$, $p < .006$).

"Total adjustment" (TOTADJ), a composite of POSADJ and NEGADJ, was strongly related to both criteria ($\rho = .67$ and .76, $p < .001$, for social competence and sociometric status, respectively). Although these latter composites contain items that are not solely affective, they do represent summary observations of the way the child manages impulses and feelings, a central aspect of emotional development. It is important to point out that these molar items were composited a priori, without references to the social-competence data. Further research will be required to confirm these findings, including data from a sufficient number of subjects to allow factor analysis of the Affect Checklist. Nonetheless, we suggest that different aspects of behavior may underlie teacher judgments of social competence and status with peers. Peer status (popularity) may be more strongly influenced by the infrequency of negative affect than by the frequency of positive affect, though both are, no doubt, important. In contrast, teacher judgments of social competence (and perhaps competent interaction) may be more influenced by positive affect. At the least, the two criteria appear to have somewhat different correlates.

Cross-lag correlations, which sometimes may be useful for implying causal directions, really were not possible with the present data. Teacher ranking and sociometric status were obtained only at the very end of the school term. And most of the term was required to obtain even the affect observations in sufficient quantity. Thus, one could not look at patterns of correlation across time.

Affect in action: observations on process

The empirical findings presented in the previous sections are all correlations and, admittedly, cannot demonstrate causal influences on social status or even judged social competence. Children may like other children (or look to them) for reasons other than affect expressed, and teachers may base their competence judgments on a variety of other indicators. In fact, such statements are certainly true in part. Many factors underlie social competence and social status. We found, for example, that positive sociometric nominations were heavily influenced by exposure and propinquity; children who rode to school in the same vehicle nominated each other more than they nominated other children. And teachers clearly used social involvement and social skill (timing, facility, and smoothness in social interactions) in their judgments. Commonly, social skill, social involvement, affective expressiveness, and flexible emotional modulation all go together.

Nonetheless, the more deeply we study social behavior in the free flow of the classroom, the more important affect and emotional modulation appear. With our Class 1 data we were able to suggest that sheer frequency of social participation did not account for our affect findings. And for both classes there are correlations between preschool social competence and affect measures obtained in the toddler period, a time when social competence is at a rather primitive stage (Bronson, 1981). Beyond this, we have the sheer strength of the affect-social relationships obtained in both classes, which suggests at the least that social competence and affect control/expression are integrated.

The empirical relations presented provide justification for offering what in many ways is the strongest evidence we have for the critical role of affect in social competence; namely, what we saw in our daily observations in the classroom. The centrality of affect – of emotional control and expression – is most apparent in the free flow of behavior; that is, in chains of initiations, responses, adjustments, shared delight, protests, apologies, modifications, new directions, and further shared feeling. The place of affect in promoting, guiding, and perpetuating exchanges (or disrupting, disorganizing or terminating them) is obvious to trained observers but nonetheless very difficult to quantify. While we continue to work on this measurement problem, we would like to present some narrative examples to illustrate the place of affect in the social-interaction process. The narratives and other brief examples were selected from unedited videotape records made at least weekly in the classroom.

An example drawn from late in the first class, after friendship and group interaction patterns were well formed, illustrates the multiple roles for affect in social behavior. As the scene begins, structured small-group activities are finished and the children are free to play as they wish. Seven children are present: Howard, John, Eddie, and Jerry (boys) and Tracy, Linda, and Alicia (girls).

With great positive affect Howard says, "Let's go to the movies!" Howard, John, Tracy, and Linda move off excitedly to a back corner of the room, while Jerry and Eddie watch them go. Alicia continues to work at a craft table. The four, with much shared excitement, set up a cardboard "screen" and line up chairs in front of it to "watch." John moves his chair to the front (very carefully so as not to hit anyone). When he notices that he is blocking Tracy's view, he moves his chair to the side. Led by Howard's improvised fantasies, all enjoy the "movie."

Then, at one point in response to the "movie," Howard stands up and begins to dance. His enthusiasm spreads to the others and, at his suggestion, they all move joyously to a larger play area and begin to dance. A teacher responds to their mood by providing a record player. All four children eagerly anticipate the music with broad smiles on their faces. A scene of uproarious glee follows, so affective that it cannot fully be captured with words.

At one point in the dancing, Linda pretends to fall down. Howard, at first not recognizing the pretense, stops all activity and looks on with opened mouth and concerned facial expression. He then realizes the pretense and falls down himself. Soon all are laughing and dancing again.

It is interesting to note the behavior of the other three children in the group, who all eventually wind up in the dance area. Alicia, working at a nearby craft table, turns around to watch. Soon she is smiling. In time this becomes laughter and glee. Ultimately, she is up and dancing, showing great zest and joy. Eddie and Jerry were attracted to the area too. Eddie (who was depressed during much of the quarter) watches with great interest but makes only one tentative and incomplete movement to join. He cannot even respond to a rather explicit invitation by two girls, though he clearly is interested. He does occasionally smile slightly, and by the end is tapping his foot! In stark contrast, Jerry works with construction materials at the craft table, facing away from the group the entire time. In his world, it is as though this incredible scene was not even happening.

All four central characters in this scene were ranked high on social competence, whereas Alicia, who at other times was very withdrawn from the group, and Eddie had moderate rankings. Jerry was low ranked.

Affective response in two top-ranked children

Tracy, in the above vignette, was the second-ranked child in the first class in terms of social competence. Monica was first. Both girls had delightful qualities, which included a great deal of positive affect in their social encounters. More often than any others, they initiated interaction with smiling faces and responded positively to others' initiations as well. The teachers (especially the women) were very positive about these two girls from the beginning, long before the class social structure emerged. After all, these girls were warm in their greetings, were enthusiastic about classroom activities, and shared their joy in discovery.

Other children, too, were soon attracted to these girls. Although for the first few days of the class they were exploring various aspects of the setting and became actively involved with others only after the first week, early encounters did of course occur. And encounters with these children were routinely affectively positive. Monica and Tracy were among the first names known by everyone, and they were always chosen first in group activities.

Four brief examples from Monica may illustrate the role of affect in her high status with children and teachers: (1) Tracy and Monica, playing happily in a group, move off to another area. Linda expresses concern about their departure. Monica smiles and invites her along. (2) Monica and Alice are sitting on a box listening to music. Alice begins clapping her hands. Monica watches her, smiling. Later Alice covers her ears because of the noise around them. Monica does too, smiling broadly at Alice. (3) Monica is up on the loft and calls down to three others with a big smile. All go up to join her. (4) Tracy and Monica go to an area where Linda is already playing. Linda greets them with a smile. They return warm, positive greetings. These examples, which are only a few of many, reveal the affective responsiveness and positive social orientation of Monica.

We do not mean to imply that simply walking around with a perpetual smile on your face will ensure high social status. In fact, one near-psychotic boy who smiled considerably was ranked sociometrically at the bottom of the first class. It is the appropriate display of affect that appears to be the key – the sharing of good feelings and the rewarding of others' overtures with positive affect, affect that is timely and fits the circumstances.

Tracy and Monica were not without negative affect. Tracy especially showed affect mobility. Her feelings changed with circumstances and covered the entire range from sorrow to joy and anger to pleasure. But, generally, her affect was appropriate. She did not express anger when offered a kindness.

In fact, the competence of Tracy and Monica is equally apparent in their handling of negative affect and their sharing of positive affect. Competent functioning entails the ability both to modulate negative affect – so that it does not become overwhelming or result in impulsive behavior – and to use it appropriately in social encounters. Negative affect can play an important role in warding off unwanted input and in signaling one's need or displeasure to others. Both Tracy and Monica possessed these abilities.

Although both girls showed relatively little negative affect overall, they had the capacity to signal negative affect effectively and to modulate it when it did occur. For example, while the children were sitting in a circle, listening to a story, one of the boys began to imitate Monica's movements and then to play with her hair. She became annoyed, looked at him sharply and said,

"Don't." This was firm enough to ward off further teasing, and Monica was able to return her attention to the storytelling.

At another time, Tracy was playing a board game with some other children. One of the players (Linda) began to interfere with Tracy's play, reaching across her to move the pieces on the board. Tracy stared at her directly and told her sharply to stop. This resolved the issue. Tracy then demonstrated her ability to sustain positively toned interaction, even after an unpleasant interchange. Shortly, she smiled at Linda, who returned the smile. A few minutes later Tracy cheered enthusiastically for Linda when she won a point in the game.

In contrast to the adaptive handling of negative affect by Tracy and Monica, Alicia demonstrated less ability. For example, when another child (Andrea) took the Christmas cookie that Alicia was decorating, Alicia said that it was *her* cookie: her affect however was plaintive rather than assertive, and she did not look directly at Andrea. This affective tone – unlike Tracy's and Monica's clear displays of annoyance – seemed ineffectual; the other child kept the cookie. Alicia did not say anything more to the girl who had taken her cookie, but she continued to complain in a low voice to Monica about the incident for at least 15 minutes afterward.

*Inappropriate negative affect as detracting from positive
characteristics: the case of Linda*

Linda was a beautifully expressive child. Her exuberance and flashing smile were unparalleled by any other child in her class. When she enthusiastically greeted a visitor with a "Hi! I haven't seen you in a LONG time!" (accompanied by her ear-to-ear smile), it is no wonder that the visitor was charmed. And she showed these displays to other children as well, almost as often as did Monica and Tracy. Still, she was much less successful in getting others to follow her lead, even when the invitation was accompanied by strong positive affect, and she had only a middle rank on social competence. The explanation for her less-than-top status lies, perhaps, in her inappropriate displays of negative affect, which were due in part to her relative immaturity. We discuss this in part as a counterpoint to our general conclusion concerning the power of positive affect. Four examples follow:

1. Linda teases John in an unfriendly fashion. She holds out a puzzle piece in her hand, as if to show it to him, but when he reaches for it, she gets angry and pulls the piece away. She gestures as if to hit him.
2. A bit later she is at the table playing with a teacher. Eddie comes over and tries to join her. She grabs the box of puzzle pieces and yells, "No!" She teases Eddie by holding out puzzle pieces, then protesting when he takes one. Later, when she returns to the table where Eddie is now playing, he sees her coming and says, "I'm not playing anymore. You can have all of mine." He dumps all the pieces in a box and pushes it toward her, evidently having had enough of her negativism.

3. Tracy, John, and Linda had been playing happily on a couch. When the three of them leave, Jerry climbs onto the couch. Linda returns to the couch and shouts at him "You get off my couch!" She climbs on the couch and pushes him, trying to grab the pictures he is holding.

4. Linda has been building an "apartment building." With positive affect, she shows her building to a teacher. Attracted by the positive affect, Howard approaches. But she rebuffs him, shouting "No!" in a sharp voice, even though Howard had been showing control and was approaching in a friendly, curious way. Zeke also looks at it and asks Linda a question. Linda frowns at him with an exaggerated grimace and he walks off. John comes by to look, and again she yells, "No!" with an angry face and gestures as if she would hit him. He goes to a box of blocks a few feet away and starts to take out some blocks. Although Linda is not using them, and a large number of blocks is available, she again yells, "No!" and runs to cover the box with her arms to prevent John from taking them.

Despite her considerable capacities to attract and engage other children, Linda did just as much to alienate them. In fact, her relative acceptance, given this negative behavior, is testimony to both the power of positive affect and role of negative affect.

Affective "attractiveness" as distinguished from other qualities: the case of John

John provides a very interesting case, because, unlike Monica, Tracy, and Linda, he was not a *physically* attractive child based on photographic ratings. And he was one of the lowest (if not the lowest) cognitively functioning children in the classroom, based on teacher judgments, his 24-month Bayley score, and subsequent testing in the Minneapolis Preschool Screening Program. Yet he was rated high on social competence by teachers and was well liked by the children, having several close and warm friendships. His uniformly positive initiations and response to other children – his "sweet nature" as one teacher put it – quite obviously played an important role in his social success.

John was the child mentioned earlier who had moved his chair so that Tracy could see the "movies." Such examples of empathy and caring abound in his record. And he was *never* observed to engage in a hostile or mean act. When appropriate, he stood up for himself, and he never allowed himself to be abused. But he was an extraordinarily kind and caring child. Three typical examples of his behavior follow:

1. Eddie and John play together with blocks for more than 15 minutes. During the entire time, they smile frequently at each other. As the tower they build approaches the point at which its collapse becomes inevitable, they look at each other in mock alarm. Then they chortle gleefully as it succumbs to the force of gravity. This activity stops only when the teachers say it's time to go outside.

2. Tracy is playing with toy animals and the toy barn. She tells the others in a whisper, "The animals are asleep." John smiles his appreciation of her construction.

3. Howard and John are chasing each other, a common activity for this pair. They take turns being pursuer and pursued, laughing and smiling all the while. John interrupts his running briefly, greets one of the teachers affectionately, then chases after Howard again.

Affective displays of low-ranked children

Various patterns of affective display were observed to be related to low social status and lack of social effectiveness. The extreme affective lability (unpredictability) of some children served them poorly in the peer group. Associated with the low rank of other children was rather uniformly flat affect or *affectlessness*. Still others of low rank were chronically whining and complaining or hostile and vitriolic.

Children of the first sort were generally characterized by an inability to modulate affect, with even positively toned excitement spilling over into impulsive, disorganized behavior, which alienated others. Linda at times showed this type of behavior. In one interaction with a teacher, which began with very positive affective exchanges in the course of playful banter, Linda lost control. She began clowning and holding her glass aloft. She spilled her juice in her eye and had to be helped. She wound up going off angrily.

Dirk had trouble modulating both positive and negative affects. His pleasure could often turn quickly to excitement and hyperactivity (disorganization), and his negative affect could lead to angry, aggressive behavior. For example, the events of just one tape: Dirk was sitting behind the steering wheel of a toy "car." When Marilyn came to take her turn at the car, he got off, but then began waving his arms and had to be calmed by a teacher. A few minutes later it was announced that the class would be moving to another room across the hall. Following the other children who were walking, Dirk began to run with abandon to the next room. He skidded on a large piece of paper that was lying on the floor. (He seemed to see it in advance but perhaps he was going too fast to avoid it.) He fell down, and the paper was ripped. This struck him as funny, and he began to laugh and chortle. The teacher took him aside and told him that it wasn't funny, because he had torn the paper that was to be used for a project later that day.

The same day, Dirk spent some time playing relatively quietly by himself at the sandbox. But when Marilyn and Alex began to play "crocodiles" (lying on skateboards and proclaiming that they were "crocodiles" and that they were eating "fish and worms"), and then began to play on the monkeybars, Dirk was attracted to their activity. He began to crawl around inside a play "cage," crying, "Look, I'm a monkey, you guys!" over and over, until he finally got Alex and Marilyn to join him in the cage. He then became more and more excited, hanging upside down over the roof of the "cage" and yelling more and more loudly. After this, his activity became increasingly frenzied. He led Marilyn to the monkeybars and they both jumped on them, so that the bars shook. A teacher reprimanded them for this, but by this time Dirk was too excited to be easily calmed by the teacher. He began to run from one part of the room to another in a disorganized fashion. A little later, the teachers had managed to get him to sit down with a group for a quiet activity, but he could not tolerate this for long, and it took considerable effort to keep him from running away. Still later that day, he shut one of the children in a cabinet and hit another child. Such affective and impulsive lability was common for Dirk.

Some of the children who were among the lowest ranked by teachers and peers were frequently observed to have blank affect or expressionless faces. This was particularly true in the case of Jerry, who often seemed to be "alone in the crowd." For example, on more than one occasion, Jerry played at the same table with other children for extended periods of time without making eye contact or smiling or even seeming to notice what the others were doing (e.g., the dancing sequence above). Even when other children attempted to engage him, Jerry often was unable to make such affective response (in contrast to Eddie, who, though initially too depressed to initiate much contact, was usually pleasant when others initiated contact). Strikingly, only half the children knew Jerry from his picture at the end of the 10-week class.

One day Andrea tried to engage Jerry in play, and he did follow her lead, but he looked subdued and unenthusiastic. A little later, Linda showed him a picture. She was enthusiastic and made an effort to engage him, but he responded little. Then Howard tried to show something to Jerry and two others (Tracy and John), and only Jerry showed no affective response.

On another occasion, when Jerry and Alex (another low-ranked child) were playing at a table with cars, with little interaction or even mutual attention and no positive affect, Alex began rolling a particular car. Jerry, who also wanted this car, tries to take it from Alex. Alex says "NO, NO, NO," without looking at Jerry, and Jerry does not even look at him. Jerry takes the car away and starts playing with it. The two then continue playing as though nothing had happened. There was *no* further interaction and no affective expression.

Even on the rare occasions when Jerry showed positive affect, it typically was in the role of follower. Howard would laugh, then Jerry would laugh. Tracy and Linda would cheer. Then Jerry would cheer. *Spontaneous* affect was exceedingly rare.

Arnold was the prototypic example of the chronic whiner. Everything, even the most simple statement of fact, was said in a whining tone, and he was constantly complaining to teachers and children about the behavior of others. "Heeee won't let me plaay with that." He was one of the very few children not liked by teachers *or* children.

Finally, Vera is a case of parallel importance to John, discussed earlier. In contrast to the (in some ways) limited assets of John, Vera was a strikingly beautiful child, with fully sufficient intellectual potential. But Vera was a tragically unhappy and angry child. Many days she filled the air of the classroom with shouts of "SHUT UP! YOU SHUT UP OR I'M GONNA SMASH YOU."

She matched her words with aggressive behavior, and, ultimately, was ranked at the very bottom (of 24) of the sociometric rank in the second class. Space will permit only one example:

Leonard, Peter, and Alvin are sitting in the back of the school van, making up words that sound similar and laughing uproariously over their creations. Vera climbs into the van, scowling and ignoring the other children's greetings. She throws herself into the seat just in front of the boys and stares out the window, arms folded, jaw set. The boys continue their game. Soon, Vera turns around and demands angrily that they stop saying these words. The boys ignore her, continue to play, and pointedly repeat the words even more loudly. The more she asks them to stop, the more they ignore her and the louder they play. The chaperon tries to quiet Vera, who by now is screaming. Vera screams at the chaperon that she doesn't have to keep quiet, but that THEY have to keep quiet. Vera turns around and tells the boys to stop looking at her. (They looked only after she turned her head.)

Later, she addresses herself to Leonard, "I want you to tell me you are sorry and you won't hurt me again." Leonard glares at her. Vera insists: "Tell me you are very sorry you pushed me; you pushed me and I won't forget " (the chaperon finds out that Leonard had pushed her in the classroom the week before). Vera mutters to herself that Leonard shouldn't have done it and that people shouldn't hurt her. She screams angrily again at Leonard that he hurt her. Then she turns to him, pleading, "Leonard tell me you are sorry that you pushed me and you won't do it again – and then we can play together. OK?" Leonard just glares at her – says nothing.

The boys continue to play their word game, pointedly and loudly repeating the words. She still demands that they stop – the more she asks, the worse it gets. The van driver tells them to stop it. Vera turns to the driver and tells him to shut up too. The episode ends when the driver stops the van at the side of the street and tells them that they have to stop talking until they get to school.[4]

We cannot detail the history of this child, who once dreamed that her beloved teacher had thrown her against a wall and who asked the teacher to explain why she liked her. Nor can we detail how we think her inner feelings were converted into the displays we saw. Still, it should be clear that such a child would not be esteemed by other children nor be viewed as competent by teachers, despite her frequent demonstrations of insight into social behavior.

Conclusion: affect, cognition, and social behavior

In these days of the ascendancy of cognition, it sometimes seems as though affect is considered almost superfluous. It has been argued recently, for example, that affect is the mere outcome of an important cognitive process (e.g., Mandler, 1975). It may have communicative value, but beyond this, it plays little role in individual or social behavior. Cognition, on the other hand, is granted major importance. As one illustration, there is a vast literature on social cognition, which derives from the belief that a child's understanding of the social world will strongly influence his or her social competence. In contrast, there is a very limited literature on the role affect may play in social competence. Such an imbalance is unfortunate.

It has often been argued that cognition *precedes* affect, in the sense that affect is the result of a cognitive process. Recently, however, a number of writers have called attention once again to the interdependence of affect and cognition (Cicchetti & Sroufe, 1978; Fiske, 1981; Haviland, 1975; Pogge-Hesse & Cicchetti, in press; Sroufe, 1979b; Zajonc, 1980). Attention cannot be distributed in all directions at once, nor can every event be given thorough processing. Rather, such activities are guided, in part, by interest and other affects (Piaget & Inhelder, 1969). Moreover, the *meaning* of an event, in large part, has to do with previous affective experiences. As Arnold (1960) and later Fiske (1981) have written, an immediate intuitive appraisal of an event (its valence) is cued by earlier affective experiences. This immediate affective response moves one toward or away from the person involved before complex cognitive processing can be completed.

We would, of course, not argue against the importance of cognitive factors in social behavior. In emphasizing, as we have, the importance of the timing and pacing of affective response, there is an obvious role for cognition. Moreover, recognizing the other's readiness for interaction, intentions, displeasures, interest, and so forth is based upon cognitive processes. It is impossible to examine the role of affect in social behavior without encountering the fundamental importance of cognitive variables.

Still, social competence is much more than "knowing what to do" or "understanding the intentions of others." Some children, despite considerable understanding of the wishes and intentions of others, do not respond in an empathic way. In fact, as much recognition of the other's perspective and experience is required for exquisite hostility as is required for empathy (Sroufe, 1983). A child wearing a mask approached children one by one and growled at them. Inevitably, he came upon a child who, quite frightened, backed away and asked him to stop. Although he had approached other children only briefly, the boy did not stop now. He pursued the frightened child around the room until she was quite upset. Clearly, he *recognized* her reaction, but the recognition per se was not sufficient to ensure an empathic reaction.

Other children are "emotionally handicapped"; that is, their intellectual potential is not free to engage in gratifying social encounters. The contrasting cases of Vera and John illustrated this well. Vera was quite bright and showed instances of impressive social *skill* (as when she suggested to Leonard that an apology from him would clear the slate and they could be friends). But she was uncontrollably angry, and her hostility was expressed frequently and indiscriminately. Rarely could she sustain positive interactions with anyone, and even her initiations were often negative. John, on the other hand, while intellectually limited, had all his cognitive resources available. He experienced little "affective interference." He showed far more empathy than the intellectually superior Vera. And his affective responsiveness to others elicited continued positive engagement from them. John developed true, reciprocal friendships with other children, was well liked by teachers and peers and was effective within the peer group. Vera was strongly disliked by the other children and was commonly isolated.

To be effective in the peer group, children have to *want* to be involved with others. And to maintain effective involvement, they have to find such encounters enjoyable. That is, beyond skills such as the recognition of the affective expressions of others, there are important motivational variables to be considered. To fully understand social competence, we need to include affective as well as cognitive variables and to broaden our conceptualization of the affective domain as well.

Summary

In this chapter we have been concerned not with emotion per se, with its causes, or its obvious ties to cognition, but with "affect in action." We assume, in general, that the children we are studying are capable of the same emotions and in certain extreme conditions (e.g., when confronted with a large, snarling dog) would show similar emotional reactions. But in their ongoing social behavior children differ widely in the frequency and quality of the affect expressed. We were interested in the implication of these individual differences for social behavior.

Based on extensive, repeated observations of children in two nursery-school classrooms, we found strong relationships between the tendency to initiate encounters with positive affect and to respond positively to the overtures of others (and more generally the control and modulation of affect) and assessed social competence. Both sociometric status and independent assessments of social competence by teachers were related to the affect variables.

The study was correlational and therefore does not permit strong conclusions concerning causality. Socially skilled children may enjoy social encounters more and therefore show more positive and less negative affect. And children may be assessed as socially competent based on nonaffective characteristics. Nonetheless, it seems likely that affect expression and control are part of a network of characteristics that contribute to competence with peers.

Appendix: MINNESOTA PRESCHOOL AFFECT CHECKLIST

Edward J. Schork and L. Alan Sroufe, Institute of Child Development, University of Minnesota

CHILD: _____ Time: _____ Activity: _____

DATE: _____ Observer: _____

Period: I   II   III

POSITIVE AFFECT

1. ____ displays positive affect in <u>any</u> manner (baseline)

2. ____ uses positive affect to initiate contact, to engage another (must begin, or restart interaction after a substantial break)

3. ____ when <u>already in interaction with someone</u>, directs positive affect at them (affect is <u>directed at specific person</u>)

4. ____ when in a social situation   displays positive affect but <u>does not direct it to any one in particular</u>

5. ____ shows <u>very positive affect</u>: exuberance, "lights up"

6. ____ shows <u>ongoing high enjoyment</u>, "has a lot of fun" (sustained continuously for 30 sec. or more)

7. ____ uses face very expressively to show <u>positive</u> affect <u>in communicating directly with another.</u>

*8. ____ uses positive affect in a way that makes a significant contribution to keeping a social interaction going (with one or more others)

9. ____ shows pride in accomplishment (usually verbal statement)

NEGATIVE AFFECT

10. ___ displays negative affect in <u>any</u> manner (baseline)

11. ____ uses negative affect <u>to initiate contact</u>, <u>to begin a social interaction</u> with someone

12. ____ directs negative affect specifically <u>at a particular other person</u> when <u>already in interaction with them</u>

---

* Eliminated from the final set

13. ____ uses face very expressively to show negative affect in communicating directly with another

14. ____ facial expression looks depressed (can be brief)

15. ____ shows very negative affect: anger, distress, protest, crying vigorously, etc.

INAPPROPRIATE AFFECT

16. ____ expresses negative affect to another CHILD in response to the other's neutral or positive overture (appears inappropriate in context)

*17. ____ fails to show positive affect when appropriate (as defined by context) (e.g., in a group when others are all laughing)

*18. ____ fails to show negative affect when appropriate (e.g., after being hit)

19. ____ takes pleasure in another's distress

20. ____ does not respond when approached affectively by another.

*21. ____ cries in the absence of physical injury

22. ____ whines in the absence of physical injury

INVOLVEMENT: PRODUCTIVE, FOCUSED USE OF PERSONAL ENERGY

23. ____ engrossed, absorbed, intensely involved in activity: emotionally invested in creative, productive, thematically organized, or other activity that has a positive emotional function (does not include intensive but unfocused activity, e.g., running around the room)

24. ____ independence: involvement in an activity that the child organizes for himself

INVOLVEMENT: UNPRODUCTIVE, UNFOCUSED USE OF PERSONAL ENERGY

25. ____ wandering: moves around the room with no/little involvement in social interaction or activities

26. ____ listless: looks fidgety and emotionally uninvested but still emotionally "present"; stays in one area, but shows little/no involvement in activities or social interaction

27. ____ vacant: very flat, unexpressive, detached face, no involvement, looks "emotionally absent."

28. ____ tension bursts: undirected motor release (one or several) (usually brief)

*29. ____ extremely high activity in comparison to context (outdoors: risk of

harm to self/others also involved)

30. ____ diffuse: looks somewhat emotionally invested but unable to sustain it

for long in any one activity, i.e., "jumps from one thing to another"

(gets slightly involved in one thing, then soon moves on, repeatedly).

LAPSES IN IMPULSE CONTROL AND NEGATIVE RESPONSES TO FRUSTRATION, CONFLICT, AND

OTHER EMOTIONALLY AROUSING PROBLEM SITUATIONS   (e.g., object struggle, teasing,

rejection, inability to solve puzzle, encountering obstacle to goal attainment)

*31. ____ context-related, physical, interpersonal aggression (someone does

something to which the child responds with aggression -- an emotionally

arousing preceding event must be observed, usually but not necessarily

provocation by another)

32. ____ hits, kicks, shoves, knocks over, or throws objects

*33. ____ ____ tantrum (pronounced upset and loss of control)

*34. ____ ____ very angry (vs. tantrum: not as sustained, loss of control

not as great and may be limited)

*35. ____ ____ inability to stop ongoing behavior

*36. ____ ____ withdrawal (=becomes withdrawn), "shut down" (whether leaves

area or not) (NB: must see the withdrawal occur)

*37. ____ ____ disorganized, non-goal-directed activity

38. ____ ____ pouty, sullen

(describe behavior, emotionally arousing events, responses of others:)

_____

_____

_____

POSITIVE REACTIONS TO FRUSTRATION, CONFLICT, AND EMOTIONALLY AROUSING PROBLEM

SITUATIONS (e.g., object struggle, teasing, rejection, inability to solve

puzzle, encountering obstacle to goal attainment)

39. ____ promptly expresses, in words, feelings arising from problem situation

then moves on to same or new activity (vs. withdrawing, displacing the

affect to others or to objects, staying upset)

39a. ____ shows primarily neutral or positive affect

39b.____ shows primarily negative affect

40. ____ shows ability to tolerate well (although does not promptly verbalize

feelings to others)

(describe emotionally arousing event and behavior:)_____

_____

_____

UNUSUAL BEHAVIOR

*41. ____ bizarre behavior (e.g., licking the wall)

42. ____ mannerisms, stereotypes (e.g., rolling the tongue around the mouth,

characteristic facial distortions, characteristic nonverbal

vocalizations) ("quirky gestures")

*43. ____ ritualistic, repetitive behaviors (more complex, organized, and

larger-scale than mannerisms, more normal than bizarre behaviors)

SOCIAL ISOLATION

44. ____ no social interaction continuously for 3 min. or more.

HOSTILITY

45a.____ unprovoked, physical, interpersonal aggression (no preceding

provocation behavior by the victim) (describe aggression and

subsequent behavior by all involved): _____

_____

_____

45b.____ hazing, teasing, or other verbal or nonverbal provocation or threat

SKILLS IN LEADING AND JOINING

46a.____ successful leadership: plays an organizing role in an activity

in which other children "follow the lead" and participate

46b.____ inept attempts at leadership: attempts to exert an organizing,

directive, or leadership influence on others, but they do not

comply (check on basis of others' noncompliance) (often includes

self-defeating use of affect, e.g., bossiness)

47a.____ smoothly approaches an already ongoing activity (does not disrupt

or antagonize) and gets actively involved

47b.____ smoothly approaches an already ongoing activity (does not disrupt or

antagonize) but does not get actively involved

EMPATHY AND PROSOCIAL BEHAVIOR

48. ____ interpersonal awareness: behavior reflecting knowledge or awareness

about another person

(describe): _____

_____

_____

49. ____ empathy: concern or other empathic response to another person's

emotional display (usually when another is distressed)

(describe): _____

_____

_____

50. ____ helping behavior (unsolicited) directed to other child

*51. ____ helping behavior (unsolicited) directed to teacher

Notes

1 Emotion is defined as a subjective reaction to a salient event, characterized by physiological, experiential, and (usually) overt behavioral change. The term *subjective* implies that emotions are the result of a person's evaluation of an event rather than the event per se. The terms *subjective*, *salient*, and *evaluation* all imply a heavy cognitive component. In this chapter we are primarily concerned not with emotion per se but with affect in the context of social interaction.
2 Affect expressed within peer interaction was classified according to its primary hedonic tone. Positive affect was coded when the initial behavior or response was expressed with unqualified enthusiasm (broad smiling, giggling, laughter). Negative affect was defined as strong expressions of fear, displeasure, or anger (crying, stamping feet, harsh commands, threats, or physical attacks were coded as negative). Observers were instructed to ignore exchanges in which the affective tone was neutral, mild, or unclear. Thus, only exchanges that were charged with emotion were coded as positive or negative. Although errors of omission occurred in the coding of hedonic tone, there were no errors of commission, that is, positive and negative affect were never confused.
3 These data will be summarized in the dissertation of the second author, Edward Schork. Unpublished doctoral dissertation, University of Minnesota, 1983
4 This example was contributed by McDonna Michaud, a van chaperon and observer.

References

Ainsworth, M., Blehar, M., Waters, E., & Wall, S. *Patterns of attachment: Observations in the strange situation and at home*. Hillsdale, N.J.: Erlbaum, 1978.
Arend, R., Gove, F., & Sroufe, L. A. Continuity of early adaptation: From attachment in infancy to ego-resiliency and curiosity at age 5. *Child Development*, 1979, *50*, 950–959.

Arnold, M. *Emotions and personality.* New York: Columbia University Press, 1960.

Asher, S. R., Singleton, L. C., Tinsley, B. R., & Hymel, S. A reliable sociometric measure for preschool children. *Developmental Psychology*, 1979, *15*, 443–444.

Birns, B., & Golden, M. Prediction of intellectual performance at three years from infant test and personality measures. *Merrill-Palmer Quarterly*, 1972, *18*, 53–58.

Brazelton, T., Koslowski, B., & Main, M. The origins of reciprocity: The early mother–infant interaction. In M. Lewis & L. Rosenblum (Eds.), *The effect of the infant on its caregiver*, New York: Wiley, 1974.

Bronson, W. Toddler's behaviors with agemates: Issues of interaction, cognition and affect. In Lewis P. Lipsitt (Ed.), *Monographs on infancy*. Norwood, N.Y.: Ablex, 1981.

Cicchetti, D., & Sroufe, L. A. An organizational view of affect: Illustration from the study of Down's syndrome infants. In M. Lewis & L. Rosenblum (Eds.), *The development of affect*, pp. 309–350. New York: Plenum, 1978.

Egeland, B., & Sroufe, L. A. Developmental sequelae of maltreatment in infancy. In R. Rizley & D. Cicchetti (Eds.), *Developmental perspectives in child maltreatment*. San Francisco: Jossey-Bass, 1981.

Fiske, S. T. Social cognition and affect. In J. H. Harvey (Ed.), *Cognition, social behavior, and the environment*. Hillsdale, N.J.: Erlbaum, 1981.

Greenson, R. R. On enthusiasm. In C. W. Sacarides (Ed.), *The world of emotions: Clinical studies of affects and their expression*. New York: International Universities Press, 1977.

Haviland, J. Looking smart: The relationship between affect and intelligence in infancy. In M. Lewis (Ed.). *Origins of infant intelligence*. New York: Plenum, 1975.

Izard, C. E. *The face of emotion*. New York: Appleton-Century-Crofts, 1971.

Izard, C. E. *Human emotions*. New York: Plenum, 1977.

Izard, C. E., & Buechler, S. Aspects of consciousness and personality in terms of differential emotions theory. In R. Plutchik & H. Kellerman (Eds.), *Emotion: Theory, research, and experience*, Vol. 1: *Theories of emotion*. New York: Academic Press, 1980.

Mandler, G. *Mind and emotion*. New York: Wiley, 1975.

Matas, L., Arend, R., & Sroufe, L. A. Continuity of adaptation in the second year: The relationship between quality of attachment and later competent functioning. *Child Development*, 1978, *49*, 547–556.

Murphy, L. *The widening world of childhood: Paths toward mastery*. New York: Basic Books, 1962.

Piaget, J., & Inhelder, B. *The psychology of the child*. New York: Basic Books, 1969.

Pogge-Hesse, P., & Cicchetti, D. Socioemotional development: Toward an integrative theory. In R. Plutchik (Ed.), *Emotions in early development*. New York: Academic Press, in press.

Rothenberg, B. Children's social sensitivity and the relationship to interpersonal competence, intrapersonal comfort and intellectual level. *Developmental Psychology*, 1970, *2*, 335–350.

Sander, L. Infant and caretaking environment. In E. J. Anthony (Ed.), *Explorations in child psychiatry*. New York: Plenum, 1975.

Sherman, L. W. An ecological study of glee in small groups of preschool children. *Child Development*, 1975, *46*, 53–61.

Sroufe, L. A. The coherence of individual development: Early care, attachment, and subsequent developmental issues. *American Psychologist*, 1979, *34*(10), 834–841. (a)

Sroufe, L. A. Socioemotional development. In J. D. Osofsky (Ed.), *The handbook of infant development*. New York: Wiley, 1979. (b)

Sroufe, L. A. The organization of emotional development. *Psychoanalytic Inquiry*, 1982, *1*, 575–599.

Sroufe, L. A. Infant–caregiver attachment and patterns of adaptation in preschool: The roots of maladaptation and competence. *Minnesota symposium in child psychology* (Vol. 16). Minneapolis: University of Minnesota Press, 1983.

Sroufe, L. A., & Waters, E. The ontogenesis of smiling and laughter: A perspective on the organization of development in infancy. *Psychological Review*, 1976, *83*, 173–189.

Sroufe, L. A. & Waters, E. Attachment as an organizational construct. *Child Development*, 1977, *48*, 1184–1199.

Stern, D. The goal and structure of mother–infant play. *Journal of the American Academy of Child Psychiatry*, 1974, *13*, 402–421.

Vaughn, B. E., & Waters, E. Social organization among preschool peers: Dominance, attention and sociometric correlates. In D. Omark, F. Strayer, & D. Freedman (Eds.), *Dominance relations: An ethological view of human conflict and social interaction*. New York: Garland, 1980.

Vine, I. The role of facial visual signalling in early social development. In M. von Cranach & I. Vine (Eds.), *Social communication and movement: Studies of men and chimpanzees*. London: Academic Press, 1973.

Waters, E., & Sroufe, L. A. A developmental perspective on competence. *Developmental Review*, *3*, 79–97, 1983.

Waters, E., Wippman, J., & Sroufe, L. A. Attachment, positive affect and competence in the peer group: Two studies in construct validation. *Child Development*, 1979, *50*, 821–829.

Zajonc, R. B. Feeling and thinking: Preferences need no inferences. *American Psychologist*, 1980, *35*, 151–175.

11   Affect, cognition, and hemispheric specialization

Richard J. Davidson

Although functional differences in the cognitive domain have been the most extensively studied of the differences between the two sides of the brain, a variety of observations from both clinical and experimental research are pointing toward important hemispheric differences in the regulation of affective behavior. The growing literature on affective lateralization highlights the complexity of hemispheric specialization in several ways. First, it raises the possibility that an entire hemisphere is not functionally specialized for a single process or type of information processing. Rather, different regions along the rostral/caudal plane may show hemispheric specialization for different functions. As will be described in detail, asymmetries in the frontal region seem to be more specifically related to affective behavior and posterior cortical asymmetries are more closely associated with cognitive function.

A second and related issue raised by the affective lateralization data indicates that different cortical regions may show different patterns of hemispheric activation at the same points in time, in response to particular stimuli. In fact, different regions may literally show opposite patterns of activation asymmetry simultaneously. This simple fact must temper models of hemispheric asymmetry that posit uniform activation of an entire hemisphere.

A third general point follows from the preceding issues. That asymmetries along the rostral/caudal plane may differ in functional significance and show opposite patterns of activation leads us to consider the possibility of reciprocal interaction between asymmetries in anterior and posterior cortical association regions. Major anatomical connections exist which reciprocally link certain regions of the parietal and temporal lobes to the frontal cortex (Nauta, 1971), thus providing an anatomical substrate for this hypothesized functional interconnection. We believe that reciprocal relations between frontal and parietal asymmetry may be crucial for at least certain affect/cognition interactions.

These three issues, among many others, underscore the complexity of hemispheric specialization implicit in contemporary research. Each issue will be

Preparation of this chapter was supported in part by grants from the John D. and Catherine T. MacArthur Foundation, the Spencer Foundation, the Foundation for Child Development, and the Research Foundation of the State University of New York. I thank Carrie Schaffer and Clifford Saron for their comments and Diana Angelini for her secretarial assistance.

320

illustrated and more fully elaborated in subsequent sections of this chapter. They are presented at the outset because of their relevance to understanding the relations between hemispheric specialization for cognition and affect.

This chapter will begin by first offering some precision to the definition of emotion and specifying the class of phenomena to which this label can be reasonably applied. The phylogenetic antecedents of cerebral asymmetry for affect will then be described. Asymmetries for affective processes in adult humans will then be reviewed, followed by a discussion of some developmental issues related to the hemispheric specialization for affect. In the final section, the relevance of hemispheric differences to the problem of affect/cognition interaction will be illustrated with examples from current research.

Some definitions of the phenomena of emotion

Before discussing the hemispheric substrates of affective behavior, it would be instructive to comment briefly on how I am using the term emotion and to delineate, albeit broadly, the class of behavior to which the category emotional applies. The perspective adopted in this chapter draws heavily on the work of a number of emotion theorists including Ekman, Izard, and Tomkins (e.g., Ekman, 1980b; Izard, 1977; Tomkins, 1980).

Emotional responses, as distinguished from other responses emitted by the organism, are brief, often quick, organized, involve complex patterning across a number of different systems, and are difficult to control. One of the most important characteristics of emotion is that it can be very brief. A person might be frightened or happy for just a few seconds and surprise is always short in duration. When an emotion is said to last for a long period of time (e.g., many hours or days), we commonly refer to this phenomenon as mood. The rise time of an emotion is also brief. Most emotions can be elicited in portions of a second.

Another hallmark of emotional behavior is the recruitment of multiple response systems and the complex and coherent patterning that inheres in these multimodal responses. The activation of emotion is usually (but not always) associated with changes in skeletal muscular activity, facial behavior, vocal responses, and in a number of biological parameters including autonomic, endocrine and central nervous system activity. An important feature of these patterned responses is that at least some of them are relatively specific for particular emotions or combinations of emotions and that at least some of the changes are common to all people and possibly certain other species.[1]

Two other features are also common to emotional behavior. First, the activation of emotion often results in the generation of coping behavior, which interacts with the expression of the emotion. Some of the behavioral manifestations of emotion that are readily observable to others include a mixture of the "pure" emotional response upon which is overlaid various coping activities.

The other feature common to at least many instances of emotional behavior in humans is the subjective experience of emotion. Although this component need not always be present or if present, consistently veridical, a subjective feeling state is often reported. The variables that govern this component are not well known. Some of the subjective components may arise as a result of feedback from skeletal-muscular and/or autonomic activity. The degree to which this component is present in young infants and the developmental course it follows are virtually unknown. Some of the data reported here have certain relevant implications for this problem.

Most empirical research on the phenomenon of emotion has not included the assessment of a large number of measures from different response systems. As a result, the richness and complexity of the coherent patterned responses typical of emotional behavior often have been unappreciated. However, the data from studies that measure certain single responses or simple combinations of a few response systems are still relevant and contribute importantly to our understanding of the nature of emotional phenomena. In studies where only one or two responses that presumably reflect affect are measured, the presence of emotion must be inferred primarily from certain contextual variables such as the elicitor of the behavior. An affect elicitor can be described as an event that is appraised quickly as the occasion for one or another emotion (e.g., Ekman, 1980b). Thus, given the presence of such an elicitor and the manifestation of certain components of what is likely to be a complex, patterned multisystem response, the presence of emotion can be reasonably inferred.

Phylogenetic antecedents

The emphasis on asymmetries associated with cognitive function and particularly language probably contributed to some early suggestions regarding the uniqueness of lateralization to humans and possibly some higher nonhuman primates (e.g., Warren & Nonneman, 1976). Mostly within the last decade, a large number of studies have reported on species-consistent functional asymmetries in a variety of animals (see review by Denenberg, 1981). Although some of these data clearly point toward the existence of asymmetries for some cognitive processes in nonhuman species, asymmetries for certain affective behaviors may indeed be more pervasive throughout various levels of phylogeny.

The first evidence for lateralization of function in animals was Nottebohm's (1970) demonstration of left-sided specialization for birdsong in the chaffinch. He observed that severing the left versus right hypoglossal nerve produced dramatic differences in the quality of the chaffinch's song. Left-sided sectioning eliminated most of the components of the song, whereas right-sided lesions had only minor effects. Interestingly, in subsequent research Nottebohm and his colleagues have found that the effects of hypoglossal surgery are age-dependent. In both chaffinches and canaries, left hypoglossal sectioning very early in life can result in a shift of specialization for song production to the right side (Nottebohm, Manning, & Nottebohm, 1979).

In a series of studies on lateralization in chicks, Rogers and her colleagues obtained evidence indicating that visual discrimination learning is preferentially subserved by the left hemisphere, whereas copulation and attack behavior are preferentially performed by the right hemisphere (Rogers & Anson, 1979; Rogers, 1980). These studies were performed by comparing the effects of left- versus right-sided injections of cycloheximide, a compound that inhibits ribosomal protein synthesis. Andrew, Mench, and Rainey (1980) have confirmed some of these findings in the absence of drug intervention. These investigators simply occluded the left or the right eye and observed behavioral differences between groups of chicks with one versus the other eye open. For example, chicks with an open left eye emitted peep calls in response to a threatening stimulus, whereas birds with an open right eye did not. This finding is consistent with the notion of right-hemisphere specialization for certain negative affects. Unfortunately, it is not possible to rule out the alternative hypothesis positing right-hemisphere specialization for affect in general.

The most extensive body of evidence on asymmetries in animal brains has been performed with rodents. Asymmetries at both the individual and population levels have been studied. Glick and his colleagues (e.g., Glick, Jerussi, & Zimmerberg, 1977) have examined the relations between neurochemical asymmetries in the nigrostriatal system and rotation behavior in rats. They observed that an injection of amphetamine induces rotation in a normal rat. Although animals differed as to direction of rotation, consistency was observed within animals. Importantly, Glick and his associates (1974) also found less dopamine in the striatum ipsilateral to the direction of rotation compared with the level on the opposite side. Subsequent work by this group demonstrated that individual differences among rats in directional preference was associated with asymmetries in dopamine with higher levels in the striatum ipsilateral to the nonpreferred side (Zimmerberg, Glick, & Jerussi, 1974).

While the work of Glick and his colleagues has emphasized asymmetries at the individual level, Denenberg (1981) reanalyzed the data from several Glick studies and found some evidence for a rightward population bias. Denenberg examined data on a total of 292 rats that were trained on a two-lever operant task and found that 57.5% preferred the right bar.

A species-consistent hemispheric asymmetry also has been found in studies of regional cerebral metabolism. Glick and his colleagues (1979) have found that both the left frontal cortex and the left hippocampus were relatively more metabolically active than corresponding right-hemisphere regions. Other studies have reported species-consistent behavioral and neurochemical changes following ligation of the left versus the right middle cerebral artery (Robinson, 1979; Robinson & Coyle, 1980; Robinson, Shoemaker, & Schlumpf, 1980). Following the ligation of the right middle cerebral artery, there is a two- to three-week period of hyperactivity and a decrease in both norepinephrine and dopamine concentrations on the side ipsilateral to the lesion. Left-sided ligation produces none of these effects. In a recent report, Pearlson and Robinson (1981) found that suction lesions on the right frontal cortex produced both hyperactivity and a bilateral decrease in norepinephrine concentrations in the cortex as well as the locus coeruleus. Again, identical lesions of the left frontal cortex produced neither hyperactivity nor catecholamine depletion.

Denenberg and his colleagues (see Denenberg, 1981) have recently performed an extensive series of experiments on the differential effects of left versus right neocortical ablation in rats. One major aim of this research program was to evaluate the impact of early experience on subsequent lateralization. A second goal was to determine the nature and extent of species-consistent functional hemispheric specialization in the rat.

To investigate the effect of early experience on lateralization, rats are randomly assigned to either a handled or nonhandled group. Whole litters are randomly assigned to one of these two groups. At birth, the newborn litter is removed from the nest and culled to eight rats. The nonhandled litters are returned to the maternity nest after culling and are not disturbed thereafter until weaning at 21 days. If a litter is to be handled, the pups are put singly into one-gallon cans containing shavings, left there for 3 minutes, and then returned to the maternity cage. The procedure is repeated daily for the first 20 days of life. Although the handling manipulation may appear to be slight, it has been found to reduce emotionality and increase exploratory behavior (see Denenberg, 1977).

In a number of studies, Denenberg (1981) has found that early handling accentuates the differences between left versus right ablations on various behavioral measures. Two of the most interesting tasks on which differences between right versus left lesioned rats have been observed include taste aversion and muricide (mouse killing). In the taste aversion study (Denenberg et al., 1980), rats were trained in a standard taste-aversion paradigm (Garcia, Hankin, & Rusiniak, 1974). Following this training, one-quarter of the rats received left neocortical ablation, one-quarter received right neocortical ablation, one-quarter received a sham operation, and one-quarter served as no-treatment controls. Following recovery from surgery, the rats were retested to assess their retention of the taste aversion.

Among rats who were not handled as infants, no differences were observed among groups. Specifically, all left lesioned, right lesioned, and control subjects exhibited equal retention of the taste aversion. However, among those rats that had been handled in infancy, Denenberg and his colleagues (1980) found that removal of the right hemisphere resulted in significantly less retention of the taste aversion than did removal of the left hemisphere. In other words, the right hemisphere is more involved than the left in retaining the taste aversion. These findings are consistent with the hypothesis of right-hemisphere involvement in affect (and particularly negative affect).

As a second measure of emotionality in the rat, Garbanati and his colleagues (1983) used muricide. Mouse killing is a spontaneous species-specific act that is not dependent upon food deprivation for its occurrence. The basic paradigm used in this study is similar to that used in the taste-aversion study. Rats were either handled or not and following weaning were either subjected to left or right neocortical ablations or served as controls. After recovery from surgery, a single mouse was placed in a cage containing an isolated rat. The two remained together for a maximum of five days. Handled rats with an intact right hemisphere were significantly more likely to kill the mouse than were those with an intact left hemisphere. These findings suggest that mouse killing is preferentially subserved by the right hemisphere. These results and the taste-aversion data are consistent in two important ways: (1) They both demonstrate laterality differences only for rats that were handled in infancy, and (2) they both support the hypothesis of right-hemisphere specialization in the regulation of negative affective behavior.

The Denenberg findings are also consistent with a previously mentioned hypothesis, right-hemisphere specialization for affect in general. In a study that bears on these two alternative hypotheses, Denenberg and his colleagues (1978) used a paradigm that was similar to those used in the Denenberg studies just discussed. The behavioral measure adopted in this experiment was open-field activity. Although open-field behavior has been found to be factorially complex (Whimbey & Denenberg, 1967), one dimension represented in this measure is exploratory behavior. Exploratory behavior can be thought of as associated with interest and approach. If the right hemisphere was specialized for all affect, one would expect a more significant decline in open-field activity scores following right versus left neocortical ablation. However, if the left hemisphere was more involved than the right with at least certain positive affects, we would predict that left neocortical ablation would reduce open-field activity scores more than would right-sided removal. The results of this study support the hypothesis of differential lateralization for positive versus negative affect. Specifically, handled rats who received right neocortical ablations (i.e., those with intact left hemispheres) exhibited more open-field activity than did rats having only an intact right hemisphere. Again, these findings obtained only for the handled group who were subsequently (after weaning) housed in a standard laboratory environment. Thus, emotional behavior of all types is *not* decreased following right-hemisphere removal. Rather, it appears that right-sided ablation interferes most with negative affective behavior. The open-field data suggest that positive affective behavior is decreased most following left-hemisphere ablation.

Of the various studies that have explored functional asymmetries in a number of nonhuman primates, all have focused on aspects of cognitive behavior, for example, lateralization in visual learning and memory tasks in monkeys (e.g., Doty, Negrao, & Yamaga, 1973; Doty & Overman, 1977; Gazzaniga, 1963; Hamilton, 1977; Hamilton & Lund, 1970; Hamilton, Tieman, & Farrell, 1974).

Many of these findings have been inconsistent. Less variable results have been obtained in studies of lateralization in the auditory modality. Dewson (1977, 1978, 1979) found that lesions in the left superior temporal cortex dramatically interfered with the performance of macaques on an auditory discrimination task, whereas comparable lesions in the homologous area on the right side had very little effect.

Using a behavioral monaural listening paradigm, Petersen and his colleagues (1978) found that Japanese macaques showed a right-ear advantage in discriminating between two "coo" sounds recorded from other Japanese macaques in the field. They interpret their findings as reflecting a left-hemisphere specialization for discrimination of a communicatively relevant acoustic feature.

The data on hemispheric specialization in animals clearly indicate that functional asymmetries are not found exclusively in humans. The rodent and bird findings suggest that lateralization for affective processes is present at a number of different levels across phylogeny. Although the precise dimension along which the hemispheres are lateralized in the affective domain is not unambiguously discernible from the animal data, the recent rodent work is consistent with human evidence for differential lateralization for positive and negative emotion.

Two other important issues addressed in the animal data that are currently not resolvable will require additional study. The first concerns the issue of anterior–posterior differences. Many studies reviewed in this section did not consider anterior–posterior specificity as a variable. Those studies that involved whole hemisphere removal or destruction necessarily cannot address questions concerning where along the anterior–posterior continuum the asymmetries for affect and/or cognition are most pronounced. A notable exception in the study of affective behavior is the recent data from Robinson's group (Pearlson & Robinson, 1981) on the effects of left versus right frontal lesions in rats. Dewson's (1977, 1978, 1979) work with macaques demonstrated the importance of superior temporal lesions as compared with primary auditory cortex lesions in affecting auditory discrimination behavior. Whereas those monkeys with left superior temporal cortex lesions showed a deficit in performance, the monkey who received a left primary auditory cortex lesion did not.

The second issue that needs clarification in future research concerns the chronological sequence of affective and cognitive asymmetries in phylogenetic history. It would be important to explore asymmetries for cognitive behavior in rodents to ascertain their presence, and if present, whether they are as robust as the affective asymmetries appear to be.

Asymmetries for affective processes in adult humans

Research on clinical populations

Research on affective asymmetries in adults has received less attention than the study of cognitive asymmetries. However, during the past decade, a growing interest in the psychobiological substrates of affect has helped to stimulate more research on asymmetry and affect. Data based upon a variety of methods with both normal and clinical populations are beginning to challenge an early hypothesis suggesting right-hemisphere specialization for emotion in general (e.g., Schwartz, Davidson, & Maer, 1975). The findings are more consistent with the notion of differential lateralization for at least certain positive and negative affects. More formally stated, this hypothesis holds that certain regions of the left hemisphere are specialized for the processing of certain forms of positive affect, and that certain regions of the right hemisphere are specialized for the processing of certain forms of negative affect.

The reader will note two major qualifications in the statement of this hypothesis: (1) The specific hemispheric regions associated with affective asymmetry are left unstated and (2) the precise emotions for which this asymmetry exists are not indicated. More detailed specification on these two points is lacking because of insufficient data. Regarding the second point, data are particularly meager with respect to the negative emotions. However, for the positive emotions, a variety of recent findings in the context of the theoretical perspective adopted in this chapter make it increasingly likely that the predominant emotion for which the left hemisphere (i.e., certain regions thereof) is specialized is interest. Evidence in support of this suggestion will be presented later in the chapter.

The effects of unilateral cerebral lesions on emotional processes. Alford (1933) and Goldstein (1939) were among the first to note a high incidence of negative affect and "catastrophic" reactions among patients with unilateral left-hemisphere damage. This reaction is characterized by excessive negative affect, tears, and pessimism about the future. A number of workers observed either an indifferent or euphoric reaction following unilateral right-hemisphere damage (e.g., Denny-Brown, Meyer, & Horenstein, 1952; Hecaen, Ajuriaguerra, & Massonet, 1951). The indifferent reaction is characterized by lack of emotional responsivity as well as anosognosia. The euphoric reaction is typically associated with inappropriate displays of positive affect, joking, and laughing.

Gainotti's (1969, 1972) examination of the differences in emotional behavior of patients with left- versus right-sided unilateral lesions revealed that left-hemisphere lesions produced more frequent displays of the catastrophic reaction. Joking behavior was most frequently displayed by patients with right-hemisphere lesions. Patients suffering from right-hemisphere lesions also showed a higher incidence of indifference, anosognosia, and minimization. Similar emotional differences were observed by Bear and Fedio (1977) between patients with right versus left unilateral epileptic foci.

Sackeim and his associates (1982) located 109 case reports of pathological laughing and crying (see Davison & Kelman, 1939, for an early report on this phenomenon). Each case was independently reviewed to ascertain the lateralization of the insults. In addition, each judge identified the emotional outbursts as primarily laughing, crying, or mixed symptoms. Although it was not clear from their report whether the judges were blind to the affective expression of the patient when making all of the lesion determinations, Sackeim and his colleagues (1982) found that left-sided lesions were more frequently associated with crying, whereas right-sided lesions were more frequently associated with laughing (see also Folstein, Maiberger, & Meutsch, 1977; Hall, Hall, & LaVoie, 1968). These data challenge the simple view that has argued for right-hemisphere specialization of emotion (Gardner et al., 1975; Heilman, Scholes, & Watson, 1975; Lishman, 1971; Ross & Mesulam, 1979; Tucker, Watson, & Heilman, 1977; Wechsler, 1973). Unfortunately, these latter studies did not specifically examine the effects of left- versus right-hemisphere lesions on positive and negative affective processes.

An important recent series of studies evaluated the effects of location of lesion within the left hemisphere and its relation to the severity of depression (Benson, 1973, 1979; Robinson & Benson, 1981; Robinson & Szetela, 1981). Benson (1973) found that depression was more severe in patients with anterior aphasias, and Robinson and Szetela (1981) reported that proximity of injury to the frontal lobe was strongly correlated with the severity of depression. Robinson and Benson (1981) have recently observed that depression among nonfluent aphasic patients was both more frequent and more severe compared with both fluent and global aphasics. The lesions of patients with nonfluent aphasias were more anterior than those of the other two groups, as assessed by CT scan. All patients with nonfluent aphasias had frontal lobe lesions. Importantly, lesion size was equivalent in the nonfluent and fluent aphasic groups. These findings indicate that depression is most likely to be associated with damage to the left frontal region rather than to the left posterior region.

Ross and Rush (1981) have recently presented a more complicated argument regarding the anatomical loci underlying depressive disorders. They decompose depression into specific symptom clusters, such as verbal-cognitive set, depressive affect, and vegetative anomalies, and propose specific cortical structures that may mediate each group of symptoms. However, they also suggest that endogenous depression may be initiated by structures in the right hemisphere, although a particular region is not specified.

Two important conclusions emerge from the unilateral lesion literature: (1) Left-hemisphere damage is more likely than right to accentuate negative affect and the display of a catastrophic-depressive reaction, whereas right-hemisphere damage is more often associated with indifference or euphoria; and (2) these hemispheric differences were most apparent for frontal-lobe lesions.

The association of frontal-lobe damage with affective change is, not surprisingly, based upon the anatomical situation of this brain region as well as previous empirical findings relating the frontal lobes to affective regulation. The frontal lobes have more extensive anatomical reciprocity with limbic structures than any other cortical region (e.g., Nauta, 1964, 1971; Kelly & Stinus, in press). A variety of neuropsychological evidence links damage to particular frontal-lobe areas to deficits in affective regulation (e.g., Akert, 1964; Baranovskaya & Homskaya, 1973; Luria, 1966, 1973; Pribram, 1973; Simernitskaya, 1973). In recent research, frontal-lobe lesions have been found to impair both voluntary and spontaneous facial expressions (Kolb & Milner, 1981a, 1981b). Interestingly, although they failed to comment on this, Kolb and Milner (1981b) found that left-sided frontal lesions resulted in significantly less spontaneous smiling than did right-sided lesions. Again, these findings support the hypothesis of differential lateralization for positive versus negative affect.

Effects of unilateral injections of sodium amytal on emotional processes. Since the early reports by Wada and others (Wada, 1949; Wada & Rasmussen, 1960; Werman, Anderson, & Christoff, 1959) on the selective barbiturization of a single hemisphere via carotid injection of sodium amytal, a number of investigators have noted differences in emotional state following disturbance of the left versus the right hemispheres (e.g., Hommes & Panhuysen, 1971; Perria, Rosadini, & Rossi, 1961; Rossi & Rosadini, 1967; Serafetinides, Hoare, & Driver, 1965; Terzian, 1964). Rossi and Rosadini (1967) have conducted the most extensive examination of the affective sequelae of intracarotid barbiturization.

In 65 intracarotid injections that were followed by an emotional reaction (Rossi & Rosadini, 1967), 68% of the injections to the dominant hemisphere produced depression and 32% were associated with euphoria. When the emotional sequelae of nondominant barbiturization were examined, 84% of the injections were associated with euphoria and 16% were associated with depression ($\chi^2[1] = 17.96$, $p = .00002$). It is unlikely that the depression associated with selective sedation of the left hemisphere can be solely attributed to the loss of language, as Rossi and Rosadini have noted that the identical emotional changes were observed in a subset of their patients given a dose of sodium amytal sufficiently low so as not to produce even mild sensorimotor or language impairment. In contrast to the Rossi and Rosadini findings, Milner (1967) did not observe any systematic differences between left versus right carotid injections. Significant methodological differences between the studies are likely to account for the discrepancies. Milner typically used a higher dosage of sodium amytal and injections were to the common carotid. Moreover, Milner's sample contained a large number of individuals who had suffered significant brain dysfunction at an early age. Similar findings have recently been reported by Kolb and Milner (1981b).

Lateralized dysfunctions in affective disorders. The literature reviewed in the two preceding sections was concerned with the study of brain-damaged populations. The degree to which the association of dysphoric mood with the right hemisphere is generalizable to patients with no obvious structural damage requires the examination of other populations. Individuals exhibiting depressive disorders are an important population to study in this regard, as they do not present with any obvious neurological anomaly. Studies addressing the differences in asymmetrical brain activation in depressed subjects have used, in most cases, electrophysiological methods.

The basic strategy in the use of the spontaneous EEG to assess asymmetrical brain activation is to record from homologous scalp regions and compare the relative differences between the regions in alpha power. A variety of evidence suggests that alpha-power suppression is related to activation (e.g., Shagass, 1972) and can be used to index asymmetries in relative activation in different scalp regions (Davidson & Ehrlichman, 1980). Alternatively, differences between homologous sites in the distribution of beta activity can provide a related index of differential activation. The more beta activity present, the greater the degree of activation underlying a particular scalp region.

EEG measures of differential hemispheric engagement can be used to assess asymmetries in activation in response to various tasks or to measure more tonic differences among individuals during resting situations. A variety of data suggest that posterior cortical asymmetries are closely associated with cognitive task performance. Recent evidence suggests that temporal and frontal EEG asymmetry may be particularly related to affective processes (see Davidson, in press, for a review).

Flor-Henry and his colleagues (1979) compared the EEGs of psychotically depressed patients with those of normal controls. The depressed patients showed a bilateral increase in temporal power in the 13–20 Hz (beta) band while at rest with eyes closed relative to the controls. The energy distribution was lateralized to the right hemisphere, indicated by a larger increase in right temporal beta power than in left relative to controls. Other investigators have also observed a greater proportion of right- versus left-sided EEG abnormalities among depressed patients (e.g., Abrams & Taylor, 1979; Shagass et al., 1979). Perris and Monakhov (1979) have recently found positive correlations between right precentral activation and ratings of depressive mood. Karlin and his colleagues (1978) studied four right-handed patients suffering from organically based pain syndromes, with the pain being perceived as along the midline of the body. In three of the four cases, right temporal activation was significantly greater than that of the left while patients were resting. When hypnotic analgesia was administered, a laterality shift toward greater relative left-sided activation was observed.

Schaffer, Davidson, and Saron (1983a) have recently studied resting frontal and parietal EEG asymmetry in groups of subclinically depressed subjects and matched normal controls. The Beck Depression Inventory (BDI; Beck et al., 1961) and a number of other psychometric tests were administered to 415

Table 11.1 *Psychometric characteristics of depressed and nondepressed groups*

	Initial BDI	Trait BDI	State BDI	MC
Depressed (N = 6)				
X̄	29.70	25.70	18.00	12.80
SD	7.84	8.26	5.90	0.84
Nondepressed (N = 9)				
X̄	4.20	4.80	4.30	8.40
SD	1.39	2.11	2.35	2.65

Note: The initial Beck Depression Inventory (BDI) was administered 3 to 6 months before the lab session. The trait and state BDIs were administered at the lab session. The state form was given with instructions to answer according to "how you feel at the moment," whereas the trait form was administered in the normal fashion. The Marlowe-Crowne (MC) scale was administered with the initial BDI.
Source: C. E. Schaffer, R. J. Davidson, and C. Saron, "Frontal and parietal EEG asymmetry in depressed and non-depressed subjects," *Biological psychiatry*, 1983, *18*, 753–762. Copyright 1983 by the Society of Biological Psychiatry. Reprinted by permission.

individuals. Depressed and nondepressed subjects who fell at the extremes of the distribution on the BDI were asked to participate. Subjects scoring 20 or above came to the laboratory as potential depressed subjects. They were re-administered the BDI in two forms: one assessing trait characteristics and the other assessing state characteristics (i.e., according to how they felt at the moment). To participate further, the depressed subjects were required to score 14 or above on the trait scale. After excluding subjects for failing to meet these criteria and for excessively confounded EEG records, six depressed individuals were selected for further participation. These subjects had a mean score of 29.7 (*SD* = 7.84) on the initial BDI, 25.7 (*SD* = 8.26) on the trait scale, and 18.0 (*SD* = 5.9) on the state scale, the latter two administered just before the experimental sessions.

The control group of truly nondepressed subjects was to be matched to the depressed group on sex, age, and marital status. Individuals were required to score 6 or below on the BDI to meet the initial criterion of nondepression. To screen out subjects who were defensively denying depression in their self-reports, we administered the Marlowe-Crowne Scale of Social Desirability (MC) (Crowne & Marlowe, 1964). By thus eliminating subjects who scored low on the BDI and high on the MC, the nondepressed sample was restricted to individuals who were nondefensively reporting nondepression. Subjects had to score 11 or below on the MC to meet the criterion for nonrepression. Subjects scoring 6 or below on the BDI *and* 11 or below on the MC who met the other subject characteristic criteria (i.e., sex, age, marital status) were invited to the laboratory. At the time of the laboratory session, the BDI was

Table 11.2. *Means and standard deviations for EEG laterality ratio scores for an eyes-closed resting period, split by group and by scalp region*

	Depressed		Nondepressed	
	F-ratio	P-ratio	F-ratio	P-ratio
X̄	$-.015^a$	.158	$.034^a$	.072
SD	.059	.110	.031	.080

Note: The ratio scores were computed with the formula $R - L/R + L$ alpha power. Higher numbers on this ratio are indicative of greater relative left-sided activation. The F-ratio was derived from F3 and F4 leads and the P-ratio was derived from P3 and P4 leads.
$^a p = .05$.
Source: C. E. Schaffer, R. J. Davidson, and C. Saron, "Frontal and parietal EEG asymmetry in depressed and non-depressed subjects," *Biological Psychiatry*, 1983, *18*, 753–762. Copyright 1983 by the Society of Biological Psychiatry. Reprinted by permission.

again readministered in both forms and subjects had to score 8 or below on the trait scale to be tested. After eliminating subjects who failed to meet the criteria presented above and subjects whose EEG records were excessively confounded, nine nondepressed subjects remained in the control group. All subjects were right-handed as assessed by the Edinburgh Inventory (Oldfield, 1971). The psychometric characteristics of the final groups are summarized in Table 11.1.

Resting EEG was recorded for both eyes open and eyes closed for 30-sec periods prior to the administration of various cognitive and affective tasks. Alpha activity from left and right frontal and left and right parietal regions (F3, F4, P3, and P4) referenced to a common vertex (Cz) was extracted for all artifact-free epochs. The results revealed no group differences for either frontal or parietal EEG during the eyes-open base-line period. However, for the eyes-closed resting period, a significant ($p = .05$) group effect was obtained on a measure of frontal alpha asymmetry ($R - L/R + L$ alpha; higher numbers on this index reflect greater relative left-sided activation). The relevant means are presented in Table 11.2 and indicate that depressed subjects show greater relative right-frontal activation than do nondepressed subjects. Importantly, no significant group effects were obtained on the parietal ratio score, indicating that the group difference was specific to the frontal recordings.

Figure 11.1 presents the individual subject means for the frontal ratio score derived from the eyes-closed base-line, separately for each group. As this figure indicates, all nondepressed subjects showed frontal ratio scores indicative of relative left-sided activation, whereas 5 out of 6 depressed subjects showed the opposite pattern. This difference is significant ($\chi^2[1] = 7.81$, $p < .01$ with Yates's correction for continuity).

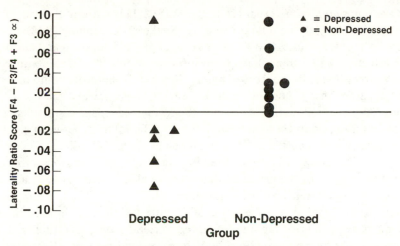

Figure 11.1. Frontal laterality ratio (R − L/R + L alpha power) scores for individual subjects split by group. Positive numbers on this score are indicative of left-sided frontal activation, and negative numbers are indicative of right-frontal activation. (From C. E. Schaffer, R. J. Davidson, and C. Saron, "Frontal and parietal EEG asymmetry in depressed and non-depressed subjects, *Biological Psychiatry*, 1983, *18*, 753–762.) Copyright 1983 by the Society of Biological Psychiatry. Reprinted by permission.

The separate contributions of the left and right hemispheres to the frontal ratio score difference between groups was also examined. A significant Group X Hemisphere interaction ($p = .007$) was obtained in which depressed subjects showed less alpha activity in the right- versus left-frontal region ($p = .004$), whereas nondepressed subjects showed slightly less alpha in the left- versus right-frontal regions ($p < .02$). Thus, the major difference between groups is that the depressed subjects showed right-frontal activation, whereas the non-depressed subjects showed slight left-frontal activation.

Most studies using behavioral and neuropsychological measures of hemispheric involvement (e.g., Bruder & Yozawitz, 1979; Flor-Henry, 1976; Flor-Henry & Yeudall, 1979; Kronfol et al., 1978; Yozawitz et al., 1979) have revealed a deficit in right-hemisphere sensorimotor and cognitive skills among individuals who are depressed as compared with normal controls. For example, Flor-Henry (1976) found that patients with affective disorders showed evidence of right-sided dysfunction on a standardized battery of neuropsychological tests. Kronfol et al. (1978) administered eight neuropsychological tests, four tapping left-sided functioning and four tapping right-sided functioning, to a group of 18 right-handed depressed patients. Before treatment with ECT, performance on right-hemisphere tests was inferior to that on left-hemisphere tests. Goldstein et al. (1977) found a similar pattern.

In an examination of the neuropsychological test performance of children born to at least one parent with bipolar manic-depressive illness (Kestenbaum, 1979), it was found that the children exhibited significantly worse performance

IQ as compared with verbal IQ on the WISC. This pattern of results has been replicated recently on a larger sample (Sackeim & Decina, 1982).

The neuropsychological findings from depressed subjects and children born to affectively ill parents have been interpreted to reflect deficits in cognitive and perceptual skills subserved by the right hemisphere. It should immediately be apparent that a possible inconsistency exists between the data on right-sided hyperactivation (particularly in the frontal leads) and right-sided cognitive dysfunction in depressed subjects. What is the relation between right-frontal hyperactivation and the deficits in right-hemisphere-mediated cognitive processes? This issue will be examined in detail in the final section of this chapter. Suffice to say, for the moment, that reciprocal relations between anterior and posterior activation within a hemisphere might exist. Thus, a hyperactivated right-frontal region may be associated with a reciprocal inhibition in right-hemisphere posterior regions (e.g., the parietal lobe), resulting in deficits in certain right-hemisphere controlled cognitive and perceptual activities.

Effects of lateralized electroconvulsive therapy (ECT). Since its introduction in 1938, electroconvulsive therapy (ECT) has been a widely used psychiatric intervention, particularly in the treatment of depression. Originally, ECT was administered bilaterally. In an attempt to produce focal seizures in patients for whom generalized seizures were believed to be too stressful, Parcella and Impastato (1954) introduced unilateral ECT. The introduction of unilateral ECT has led to the comparison of the therapeutic efficacy of left versus right ECT. Given that ECT slows brain electrical activity, unilateral right ECT would be expected to be more effective than unilateral left, as depression is often associated with hyperactivation in certain regions on the right side.

Studies that directly compared the therapeutic efficacy of left versus right ECT (Cohen, Penick, & Tarter, 1974; Cronin et al., 1970; Deglin & Nikolaenko, 1975; Halliday et al., 1968; Zinkin & Birthnell, 1968) indicate that right-sided ECT is clearly more effective than left-sided ECT.

In a unique study, Deglin and Nikolaenko (1975) subjected 40 patients with a heterogeneous mixture of various forms of psychopathology to alternate right and left ECT on alternate days. Clinical analysis of the patients' emotional state was performed after ECT-induced seizures. These investigators found that nondominant ECT was associated with smiling, joking, laughter, and exclamations of joy. Dominant ECT, on the other hand, led to anxiety, dysphoria, and an intensification of preexisting melancholia or delusional anxiety. These emotional shifts typically lasted for several days.

These findings suggest that psychotic depression may be associated with hyperactivation of right-hemisphere areas, which become more normalized following ECT. Moscovitch, Strauss, and Olds (1981) examined the performance of right-handed depressed subjects on a dichotic listening task before and after nondominant ECT. Dichotic assessment was performed approximately one day prior to receiving ECT, 4 hours following the second ECT (the average number of treatments was 10), and again 3 to 4 months post ECT. Before treatment, 5 of the 6 patients in the ECT group failed to show the normal pattern of right-ear scores. Interestingly, the one patient who failed to show the normal right-ear advantage following ECT was the only subject in the group to have relapsed within 3 to 4 months. Five patients were available for dichotic retesting 3 to 4 months following ECT. All of these patients were judged by physicians to have made significant clinical improvements and all maintained a significant right-ear advantage at this third testing occasion.

A much larger group of studies has compared the effectiveness of bilateral versus right ECT (most of the studies have been reviewed by d'Elia & Raotma, 1975 and Stromgren, 1973). The majority of investigators in this area found no difference between these two modes of treatment. Given the association between the right hemisphere and at least certain negative affects, it is not entirely clear why bilateral and unilateral right ECT should not differ in therapeutic effectiveness. One critical element that has not received very much attention concerns the placement of ECT electrodes along the rostral-caudal plane. It may be that different placements would alter the therapeutic efficacy by shifting the location of the focal seizures.

Research on normal populations

The data reviewed in the preceding section were derived from the study of various clinical populations. Although the data provide important information on hemispheric involvement in affective regulation, such information is not always generalizable to the intact organism. In the study of lesion cases, the damage is often not discretely localized, which probably introduces variability to the phenomena under study. Generalizing to normals from the study of psychiatric patients is occasionally problematic because of diagnostic heterogeneity and the complexity of certain disorders. For example, as Ross and Rush (1981) have recently pointed out, only certain components of the depressive syndrome may be associated with right-hemisphere dysfunction. The findings from the clinical literature have helped to pose the key questions for study in normals. The remainder of this section will review both behavioral and electrophysiological studies of hemispheric asymmetries in affective behavior, emphasizing those performed in our laboratory over the past several years.

Lateral gaze shifts in response to affective stimuli. Lateral gaze shifts have been employed as a gross index of asymmetrical hemispheric engagement by numerous investigators (see Ehrlichman & Weinberger, 1978; Gur, 1975; Gur & Gur, 1977; Kinsbourne, 1972; Kocel et al., 1972; Schwartz et al., 1975). Considerable controversy has been generated concerning the validity of lateral gaze shifts as an index of hemispheric asymmetry. Ehrlichman and Weinberger

(1978) have reviewed 19 published experiments that examined the effects of reflective questions designed to differentially activate the left versus the right hemisphere on lateral eye movements (LEMS). They observed that only 9 of those experiments obtained significant effects in the predicted direction, that is, that "left hemisphere" questions elicited a significantly greater proportion of right LEMs that did "right hemisphere" questions. Numerous methodological inadequacies have plagued research using LEMs as a dependent measure (see Ehrlichman & Weinberger, 1978). In our previous work using this measure, we reasoned that, despite its methodological limitations, it may be particularly useful in the study of affective processes, as Ehrlichman and Weinberger (1978) have acknowledged. A significant component of eye-movement control resides in the frontal cortex (Robinson & Fuchs, 1969). This cortical region has been implicated in the regulation of affective processes (Luria, 1973; Nauta, 1971; Pribram, 1973), and we have obtained EEG evidence suggesting that this region specifically discriminates between positive versus negative affect.

In our earlier work, we sought to examine whether greater right-hemisphere involvement was associated with the processing of affective versus nonaffective questions (Schwartz et al., 1975). We found significantly more left and fewer right-eye movements in response to emotional versus non-emotional questions. (The first eye movement following the presentation of the question was scored; Ehrlichman [1979] found this to be the most discriminating measure in a comparison of verbal versus spatial questions.) These data have been successfully replicated in our laboratory with simultaneous measures of electrodermal activity (Davidson, Schwartz, & Weinberger, 1977), in which it was confirmed that affective questions elicited significantly more skin resistance responses (defined as a change of at least 1000 ohms following presentation of the question), as compared with nonaffective questions. Two independent laboratories have also replicated our eye-movement findings using the set of questions we developed (Hasset & Zelner, 1977; Tucker et al., 1977).

Interestingly, when we reexamined the eye-movement data we found that more negative than positive questions were employed and that the negative questions elicited more left-eye movements (indicative of greater right-hemisphere activation), as compared with the positive questions. The relative paucity of questions in these two categories did not permit a rigorous analysis of these differences.

To more systematically explore these preliminary observations, we designed an experiment to explicitly examine lateral gaze shifts in response to positive, negative, and neutral questions of a verbal and spatial nature (Schwartz et al., 1979). Examples of each question type are:

> *Verbal-positive*: "What is the primary distinction between pleasure and ecstasy?"
> *Verbal-neutral*: "What is the primary distinction between logical and rational?"
> *Verbal-negative*: "What is the primary distinction between anger and hate?"

Spatial-positive: "Try to picture and describe the first situation in which you fell in love."
Spatial-neutral: "Try to picture and describe the blandest situation in which you have been."
Spatial-negative: "Try to picture and describe the first situation in which you experienced hatred."

If the asymmetrical hemispheric engagement seen in response to positive and negative affective stimuli is in part a function of the differential contribution of the left- and right-frontal regions, then one might expect LEMs to reflect this asymmetry. Twenty-four right-handed subjects were presented with 48 questions, with each cell of a 2×3 matrix (verbal-spatial $\times$ positive-neutral-negative emotion) containing 8 questions. The findings revealed a significant Emotion (positive, negative, neutral) $\times$ Eye Movement Direction interaction. Negative questions elicited more left and fewer right-eye movements, compared with positive questions for both the verbal and spatial subsets.

Visual field asymmetry in response to affective stimuli. The issue of hemispheric activation in response to affective visual stimuli has been addressed by many studies. In studying recognition memory for emotional and non-emotional faces in each visual field, Suberi and McKeever (1977) found a greater left visual field (LVF) advantage (faster reaction time) in the recognition of emotional, as compared with non-emotional, faces. Importantly, they also observed that sad faces produced the greatest left-visual-field (right-hemisphere) advantage, whereas happy and angry faces were associated with the least LVF superiority.

In a similar vein, Ley and Bryden (1979) reported that subjects required to recognize schematic emotional faces that were tachistoscopically exposed to each visual field showed, on the average, a left-visual-field advantage for this task across all emotions. However, when separate emotions were examined, subjects made more errors when extremely positive expressions, as compared with extremely negative expressions, were presented to the LVF.

In studies by Sackeim and his colleagues (Sackeim & Gur, 1978; Sackeim, Gur, & Saucy, 1978), subjects were asked to judge the intensity of emotional expression of left-side and right-side composites of human faces posing six different emotions. In general, the left-side composites were judged as expressing emotions more intensely than the right-side composites. However, a post-hoc analysis revealed that this effect held more strongly for the negative emotions. Overall, in 73% of the instances of negative emotions, mean judgments of emotional intensity were higher for left-side composites, whereas this held in only 45% of the instances of positive emotions ($p < .05$, by χ^2). However, Ekman (1980a) has pointed out that the faces depicting negative emotions were all posed, whereas the positive facial expressions were spontaneous. This difference could have contributed significantly to the finding by Sackeim and his colleagues of asymmetric differences between positive versus negative facial expressions.

To examine left- versus right-hemisphere specialization for positive and negative affect, Dimond and his colleagues (Dimond & Farrington, 1977; Dimond, Farrington, & Johnson, 1976), developed a contact-lens system whereby prolonged visual input can be projected to either the left or the right visual fields. Using such a system, films were projected separately to each visual field and were then subsequently rated on the nature of the affect elicited. Heart rate was recorded as a measure of autonomic reactivity. Dimond and his colleagues (1976) found that films projected to the right hemisphere first (LVF) were judged to be significantly more unpleasant than the same films initially projected to the left hemisphere (RVF). Moreover, Dimond and Far- rington (1977) found that cartoons produced the greatest change in heart rate when projected to the left hemisphere, whereas more unpleasant or threatening films evoked the greatest heart-rate changes when projected to the right hem- isphere.

These findings suggest that each hemisphere may differ with respect to the valence of its affective bias. The similarities between these perceptual findings and the data on the effects of cerebral insult on the experience of emotion suggest some important similarities in the perception and experience/expression of emotion. This hypothesis is consistent with cognitive theory, which suggests that perceptual activity calls upon certain neural mechanisms that are centrally involved in the production of that class of behavior (e.g., speech perception depends critically on the structures involved in speech production; see Liberman et al., 1967; Turvey, 1977; Weimer, 1977).

We have recently completed an experiment (Davidson et al., 1983) in which 19 right-handed subjects were presented with affective or neutral faces uni- laterally to either the left or right visual field for a prolonged 8 sec exposure. This duration was established during pilot work, which indicated that shorter durations did not allow subjects to make the kinds of complex judgments required. To ensure that subjects were centrally fixating throughout stimulus exposure, EOG was recorded and any trial associated with an eye movement of greater than 1° was omitted. Following presentation of the faces, subjects were asked to rate each face on the degree to which it expressed various emotions as well as on the degree to which it evoked various emotions in themselves (on 7-point scales). Both types of questions were asked because we believed that the asymmetry would be much stronger for ratings of subjects' emotional *experience*, as compared with ratings of the stimulus.

Subjects' ratings of the degree to which each face *expressed* various emotions was uninfluenced by the hemifield to which the face was presented. However, when subjects were asked to rate the degree to which the face evoked various emotions in *themselves*, significant visual-field effects emerged. Specifically, when asked to rate how happy they felt in response to the stimuli, subjects reported experiencing significantly more happiness in response to faces presented to the RVF (i.e., initially to the left hemisphere), as compared with responses to the *identical faces* when presented to the LVF. This effect held irrespective

Table 11.3. *Mean and standard deviations of Ss ratings of happiness and sadness evoked by the unilateral presentation of faces*

	Rating of happiness		Ratings of sadness	
	Happy face	Sad face	Happy face	Sad face
Left hemifield				
X̄	3.19	1.95	1.98	2.65
SD	1.26	.91	.91	.86
Right hemifield				
X̄	3.26	2.31	1.92	2.59
SD	1.30	.86	.82	1.06

Note: A 7-point scale was used. $N = 19$.
Source: R. J. Davidson, E. Moss, C. Saron, and C. E. Schaffer, Self-reports of emotion are influenced by the visual field to which affective information is presented. Manuscript submitted for publication, 1983.

of the valence of the face. That is, more happiness was reported in response to RVF presentations of all faces, as compared with LVF exposures. The data on ratings of happiness and sadness in response to happy and sad faces exposed to the RVF and LVF are presented in Table 11.3. As can be seen from this table, subjects report more happiness in response to RVF presentations of happy and sad faces, as compared with LVF presentations of the identical faces. The data on sadness ratings are in the predicted direction, that is, higher ratings of sadness in response to LVF presentations. However, these latter findings are clearly nonsignificant.

In a recent experiment, we have replicated this basic pattern of effects (Schaffer, Davidson, & Saron, 1983b). Subjects were again exposed to 8-sec lateralized presentations of happy, sad, and neutral faces and asked to rate their experience on various dimensions of affect. In response to happy, sad, and neutral faces, subjects rated their experience as containing more intense happiness when these faces were exposed to the RVF, as compared with the LVF. When asked to rate the degree to which they experienced sadness, subjects consistently reported more intense sadness following LVF presentations of all three face types.

In another type of study (Reuter-Lorenz & Davidson, 1981), we have obtained additional evidence suggesting that the left and right hemispheres are differentially specialized for the perception of happy and sad faces. Twenty-eight right-handed subjects were tachistoscopically exposed to a neutral and an emotional face of the same individual presented unilaterally, one to the RVF and one to the LVF simultaneously. On each trial, subjects were required to indicate on which side the emotional face had been presented. Reaction time and accuracy were both recorded. Figure 11.2 presents the results. As can be

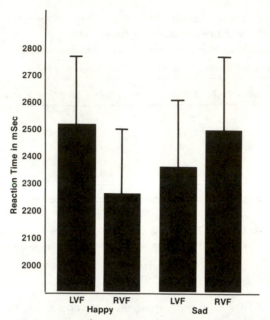

Figure 11.2. Mean reaction time (bars indicate standard errors) for happy and sad stimulus presentations, separately for each visual field. (From P. Reuter-Lorenz and R. J. Davidson, "Differential contributions of the two cerebral hemispheres to the perception of happy and sad faces," *Neuropsychologia*, 1981, *19*, 609–613.) Copyright 1981 by Pergamon Press, Ltd. Reprinted by permission.

seen from this graph, happy faces were responded to more quickly when presented to the RVF than when presented to the LVF. The opposite pattern of results was obtained in response to the sad faces.

The data reviewed in this section call into question the notion of right-hemisphere involvement in all emotional behavior and support the suggestion of differential lateralization for certain positive and negative affects. The perceptual data indicate that the left-visual-field advantage for recognition of faces varies as a function of emotional expression and that in certain task situations it actually disappears in favor of a right-visual-field advantage. Interestingly, in the Suberi and McKeever (1977) study, both happy and angry faces produced the smallest LVF advantage. The finding for angry faces calls into question the positive–negative basis for the asymmetry that has been discussed. A possible resolution of this apparent inconsistency may lie in classifying the emotions according to their association with approach or avoidance. In a later section of this chapter, approach–avoidance as a basis for the affective asymmetry will be considered. If particular regions of the hemispheres are lateralized for approach versus avoidance behavior, we might expect that those negative emotions often associated with approach, such as anger, would be lateralized to the left side or at least not show strong right-hemisphere specialization. Although admittedly post-hoc and speculative, this would provide an explanation for the Suberi and McKeever (1977) finding.

Another important issue incompletely understood concerns the differential asymmetries present in the *perception* of positive and negative affective stimuli. It is commonly thought that right-hemisphere posterior cortical regions (i.e., the right parietal region) are involved in the perception of emotion, particularly in perceiving emotional faces (e.g., Luria, 1973). This specialization of right posterior areas for affective perception is thought to apply to the perception of all valences of emotion. Moreover, EEG data indicate that the right parietal region is activated in the perception of affective stimuli and that this asymmetry in parietal activation does *not* vary as a function of the valence of an affective stimulus (e.g., Davidson & Schwartz, 1976).

To account for the inconsistency that exists in the literature on the perception of emotion (i.e., some studies show differential lateralization effects as a function of valence and others show right-hemisphere superiority for the perception of emotion in general), the following proposal is offered. Differential lateralization as a function of affective valence in behavioral studies of the perception of affective stimuli will occur as a function of the degree to which subjects covertly (or overtly) produce the affective expression that matches the stimulus in the act of perception. As was mentioned earlier, contemporary models of speech perception are analogous in proposing an important role for speech production in the process of perceiving. Recent data on the perception of emotional faces (Dimberg, 1982) indicates that subjects tend to make a covert facial expression (as assessed with facial EMG) that mimics the expression to be perceived in a task requiring facial expression identification.

Electrophysiological studies of hemispheric activation in response to affective stimuli. The use of the spontaneous EEG recorded from homologous left and right scalp leads to infer asymmetrical patterns of brain activation has a number of important advantages in the study of asymmetries associated with affect. Because this procedure does not require special constraints on stimulus exposures as do the behavioral methods of inferring hemispheric involvement, the investigator is able to present continuous stimulation that is likely to actually elicit emotion in the observer. For example, emotional films can be presented while EEG is recorded from various scalp loci. Differences in patterns of EEG activation can then be examined as a function of subject self-reports of their affective response to the stimulation.

We have used this strategy in a number of studies, in particular, in comparing frontal and parietal EEG asymmetries in response to various positive and negative affective stimuli. Based upon the literature just reviewed, we hypothesized that greater relative left-frontal activation would be associated with epochs of positive affect than with epochs of negative affect. We also predicted that parietal EEG asymmetry would not differentiate between positive and negative epochs.

In one study (Davidson et al., 1979), 16 right-handed subjects were exposed to videotaped segments of popular television programs that were judged to vary in affective content. While viewing the videotapes, subjects were instructed to continuously rate the degree to which they experienced positive versus negative affect by pressing up and down on a pressure-sensitive gauge. The output of this pressure transducer was digitized to provide a quantitative measure of affective self-report.

EEG was recorded from the left and right frontal (F3 and F4) and left and right parietal (P3 and P4) regions referred to a common vertex (Cz). Activity in the alpha band was extracted from the EEG and integrated and digitized. EOG was also recorded and epochs confounded by eye-movement artifact were eliminated. To obtain an independent measure of the subjects' affective response to the video stimuli, two channels of facial EMG were also recorded, one from the zygomatic major region (the "smile" muscle) and one from the frontalis region (associated with tension and frowning) (Schwartz et al., 1976). EMG data were also integrated and digitized.

To test our major hypotheses, we compared the 30-sec epoch each subject judged to be most positive with one rated as most negative. This information was derived from the pressure transducer data. The positive and negative epochs deviated from the central neutral position by comparable amounts. It is important to emphasize that the positive and negative epochs were individually obtained for each subject on the basis of his or her self-reports. We believe that this methodological approach is superior to analyses based upon a priori classification of stimulus conditions.

We first compared the positive and negative epochs on the laterality alpha ratio score ($R - L/R + L$ alpha power). Higher numbers on this score indicate greater relative left-sided activation. We found that significantly greater relative left-frontal activation was elicited by positive epochs than by negative epochs ($p = .02$). Parietal asymmetry did not distinguish between conditions. These data are displayed in Table 11.4. Interestingly, parietal EEG indicated that subjects showed right-sided activation in both positive and negative epochs. Analysis of the separate contributions of the left and right frontal sites to the ratio score difference revealed that positive epochs were associated with less left hemisphere and more right hemisphere alpha, as compared with negative epochs.

To independently examine the impact of self-rated positive and negative epochs on a physiological system that has been found in previous research to discriminate between self-generated positive and negative imagery, we examined the integrated EMG recorded from the zygomatic and frontalis muscle regions. As Table 11.5 reveals, positive segments elicited more zygomatic and less frontalis activity than did negative segments ($p = .04$). The EMG data confirm

Table 11.4. *Means and standard deviations for frontal and parietal laterality ratio scores (R − L/R + L alpha)*

	Positive	Negative
Frontal ratio		
X̄	.102	−.154
SD	.358	.365
Parietal ratio		
X̄	−.046	−.119
SD	.236	.209

Note: Higher numbers on this ratio score are indicative of greater relative left-sided activation. The data are separately presented for self-rated extreme positive and negative epochs in response to affective video stimuli. *Source*: R. J. Davidson, G. E. Schwartz, C. Saron, J. Bennett, and D. J. Goleman, "Frontal versus parietal EEG asymmetry during positive and negative affect," *Psychophysiology*, 1979, *16*, 202–203.

that self-reports were indeed associated with expected changes in facial muscle activity.

In a second study, we (Bennett, Davidson, & Saron, 1982) presented affective (positive and negative) and neutral words to subjects (pretrained on generating affective imagery) who were then requested to generate affective imagery for a 45-sec period by conjuring up personal associations to the word. In response to one set of affective words, we confirmed that subjects who rated those words more positively showed greater relative left frontal activation, as compared with subjects who rated the words more negatively. Parietal asymmetry again failed to discriminate between the groups. Moreover, we found that subjects' ratings of the intensity of their affective experience were highly correlated with frontal asymmetry and uncorrelated with parietal asymmetry.

A number of other investigators have recently examined EEG asymmetry during positive and negative affective states and have obtained results consistent with ours. Karlin and his associates (1978) assessed temporal asymmetry in response to cold pressor pain bilaterally administered and found greater relative right-hemisphere activation during this condition, as compared with hypnotically induced analgesia. In a second study employing hypnotically revivified happy and sad memories, Karlin and his colleagues (1978) found that sad experiences elicited greater relative right-hemisphere activation, as compared with happy experiences. Tucker and his associates (1981) also employed hypnotically induced mood states as an independent variable and found that the induction of a depressed mood produced significantly greater relative right-hemisphere

Table 11.5. *Means and standard deviations
for zygomatic major and frontalis region
EMG*

	Positive	Negative
Zygomatic EMG		
X̄	263.63	222.19
SD	157.71	150.46
Frontalis EMG		
X̄	188.88	201.50
SD	39.52	44.68

Note: The data are separately presented for the identical
positive and negative epochs described in Table 11.4. Units
are arbitrary.
Source: R. J. Davidson, G. E. Schwartz, C. Saron, J. Bennett, & D. J. Goleman, "Frontal versus parietal EEG asymmetry during positive and negative affect," *Psychophysiology*, 1979, *16*, 202–203.

activation, as compared with a euphoric mood only at the frontal leads. Central,
parietal, and occipital asymmetry did not discriminate between these conditions.

Harman and Ray (1977) recently found differential lateralization in the
temporal region for verbally induced positive and negative affect in a direction
opposite to our findings as well as to those of others (Flor-Henry, 1979; Karlin
et al., 1978; and Tucker et al., 1981). A number of serious methodological
inadequacies in their study preclude an unambiguous interpretation of their
data. Harman and Ray (1977) examined broad-band activity (3-30 Hz) and
sampled for an epoch that apparently was prior to the actual self-generation
of affect in the subjects. The experimenter was "verbally couching" the subjects
during the entire epoch, and across the two hemispheres, negative emotions
elicited significantly more activation. Because of these methodological short-
comings it is not possible to interpret the data from this study.

*Summary: hemispheric specialization for emotion in adult
humans*

Data derived from both clinical and normal populations indicate that the two
cerebral hemispheres play different roles in the regulation of affect. Aspects
of the clinical and normal data suggest that the asymmetries for affect are
localized to particular regions along the rostral/caudal plane with the frontal
lobes and possibly the temporal lobes critically involved. The evidence indicates
that the left-frontal region is particularly involved in certain positive affects
and the right frontal region in certain negative affects. Importantly, the parietal
and other cortical regions do not discriminate between affective stimuli that
differ in valence.

A number of important questions remain to be resolved. As was discussed earlier, the precise nature of the affective asymmetry has not yet been delineated. Although the positive–negative continuum has been invoked to describe the nature of the affective asymmetry, we have seen that this is probably not quite accurate, since both anger and happiness were found to be perceptually lateralized in a similar manner (Suberi & McKeever, 1977). The type of research critically needed will use more precise measures of an individual's affective state and will examine the association between these indices and ongoing measures of brain activity. We are currently engaged in research in which subjects are exposed to films differing in emotional content. In addition to recording brain and autonomic activity, we are unobtrusively videotaping subjects' facial behavior in response to the films. We can then use the face as a flag and extract epochs of physiological activity that bracket well-defined changes in facial expression. Because of the very finely differentiated nature of facial expression, we can relate specific expressions of discrete emotions to patterns of central and autonomic nervous system activity. In this way, we allow for individual variability in responsiveness to the films and analyze the physiological data on the basis of common subject facial responses rather than common stimulus characteristics. We hope to more precisely refine our understanding of the asymmetry for affect by examining asymmetries associated with various discrete emotions.

Another important question raised by some of the data presented here is the relation between asymmetries in anterior and posterior cortical regions. We believe that this relation is central to understanding the role of hemispheric organization in affect–cognition interactions and will help to explain the exhibition by depressed subjects of selective deficits on tasks presumably subserved by right-hemisphere posterior regions. This issue will be discussed in more detail in the final section on affect-cognition interaction.

Finally, an issue not addressed by the data just reviewed is the ontogeny of the asymmetries for affect. What is the relation between the maturation of certain cerebral systems and the emergence of affective response systems over the first year of life? It is to these issues that we now turn.

Developmental issues in hemispheric specialization for affect

Although a fairly extensive body of literature has accumulated on the ontogeny of hemispheric specialization for language and other cognitive processes (e.g., Kinsbourne, 1976), virtually no published studies have appeared relating cerebral asymmetry to the development of affect. However, this is an area that I have recently begun to study in collaboration with Nathan Fox (e.g., Davidson & Fox, 1982; Fox & Davidson, in press; Fox & Davidson, 1983). In addition to collecting initial data relevant to this issue, we have begun to pose a number of questions that are fundamental to research on this topic.

Increasing attention has been devoted to the study of the development of infant affective response systems over the first year of life. Some of this work has focused on the development of facial expression, and other research has examined the developing capacity of the infant to perceive facial expressions. Still other programs of study have assessed the patterning among the various response systems that reflect emotion in an attempt to use converging measures to identify the emergence of major discrete affects over the first year of life.

The literature on the development of naturally occurring spontaneous affective expression suggests that only certain facial expressions are present in the neonate and that others appear to emerge over the course of the first year. Field and her associates (1982) have recently claimed that a number of facial expressions of affect can be imitated by neonates. Specifically, they found evidence of imitation in neonates in response to posed expressions of happy, sad, and surprise faces by a live model. Whether such facial imitation actually reflects the presence of the underlying associated affect is a difficult and currently unresolved question, which can be approached only by measuring several converging response systems.

Spontaneously produced smiles have been observed in the neonate (Emde & Harman, 1972), but smiling is more frequently observed in response to social stimuli at around 2 months of age (Sroufe & Waters, 1976). The facial expression of interest has been observed to occur in the neonate in response to certain classes of stimuli (Izard, personal communication, 1980). We have recently observed the expression of interest in a majority of newborn subjects ($N = 15$) following the oral introduction of a sucrose solution (Fox & Davidson, 1983).

Among the negative affects, distress and disgust have been observed in neonates (Izard, personal communication, 1980; Fox & Davidson, 1983). In our work, a disgust expression was reliably elicited by the taste of a citric acid solution.

The facial expressions in neonates occurring spontaneously or elicited by certain events, but not through imitation, include interest, possibly smiling, distress and disgust. Although other facial expressions might be elicited were the neonate exposed to the requisite stimuli, the absence of any reports to this effect suggests that it is unlikely.

Given that these are the major spontaneously observed facial expressions present in the newborn and that they therefore may reflect the primary emotions present at this age, the structural and functional properties of the neonatal brain are apparently sufficient to subserve these emotions. An important feature of brain organization at this age is the relative lack of functional connection between the two hemispheres (Rakic & Yakovlev, 1968). Thus, the affects present in the neonate are likely to be those that are controlled unilaterally,

Table 11.6. *Frontal (F) and parietal (P) ratio scores (R − L/R + L 3–12 Hz activity) by taste condition in neonates (N = 15)*

	Sucrose Solution		Citric Acid Solution	
	F-ratio	P-ratio	F-ratio	P-ratio
$\bar{X}$	.094	−.006	.034	−.056
SD	.143	.082	.132	.151

Note: Higher numbers are indicative of greater relative left-sided activation.
Source: N. Fox and R. J. Davidson, Frontal brain electrical asymmetry distinguishes between approach and withdrawal reactions in newborn infants. Manuscript submitted for publication, 1983.

not bilaterally.[2] Specifically, this view would predict that disgust and distress would be primarily subserved by right-hemisphere anterior regions and that interest would be subserved by corresponding left-hemisphere regions.

We (Fox & Davidson, 1983) recently tested this prediction in a study of facial and EEG responses to tastes differing in affective valence in infants 3 to 4 days old. After excluding subjects whose parents were not both right-handed and those with excessively confounded EEG, 15 subjects were exposed to plain distilled water, a sucrose solution, a citric acid solution and a quinine sulfate solution. Each trial consisted of the introduction of 4 ml of solution into the baby's mouth with a sterile pipette. The facial behavior of the infant was videotaped and EEG was recorded from the left and right frontal and parietal scalp regions (referenced to vertex).

EEG was filtered for 3–12 Hz activity and epochs confounded by eye movement and muscle artifact were excluded. EEGs from left- and right-sided leads from the parietal and frontal regions were converted to laterality ratio scores (R − L/R + L) so that higher numbers reflect greater relative left-sided activation.

Sucrose and citric acid solutions were chosen because of their reliability in producing interest and disgust expressions respectively, in the majority of infants. The laterality ratio scores for these conditions, separately for frontal and parietal scalp leads, indicate that the sucrose solution elicited higher frontal ratio scores than did the citric acid solution, and thus suggests greater relative left-sided activation (Table 11.6). Importantly, no significant difference was found for the parietal ratio score between these conditions.

These data indicate that asymmetries in frontal brain activation discriminate between tastes eliciting interest versus disgust in newborn infants. While parietal asymmetry was in the same direction, EEG from this region failed to discriminate between conditions. Thus, the frontal asymmetry for certain positive versus negative affects appears to be present from birth.

Certain affective response systems probably emerge later in the first year of life. For example, both fear on the visual cliff and fear in response to strangers appears to emerge around 9 months of age (e.g., Campos et al., 1975; Campos et al., 1978). Campos and his colleagues (1975) found that heart-rate responses elicited by the approach of a stranger tended to be predominantly acceleratory in 9-month-olds. Furthermore, those infants who were behaviorally distressed at either 5 or 9 months of age gave progressively acceleratory responses, whereas behaviorally undistressed infants did not.

Using the visual cliff as another stimulus context in which the development of fear could be studied, Campos (1978) again found a developmental shift between 5 and 9 months of age with 5-month-old infants showing little evidence of fear, whereas 9-month-old babies show both behavioral and physiological signs of fear. Other data show that the developmental shift in the expression of fear is not a function of inadequate depth perception at the earlier age (e.g., Day & McKenzie, 1973; Fields, 1976).

Campos et al. (1978) have isolated locomotor history as an important determinant of fear of heights. For example, in one study nonlocomoting and locomoting infants matched for age were compared on cardiac responses to placement over the shallow versus the deep side of the visual cliff. Cardiac responses to shallow placing did not differ between groups. In response to placing over the deep side, locomoting infants showed significant cardiac acceleration, whereas nonlocomoting infants showed a small deceleration.

It thus appears from both stranger-approach and visual-cliff studies that fear emerges around 7 to 9 months of age. Certain other negative emotions may also emerge at about this time. For example, Sroufe (1979) has reported that facial expressions of wariness and sadness do not typically emerge until this time or later. I would like to raise the possibility that those affects that emerge between 6 and 12 months of age may depend more on interhemispheric communication for the activation of the "affect program." Certain motor skills, which depend upon interhemispheric interaction such as crossing the midline and crawling, emerge at roughly the same period or just before the emergence of fear and possibly other negative affects. These emotions may still be associated with reliable patterns of cerebral asymmetry but may be less exclusively unilateral than those emotions that emerge earlier in the first year.

Despite our proposal that sadness should be less exclusively subserved by unilateral right-hemisphere regions as compared with other negative affects, we have observed reliable behavioral and electrophysiological asymmetries between happy and sad affective stimuli in adults. To determine whether frontal lobe asymmetry for happy versus sad affective information was present in the first year of life, we chose to study infants 10 months of age. This choice was based upon evidence that (a) indicated that by 9 months of age infants can discriminate among a variety of emotional faces, including those depicting positive and negative emotional expressions (e.g., Campos & Stenberg, 1981) and (b) suggested that by this age infants are capable of experiencing wariness (e.g., Sroufe, 1979). We specifically predicted that infants of this age would show a pattern of frontal asymmetry similar to that of adults in response to positive and negative affective stimuli.

A total of 38 infants 10 months of age were seen in two studies (Davidson & Fox, 1982). From these, we were able to obtain artifact-free data from 24 infants. Only infants born to right-handed parents were tested. The methods for both studies were virtually equivalent. The infant sat in her mother's lap facing a 21-inch (diagonal) video monitor. EEG was recorded from the left and right frontal and parietal regions referred to a common vertex and stored on separate channels of FM tape.

The positive and negative affective facial stimuli were embedded in a video recording of "Sesame Street." The stimulus tape was sequenced in the following manner; 10 sec of a "Sesame Street" segment followed by 90 sec of an affective face segment that was either happy or sad (counterbalanced across subjects). Following the first affective segment, the infant viewed 90 sec of "Sesame Street" after which the second 90-sec affective segment occurred. Each affective segment consisted of a female actress who maintained a neutral face for 15 sec and then spontaneously broke into either smiling and laughter (happy segment) or frowning and crying (sad segment). The audio portion was edited out so as to match the happy and sad segments.

EEG in response to each segment from each of the four leads was reviewed and edited for gross eye movement, muscle, and movement artifact. Artifact-free epochs were then filtered for 1–12 Hz activity. The filtered output was digitized and energy (in uv sec) in the 1–12 Hz band was computed for each of the four leads separately for each of the affective epochs.

In the second study, an observer blind to the affective condition coded the infant's visual fixation and EEG was examined only for artifact-free epochs during which the infant was fixating on the monitor.

Laterality ratio scores (R − L/R + L 1–12 Hz power) were computed for frontal and parietal scalp leads. Parietal asymmetry did not discriminate between the happy and sad segments. The frontal ratio score data indicate that greater relative left frontal activation was associated with happy epochs than with sad segments in both studies (Table 11.7). Across both studies, 20 of the 24 infants showed equal or greater relative left-frontal activation during happy versus sad epochs. These findings are consistent with the adult literature on frontal asymmetries in response to affective stimuli and with our data on EEG asymmetries in newborns in response to different tastes.

A number of questions raised by these data require additional research to answer. No behavioral measures of the infant's affective response to the videotapes were available. It would be very useful to obtain measures of facial behavior to determine more precisely the nature of the infant's response to the happy and sad segments. It would also be revealing to obtain data on EEG

Table 11.7. *Frontal ratio scores (R − L/R + L 1–12 Hz activity) by affect condition for Studies 1 and 2*

	Study 1 (N = 10)		Study 2 (N = 14)	
	Happy	Sad	Happy	Sad
$\bar{X}$	.021	−.001	.073	.032
SD	.051	.032	.100	.115

Note: Higher numbers on this ratio are indicative of greater relative left-sided activation.
Source: R. J. Davidson and N. A. Fox, "Asymmetrical brain activity discriminates between positive versus negative affective stimuli in ten month old infants," *Science*, 1982, *218*, 1235–1237. Copyright 1982 by the American Association for the Advancement of Science. Reprinted by permission.

asymmetries in response to a variety of different positive and negative stimuli longitudinally in a group of infants. If the hypothesis about more bilateral involvement in fear and sadness as compared with disgust is accurate we should observe more robust asymmetries in the newborn in response to citric acid as compared with asymmetries in the 10-month-old in response to a sad videotape. In this type of study it would be important to control for the intensity of the response, which could be inferred from measures of facial behavior (e.g., Ekman, 1982).

Many important issues relevant to cerebral asymmetry and the development of affect have not been addressed. I will briefly highlight three additional problem areas. The discussion will necessarily be brief since data bearing directly on these issues do not yet exist. They are discussed here in the hopes of focusing future research.

A number of investigators have noted important changes in infants' ability to recognize a variety of affective cues in the environment around 5 to 7 months of age. Campos and Stenberg (1981) have commented on the newly developed ability of 10-month-old infants to reference their mothers' facial affect and utilize this information in guiding their response to a particular situation. For example, infants were less likely to cross the deep side of the visual cliff or approach a novel toy when the mother expressed a facial affect signifying fear. The question related to hemispheric specialization concerns the neural substrates of this ability. It may be that maturation of right-hemisphere posterior regions (e.g., the parietal region) is critical for this emerging competence.

Another important milestone in affective development occurs during the latter half of the second year of life and involves the diminution of certain negative affective responses. At about this age, the young child shows a diminution of certain negative emotions in response to separation. This change in affective arousal is accompanied at this age period by increasing competency and mastery over the environment and the concomitant affective expressions of mastery, such as pride and joy (Sroufe, 1979). This time period marks a major transition in affective response from the inability to modulate affective responses to the competency to inhibit certain negative affect in the service of exploration and mastery.

I would like to raise the possibility that this transition in affective development is associated with important changes in hemispheric organization. Specifically, the maturing commissural pathways may develop the capacity to transmit inhibitory information. In this way, the growing child may have the capacity to exert inhibitory control over certain negative affective responses. This model specifically suggests that the left hemisphere is able to exert inhibitory control over the right so that negative affective information processing occurring in the right hemisphere will be inhibited.

The third problem area emerges from the preceding problem and concerns the origins and development of repression and repressive coping strategies. Needless to say, we know the least about the hemispheric substrates of this undoubtedly very complex process. Galin (1974) was the first to explicitly propose that repression may involve a functional disconnection between certain regions of the two cerebral hemispheres. When an individual represses negative affective information, it may be that this information, which is represented in particular right hemisphere regions, does not get complete access to verbal centers in the left hemisphere. Thus, individuals who habitually display this style of coping should exhibit dissociations between their verbal reports about how they feel and other indices, for example, autonomic measures, which reflect their emotional state. We have confirmed (Weinberger, Schwartz, & Davidson, 1979) that repressors indeed show heightened autonomic and skeletal muscular activation in response to mildly stressful stimuli despite their verbal reports of little anxiety.

The phenomenon of repression is relevant to a consideration of asymmetry and affective development because of the well-known fact that the corpus callosum and other commissural pathways are not fully myelinated until at least 13 years of age (Yakovlev & Lecours, 1967). To the extent that repressive coping strategies are dependent upon intact commissures, we would expect that such styles of defense would not emerge in complete form until around age 13. Furthermore, we could predict a close association between the functional integrity of the commissures and the child's ability to inhibit and/or repress negative affective information. Since noninvasive measures of interhemispheric transfer do exist (e.g., Bashore, 1981), this prediction is testable in longitudinal and cross-sectional research. Probably, the most convincing demonstration would be with children of the same age who differ in their ability to inhibit and/or repress negative emotional events. We would predict that measures of interhemispheric communication should account for at least some of the variance in ability to repress affective information.

We have tested whether the dissociation between verbal report and other indices of affective responding (e.g., autonomic measures) in adults involve deficits in interhemispheric communication (Davidson, Perl, & Saron, 1983). In one study, subjects were presented with affective faces exposed tachisto-scopically to the left and right visual fields. The subjects were required to verbally name the emotion depicted on the face. Because we required subjects to respond verbally, we can be reasonably confident that, in right-handed subjects, this response is controlled by the left hemisphere. When the stimulus is presented to the left visual field (going initially to the right hemisphere), the task requires a commissural transfer. We therefore predicted that repressors should differ from nonrepressors in their accuracy of verbally identifying faces only when the stimuli are presented to the left visual field. When the stimuli are presented to the right visual field, no commissural transfer is required because the entire task can be performed exclusively within the left hemisphere. As can be seen from Figure 11.3, repressors and controls do not differ in their accuracy of verbal identification in response to right-visual-field information. However, the repressors show significantly worse performance compared with controls in response to left-visual-field presentations.

An alternative interpretation of these data is that repressors simply show deficits in right-hemisphere mediated cognitive skills and consequently respond poorly to left-visual-field presentations. Although this alternative interpretation should be explored further, other data from our study argue against it. We ran a second task with the identical facial stimuli that were used in the task described earlier. Half the faces were male and half were female. In the second task, subjects were required to identify the face by gender verbally. We reasoned that affective judgments were not required in this task and that if the repressor's interhemispheric transfer deficit was functional and expressed only in response to affective challenges that no group difference would be observed in the gender task despite the fact that the identical stimuli were used. The results confirmed our prediction and revealed no group difference in the gender task.

Affect cognition interaction and hemispheric organization

Throughout this chapter, references have been made to relations between affective and cognitive asymmetries. These relations and interactions will be

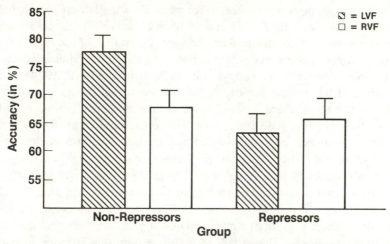

Figure 11.3. Mean accuracy (bars indicate standard errors) for verbal identification of the emotional expression of faces presented unilaterally to the LVF and RVF for non-repressors and repressors. $N = 13$ for nonrepressors; $N = 11$ for repressors. (From R. J. Davidson, J. Perl, and C. Saron, *Hemispheric interaction in repressors and non-repressors*. Manuscript submitted for publication, 1983.

considered more systematically here. One of the most important questions to address initially is why certain positive affects should be localized to the left hemisphere and certain negative affects to the right. I am confident that the quality of response to this question will improve over the next few years as more relevant research is performed. An interim, tentative consideration of this problem will be attempted here.

At a number of points in the chapter, the basis for the affective asymmetry was considered. A sufficient number of anomalous findings have questioned the positive–negative dichotomy as the essential basis for the affective asymmetry. I have proposed (e.g., Davidson, in press) that approach–avoidance may be a more plausible dimension for the affective lateralization. Since certain negative emotions may be associated with approach (e.g., anger), we would expect these particular affects to violate the positive–negative left–right association.[3]

If approach–avoidance is viewed as a candidate for the basis of affective lateralization, we must question why approach should be lateralized to the left anterior region and avoidance to the right anterior region. Approach behavior often involves the sequential execution of action, an important component of which is fine motor behavior. The nature of action associated with withdrawal is usually more gross and less differentiated. A considerable body of data has been generated recently that indicates the left hemisphere motor region is specialized for the control of fine manual behavior and sequentially executed movements on both the contralateral as well as ipsilateral sides of the body (e.g., Geschwind, 1975; Kimura & Archibald, 1974). Alternatively, other investigators have commented on the specialized role of the right hemisphere in the control of more automatic action (e.g., Luria & Simernitskaya, 1977; Luria, Simernitskaya, & Tubylevich, 1970; Simerniskaya, 1974). One interpretation of the association of approach behavior and certain positive affects with the left hemisphere is based upon its known specialization for voluntary, sequential, and fine motor behavior. However, the extent to which this type of action is indeed characteristic of approach and certain positive emotions needs to be more fully explored. Avoidance or withdrawal is often performed more automatically than is approach. Fine manual activity probably plays a less significant role in avoidance than in approach. It is also the case that situations engendering avoidance are often stressful and do not permit a voluntarily initiated sequential strategy to develop. Rather, the goal is to withdraw and to do it quickly. Therefore, an action system that is more automatic and reflexive, albeit less differentiated, is probably adaptive for these situations.

The association of approach and avoidance with the differential motor specializations of two cerebral hemispheres may account for the usual anterior localization of the affective asymmetries. It would be interesting to explore whether these asymmetries might be detected more prominently over the motor regions themselves. This type of topographic mapping for affective asymmetries has not yet been performed, although the requisite tools are available.

The data presented in this chapter indicate that affective asymmetries are most often observed in the frontal region. Anatomical evidence suggests that important cortico-cortical connections exist between frontal and temporal and frontal and parietal regions (e.g., Nauta, 1971). The temporal and parietal regions specifically have been implicated in the major cognitive asymmetries that have been observed in various perceptual tasks (e.g., Luria, 1973). In our EEG data, we have observed consistently reliable parietal asymmetries in response to various cognitive tasks, along with an absence of systematic frontal asymmetries. Conversely, we have found reliable frontal asymmetries in response to particular affective stimuli in the absence of reliable parietal differences between stimuli. However, we have found right-sided parietal activation in response to most affective tasks with little difference in parietal asymmetry between affective stimuli that differ in valence (Davidson & Schwartz, 1976; Davidson et al., 1979).

The relation between the posterior asymmetries associated with certain cognitive processes and the anterior asymmetries associated with affect remain to be carefully elucidated. However, a number of recent findings provide the foundation for a deeper understanding of this important relation. In the discussion of affective disorders in the preceding section, it was noted that depressed subjects exhibit selective impairments on certain right-hemisphere cognitive tasks, such as shape recognition and other tests of visuospatial ability. It is likely that these tasks critically depend upon right-parietal involvement. Since it was also found that depressed subjects show greater relative right-frontal activation, as compared with controls, it appears that a reciprocal relation might exist between activation asymmetries in the anterior and posterior cortical regions. In the depressed subjects, relative right-frontal activation may be associated with relative left-parietal activation. In the Schaffer, Davidson, and Saron (1983a) study the parietal EEG data were in the expected direction but were not significant.

We recently have examined the relations between frontal and parietal EEG asymmetry during a resting state in 14 right-handed subjects. Data were collected every 3 sec for a 30-sec epoch. Within-subject correlations were computed between frontal and parietal asymmetry across the 3-sec periods. In 10 out of 14 subjects, the correlations between frontal and parietal activation asymmetry were negative, indicating an inverse relation. The mean correlation for the 10 subjects showing inverse correlations was .42 (range: .18 to .72).

These findings support our hypothesis of reciprocal relations between frontal and parietal activation asymmetry. They suggest that relatively left-sided frontal activation is balanced by relatively right-sided parietal activation and vice versa. The significance of this pattern of hemispheric organization is unclear at the present time. However, the findings do suggest that spatial cognition and certain positive affects (most likely interest) are more likely to occur concurrently than are, for example, verbal cognition and positive affect. The capacity to simultaneously activate centers concerned with visuospatial function and the left-frontal region (associated with particular positive affects, such as interest) may serve an important adaptive function in controlling approach behavior, which can be thought of as a complex affective-cognitive combination. Spatial analysis of the environment is often required in approach. When an organism approaches, it usually approaches a particular location or place within a larger gestalt. The spatial cognition required for these activities might critically depend upon right-hemisphere posterior regions. The approach and associated positive affect may preferentially involve left-hemisphere anterior regions.

This model of reciprocal relations between anterior and posterior hemispheric asymmetries not only helps to explain the cognitive deficits associated with depression but also may provide an explanation for an apparent exception to the general claim that left-hemisphere damage is likely to produce a dysphoric, depressive reaction. Geschwind (personal communication) has noted that Wernicke's aphasics are often euphoric, with a display of excessive jocularity and inappropriate positive affect. In Wernicke's aphasics, certain posterior left-hemisphere regions have been damaged. It is possible that this posterior damage releases the left-frontal region from reciprocal inhibition and therefore results in hyperactivation in this area. This left-anterior overactivation has been implicated in the expression of certain positive affects. In a similar vein, Robinson and Benson (1981) have observed an inverse correlation between the size of the posterior brain lesion in fluent aphasics and the severity of depression. Whether any of their patients were actually euphoric is not stated in the report.

Summary and conclusions

A growing body of data indicates that reliable species-consistent functional asymmetries exist in animals. The evidence on rodent asymmetries suggests that differences between the hemispheres in the regulation of certain components of affective behavior are quite prominent and may be more robust than hemispheric differences for cognition. This raises the possibility that asymmetries for affect are phylogenetically older than are the asymmetries for cognition. Cognitive asymmetries may be a more recent evolutionary development, associated with the emergence of complex communication and language.

The evidence for affective asymmetries in adults indicates that certain regions of the two hemispheres are specialized for the regulation of certain positive and negative emotions. The frontal region has displayed this asymmetry most consistently, and the findings indicate that the left-frontal region is more involved with certain positive affects (particularly interest) and the right-frontal region with certain negative affects. A more precise basis for this asymmetry awaits additional research, but approach–avoidance may provide a suitable description.

Little is known about the ontogeny of lateralization for affect. I proposed that those affects seen very early in life, that is, in the neonate, may be predominantly under unilateral control since the commissural pathways are quite undeveloped at birth and myelination of these fibers is far from complete. Data were presented indicating that frontal EEG asymmetries in newborn infants distinguished between the taste of a sweet and sour solution, which elicited predominantly the facial expressions of interest and disgust, respectively. Parietal asymmetry failed to discriminate between these conditions.

Evidence was presented suggesting that other negative affective response systems do not develop until the second half of the first year of life. Because 10-month-old infants can discriminate and express a wide range of both positive and negative facial affects, it was proposed that the frontal asymmetry for happy versus sad affective stimuli should be present by this age. Two of our recent studies that support this hypothesis were described.

The role of the corpus callosum and other commissural pathways was considered in relation to their potential role in the inhibition of negative affect and the development of repression. We proposed that increasing ability to inhibit negative affect (manifested during the second half of the first year of life) may be associated with important maturational changes in commissural connections. Data were presented indicating that deficits in interhemispheric transfer of affective information were present in adult individuals who characteristically exhibit a repressive coping style.

Speculations about why the left and right frontal regions might be differentially specialized for certain positive and negative affects were provided. The left-frontal region may be involved with approach behavior and associated positive affects as a function of its specialization for voluntary, fine manual behavior, which may be predominant during approach. Conversely, withdrawal is often reflexive and automatic and involves less-differentiated action sequences. Some investigators have proposed that right-hemisphere anterior regions are specialized for this form of action.

The relation between anterior and posterior cerebral asymmetries was considered in the context of accounting for certain interactions between affect and cognition. Reciprocal relations exist between anterior and posterior activation asymmetries. This reciprocal interaction might account for the cognitive anomalies associated with depression and the affective dysfunctions associated with Wernicke's aphasia.

It should be evident that the study of functional asymmetries between the hemispheres has much to contribute to our understanding of cognition and affect and their development and interaction. We now have the behavioral and biological tools to answer many of the outstanding questions in this area. Future research should be extremely exciting in further illuminating the hemispheric substrates of cognition and affect.

Notes

1 In a recent experiment, Ekman, Levenson, and Friesen (1983) obtained very compelling evidence for autonomic discrimination among a number of emotions, including certain negative emotions (i.e., disgust, sadness, anger, and fear). In assessing heart rate, skin resistance, left and right finger temperature, and forearm muscle tension, they observed complex patterns for each emotion and found that the patterns reliably discriminated among the emotions tested. They used measures of facial behavior to restrict data analysis to only those epochs during which expressions of "pure" emotion were present. This methodological advance probably contributed greatly to their findings. The data provided by Ekman and his associates should finally put to rest those theories of emotion based upon anachronistic conceptions of undifferentiated arousal (e.g., Schachter & Singer, 1962; see Davidson, 1978, for a more general critique of the concept of undifferentiated arousal).

2 I am referring here to the control of the affective central state and not specifically to the facial expression of emotion, which presumably requires the involvement of other brain regions.

3 Approach–avoidance may seem problematic as the basis for affective lateralization, as one might imagine that certain negative emotions usually associated with withdrawal occasionally involve an approach component as well. For example, a person might first approach a disgusting object and then subsequently get rid of it or withdraw from it. I would propose that in this situation a complex sequence of emotions may occur over time with interest initially predominating and thus tipping the approach–avoidance gradient toward approach. However, as the person draws closer to the object, disgust becomes more prominent and the direction of the approach–avoidance gradient is reversed. Since emotions do come and go rather quickly, it is entirely possible for these changes to occur quite rapidly.

References

Abrams, R., & Taylor, M. A. Differential EEG patterns in affective disorder and schizophrenia. *Archives of General Psychiatry*, 1979, *36*, 1355–1358.

Akert, K. Comparative anatomy of frontal cortex and thalamofrontal connections. In J. M. Warren & K. Akert (Eds.), *The frontal granular cortex and behavior*. New York: McGraw-Hill, 1964.

Alford, L. B. Localization of consciousness and emotion. *American Journal of Psychiatry*, 1933, *12*, 789–799.

Anderson, S. W. Language-related asymmetries of eye movement and evoked potentials. In S. Harnad, R. W. Doty, L. Goldstein, J. Jaynes, & D. Krauthamer (Eds.), *Lateralization in the nervous system*. New York: Academic Press, 1977.

Andrew, R. J., Mench, J., & Rainey, C. Right-left asymmetry of response to visual stimuli in the domestic chick. In D. J. Ingle, R. J. W. Mansfield, & M. A. Goodale (Eds.), *Advances in the analysis of visual behavior*. Cambridge, Mass.: MIT Press, 1980.

Baranovskaya, Q. P., & Homskaya, E. B. Changes in the electroencephalogram frequency spectrum during the presentation of neutral and meaningful stimuli to patients with lesions of the frontal lobe. In K. H. Pribram & A. R. Luria (Eds.), *Psychophysiology of the frontal lobes*. New York: Academic Press, 1973.

Bashore, T. R. Vocal and manual reaction time estimates of interhemispheric transmission time. *Psychological Bulletin*, 1981, *89*, 352–368.

Bear, D. N., & Fedio, P. Quantitative analysis of interietial behavior in temporal lobe epilepsy. *Archives of Neurology*, 1977, *34*, 454–467.

Beck, A. T., Ward, C. H., Mendelson, M., Mock, J., & Erbaugh, J. An inventory for measuring depression. *Archives of General Psychiatry*, 1961, *4*, 561–571.

Bennett, J., Davidson, R. J., & Saron, C. Patterns of self-rating in response to verbally elicited affective imagery: Relation to frontal vs. parietal EEG asymmetry. Unpublished manuscript, 1982.

Benson, D. F. Psychiatric aspects of aphasia. *British Journal of Psychiatry*, 1973, *123*, 555–566.

Benson, D. J. *Aphasia, alexia and agraphia*. New York: Churchill-Livingstone, 1979.

Bruder, G. E., & Yozawitz, A. Central auditory processing and lateralization in psychiatric patients. In J. Gruzelier and P. Flor-Henry (Eds.), *Hemisphere asymmetries of function in psychopathology*. New York: Elsevier/North Holland, 1979.

Campos, J. J., Emde, R. N., Gaensbauer, T., & Henderson, C. Cardiac and behavioral inter-relationships in the reactions of infants to strangers. *Developmental Psychology*, 1975, *11*, 581–601.

Campos, J. J., Hiatt, S., Ramsay, D., Henderson, C., & Svejda, M. The emergence of fear on the visual cliff. In M. Lewis and L. Rosenblum (Eds.), *The development of affect*. New York: Plenum, 1978.

Campos, J. J., & Stenberg, C. R. Perception, appraisal and emotion: The onset of social referencing. In M. Lamb and L. Sherrod (Eds.), *Infant social cognition*. Hillsdale, N.J.: Erlbaum, 1981.

Cohen, B. D., Penick, S. B., & Tarter, R. I. Antidepressant effects of unilateral electric convulsive shock therapy. *Archives of General Psychiatry*, 1974, *31*, 673–675.

Cronin, D., Bodley, P., Potts, L., Mather, M. D., Gardner, R. K., & Tobin, J. C. Unilateral and bilateral ECT: A study of memory disturbance and relief from depression. *Journal of Neurology, Neurosurgery, and Psychiatry*, 1970, *33*, 705–713.

Crowne, D. P., & Marlowe, D. *The approval motive: Studies in evaluative dependence*. New York: Wiley, 1964.

Davidson, R. J. Specificity and patterning in biobehavioral systems: Implications for behavior change. *American Psychologist*, 1978, *33*, 430–436.

Davidson, R. J. Hemispheric specialization for cognition and affect. In A. Gale & J. Edwards (Eds.), *Physiological correlates of human behavior*. London: Academic Press, in press.

Davidson, R. J., & Ehrlichman, H. Lateralized cognitive processes and the electroencephalogram. *Science*, 1980, *207*, 1005–1006.

Davidson, R. J., & Fox, N. A. Asymmetrical brain activity discriminates between positive versus negative affective stimuli in ten month old infants. *Science*, 1982, *218*, 1235–1237.

Davidson, R. J., Moss, E., Saron, C., & Schaffer, C. E. Self-reports of emotion are influenced by the visual field to which affective information is presented. Manuscript submitted for publication, 1983.

Davidson, R. J., Perl, J., & Saron, C. Hemispheric interaction in repressors and non-repressors. Manuscript submitted for publication, 1983.

Davidson, R. J., & Schwartz, G. E. Patterns of cerebral lateralization during cardiac biofeedback versus the self-regulation of emotion: Sex differences. *Psychophysiology*, 1976, *13*, 62–68.

Davidson, R. J., Schwartz, G. E., Saron, C., Bennett, J., & Goleman, D. J. Frontal versus parietal EEG asymmetry during positive and negative affect. *Psychophysiology*, 1979, *16*, 202–203.

Davidson, R. J., Schwartz, G. E., & Weinberger, D. Eye movement and electrodermal asymmetry during cognitive and affective tasks. Paper presented at the Annual Meeting of the American Psychological Association, San Francisco, August 1977.

Davison, C., & Kelman, H. Pathological laughing and crying. *Archives of Neurology and Psychiatry*, 1939, *42*, 595–643.

Day, R., & McKenzie, B. Perceptual shape constancy in early infancy. *Perception*, 1973, *2*, 315–320.

Deglin, V. L., & Nikolaenko, N. N. Role of the dominant hemisphere in the regulation of emotional states. *Human Physiology*, 1975, *1*, 394–402.

d'Elia, G., & Raotma, H. Is unilateral ECT less effective than bilateral ECT? *British Journal of Psychiatry*, 1975, *126*, 83–89.

Denenberg, V. H. Assessing the effects of early experience. In R. D. Myers (Ed.), *Methods in psychobiology* (Vol. 3). New York: Academic Press, 1977.

Denenberg, V. H. Hemispheric laterality in animals and the effects of early experience. *Behavioral and Brain Sciences*, 1981, *4*, 1–49.

Denenberg, V. H., Garbanatti, J., Sherman, G., Yutzey, D. A., & Kaplan, R. Infantile stimulation induces brain lateralization in rats. *Science*, 1978, *201*, 1150–1152.

Denenberg, V. H., Hofmann, M., Garbanatti, J. A., Sherman, G. F., Rosen, G., & Yutzey, D. A. Handling in infancy, taste aversion and brain laterality in rats. *Brain Research*, 1980, *200*, 123–133.

Denny-Brown, D., Meyer, S. T., and Horenstein, S. The significance of perceptual rivalry resulting from parietal lesion. *Brain*, 1952, *75*, 433–471.

Dewson, J. H., III. Preliminary evidence of hemispheric asymmetry of auditory function in monkeys. In S. Harnad, R. W. Doty, L. Goldstein, J. Jaynes, & G. Krauthamer (Eds.), *Lateralization in the nervous system*. New York: Academic Press, 1977.

Dewson, J. H., III. Some behavioral effects of removal of superior temporal cortex in the monkey. In D. Clivers & J. Herbert (Eds.), *Recent advances in primatology*, Vol. 1: *Behaviour*. London: Academic Press, 1978.

Dewson, J. H., III. Toward an animal model of auditory cognitive function. In C. L. Ludlow & M. E. Doran-Quine (Eds.), *The neurological bases of language disorders in children: methods and directions for research, National Institute of Neurological and Communicative Diseases and Stroke Monograph No. 22*. Washington, D.C.: U.S. Government Printing Office, 1979.

Dimberg, U. Facial reactions to facial expressions. *Psychophysiology*, 1982, *19*, 643–647.

Dimond, S., & Farrington, L. Emotional response to films shown to the right or left hemisphere of the brain measured by heart rate. *Acta Psychologica*, 1977, *41*, 255–260.

Dimond, S., Farrington, L., & Johnson, P. Differing emotional response from right and left hemispheres. *Nature*, 1976, *261*, 690–692.

Doty, R. W., Negrao, N., & Yamaga, K. The unilateral engram. *Acta Neurobiologiae Experimentalis*, 1973, *33*, 711–728.

Doty, R. W., & Overman, W. H. Mnemonic role of forebrain commissures in macaques. In S. Harnad, R. W. Doty, L. Goldstein, J. Jaynes, & G. Krauthamer (Eds.), *Lateralization in the nervous system*. New York: Academic Press, 1977.

Ehrlichman, H. EOG recording of gaze direction and eye movement rate in response to verbal and spatial questions. Paper presented at the Society for Psychophysiological Research, Cincinnati, October 1979.

Ehrlichman, H., & Weinberger, A. Lateral eye movements and hemispheric asymmetry: A critical review. *Psychological Bulletin*, 1978, *85*, 1080, 1101.

Ekman, P. Asymmetry in facial expression. *Science*, 1980, *209*, 833–834. (a)

Ekman, P. Biological and cultural contributions to body and facial movement in the expression of emotions. In A. O. Rorty (Ed.), *Explaining emotion*. Berkeley: University of California Press, 1980. (b)

Ekman, P. Methods for measuring facial action. In K. R. Scherer & P. Ekman (Eds.), *Handbook of methods in nonverbal behavior research*. Cambridge: Cambridge University Press, 1982.

Ekman, P., Levenson, R. W., & Friesen, W. V. Autonomic nervous system activity distinguishes among emotions. *Science*, 1983, *221*, 1208–1210.

Emde, R. N., & Harmon, R. Endogenous and exogenous smiling systems in early infancy. *Journal of the American Academy of Child Psychiatry*, 1972, *11*, 177–200.

Field, T. M., Woodson, R., Greenberg, R., & Cohen, D. Discrimination and imitation of facial expressions by neonates. *Science*, 1982, *218*, 179–181.

Fields, J. The adjustment of reaching behavior to object distance in early infancy. *Child Development*, 1976, *47*, 304–308.

Flor-Henry, P. Lateralized temporal-limbic dysfunction and psychopathology. *Annals of the New York Academy of Sciences*, 1976, *280*, 777–795.

Flor-Henry, P. On certain aspects of the localization of the cerebral systems regulating and determining emotion. *Biological Psychiatry*, 1979, *14*, 677–698.

Flor-Henry, P., Koles, Z. J., Howarth, B. G., & Burton, L. Neurophysiological studies of schizophrenia, mania and depression. In J. Gruzelier & P. Flor-Henry (Eds.), *Hemisphere asymmetries of function in psychopathology*. New York: Elsevier North-Holland, 1979.

Flor-Henry, P., & Yeudall, L. T. Neuropsychological investigation of schizophrenia and manic-depressive psychoses. In J. Gruzelier & P. Flor-Henry (Eds.), *Hemisphere asymmetries of function in psychopathology*. New York: Elsevier North-Holland, 1979.

Folstein, M. F., Maiberger, R., & Meutsch, P. R. Mood disorder as a specific complication of stroke. *Journal of Neurology, Neurosurgery and Psychiatry*, 1977, *49*, 1018–1020.

Fox, N. A., & Davidson, R. J. (Eds.). *The psychobiology of affective development*. Hillsdale, N.J.: Erlbaum, in press.

Fox, N., & Davidson, R. J., Frontal brain electrical asymmetry distinguishes between approach and withdrawal reactions in newborn infants. Manuscript submitted for publication, 1983.

Gainotti, G. Reactions "Catotrophiques" et manifestations d'indifference au cours des atteintes cerebrais. *Neuropsychologia*, 1969, *7*, 195–204.

Gainotti, G. Emotional behavior and hemispheric side of lesion. *Cortex*, 1972, *8*, 41–55.

Galin, D. Implications for psychiatry of left and right cerebral specialization. *Archives of General Psychiatry*, 1974, *31*, 572–583.

Garbanati, J. A., Sherman, G. F., Rosen, G. D., Hofmann, M., Yutzey, D. A., & Denenberg, V. H. Handling in infancy, brain laterality and muricide in rats. *Behavioural Brain Research*, 1983, *7*, 351–359.

Garcia, J., Hankin, W. G., & Rusiniak, K. Behavioral regulation of the milieu interne in man and rat. *Science*, 1974, *185*, 824–831.

Gardner, H., Ling, P. K., Flamm, L., & Silverman, J. Comprehension and appreciation of humorous material following brain damage. *Brain*, 1975, *98*, 399–412.

Gazzaniga, M. S. Effects of commissurotomy on a preoperatively learned visual discrimination. *Experimental Neurology*, 1963, *6*, 340–353.

Geschwind, N. The apraxias: Neural mechanisms of disorders of learned movement. *American Scientist*, 1975, *63*, 188–195.

Glick, S. D., Jerussi, T. P., Waters, D. H., & Green, J. P. Amphetamine-induced changes in striatal dopamine and acetylcholine levels and relationship to rotation (circling behavior) in rats. *Biochemical Pharmacology*, 1974, *23*, 3223–3225.

Glick, S. D., Jerussi, T. P., & Zimmerberg, B. Behavioral and neuropharmacological correlates of nigrostriatal asymmetry in rats. In S. Harnad, R. W. Doty, J. Jaynes, L. Goldstein, &

G. Krauthamer (Eds.), *Lateralization in the nervous system*. New York: Academic Press, 1977.

Glick, S. D., Meibach, R. C., Cox, R. D., & Maayani, S. Multiple and interrelated functional asymmetries in rat brain. *Life Sciences*, 1979, *25*, 395–400.

Goldstein, K. *The Organism*. New York: Academic Book, 1939.

Goldstein, S. G., Filskov, S. B., Weaver, L. A., & Ives, J. O. Neuropsychological effects of electroconvulsive therapy. *Journal of Clinical Psychology*, 1977, *33*, 798–806.

Gur, R. E. Conjugate lateral eye movements as an index of hemispheric activation. *Journal of Personality and Social Psychology*, 1975, *31*, 751–757.

Gur, R. E., & Gur, R. C. Correlates of conjugate lateral eye movements in man. In S. Harnad, R. W. Doty, L. Goldstein, J. Jaynes, & G. Krauthamer (Eds.), *Lateralization in the nervous system*. New York: Academic Press, 1977.

Hall, M. M., Hall, G. C., & LaVoie, P. Ideation in patients with unilateral or bilateral midline brain lesions. *Journal of Abnormal Psychology*, 1968. *73*, 526–531.

Halliday, A. M., Davison, K., Browne, M. W., & Kreeger, L. C. A comparison of the effects on depression and memory of bilateral E.C.T. and unilateral E.C.T. to the dominant and non-dominant hemispheres. *British Journal of Psychiatry*, 1968, *114*, 997–1012.

Hamilton, C. R. Investigations of perceptual and mnemonic lateralization in monkeys. In S. Harnad, R. W. Doty, L. Goldstein, J. Jaynes, & G. Krauthamer (Eds.), *Lateralization in the nervous system*. New York: Academic Press, 1977.

Hamilton, C. R., & Lund, J. S. Visual discrimination of movement: Mid-brain or forebrain? *Science*, 1970, *170*, 1428–1430.

Hamilton, C. R., Tieman, S. B., & Farrell, W. S. Cerebral dominance in monkeys. *Neuropsychologia*, 1974, *12*, 193–197.

Harmon, D. W., & Ray, W. J. Hemispheric activity during affective verbal stimuli: An EEG study. *Neuropsychologia*, 1977, *15*, 457–460.

Hassett, J., & Zelner, B. Correlations between measures of cerebral asymmetry. *Psychophysiology*, 1977, *14*, 79.

Hécaen, H., Ajuriaguerra, J. D., & Massonet, J. Les troubles visuo, constructifs par lesions parieto-occipitales droctes. Role des perturbations vestibulaires. *L'Encephale*, 1951, *1*, 122–179.

Heilman, K. W., Scholes, R., & Watson, T. R. Auditory affective agnosia: Disturbed comprehension of affective speech. *Journal of Neurology, Neurosurgery, and Psychiatry*, 1975, *38*, 69–72.

Hommes, O. R., & Panhuysen, L. H. H. M. Depression and cerebral dominance: A study of bilateral intracarotid amytal in eleven depressed patients. *Psychiatrica, Neurologia, and Neurochirica*, 1971, *74*, 259–274.

Izard, C. E. *Human emotions*. New York: Plenum, 1977.

Izard, C. E. Personal communication, 1980.

Karlin, R., Weinapple, M., Rochford, J., & Goldstein, L. Quantitative EEG features of negative affective states: Report of some hypnotic studies. Paper presented at the Society of Biological Psychiatry, Atlanta, Georgia, 1978.

Kelly, A. E., & Stinus, L. Neuroanatomical and neurochemical substrates of affective behavior. In N. Fox & R. J. Davidson (Eds.), *The psychobiology of affective development*. Hillsdale, N.J.: Erlbaum, in press.

Kestenbaum, C. J. Children at risk for manic-depressive illness: Possible predictors. *American Journal of Psychiatry*, 1979, *136*, 1206–1208.

Kimura, D., & Archibald, Y. Motor functions of the left hemisphere. *Brain*, 1974, *97*, 337–350.

Kinsbourne, M. Eye and head turning indicates cerebral lateralization. *Science*, 1972, *76*, 539–541.

Kinsbourne, M. The ontogeny of cerebral dominance. In R. W. Rieber (Ed.), *The neuropsychology of language*. New York: Plenum, 1976.

Kocel, K., Galin, D., Ornstein, R., & Merrin, E. L. Lateral eye movement and cognitive mode. *Psychonomic Science*, 1972, *27*, 223–224.

Kolb, B., & Milner, B. Performance of complex arm and facial movements after focal brain lesions. *Neuropsychologia*, 1981, *17*, 491–503. (a)

Kolb, B., & Milner, B. Observations on spontaneous facial expression after focal cerebral excisions and after intracarotid injection of sodium amytal. *Neuropsychologia*, 1981, *19*, 505–514. (b)

Kronfol, Z., Hamsher, K. deS., Kigre, K., & Waziri, R. Depression and hemispheric functions: Changes associated with unilateral ECT. *British Journal of Psychiatry*, 1978, *132*, 560–567.

Ley, R., & Bryden, M. Hemispheric differences in processing emotions and faces. *Brain and Language*, 1979, *7*, 127–138.

Liberman, A. M., Cooper, F. S., Shankweiler, D., & Studdert-Kennedy, M. Perception of the speech code. *Psychological Review*, 1967, *74*, 431–461.

Lishman, W. A. Emotion, consciousness and will after brain bisection in man. *Cortex*, 1971, *7*, 181–192.

Luria, A. R. *Higher cortical functions in man*. New York: Basic Books, 1966.

Luria, A. R. *The working brain*. New York: Basic Books, 1973.

Luria, A. R., & Simernitskaya, E. G. Interhemispheric relations and the functions of the minor hemisphere. *Neuropsychologia*, 1977, *15*, 175–178.

Luria, A. R., Simernitskaya, E. G., & Tubylevich, D. The structure of psychological processes in relation to cerebral organization. *Neuropsychologia*, 1970, *8*, 13–18.

Milner, B. Discussion of "Experimental analysis of cerebral dominance in Man." In C. H. Millikan & F. L. Darley (Eds.), *Brain mechanisms underlying speech and language*. New York: Grune & Stratton, 1967.

Moscovitch, M., Strauss, E., & Olds, J. Handedness and dichotic listening performance in patients with unipolar endogenous depression who received ECT. *American Journal of Psychiatry*, 1981, *138*, 988–990.

Nauta, W. J. H. Some efferent connections of the prefrontal cortex in the monkey. In J. M. Warren & K. Akert (Eds.), *The frontal granular cortex and behavior*. New York: McGraw-Hill, 1964.

Nauta, W. J. H. The problem of the frontal lobe: A reinterpretation. *Journal of Psychiatric Research*, 1971, *8*, 167–187.

Nottebohm, F. Ontogeny of bird song. *Science*, 1970, *167*, 950–956.

Nottebohm, F., Manning, E., & Nottebohm, M. E. Reversal of hypoglossal dominance in canaries following unilateral syringeal denervation. *Journal of Comparative Physiology*, 1979, *134*, 227–240.

Oldfield, R. C. The assessment and analysis of handedness: The Edinburgh Inventory. *Neuropsychologia*, 1971, *9*, 97–113.

Parcella, B. L., & Impastato, D. J. Focal stimulation therapy. *American Journal of Psychiatry*, 1954, *110*, 576–578.

Pearlson, G. D., & Robinson, R. G. Suction lesions of the frontal cerebral cortex in the rat induce asymmetrical behavior and catecholamingeric responses. *Brain Research*, 1981, *218*, 233–242.

Perria, L., Rosadini, G., & Rossi, G. F. Determination of side of cerebral dominance with amobarbital. *Archives of Neurology*, 1961, *4*, 173–181.

Perris, C., & Monakhov, K. Depressive symptomatology and systemic structural analysis of the EEG. In J. Gruzelier & P. Flor-Henry (Eds.), *Hemisphere asymmetries of function in psychopathology*. New York: Elsevier North-Holland, 1979.

Peterson, M. R., Beecher, M. D., Zoloth, S. R., Moody, D. B., & Stebbins, W. C. Neural lateralization of species-specific vocalizations by Japanese macaques (*Macaca fuscata*). *Science*, 1978, *101*, 324–327.

Pribram, K. H. The primate frontal cortex – executive of the brain. In K. H. Pribram & A. R. Luria (Eds.), *Psychophysiology of the frontal lobes*. New York: Academic Press, 1973.

Rakic, P., & Yakovlev, P. I. Development of the corpus callosum and the cavum septi in man. *Journal of Comparative Neurology*, 1968, *132*, 45–72.

Reuter-Lorenz, P., & Davidson, R. J. Differential contributions of the two cerebral hemispheres to the perception of happy and sad faces. *Neuropsychologia*, 1981, *19*, 609–613.

Robinson, D. A., & Fuchs, A. F. Eye movements evoked by stimulation of frontal eye fields. *Journal of Neurophysiology*, 1969, *32*, 637–648.

Robinson, R. G. Differential behavioral and biochemical effects of right and left hemispheric cerebral infarction in the rat. *Science*, 1979, *105*, 707–710.

Robinson, R. G., & Benson, D. F. Depression in aphasic patients: Frequency, severity and clinical-pathological correlations. *Brain and Language*, 1981, *14*, 282–291.

Robinson, R. G., & Coyle, J. T. The differential effect of right versus left hemispheric cerebral infarction on catecholamines and behavior in the rat. *Brain Research*, 1980, *188*, 63–78.

Robinson, R. G., Shoemaker, W. J., & Schlumpf, M. Time course of changes in catecholamines following right hemispheric cerebral infarction in the rat. *Brain Research*, 1980, *181*, 202–208.

Robinson, R. G., & Szetela, B. Mood change following left hemispheric brain injury. *Annals of Neurology*, 1981, *9*, 447–453.

Rogers, L. J. Lateralization in the avian brain. *Bird Behaviour*, 1980, *2*, 1–12.

Rogers, L. J., & Anson, J. M. Lateralisation of function in the chicken fore-brain. *Pharmacology, Biochemistry and Behavior*, 1979, *10*, 679–686.

Ross, E. D., & Mesulam, M. M. Dominant language functions of the right hemisphere? *Archives of Neurology*, 1979, *36*, 144–148.

Ross, E. D., & Rush, A. J. Diagnosis and neuroanatomical correlates of depression in brain-damaged patients: Implications for a neurology of depression. *Archives of General Psychiatry*, 1981, *38*, 1344–1354.

Rossi, G. F., & Rosadini, G. Experimental analysis of cerebral dominance in man. In C. H. Millikan & F. L. Darley (Eds.), *Brain mechanisms underlying speech and language*. New York: Grune & Stratton, 1967.

Sackeim, H. A., & Decina, P. Lateralized neuropsychological abnormalities in bipolar adults and in children of bipolar probands. Paper presented at the Second International Conference on Laterality and Psychopathology, Banff, Alberta, Canada, April 1982.

Sackeim, H. A., & Gur, R. C. Lateral asymmetry in intensity of emotional expression. *Neuropsychologia*, 1978, *16*, 473–481.

Sackeim, H. A., Gur, R. C., & Saucy, M. C. Emotions are expressed more intensely on the left side of face. *Science*, 1978, *202*, 434–436.

Sackeim, H. A., Weinman, A. L., Gur, R. C., Greenberg, M., Hungerbuhler, J. P., & Geschwind, N. Pathological laughing and crying: Functional brain asymmetry in the expression of positive and negative emotions. *Archives of Neurology*, 1982, *39*, 210–218.

Schachter, S., & Singer, J. E. Cognitive, social and physiological determinants of emotional state. *Psychological Review*, 1962, *69*, 379–399.

Schaffer, C. E., Davidson, R. J., Saron, C. Frontal and parietal EEG asymmetry in depressed and non-depressed subjects. *Biological Psychiatry*, 1983, *18*, 753–762. (a)

Schaffer, C. E., Davidson, R. J., & Saron, C. *Affective responses to faces: Visual field asymmetries in depressed and non-depressed subjects*. Manuscript submitted for publication, 1983. (b)

Schwartz, G. E., Ahern, G., Davidson, R. J., & Pusar, J. Differential eye movement asymmetry in response to positive and negative affective questions. Unpublished manuscript, 1979.

Schwartz, G. E., Davidson, R. J., & Maer, F. Right hemisphere lateralization for emotion in the human brain: Interaction with cognition. *Science*, 1975, *190*, 286–288.

Schwartz, G. E., Fair, P. L., Salt, P., Mandel, M., & Klerman, G. L. Facial muscle patterning to affective imagery in depressed and non-depressed subjects. *Science*, 1976, *192*, 489–491.

Serafetinides, E. A., Hoare, R. D., & Driver, M. V. Intracarotid sodium amylobarbitone and cerebral dominance for speech and consciousness. *Brain*, 1965, *68*, 107–130.

Shagass, C. Electrical activity of the brain. In N. S. Greenfield & R. H. Sternbach (Eds.), *Handbook of psychophysiology*. New York: Holt, Rinehart and Winston, 1972.

Shagass, C., Roemer, R. A., Straumanis, J. J., & Amadeo, M. Evoked potential evidence of lateralized hemispheric dysfunction in the psychoses. In J. Gruzelier & P. Flor-Henry (Eds.),

Hemisphere asymmetries of function in psychopathology. New York: Elsevier North-Holland, 1979.

Simernitskaya, E. G. Application of the method of evoked potentials to the analysis of activation processes in patients with lesions of the frontal lobes. In K. H. Pribram & A. R. Luria (Eds.), *Psychophysiology of the frontal lobes*. New York: Academic Press, 1973.

Simernitskaya, E. G. On two forms of writing defects following focal brain lesions. In S. J. Dimond & J. G. Beaumont (Eds.), *Hemisphere function in the human brain*. New York: Halsted, 1974.

Sroufe, L. A. Socioemotional development. In J. Osofsky (Ed.), *Handbook of infant development*. New York: Wiley, 1979.

Sroufe, L. A., & Waters, E. The ontogenesis of smiling and laughter: A perspective on the organization of development in infancy. *Psychological Review*, 1976, *83*, 173–189.

Stromgren, L. S. Unilateral versus bilateral electroconvulsive therapy: Investigations into the therapeutic effect in endogenous depression. *Acta Psychiatrica Scandinavica*, 1973, *Suppl. 240*, 1–65.

Suberi, M., & McKeever, W. F. Differential right hemispheric memory storage of emotional and non-emotional faces. *Neuropsychologia*, 1977, *15*, 757–768.

Terzian, H. Behavioral and EEG effects of intracarotid sodium amytal injection. *Neurochirica*, 1964, *12*, 230–239.

Tomkins, S. S. Affect as amplification: Some modifications in theory. In R. Plutchik & H. Kellerman (Eds.), *Emotion: Theory, research and experience*, Vol. 1: *Theories of emotion*. New York: Academic Press, 1980.

Tucker, D. M., Roth, R. S., Arneson, B. A, & Buckingham, V. Right hemisphere activation during stress. *Neuropsychologia*, 1977, *15*, 697–700.

Tucker, D. M., Stenslie, C. E., Roth, R. S., & Shearer, S. L. Right frontal lobe activation and right hemisphere performance decrement during a depressed mood. *Archives of General Psychiatry*, 1981, *38*, 169–174.

Tucker, D. M., Watson, R. T., & Heilman, K. M. Discrimination and evocation of affectively intoned speech in patients with right parietal disease. *Neurology*, 1977, *27*, 947–950.

Turvey, M. T. Preliminaries to a theory of action with reference to vision. In R. Shaw and J. Bransford (Eds.), *Perceiving, acting and knowing*. Hillsdale, N.J.: Erlbaum, 1977.

Wada, J. A. A new method for the determination of the side of cerebral speech dominance: A preliminary report on the intracarotid injection of sodium amytal in man. *Medicine and Biology*, 1949, *14*, 221–222.

Wada, J. A., & Rasmussen, T. Intracarotid injection of sodium amytal for the lateralization of cerebral speech dominance: Experimental and clinical observation. *Journal of Neurosurgery*, 1960, *17*, 266–282.

Warren, J. M., & Nonneman, A. J. The search for cerebral dominance in monkeys. *Annals of the New York Academy of Sciences*, 1976, *280*, 732–744.

Wechsler, A. F. The effect of organic brain disease on recall of emotional charged versus neutral narrative tests. *Neurology*, 1973, *23*, 130–135.

Weimer, W. A conceptual framework for cognitive psychology: Motor theories of mind. In R. Shaw & J. Bransford (Eds.), *Perceiving, acting and knowing*. Hillsdale, N.J.: Erlbaum, 1977.

Weinberger, D. A., Schwartz, G. E., & Davidson, R. J. Low anxious, high anxious and repressive coping styles: Psychometric patterns and behavioral and physiological responses to stress. *Journal of Abnormal Psychology*, 1979, *88*, 369–380.

Werman, R., Anderson, P. J., & Christoff, N. Electroencephalographic changes with intracarotid megimide and amytal in man. *Electroencephalography and Clinical Neurophysiology*, 1959, *11*, 267–274.

Whimbey, A. E., & Denenberg, V. H. Two independent behavioral dimensions in open-field performance. *Journal of Comparative and Physiological Psychology*, 1967, *63*, 500–504.

Yakovlev, P. I., & Lecours, A. The myelogenetic cycles of regional maturation of the brain. In A. Minkowski (Ed.), *Regional development of the brain in early life*. London: Blackwell, 1967.

Yozawitz, A., Bruder, G., Sutton, S., Sharpe, L., Gurland, B., Fleiss, J., & Costa, L. Dichotic perception: Evidence for right hemisphere dysfunction in affective psychosis. *British Journal of Psychiatry*, 1979, *135*, 224–237.

Zimmerberg, B., Glick, S. D., & Jerussi, T. P. Neurochemical correlates of a spatial preference in rats. *Science*, 1974, *185*, 623–625.

Zinkin, S., & Birthnell, J. Unilateral electroconvulsive therapy: Its effects on memory and its therapeutic efficacy. *British Journal of Psychiatry*, 1968, *114*, 973–988.

12   Theoretical and empirical considerations in the investigation of the relationship between affect and cognition in atypical populations of infants

Dante Cicchetti and Karen Schneider-Rosen

Pathology and developmental biology must be reintegrated so that our understanding of the "abnormal" will become but an extension of our insight into the "normal," while . . . the study of the "abnormal" will contribute to the deepening of that very insight. Their common problems should provide foci for common orientation, so that, as they advance in joint directions, their efforts may supplement and reinforce each other to mutual benefit. (Weiss, 1961)

Historically, scientists in a variety of disciplines, such as biology, embryology, and psychology, have emphasized the need for examining the relationship between normal and deviant patterns of development (e.g., Darwin, 1872; Freud, 1937/1955; Goldstein, 1939, 1940; James, 1917, 1920; Waddington, 1966; Weiss, 1969). Implicit in this orientation is an underlying commitment to understanding normal developmental patterns so that we may begin to investigate the ways in which deviant development may eventuate. Furthermore, examination of abnormal ontogenetic principles and of the deviations from normal pathways of development may illuminate the range of individual variation inherent in the human organism. The ultimate goal of this enterprise is the formulation of an integrative developmental theory that can account for both normal and abnormal processes of ontogenesis.

Within the field of psychology, the examination of normal and atypical patterns of development requires a consideration of the different behavioral systems within which advances are proceeding in parallel and exerting mutual

We would like to thank Ellen Bressler for typing this manuscript. We also extend our appreciation to Dr. Carroll Izard and Dr. Peter Read for their support and encouragement during the preparation of this chapter.

Dante Cicchetti's work on this chapter was supported by a grant from the National Center for Child Abuse and Neglect (No. 90-C-1929) and by an award from the Foundation for Child Development Program for Young Scholars in Social and Affective Development. Karen Schneider-Rosen would like to acknowledge the support that she has received from the National Science Foundation Graduate Fellowship Program. Dante Cicchetti would like to express his affection, appreciation, and gratitude to Dr. Jules Bemporad and Dr. Sanford Gifford.

influences upon each other. An accumulating body of empirical work and theoretical formulation has focused on normal processes of development in the cognitive, affective, and social domains and on the relationship between development in childhood and later adaptation (e.g., Arend, Gove, & Sroufe, 1979; Cicchetti & Pogge-Hesse, 1981; Cicchetti & Sroufe, 1976, 1978; Decarie, 1965; Emde, Gaensbauer, & Harmon, 1976; Londerville & Main, 1981; Sroufe, 1979a, 1979b; Zigler & Trickett, 1978). Much of this work has been guided by the organizational perspective of development (Santostefano & Baker, 1972; Spitz, 1959; Sroufe, 1979b; Werner, 1948; Werner & Kaplan, 1963) and has proceeded in an effort to expand our knowledge of normal developmental processes. However, there has been only limited systematic investigation of development in atypical populations of infants.

The adoption of this perspective reflects a commitment to characterizing behavior and development in terms of the changing integration and organization of capacities in the social, affective, and cognitive domains. An attempt is made to discover the ways in which less complex behaviors become hierarchically integrated within more differentiated developmental systems and to illuminate the manner in which later modes of functioning evolve from earlier precursors. Additionally, the relationships among behavioral systems are examined so as to understand the consequences and implications of advances or lags in the functioning of one behavioral system for the operation of another. Thus, the underlying assumption of the organizational perspective is that an examination of only one domain of development, to the relative neglect of the others, would lead to a diminished view of the complexity of the developmental process.

Similarly, to theorize about development without considering deviations that might be expected as a result of prominent and pervasive intra- or extraorganismic disturbances would lead to incomplete or ambiguous accounts of development that do not adequately consider individual differences, the continuity and quality of adaptation, and the different processes by which the same developmental outcomes may be achieved. Therefore, it is imperative that researchers move away from delineating symptoms and behavioral characteristics of deviant populations and attempt, instead, to illuminate the factors that shape the course of development. To achieve this goal, it is necessary to adopt a model that transcends the simple, linear, "main effects" developmental model prevalent in the psychological literature (Reese & Overton, 1970; Sameroff & Chandler, 1975). Researchers must consider the complex, multifaceted ways in which constitutional, organismic, and environmental factors interact to affect development. Therefore, any consideration of atypical patterns of development needs to take into account the unique characteristics of the individual, the age and stage-level of functioning, the experiences to which the infant has been exposed, and the stability of environmental conditions (Greenspan & Lourie, 1981). In addition, the characteristics of the care-giving environment, the compatibility of the infant–care-giver dyad, the continuity or discontinuity of adaptive or maladaptive behavioral patterns, and the advances or lags in different developmental domains must be considered. Within this framework, atypical developmental patterns may be best conceptualized as resulting from the lack of integration, organization, or differentiation of cognitive, social, and emotional development when considered in terms of the psychologically relevant competencies that are expected to emerge in the different domains and the salient developmental tasks that need to be accomplished.

Reasons for the limited systematic investigation of the relationship between affect and cognition

Despite the appeal of the theoretical propositions emanating from the organizational perspective, it is only recently that empirical work on both normal and atypical infant development has attempted to examine concurrently the mutually interacting nature of affect and cognition. The reasons for the paucity of systematic investigations that bear on the interrelationship between affective and cognitive capacities in infancy include: the confluence of the impact of historical factors, problems in contemporary research on emotional development, trends in the definition, diagnosis, and treatment of deviant patterns of development, and limitations in current empirical work.

There are historical factors that have impeded the study of the relationship between affect and cognition in infancy. Within Freud's classic closed hydraulic model, affects were defined in terms of quantities of energy. They were viewed as having a disorganizing effect on behavior and as the forces that impelled the infant to discharge tension (Freud, 1895/1955, 1895/1962). In this "conflict" theory, affects were thought to act as safety valves, ridding the organism of excessive drive tension (Rapaport, 1953, 1960). Moreover, the classic Freudian psychoanalytic viewpoint paid little attention to the role of cognitive factors in motivating human behavior.

In later elaborations of the primary model of affect, Freud (1923–4/1961, 1926/1959) argued that the drive tension brought about by the absence of the need-reducing object did not bring about affective discharge (Green, 1977; Rapaport, 1953). Rather, in the secondary model of affect Freud claimed that the affect became subordinated to, or controlled by, the ego. The ego could permit small anticipatory quantities of affect to be discharged. These acted as signals of the drive tension. Although this revised model paid more attention to cognitive ("ego") factors, affects were still not given a prominent role in cognition; they were seen, rather, as signals originating in the ego (or superego) and hence lacked the power to control consciousness.

Common to both Freud's primary and secondary theories, affects were depicted as something negative, needing to be eliminated or sublimated. They were described in terms of their quantitative aspects, and the qualitative aspects were ignored, that is, a differentiation between other possible "signaling-affects," such as depression or anger, was not made. Furthermore, because of the corresponding emphasis on the organism's tendency to seek pleasure and to avoid tension, study was focused on negative affects to the relative neglect of the more positive "organizing" affects. Behavior was felt to be motivated by the need-reducing drives. This conception of affects and behavior was difficult to subject to empirical investigation, as many of its defining constructs defied operationalization and thereby limited the ability to examine systematically psychoanalytic hypotheses about the nature of affect.

In part stimulated by criticisms of the psychoanalytic paradigm, behaviorism came into prominence in psychological theory and research. The rise of the behaviorist movement, with its emphasis on the manipulation of environmental conditions and on observable behavioral responses to specific stimuli, led to the relative neglect of the study of emotions. Affects were conceptualized as tendencies to respond to stimuli in particular ways (Berlyne, 1978; Skinner, 1953). Thus, attempts to understand the unconscious aspects of the mind, and the use of introspection as a method for gaining access to emotional phenomena (Brentano, 1924; Wundt, 1912), were relegated to an inferior position. This historical trend represented a movement toward investigating only that which could be observed and measured by objective, scientific, reliable techniques. The imprecision in the definition and assessment of emotions led to a reduction in their examination and systematic investigation (see Duffy, 1941).

Piagetian theory, with its focus on the understanding of cognitive development, led to a proliferation of research and theorizing about the emerging cognitive capacities of the infant and a corresponding neglect of the emotional domain (Piaget, 1952, 1954, 1962). Even though Piaget wrote about the nature of the relationship between affect and cognition (Piaget 1954/1981), he viewed affects as the energy and cognition as the structure underlying intelligence, thereby imputing more causal import and explanatory power to the cognitive realm. Piaget utilized his own infants' emotions and emotional behaviors for inferring their underlying cognitive competence and as a primary basis for constructing his theory of sensorimotor development (Cicchetti & Hesse, 1983). Nonetheless, he is viewed as a "cold" theorist of infant development (Kessen, 1971) because the enormous surge of interest engendered by his work led to a preoccupation with cognitive development and the creation of appropriate assessment and research techniques to evaluate the cognitive advances of the infant.

Thus, the methodological problems inherent in the psychoanalytic view, the influence of the behaviorist movement, and the power of Piaget's work conspired to minimize the study of emotional development during infancy. These historical factors led to a somewhat exclusive focus on cognitive development during infancy and thus portrayed an incomplete picture of the complexity of advances that are made across domains.

It is only recently that methodological advances in the measurement of facial expression (Ekman & Friesen, 1978; Izard, 1979b; Oster, 1978) and in the recording of psychophysiological correlates of emotions (Campos, 1976; Sroufe & Waters, 1977b) have contributed to our ability to better understand emotions in infancy. Emotions are studied as the infant's primary means of communicating with the outside world (Emde, 1980a). Affective expressions are seen as influencing and reflecting the quality of the infant's interaction with its social and nonsocial environments; actions, feelings, and sensations represent available vehicles for communication in the absence of thought and language (Stechler & Carpenter, 1967; Vygotsky, 1962). The infant's facial expressions, vocalizations, direction of gaze, and capacity for affective involvement serve to initiate, maintain, and terminate interactions with others (Brazelton, Koslowski, & Main, 1974; Oster, 1978; Stern, 1977). However, there is a persistence of problems inherent in the objective examination of emerging emotional expressions, especially those that relate to definition and classification (see Hesse & Cicchetti, 1982, for an elaboration). Theoretical controversy surrounds the issue of the way in which discrete emotional expressions evolve (see, e.g., Izard & Buechler, 1979; Sroufe, 1979b). Additionally, there is lack of agreement as to the appropriate taxonomy for classifying emotions and an absence of understanding of the correspondence between internal emotional experiences and overt affective displays. Thus, the investigation of the development of emotions and of the ways in which infants learn to express affective states selectively and in the proper environmental contexts has been relatively less comprehensive and substantial than has been the empirical investigation of cognitive development in infancy.

Furthermore, the paucity of work on the development of emotions and on the relationship between affect and cognition is apparent in current investigations of atypical populations. Despite Bleuler's (1932) claim that "affective factors play such a dominant role in psychopathology . . . that practically everything else is incidental," current examinations of psychopathology and of deviant developmental patterns in infancy have emphasized the cognitive deficits that are manifested in these populations of infants. Although the role of emotions has been recognized, for example, in investigations of depression (Beck, 1967; Becker, 1977), schizophrenia (Bleuler, 1950), autism (Kanner, 1943), and Down syndrome (Cicchetti & Sroufe, 1976, 1978), contemporary conceptualizations of atypical development fail to focus on the affective concomitants to the cognitive dysfunctions that underlie the etiology and the sequelae of various disorders. The emphasis has been on describing deviant behavioral patterns in terms of the cognitive deficits that are characteristic at different developmental stages. For example, the delay in the emergence of communicative skills, the prevalence of disordered thought, and the inability to direct attention to, or maintain focus on, relevant task demands represent common descriptors of atypical patterns manifested as a result of various forms of pathology. The predominance of the assessment of cognitive factors in the evaluation of deviant developmental processes may reflect the relative ease with which these aspects may be identified and measured. Cognitive assessment techniques are available that enable individuals to be compared to normative standards for appropriate behavior and performance at different ages, thereby facilitating the identification of delays or aberrations in the normal process of development. In addition, intervention programs may be directed toward remediating specific cognitive deficits (DesLauriers, 1978; Keogh & Kopp, 1978). Thus, it is not surprising that the concern for cognitive aspects of atypical developmental patterns, as opposed to affective characteristics, has received greater attention by those professionals who work directly with infants.

It is only recently that researchers have begun to acknowledge implicitly the reciprocal relationship between affective and cognitive capacities in their work with infants. Theoretical attempts at integrating the psychoanalytic literature on affect with the empirical literature in developmental psychology (Arieti, 1967; Emde, 1980b; Greenspan, 1979; Rapaport, 1960) have provided some of the impetus for the recognition of the relationship between emotional and cognitive development. Research in the domain of human ethology has stimulated a renewed search for the evolutionary underpinnings of affective expression (Eibl-Eibesfeldt, 1979; Ekman, 1972; Izard, 1977, 1978, 1979a; Plutchik, 1980; Tomkins, 1962, 1963, 1980). Theoretical reformulations of Freud's original psychoanalytic position by the object-relations theorists (Bowlby, 1969; Fairbairn, 1949) have recognized the infant's need for stimulation as well as the importance of affective growth in terms of its effect upon the bond that develops between the infant and the care giver (Emde, 1980b). Stechler and Carpenter (1967) have noted that cognitive-informational constructs such as discrepancy could not provide completely accurate accounts of behavior. Loevinger (1976) and Sroufe (1979b) subsequently have reiterated this position. With the demise of drive reduction and conservation of energy as acceptable explanatory concepts (Bowlby, 1969; Mandler, 1964, 1975; White, 1959), newer ideas have been generated about the roles played by motivation, feelings, and tension in modulating and controlling behavior (Izard, 1979a; Sroufe & Waters, 1976). For example, researchers interested in infant–care-giver attachment have underscored the *affective* as well as the cognitive components underlying this enduring relationship (Ainsworth, 1973; Engel, 1971; Sroufe & Waters, 1977a).

These alternative conceptions of the role of affect represent modifications of the classic psychoanalytic view; however, they continue to ascribe a central role to affective growth and to the role of affects in guiding and influencing behavior. Furthermore, they have stimulated research on affective, as well as cognitive, development during infancy while encouraging empirical work that recognizes the relationship between emotional and cognitive capacities. For example, there has been a proliferation of research that has relied upon the overt emotional responses of the infant to account for the degree of attentiveness that is directed toward particular stimuli (Berlyne, 1960; Kagan, 1971; McCall

& McGhee, 1977; Thomas, 1971). Thus, boredom to highly familiar stimuli, distress to highly discrepant stimuli, and pleasure and interest to moderately discrepant stimuli are emotional responses that serve to indicate the presence and the complexity of the mental representations that the infant possesses. Distress and sadness that result when the infant is separated from its care giver during the end of the first year of life reflects the enhancement of retrieval memory that enables the infant to experience uncertainty over the care giver's absence (Kagan, Kearsley, & Zelazo, 1978). Perceptual and cognitive competence have been assessed by the emotional reactions of infants to placement on the "visual cliff" (Campos et al., 1978; Cicchetti & Sroufe, 1978). In addition, the Uzgiris-Hunt and Bayley scales for assessing cognitive development during infancy employ affective reactions as indices of underlying cognitive abilities (Haviland, 1976). Thus, there has been an emphasis in empirical work with infants on using emotional responses to assess cognitive competence (Charlesworth, 1966, 1969; Shultz & Zigler, 1970; Sroufe & Wunsch, 1972; Zelazo & Komer, 1971). The underlying assumption of these studies is that they are capable of illuminating the emerging cognitive capacities that could not be communicated verbally by the infant but may be inferred by the overt affective expression.

However, in spite of this recognition that one may rely upon affect as the "signaling system" by which the infant's cognitive advances may be gauged, there are limitations in the degree to which it yields an accurate appraisal of both normal and atypical infants' capabilities. For example, 18-month-old infants who display a mastery smile upon the completion of a task at which they have been persisting for several minutes may be communicating to those around them that they are experiencing a sense of completion of a goal that they have conceptualized, planned, executed, and achieved. Yet this inference may be made only after the observer has considered several important factors, including the intensity and duration of the emotional expression (e.g., are there qualitative differences in the smile displayed following the completion of simple and complex tasks?), the situation or the environmental circumstances in which it was expressed (e.g., is the smile displayed only when the task is completed in the presence of others?), the eliciting conditions and the manner of termination of the task (e.g., did somebody suggest the task the infant carried out or was the task actually initiated by the infant?), and the infant's prior experience or familiarity with the stimulus material and the task demands (e.g., has the infant ever seen or played with the objects before?). Thus, although the emotional expressions of the infant may be useful indicators to gauge the advances that have been made in the cognitive domain, the interpretation of these affective displays must be considered carefully before valid inferences about the infant's cognitive capacities may be made. This point becomes especially relevant when one studies atypical populations of infants for whom there may be delays, aberrations, mutations, or absences of particular affective expressions.

In addition, for both normal and atypical infants, the possible absence of an emotional reaction may not be indicative of the failure to achieve a particular level of cognitive competence. There may be many factors that interfere with, mute, or inhibit the affective expression that another infant in the same situation might display (e.g., individual differences in arousal thresholds, in reactivity to external stimulation). Therefore, it would be erroneous to reason that the lack of an emotional display upon the completion of a task or the absence of overt distress upon separation from the primary care giver, in either normal or atypical infants, indicates conclusively that the infant has not acquired the requisite cognitive capacities that are thought to underlie these typical emotional reactions.

These problems that are prevalent in the empirical work on normal processes of development represent some of the obstacles that hinder our understanding of the integration and organization of affective and cognitive development during the first two years of life. Additionally, there is a paucity of empirical work that examines the organization of development in atypical populations. The investigation of populations of infants for whom differing patterns of social, emotional, and/or cognitive development may be expected, as a consequence of enduring and prominent influences that characterize the transaction between the infant and the environment, provides a means for establishing a model of development that is integrative and applicable to both normal and atypical populations. There are several empirical questions that preclude our complete understanding of the nature of the relationship between cognitive and affective development in infancy. In the following sections, we will delineate some of the major theoretical and empirical issues that need to be addressed, and we will attempt to provide empirical documentation, where evidence is available, to illustrate the relevance and importance of these issues. In the course of our discussion, we will propose some suggested avenues for future research that will enhance our understanding of the relationship between affect and cognition in both normal and atypical populations of infants. In the final section, we will outline some of the theoretical issues that need to be considered before an integrative and comprehensive model of development can be formulated.

We believe that the investigation of the relationship between the affective and cognitive domains is dependent upon a carefully defined concept of emotions as they exist independently from the cognitive processes that influence, and are influenced by, them (Cicchetti & Pogge-Hesse, 1981). However, we also acknowledge that emotions are complex phenomena that may not be simply described by a concrete and parsimonious definition. Rather, we feel that it is essential to consider the many components of emotions as they are experienced internally by the individual, as they impact upon one's physiological response mechanisms, and as they are overtly expressed through facial expressions and nonverbal movements. Therefore, in our discussion of the relationship between affective and cognitive development, we will consider these multiple characteristics of emotions and identify the specific definition of emotion that is being examined by the research that is reviewed or by the empirical or theoretical questions that are addressed.

The development of emotional expressions

Although advances have been made in our understanding of the normal ontogenesis of the range of facial expressions exhibited at different developmental periods, there are many controversial problems that have not been solved. Any investigation into the organization of affective development must grapple with the fundamental question of what constitutes an emotion. Many researchers rely heavily on facial expressions as the major criterion for inferring the presence of an underlying emotion (Izard, 1977, 1978). Moreover, facial expressions are necessarily the primary index of emotion in infants because of their lack of verbal ability. However, investigators are not in complete agreement about such important issues as the exact age of onset of different emotions or the eliciting conditions and contexts in which emotional expressions occur (e.g., cf. Izard & Buechler, 1979, with Sroufe, 1979b). Similarly, it is not known whether there are qualitative differences that become manifest with age in the overt phenotypic expressions of particular emotions.

There is general consensus as to the order in which the various emotional expressions emerge. Thus, pleasure, rage, disgust, wariness, interest, distress, and startle are present in the early months of life, and expressions such as surprise, anger, and fear emerge in the second half of the first year of life (Bridges, 1932; Campos & Stenberg, 1981; Charlesworth, 1969; Izard & Buechler, 1979; Sroufe, 1979b). Shame, shyness, and guilt (the "self-conscious" reactions), as well as affection and defiance, can be observed in the second year of life (Erikson, 1950; Kagan, 1981; Sroufe, 1979b). Feelings of justice, pride, jealousy, envy, love, depression, and contempt do not appear to emerge until much later in development (Arieti, 1967; Piaget, 1954/1981). In addition to their larger, more differentiated emotional repertoires, adults display these emotions in more contexts than do infants and children.

An important question that must be addressed is whether or not some emotions have universal facial expressions. One way of answering this question is to observe and to compare a variety of populations of infants, including those who are developmentally deviant. If it is found that all samples of infants studied, regardless of differences in constitution and environment, reveal the same facial expressions, then this would provide compelling evidence for the universal existence of discrete affects. For example, Eibl-Eibesfeldt's (1979) work with blind and deaf children and congenitally deaf and blind thalidomide children found that the basic facial expressions, such as smiling, laughter, anger, and fear, occurred in the same situations as with normal children. Charlesworth (1970), in a study of blind and sighted children, found that there were no major quantitative or qualitative differences in their facial expressions to a variety of surprise tasks.

However, it is likely that differences in facial musculature, aberrant neural programs, or variations in speed of information processing may affect the actual appearance or delay the emergence of certain facial expressions. In Cicchetti and Sroufe's (1976, 1978) work with Down syndrome infants, it was found that these infants laughed far less to the incongruous stimulus items presented by their mothers than did their mental-age matched normal counterparts. Emde, Katz, and Thorpe (1978) demonstrated that the onset of the social smile in Down syndrome infants, though only slightly delayed in emergence, was characterized by dampened intensity, poor eye-to-eye contact, absence of crescendoing, and lack of activation of the arms and legs. Furthermore, Emde and his colleagues (1978) have shown more uncertainty or "noise" in the emotional signaling system of the Down syndrome infant. The signals of Down syndrome infants may be less clear and more difficult to read as a result of their neuromuscular hypotonia (Cicchetti & Sroufe, 1978; Emde & Brown, 1978). Additionally, the range of facial expressions that these infants are capable of displaying may be limited and/or may appear in distorted form. Cicchetti and Sroufe (1978) found an inverse relationship between degree of hypotonia and both speed and amount of responding with laughter to visually presented stimuli. Gallagher, Jens, and O'Donnell (in press), studying a group of mentally retarded and multiple-handicapped infants, including hydrocephaly, microcephaly, cerebral palsy, and seizure disorders of unknown etiology, found a decrement in laughter responses in both hypotonic and hypertonic babies.

In addition, the characteristic slower rate of information processing in Down syndrome infants may result in longer latencies to smile, to laugh, or to exhibit negative reactions such as distress or crying. It may also result in the infrequent production of certain emotions (e.g., surprise and fear) that require fast information processing and thus a strong arousal component (see, e.g., Tomkins, 1962, 1963, 1980). These infants may express particular emotions in a qualitatively different way; that is, they may display fear, surprise, happiness, and so on by means of different facial and gestural features or only in terms of biologically based facial features but never via characteristics that presuppose the acquisition of what Ekman (1972, 1977) has called "social display rules." To date, no research has addressed this important issue.

Several critical issues that are relevant to our understanding of the development of emotional expressions must be addressed by future research. Investigations of the different situations in which particular affects are expressed by normal and atypical populations of infants would enable us to understand the importance of contextual cues in eliciting certain emotions. Additionally, the examination of atypical populations would enable us to see whether these infants express particular discrete emotions in fewer or different contexts than do normals. Furthermore, longitudinal investigations of atypical populations of infants would enable us to ascertain whether discrete affects emerge in the same sequence but at a slower rate relative to normals, or whether there are qualitative differences in the actual emotional expressions that appear over time. Sampling among a wide range of early environmental experiences, such as those to which maltreated infants, institutionalized infants, infants of psychotic parents, or handicapped infants are exposed, may reveal certain extraorganismic factors that serve to speed up, slow down, or prevent certain affects from appearing or that cause irregular or atypical patterns of emotional expressions.

Whether facial expressions should be equated with emotional *experience* remains a controversial issue and an area ripe for empirical investigation (Sroufe, 1979b). According to Izard's theory (1977), facial expressions provide sensory data to the brain for cortical-integrative activity and are implicated in the production of the emotional experience itself. What is critical here is the feedback from the face to the neural mechanisms of the somatosensory system. Research suggests that the intensification or deintensification of *facial expression per se* amplifies or attenuates the experiences of the affect itself (Lanzetta, Cartwright-Smith, & Kleck, 1976). The implication is that emotional experience is to some extent under voluntary control, at least on a phenomenological level. Down syndrome infants would be a particularly intriguing sample to study in this regard. Since their facial expressions are often muted and less emotionally intense than those of normal babies, a result of, in part, arousal modulation problems, it would be interesting to see if intensifying the overt facial expressions of these infants (e.g., through behavior modification techniques) would, in turn, quantitatively enhance arousal levels.

The relationship between emotional expressions and affective experiences may also be studied by examining morphological changes in facial musculature to see how these alterations will impact on the way in which the same emotion expression is communicated over time. It is likely that facial musculature must be more refined before the infant can communicate more differentiated or subtle emotions, but does this mean that the infant does not experience these emotions until able to communicate them? Clearly, the belief in the isomorphism of facial expressions and affective experience is problematic. There is insufficient empirical longitudinal data documenting the development of facial expressions; however, numerous impressionistic accounts describe a tendency in infancy for diffuse, global, and highly undifferentiated motoric expressions to become more differentiated, integrated, organized, and subdued as the infant matures (Charlesworth & Kreutzer, 1973; Peiper, 1963). Furthermore, Ekman and Oster (1979) have found that all but one of the discrete facial movements that comprise the later-developing full configurations of emotional expressions in adulthood can be observed in full-term and premature newborns. What then accounts for the emergence of qualitatively different facial expressions in infancy? While it is reasonable to assume that fine muscular control is a prerequisite for the ability to express more subtle emotions (e.g., smirks), it is also possible that certain cognitive developments must take place before the infant can respond to more complex stimuli and actually express and experience these emotions (see Lewis & Brooks, 1978; Sroufe, 1979b).

Research on deaf infants could provide insight on the role that verbal cues play in emotional expression. For example, "positive sensory feedback loops" (Izard, 1978) in normal infants may explain how infants perpetuate their own emotional reactions. In effect, infants are aware of their own reactions and this may contribute to their perpetuation and perhaps intensification of the emotion analogous to a primary circular reaction (e.g., "distress induced distress," Sagi & Hoffman, 1976; Simner, 1971). That most infants can hear themselves laugh or cry may play a role in prolonging the experience or abating it. An important question to address would be whether particular contexts facilitate or deter the perpetuation of emotional experience. By studying affective expressions and emotional control in deaf infants, we would begin to illuminate the role of hearing in the elicitation and control of emotional expression.

In addition, infants' ever-increasing capacities to monitor their own emotional states ("arousal modulation," Cicchetti & Sroufe, 1978; or "self-regulation," Kopp, 1982) may play a role in the inhibition of what would previously have been an uncontrolled and disorganized outburst (see also Gunnar, 1980). For example, it is possible for toddlers to reassure themselves by repeating "I'm okay, I'm okay" during an anxiety-arousing experience. How toddlers arrive at a particular emotional expression may be due primarily to their muscular ability to control affects and to their capacity to identify their internal states or to their cognitive and linguistic sophistication. Most likely, all of these factors are implicated in the process and interact in complex ways. Research on populations showing deviant development can shed light on these issues by providing "natural" controls for these variables that may not be possible to attain with normal populations.

For example, research on Down syndrome infants can help tease apart the role of cognition from the role of arousal modulation. Cicchetti and Sroufe (1978) found that even when Down syndrome and normal infants were matched on level of cognitive development (mental age), the Down syndrome infants showed less fear (crying, heart-rate acceleration) on the "visual cliff" or to looming objects than did their normal counterparts. Moreover, when Down syndrome infants did show fear reactions, they had greater difficulty calming themselves than did the nonhandicapped infants. These data suggest that Down syndrome infants may have basic arousal modulation problems and underscore the importance of arousal factors in emotional expression. A likely explanation for these results is that Down syndrome infants have difficulties with forebrain inhibitory control. This raises the question as to the role that inhibitory mechanisms play in emotional expression in general. The answer possibly may be found through research on infants with localized brain damage. For example, expressions of disgust have been found in anencephalic and hydrocephalic infants, suggesting that they originate in the brainstem (Steiner, 1973). Whether specific sites are associated with certain emotional functions and whether particular areas of the brain are implicated in emotional expression and behavior is an important question (Pribram, 1967, 1980).

While Cicchetti and Sroufe's (1976) results on smiling and laughter in Down syndrome infants again illuminate the role arousal factors play in emotional expression, several other issues are brought to the fore by this work. Even though the Down syndrome infant could not generate enough *tension* ("cognitively produced arousal," Cicchetti & Sroufe, 1978) to laugh, information-processing factors were clearly implicated, as was neuromuscular hypotonia. Cicchetti and Sroufe (1976) argued that the Down syndrome babies could not process the incongruity of the stimulus presentations with sufficient speed to generate the "arousal jag" (Berlyne, 1969) needed for laughter. Moreover, the Down syndrome babies who smiled and laughed least and latest to the incongruous stimuli were the most hypotonic. Thus, these experiments point out that all three factors – cognition, physiology, and muscle tone – played an important role in producing the results and underscore the intricate relationship that exists among these three systems. Clearly, the individual differences and developmental heterogeneity of Down syndrome infants have helped us to gain insight into a difficult issue that might not be as readily apparent by studying normal populations.

Patterns of affective-cognitive interaction between infants and their care givers

Both qualitative and quantitative differences in affective expressions and emotional responses in infants may affect the cognitive processing and interpretation of these signals by the care giver and may lead to communication problems in the dyad. Variations in the infant's facial signals, eye contact, and crying, and differences in the tendency for, and style of, initiating and maintaining interactions, may impact upon the care giver's perception and processing of the infant's signals and may have implications for the nature of the communicative patterns that are established in the dyad. An examination of these diverse factors is essential for our understanding of the ways in which infants influence their care givers, the alternative styles of interaction that may be necessitated by particular developmental deviations in infants, the role that developmental changes in the cognitive domain have on the expression of particular emotions, the dynamic nature of the interactional process, and the flexibility of care-giver responsiveness that is crucial for the development of competence in infants.

When there are prominent deviations in the interaction between care givers and infants, the quality of affective behavioral responses and the amount of reciprocal communication may be altered in significant ways. Therefore, an examination of deviant developmental patterns of communication that result from intra- or extraorganismic disturbances is essential for investigators interested in the implications of such atypical patterns for the growth and adaptation of the infant.

Care-giver responsivity to the infant may be determined by the anatomical features and facial expressions of the infant or by behavioral acts such as smiling, crying, or gaze (Stern, 1977). The degree to which the infant's capacity for eliciting certain behaviors in others is biologically determined is unknown. Similarly, the relative importance of affective expressions, anatomical features, and emotional responses (e.g., crying or laughter) for motivating attention or care is unclear. It might be, for example, that the exaggerated features of the infant with Down syndrome may elicit nurturance from the care giver for an extended period of time (Serafica & Cicchetti, 1976). The role that smiling plays in the initiation of social contact or the modulation of arousal in face-to-face interactions (Brazelton et al., 1974; Robson, 1967; Sroufe & Waters, 1976) implicates the importance of examining smiling behavior in populations of infants who might be expected to display aberrations in the development or appropriate use of this affective response. For the blind infant, smiling has been found to develop at the same time as in sighted infants, but its use tends to be erratic, showing a muting over time (Fraiberg, 1977; Freedman, 1964). In infants with Down syndrome, smiling has been found to be delayed in its emergence, and even when it has developed, it tends to be less engaging than that of normal infants (Cicchetti & Sroufe, 1976). Inadequacies or unusual characteristics of the signaling system that is employed by the infant may result in the lack of adequate stimulation to the care giver and consequent aberrations in the infant–care-giver relationship. Similarly, inappropriate responsiveness on the part of the care giver, or the lack of synchronization or regulation of dyadic behaviors, may result in a disruption of the reciprocal communication systems between the infant and the care giver.

Congenitally blind infants, beset with the inability to monitor their environments visually, may have difficulties in establishing interpersonal relationships since they are incapable of employing the sensory modality that possesses its own means for modulating and regulating interaction (i.e., by closing one's eyelids or averting, maintaining, or redirecting gaze) (Robson, 1967). The study of blind infants facilitates an understanding of the relative importance of compensatory mechanisms that promote interaction between blind infants and their care givers and the nature of the developmental process in blind infants (i.e., whether it is a slow version of the normal developmental process, as is suggested by Als, Tronick, & Brazelton, 1980, or whether it is actually different from that of sighted infants). For example, the blind infant's smiles are not elicited automatically by the care giver's voice or face as they are in sighted infants. Instead, the blind infant's most reliable stimulus is gross tactile or kinesthetic stimulation (Fraiberg, 1977). The muting or dampening of facial expressiveness and the less captivating quality of the smiling response in blind infants that occurs by about 4 to 6 months of age imply that some visual feedback is necessary to maintain full displays of smiling behavior following the initial unfolding of the infant's innate tendencies. The absence or muting of the smile or other facial expressions does not imply that the blind infant is not experiencing emotions; rather, because the blind infant is limited in the traditional means of expressing affective states (Fraiberg, 1977), alternative channels of communication, such as the signaling system of the hands, must be used to convey emotional states (Fraiberg, 1974).

Similarly, communication problems may result from both qualitative and quantitative differences in emotional expression in Down syndrome infants. As a result of their demonstrated difficulties with visual proprioceptive feedback (Butterworth & Cicchetti, 1978), their delays in information processing (Hoffman, Salapatek, Kuskowski, & Cicchetti, 1979), and their problems with arousal modulation (Bridges & Cicchetti, 1982; Cicchetti & Sroufe, 1976, 1978; Emde & Brown, 1978; Emde et al., 1978), infants with Down syndrome display delayed or weak affective responses. This may affect the care giver's cognitive perception or interpretation of the infant's cues, causing care givers to misread the emotional messages of these infants or to react with less affective involvement to their less arousable infants.

Either possibility may in turn bring about further delays or distortions in the Down syndrome infant's repertoire of behaviors that express affective states. For example, they may account for the decreased rate of referential eye contact in Down syndrome infants (Jones, 1977). Furthermore, if eye contact is associated with the frequency of smiling and vocalizations, it may be that less eye contact produces fewer signaling behaviors in the infant with Down syndrome. The communication patterns between Down syndrome infants and their care givers may be affected further by the vocalization behavior of these infants that suggests an inability to take turns in early communication. Studies by Jones (1977), Buium (1974), and Buckhalt, Rutherford, and Goldberg (1978) document the Down syndrome infants' tendency to vocalize continuously throughout interaction, thereby diminishing the capacity for early turn-taking skills that are a precursor to the development of social communication and language (Bates, 1976; Stern, 1977).

The decreased responsivity of Down syndrome infants and the dampened affective tone displayed by these infants (Cicchetti & Sroufe 1976, 1978; Cytryn, 1975; Freudenberg, Driscoll, & Stern, 1978) necessitate adequate compensatory mechanisms on the part of the care giver to initiate or maintain interactions or to be successful in the interpretation of, and response to, affective states. The impairment of the Down syndrome infant's visual proprioceptive feedback system may be such that these infants may be restricted in the range of emotional expressions that they can encode and decode. These signaling and interpretive difficulties may place the Down syndrome infant "at risk" for communicative problems. The psychophysiological and neuromuscular defects characteristic of this disorder may interfere with or disrupt the normal interactional process between the infant and the care giver.

Several investigators have speculated that deaf infants and their care givers may have difficulties in developing a system of communication (Meadow, 1975; Schlesinger, 1978; Schlesinger & Meadow, 1972). Although compensatory mechanisms, such as increased use of gestures, eye contact, body contact, and facial expressions (Ling & Ling, 1974), may facilitate the development of an adequate signaling system in hearing-impaired infants, their expression of particular emotions may be aberrant. While they possess adequate proprioceptive and visual feedback cues about the affective expressions of themselves and others, they may display deficiencies in the mediation, control, or interpretation of emotions because of their inability to respond to an environment rich in verbalization. If infants' capacities to express emotions are augmented by attention to the emotional language repertoire of their care givers, then deaf infants may be at a disadvantage. It is essential for researchers to examine the importance of early auditory experience for the capacity to display emotions in congenitally deaf infants. If audition plays a primary role in encouraging exploration and in the generalization of schemes, as suggested by Liben (1978), then it is crucial that an investigation be made of the effect of auditory feedback upon the infant's action upon, and response to, social and nonsocial objects.

Abnormalities in the development of affective communication patterns of infants who have been maltreated have been identified by recent empirical investigations. Gaensbauer and Sands (1979) delineated six patterns of distorted emotional communication from infant to care giver including affective withdrawal, lack of pleasure, inconsistency or unpredictability, shallowness, ambivalence/ambiguity, and negative affective responses (distress, anger, or sadness). In a later study, Gaensbauer, Mrazek, and Harmon (1980) described four affective patterns that appeared to be relatively consistent and that represented the predominant communicative pattern of the mother–infant dyad. These four types were labeled as developmentally and affectively retarded (characterized by lack of social responsiveness, emotional blunting, and inattentiveness to the environment), depressed (exhibiting inhibition, withdrawal, aimless quality of play, and sad and depressed facial expressions), ambivalent/affectively labile (showing sudden shifts from engagement and pleasure to withdrawal and anger), and angry (characterized by active, disorganized play and low frustration tolerance, with frequent angry outbursts). Although the direction of causality of these atypical communication patterns remains ambiguous, it is apparent that deviant styles of affective displays, decreased responsivity and reciprocal interactions, aberrations in the patterns of initiating, maintaining, or terminating interaction, and deviations in the capacity to express emotional states tend to characterize the dyad. The work of Frodi and Lamb (1980) suggests that maltreating parents have different psychophysiological responses to the cries of infants and are thus less effective in responding to the affective expressions of their infants. However, the mutually reinforcing nature of the inadequacies in the infant's communicative system and the differential impact of emotional displays upon the contingent, sensitive responsiveness of the care giver may serve to perpetuate the deviant patterns of interaction in this dyad and result in atypical developmental outcomes in the emotional and behavioral repertoire of the maltreated infant. Thus, it is essential that research be directed toward illuminating the transactional nature of maltreatment (Cicchetti & Rizley, 1981), focusing on the developmentally salient emergence, expression, mediation, and control of affective states. The contribution of both the care giver and the infant to the maintenance or remediation of early developmental deviations must be considered.

Atypical infants, because of the nature of their difficulties, may disrupt the care-giver–infant relationship and place excessive demands upon their care givers (Als, Tronick, & Brazelton, 1980; Emde & Brown, 1978; Fraiberg, 1977; Ulrich, 1972). By examining the process of development in infants with deviations that are apparent at birth or soon thereafter, a better understanding may be obtained of the alternative methods that may be employed to achieve relatively harmonious care-giver–infant interactions. Temperamental differences in normal and atypical infants require parents to adapt their style to accommodate to their infant's predisposition toward inhibition or excitability, threshold of responsivity, degree of attentiveness and so on (Bell, 1968; Thomas & Chess, 1977; Thomas, Chess, & Birch, 1968). Individual differences in infants necessitate modifications by care givers to achieve successful patterns of communication (Bell, 1968). For example, care givers of preterm newborns have been observed to be initially less active, more distant, and less likely to engage in face-to-face interactions than are parents of full-term infants (e.g., DiVitto & Goldberg, 1979). However, observations of care givers interacting with their preterm infants later in the first year of life indicate that although the infants were less likely to be attentive and active participants in the dyadic interchange, the care givers were more likely to be in closer contact with their infants, to engage in more physical contact, and to offer to demonstrate more objects and toys (e.g., Brachfeld, Goldberg, & Sloman, 1980; Field, 1977). These data suggest that care givers learn to adapt to, and to make adjustments for, the decreased attentiveness and affective involvement of their preterm infants by investing more energy and effort into their interactions with their less responsive and less active infants. Furthermore, they provide evidence for the existence of individual differences in infants that necessitate modifications by care givers to achieve successful patterns of communication.

It is only recently that investigators have begun to appreciate the compensatory adjustments that parents of handicapped infants may adopt (Sorce & Emde, 1982). Cicchetti and Sroufe (1976, 1978) suggest that mothers of Down syndrome infants appear to be able to compensate for morphological and psychophysiological deviations by exerting themselves more strenuously to initiate interaction and to elicit affective responses from their infants. Bridges and Cicchetti (1982) demonstrate that maternal ratings of infants with Down syndrome do not ascribe a greater degree of difficulty in interacting with these infants, although classification of infants according to Carey's (1970) criteria for assigning infants to different types of temperament categories reveals that more of the Down syndrome infants are difficult to manage relative to Carey's original standardization sample. This finding indicates that the care giver is successful in altering perceptions of, and attitudes toward, the infant in a manner that promotes harmonious interaction within the dyad (see Gunn, Berry, & Andrews, 1980, for similar evidence).

It is possible for care givers to have rewarding, reciprocal relationships with infants who manifest atypical patterns of development (see, e.g., Bell & Harper, 1977; Goldberg, 1977, in press). Lower intelligence, such as that exhibited by Down syndrome infants, does not necessarily result in different sequences of development in the social, affective, or cognitive domains (Cicchetti & Mans, in press; Cicchetti & Serafica, 1981; Cicchetti & Sroufe, 1978; Serafica & Cicchetti, 1976). Care givers must be aware of the need to employ compensatory mechanisms, such as substituting vocal contact for the missing visual channel in congenitally blind infants (Fraiberg, 1974). Mothers of deaf infants may compensate for their infant's greater passivity, diminished responsiveness, and less active involvement by being more dominant (Wedell-Monning & Lumley, 1980). What may appear to the observer to be overstimulation or intrusiveness in the behavior and affective responsiveness of a parent interacting with an atypical infant may actually be the overt manifestation of a sensitive and contingently responsive care giver who is employing compensatory adjustments to encourage the harmony of the interaction and the adaptation of the infant.

The additional stressors and emotional burdens that are placed upon the care giver of atypical infants certainly influence the care-giving process. A parent whose infant initiates few mutual interactions, responds less, if at all, to parental initiations, expresses fewer affective reactions, and inhibits rewarding and stimulating parental experiences must learn to understand, to interpret, and to respond to their muted or less differentiated emotional expressions. However, parents will differ in the extent to which they are capable of successfully adapting and adjusting their behaviors and responses. For example, care givers who are less proficient at decoding affective expressions in infants or who misattribute emotional expressions because of a lack of knowledge about development or appropriate parental responsiveness may contribute to, or exacerbate, the deviant developmental patterns exhibited in these infants. Thus, an examination of patterns of affective expressiveness in infants and the cognitive processing and responsivity of the care giver to these signals is crucial for the understanding of the interaction between affect and cognition in dyadic relationships.

Socialization of affect and the affective-cognitive interaction

The role played by the care giver in modifying, influencing, and altering the expression and appropriate display of affective reactions has not been adequately addressed to date. The influence of qualitative differences in the way interactive behaviors become organized (e.g., in the development of the attachment relationship) and then impact upon later social and cognitive development has been investigated (e.g., Arend, Gove, & Sroufe, 1979; Matas, Arend, & Sroufe, 1978; Waters, Wippman, & Sroufe, 1979). However, the effect of qualitative differences in early dyadic interactions upon emotional experiences and affective expressions in infancy and upon later emotional development may be significant in the way that these early socialization experiences influence the type of affects expressed, the range or variation of expressions, the context in which affects are expressed, the frequency with which emotions are exhibited, the intensity and duration of discrete expressions, and the capacity to modulate or to regulate the affective displays. Additionally, when one examines populations of infants characterized by developmental deviations, it becomes necessary to question whether the alleged influence of early socialization practices upon, for example, the suppression of overt emotional displays with age (see Ekman, Friesen, & Ellsworth, 1972; Malatesta & Haviland, 1982; Saarni, 1978) is operative in a similar manner as in normal infants or whether there are alternative socialization processes that lead to the same or different developmental outcomes in affective growth and experiences. Thus, a consideration of the processes involved in the socialization of affect during infancy is crucial for an understanding of the reciprocal relationship between emotional signaling and expressiveness of the infant and the cognitive processing, interpretation, and selective responsivity of the care giver.

The investigation of the way in which care givers socialize affect in their infants requires an understanding of the normal developmental course of the expression of affect. That is, it is necessary to examine the normal structural changes in the overt display of emotional states and in the eliciting conditions and cognitive capacities that underlie the expression of appropriate affects. Furthermore, it is only when we know what *kinds* of emotions and emotional patterns infants express nonverbally and the processes by which new and more complex emotional expressions (e.g., blends) are acquired or extant affective displays are modified or controlled that it will be possible to help infants who are deficient in the display of nonverbal emotional expressions. Similarly, the role played by the care giver's emotional language in the modulation of the infant's affective responses, and the importance of assigning emotional labels to affective behaviors and states for later emotional development, may be understood better by examining populations of infants for whom particular deficiencies may inhibit or disrupt the normal process of affective development.

The characteristic emotional style of the care giver, the cognitive interpretation of, and responsivity to, the infant's signals, the pattern of verbal and nonverbal emotional expressiveness and of affective responsiveness displayed by the care giver, and the nature of the care giver's expectations for the infant exert an influence upon the way affect is socialized in the infant. For example, if a parent is affectively expressive and responds sensitively and contingently to the infant's emotional displays, it is more likely that the dyadic interaction will be harmonious and affectively positive. Conversely, care givers who are less responsive or who display more anger, irritation, and rejection toward their infants may be fostering less emotional communication and greater disharmony in the interaction. This relationship between emotional expressivity and the quality of the dyadic interaction has been investigated with regard to the attachment relationship that develops between the infant and the primary care giver. Research on qualitative differences in maternal responsivity, sensitivity, and acceptance and the way attachment behaviors are organized (e.g., Ainsworth, Bell, & Stayton, 1974; Main, 1977; Main, Tomasini, & Tolan, 1979) indicates that the nature of the attachment relationship may reflect the infant's adaptation to the care giver's affective responsiveness (or lack thereof) such that infants who are avoidant of, or resistant to, their care givers may be displaying appropriate coping responses that reflect an inner organization that guides and determines overt behavior. The congruence between maternal affective style and quality of attachment may in turn impact upon the infant's emotional development such that the infant's later expression and experience of affects reflects the nature of the early infant–care-giver relationship. Qualitative differences in the way in which affects are socialized through the characteristic nonverbal emotional expressiveness of the care giver, and the correspondence between quality of attachment and differential affective responsiveness in the infant, represent two major areas that need to be examined to illuminate the processes underlying the socialization of affect.

Although most of the research on attachment has focused on the first two years of life, with a consequent lack of emphasis on the role of language in the development of attachment, it is likely that maternal language and infant communicative skills affect the nature of the attachment relationship. Therefore, it would be important to examine the development of attachment between deaf infants and their care givers in an attempt to better understand the importance of sound in the attachment process. Then, the influence of language and, more specifically, of the care giver's emotional language upon the degree of expressivity, the range of emotions displayed, and the control and modulation of affects in deaf toddlers should be explored.

Blind infants, too, may have difficulties controlling their emotions. The absence of eye contact and the lack of automatic smiling when in the presence of the care giver may influence the care giver's response to the blind infant and exert some effect upon the organization of attachment behaviors. The inability of blind infants to see others' facial expressions may make it difficult for them to realize the impact they have on other persons. Their inability to use vision to monitor others' responses to their behavior may cause their emotional responses and affective displays to be disorganized, noncontingent, inappropriate, and less controlled. This places an additional burden on their care givers to respond sensitively to their infants' emotional states. Otherwise, it is conceivable that blind babies may feel a sense of helplessness and confusion when dealing with affective arousal and emotional behavior. Certainly, research on how affects are socialized in blind infants will contribute to our understanding of emotional development in both normal and atypical populations.

Research with Down syndrome infants demonstrates that a relationship similar to that exhibited in normal infants may be found between early attachment with the primary care giver and the control of emotions. Cicchetti and Serafica (1981) found the attachment, affiliation, and fear/wariness systems of Down syndrome infants to be organized in a manner similar to that in normal infants (Bretherton & Ainsworth, 1974). In particular, the intensity of emotional responses in the Down syndrome infants varied with the context and the behaviors of both mother and stranger, thereby suggesting an awareness of, and sensitivity to, different eliciting conditions, and a capacity for the modulation and control of emotional states. Cicchetti and Serafica's (1981) analysis of qualitative and quantitative differences in responsiveness to mother and stranger for the fear/wariness, affiliation, and attachment behavioral systems allowed for a better understanding of the complexity of the potential conclusions that could be drawn with regard to the Down syndrome infants' emotional control. Thus, for example, the increased latency to crying during separation from the mother and the greater difficulty in soothing and calming the distressed Down syndrome infant reflect the influence of the higher arousal threshold in these infants. This psychophysiological disturbance mediates the overt display of affective responsiveness but does not minimize the need for attributing importance to the control that infants with Down syndrome must learn to exert over their emotional displays. Berry, Gunn, and Andrews (1980) found the Down syndrome babies observed in a sequence of episodes similar, though not identical, to the "Strange Situation" (Ainsworth et al., 1978) to display greater distress upon separation from the mother than those infants studied by Cicchetti and Serafica

(1981). However, the infants in the investigation by Berry and his colleagues (1980) were younger in mental and chronological age than those included in the Cicchetti and Serafica (1981) sample, thereby indicating the potential influence of increased socialization experiences upon the capacity for emotional control.

Infants' observations of parents' characteristic emotional styles may significantly affect their subsequent control of emotional displays. The greater proportion of insecurely attached maltreated infants that were found in investigations by Egeland and Sroufe (1981) and by Schneider-Rosen and Cicchetti (in press), and the observations of Main (1977), and Main and her associates (1979) lead to the conclusion that maltreated infants may be at a greater risk for delays or deviations in their acquisition of emotional control as a result of their care giver's decreased affective responsiveness and sensitivity. Cummings, Zahn-Waxler, and Radke-Yarrow (1981) found that expressions of anger by normal infants' care givers frequently caused distress in the infants. Repeated exposures to anger between the parents increased the likelihood of a negative emotional reaction by the infants, as well as the active involvement of the infants in their parents' conflict. By about 1 year of age, infants not only were aware of angry interactions between persons important to them but were also likely to evidence an emotional reaction to them. These results suggest that infants' sense of security and feelings about self, as well as their capacity to display certain positive and negative emotional responses, may be affected by constant conflict or harmony of others in their environment.

If infants must rely on emotional cues provided by their care givers to help to regulate their emotional behaviors, then the examination of atypical populations of infants is crucial to the understanding of the role that *social referencing* (Campos & Stenberg, 1981) plays in the emerging capacity for emotional control. The perceptual, emotional, and cognitive factors involved in the evaluation of, and response to, environmental stimuli implicates the importance of examining the development of social referencing in infants who are characterized by sensory or cognitive deficits or the inability to trust and respond to their care givers (especially infants of "psychologically unavailable" care givers, Egeland & Sroufe, 1981). Parents who unconsciously display mixed or contradictory messages to their infants (e.g., when vocal and visual channels are incongruous) may foster inappropriate or developmentally immature social-referencing skills that inhibit infants' capacity to learn about affectively arousing stimulus situations. Investigations of blind and deaf infants would help to illuminate the relative contributions of visual and verbal cues for the development of social referencing. Similarly, examinations of Down syndrome infants would elucidate the importance of cognitive appraisal and mediation for the interpretation of affective cues. Future investigations of social referencing in both normal and atypical populations of infants would enhance our understanding of the infant's emerging capacity to decode emotional expressions, to employ differential affective cues in the interpretation of environmental stimulation, and to respond to various situations in qualitatively different ways.

The study of emotional language will provide further evidence for the influence of parental socialization techniques upon the intensity, frequency, duration, and type of affective displays in their infants. The role that language plays, for example, in the infant's developing capacity to control and to mediate emotional responses cognitively has not been explored to date. Additionally, qualitative differences in the way in which parents employ emotional language, by encouraging or discouraging affective experiences or by assigning verbal labels to affective states, may impact upon the infant's ability to modulate internal emotional experiences or to respond appropriately and differentially to specific eliciting stimuli in the environment. The examination of the effect of the care giver's use of emotional language upon the development of emotional control in normal populations of infants will illuminate the importance of cognitive-linguistic factors for affective growth and the influence of these factors even before the infants are capable of employing emotional labels or of verbalizing about their own emotional states.

Furthermore, the investigation of infants who exhibit atypical developmental patterns may contribute to our understanding of the role that language plays in the socialization of affect. For example, it would be interesting to examine emotional growth in blind infants to determine whether they will be competent in the culture-specific characteristics for the appropriate display and control of emotions. It may be that the rules for emotional expressions can be transmitted verbally, without the need for visual and proprioceptive feedback. Conversely, the study of deaf infants would allow for an examination of the relative importance of hearing for the development of socially and universally appropriate rules for emotional expressivity. In addition, it would provide evidence for the question of whether deaf infants show greater deficiencies in the acquisition of emotional language as a result of their hearing impairment. It would also allow for the examination of the importance of the emotional language system for the control of emotions.

Similarly, the study of Down syndrome infants would enhance our understanding of the role that emotional language skills play in the cognitive control and modulation of affective states. Down syndrome infants may show deficiencies in their emotional language system as a result of socialization experiences. Care givers may be less adept at labeling their Down syndrome infants' emotions because of morphological differences in their infants' facial expressions or because of the infants' neurological abnormalities (e.g., higher response thresholds) that interfere with the display of particular affects. Subsequently, these infants may be less capable of correctly labeling their own or others' emotions if they ever acquire a language system at all. This decreased capacity to verbalize about affective states may lead to decreased competence in controlling, mediating, or interpreting their internal affective experiences.

The care givers' role in socializing affect in their infants implicates the importance of examining the synchrony of emotional responsiveness to infants' nonverbal expressions. If care givers respond adequately and appropriately to their infants' emotional displays, for example, by calming a distressed infant or laughing when the infant laughs while performing a funny act, then their infants will be more likely to be able to deal with emotions effectively and adaptively. These infants will have a greater capacity to integrate affects into their own lives and to understand the consequences of certain emotional expressions. However, care givers are not always attuned to, and adept at responding to, their infants' affective states. There may be several reasons for asynchronous emotional responsivity on the part of the parent; each may lead to particular outcomes that will influence the infant's control and subsequent display of certain emotions. For example, a parent may not be able to tolerate certain specific affects, such as fear, because of problems, frustrations, or lack of knowledge about what is an appropriate response for an infant to exhibit in a particular situation. Additionally, certain parental personality characteristics may lead to rigid or inflexible expectations for appropriate emotional behaviors to be exhibited by their infants. Unfulfilled needs and unconscious motivating factors in the parent may lead to frustration or disappointment in care givers whose infants do not display the "appropriate" affective responses that they expect and desire. As a result, the parent may be nonresponsive or display a negative affective response to the infant's expression of a particular emotion. The infant may, in turn, learn to control this emotion by muting or suppressing its expression or by avoiding those situations that might elicit the affect. Similarly, as a result of the parent's ignoring or responding negatively to the infant, the infant might learn to fear the parent, to become withdrawn, inhibited, and nonexpressive, or to "act-out" when in the presence of other adults.

If a care giver responds asynchronously to a particular class of affects (e.g., negative but not positive affects), then the infant may be more likely to inhibit those affects that the parent does not respond to in an appropriate manner. Additionally, if parents display egocentrism by responding only to their own affect that a situation elicits and not to that which is expressed by the infant, then there may be an inconsistency in parental responsiveness that may lead to the infant's sense of helplessness with regard to the availability or the sensitivity and contingent responsivity of the care giver. This could also lead to the muting or inhibition of certain affective displays or to the ignoring of the care giver as an adaptive mechanism for the infant.

These potentially deleterious consequences for affective growth may be more apparent in populations of infants who manifest deviations or delays in emotional expressiveness as a result of the operation of intra- or extraorganismic factors. If parents of blind, deaf, or premature infants or of infants with Down syndrome or other forms of mental retardation are not capable of adequately compensating for the deficiencies in affective expressiveness that result from these various handicaps, then the nature of the dyadic interaction may be more likely to be asynchronous. If infants are maltreated or are being reared by depressed or psychotic parents or "psychologically unavailable" care givers, then these environmental factors may exert a negative influence on the inter-action, thereby decreasing the possibility for emotional synchrony. The con-sequences of such patterns for later affective growth may be evident in the intensity, frequency, and duration of the infant's emotional expressions, the type and range of affects displayed, and the specific contexts in which affects are elicited. For example, the asynchronous nature of emotional responsivity may interact with the temperamental characteristics of the infant to influence the frequency of expression of certain affects such that these emotions may be displayed excessively, and particular environmental conditions may elicit only these discrete affects. Alternatively, particular emotions may be expressed intensely across a variety of contexts, thereby fostering an expectation that this may be the only way to express the affect. If the infant does not learn to be flexible or adaptive in dealing with the variety or intensity of emotions, as a consequence of early socialization processes, then the experience of particular emotions at a later age may be disorganizing, overwhelming, or unmanageable to the infant.

Furthermore, flexible emotional responsivity of the care giver is necessary for the gradual acquisition of greater selectivity in the display of certain emotions that emerges with cognitive advances during infancy and early childhood. Without this flexibility, the infant is likely to adopt a rigid rule structure and to learn to express only certain emotions in specific contexts. Future research must be directed toward illuminating the various developmental outcomes that may eventuate as a result of early asynchronous emotional experiences or socialization practices that inhibit the acquisition and expression of a variety of affective states. Additionally, the impact of other significant figures in the infant's early social environment who may mitigate against the deleterious effects of an insensitive and nonresponsive care giver and influence the infant's affective experiences needs to be examined to obtain a more complete account of the processes underlying the socialization of affect in both normal and atypical populations of infants.

The relationship between affective and cognitive development

Unfortunately, very few studies have examined the interrelationship between affective and cognitive development in atypical infants. Moreover, the majority of the empirical investigations have focused on Down syndrome infants. In a longitudinal investigation of the development of smiling and laughter, Cicchetti and Sroufe (1976, 1978) studied 25 Down syndrome infants from 4 through 24 months of age. These infants were seen in their homes twice monthly and were presented with a standard series of incongruous stimuli by their mothers. In addition, each infant was administered the Bayley and Uzgiris-Hunt scales of cognitive development several times during the course of this investigation by experimenters unaware of the infant's performance on the affect-eliciting items. Cicchetti and Sroufe (1976, 1978) found that, even though Down syndrome infants showed a later onset of laughter, these babies laughed at the incongruous stimulus items *in the exact order as normal infants*: first to intrusive auditory and tactile items and, next, during the second year of life, to the more complex social and visual items (such as mother taking pretend sucks on a baby bottle or crawling like a baby). Such an ordering suggests a tie between cognitive development and laughter at the more sophisticated items. Moreover, just as had been found with nonhandicapped infants, with increasing cognitive sophistication it was the Down syndrome infant's effortful assimilation of the stimulus content or participation in the event that generated the *tension* necessary for laughter and smiling, rather than mere quantity of stimulation (such as loud noises, being tickled, or being bounced on the knee). In other words, as schema formation becomes increasingly important in the elicitation of positive affect, it is no longer stimulation per se that produces the affective response but the babies' *effort* in processing the stimulus content. Down syndrome and normal infants progress from smiling and laughing to intrusive stimulation, to stimulation mediated by active attention, to smiling and laughing in response to stimulus content, and, finally, toward an *ever more active participation* in producing affectively effective stimulation.

The most compelling data on the affect-cognition interchange can be found in the cognitive test results. Level of cognitive development paralleled the level of affective development. For example, infants who laughed earliest or smiled and laughed most to the more cognitively sophisticated social and visual items were those who attained the highest level of cognitive development on the Uzgiris-Hunt and Bayley scales. Laughter was also found to be an excellent predictor of later cognitive development. The Down syndrome babies who laughed before 10 months had higher developmental quotients at age 2 years on the Bayley scales than did those babies who did not begin to laugh until later. Even more interestingly, early laughter was a better predictor of later cognitive development than was the infant's early level of cognitive development. In other words, affect predicted cognition better than cognition predicted cognition.

Gallagher and his associates (in press), in a cross-sectional study of a group of multiple-handicapped infants, found that the smiling responses of these babies to the same stimulus presentations used by Cicchetti and Sroufe (1976, 1978) were significantly related to their mental age. Gunn, Berry, and Andrews (1981) likewise provide evidence for a close association between affective and cognitive development. They followed ten Down syndrome babies longitudinally, assessing their affective reactions to a repeated auditory-visual event, the squeaking of a baby doll. They found that the majority of affective responses were elicited after the first year of life. Moreover, the onset of affective responsiveness was significantly positively correlated with level of cognitive development on the Bayley scales.

Cicchetti and Sroufe (1978) have also studied the ontogenesis of negative reactions in Down syndrome infants. They found that Down syndrome infants showed negative emotions (crying, heart-rate acceleration, and so on) later, both to direct placement on the "visual cliff" and in response to looming shadows approaching them on a "collision" course. Just as they had found in their studies of positive affect, Cicchetti and Sroufe (1978) showed that there was a close relationship between negative reactions and cognitive development. Thus, Down syndrome babies who showed early fear and distress reactions were similarly differentiated in their cognitive development, obtaining higher Bayley and Uzgiris-Hunt scores.

In a further examination of affect and cognition in Down syndrome babies, Mans, Cicchetti, and Sroufe (1978) examined the visual self-recognition of these infants. In normal infants, at approximately 18 to 24 months, visual self-recognition and the development of shame have been found to coincide with the emergence of the autonomous self and positive valuation of the self (Lewis & Brooks-Gunn, 1979). When shown their rouge-marked noses in a mirror, most normal infants evidence their self-knowledge by touching their own noses while examining their reflections in the mirror. The emergence of self-directed behaviors is first observed at 15 to 18 months and is common by 21 to 24 months of age. Mans, Cicchetti, and Sroufe (1978) found that the emergence of self-recognition was shown as well by Down syndrome babies when they achieved the appropriate cognitive developmental level. Thus, self-recognition was not the coincidental result of a particular chronological age but, rather, was closely tied to, and emerged with, cognitive development. For example, only those Down syndrome infants with a nearly normal level of cognitive functioning showed evidence of self-recognition by touching their rouge-marked noses when observing themselves in a mirror before 23 months of age. It was not until the age of 34 months and beyond that virtually all Down syndrome toddlers showed self-recognition. Similarly, the affective reactions of these infants to their rouge-marked visages paralleled those shown by normal infants. The predominant affective reaction of the younger Down syndrome infants was a change from positive affect before the application of the rouge to being sober or puzzled afterward. Older Down syndrome toddlers generally showed surprise reactions or an increase in positive affect after the application of rouge. Thus, their affective reactions, like nose touching, reflected their differential understanding of this event.

Hill and Tomlin (1981) observed the responses of two groups of preverbal retarded toddlers to watching marked or unmarked television images of themselves. One group was comprised of Down syndrome toddlers, and the other was a multihandicapped group, including toddlers with anoxia, rubella, and seizure disorders. Hill and Tomlin (1981) found that all the Down syndrome toddlers showed the curiosity and self-conscious behaviors that characterize nonhandicapped babies during the second year of life. Moreover, 11 of the 12 Down syndrome toddlers recognized their television images. In contradistinction, fewer than half of the multihandicapped group evinced self-recognition and their affective reactions were like those of normal 1-year-olds. In both groups of toddlers, Hill and Tomlin (1981) reported that all those who could recognize themselves had reached mental ages comparable to normal toddlers who manifested that aspect of self-knowledge. Only 1 of the toddlers studied by Hill and Tomlin (1981) could speak in sentences, and 10 could say a few words or phrases. Neuman and Hill (1978) likewise found that 6 of 7 preverbal autistic children recognized themselves, although the investigators did not observe the self-conscious affective reactions typically found in normal children.

Using the mirror-and-rouge paradigm, Spiker and Ricks (in press) examined the visual self-recognition of 52 autistic toddlers and children. Thirty-six (69%) of these children evinced self-recognition, whereas 16 (31%) did not. Although these two groups of autistic children did not differ in chronological age, several factors discriminated between those children who did and those who did not evidence the capacity for self-recognition. Severity of language impairment was the major factor that differentiated the two groups, such that those children who did not recognize themselves were more likely to be mute or to lack communicative speech. Those autistic children who recognized themselves also were rated higher on a global measure of overall functioning level, including: (1) appropriateness of social interaction; (2) differentiation of significant others; (3) self-care skills; (4) communicative skills; (5) academic skills; and (6) degree of bizarre psychotic behaviors. Congruent with the results of Neuman and Hill (1978), Spiker and Ricks (in press) found that the majority of the autistic children (79%) displayed completely neutral affective expressions throughout the course of the mirror-and-rouge procedure. Only 8 (15%) children showed any positive affect and each of these children demonstrated self-recognition. However, there were very few instances of the embarrassed, self-conscious, or coy emotional expressions typically displayed by normal or Down syndrome children (Hill & Tomlin, 1981; Lewis & Brooks-Gunn, 1979; Mans et al., 1978). None of the 16 autistic children who did not display the capacity for self-recognition showed any positive affect. The results of the Spiker and Ricks (in press) study are intriguing, as they document the intimate interaction among social, cognitive, affective, and linguistic competencies.

In an examination of 18 maltreated and 19 matched lower-class comparison infants, Schneider-Rosen and Cicchetti (in press) demonstrated the importance of the quality of the early attachment relationship for explaining individual differences in the development of the capacity for self-recognition. They hypothesized that the emergence of similar cognitive and affective advances underlie the achievement of these salient developmental tasks and, therefore, that the finding of a significant relationship between attachment and self-recognition would provide evidence for the mutually interacting nature of affective and cognitive development. Of the 37 19-month-old infants, 41% displayed self-recognition as assessed by the standard mirror-and-rouge paradigm. When data for the entire sample of infants were analyzed, it was found that those infants who recognized themselves were significantly more likely to be securely attached to their mothers (as assessed by Ainsworth & Wittig's, 1969, "Strange Situation"). However, a separate analysis of the maltreated and comparison groups of infants revealed a different pattern of results. Of the comparison infants who recognized themselves, 90% were securely attached to their care givers. In contrast, for those maltreated infants who recognized themselves, there was no significant relationship between this capacity and qualitative differences in the security of attachment.

An analysis of the infants' affective responses to their rouge-marked noses revealed a different pattern of results for the maltreated and nonmaltreated infants. A significantly greater percentage of the nonmaltreated infants (74%) showed an increase in positive affect following the application of rouge, whereas a greater proportion of the maltreated infants (78%) manifested neutral or negative reactions. One would expect to observe qualitatively different affective reactions to observing their rouge-marked noses in infants of various ages (Bertenthal & Fischer, 1978; Lewis & Brooks-Gunn, 1979). Younger infants typically manifest the response observed in the sample of maltreated infants, whereas older infants characteristically show a response similar to the non-maltreated infants. Thus, these results indicate that maltreated infants possess a differential understanding of this event and tend to be developmentally delayed in their affective reactions to their mirror images when assessed using the standard mirror-and-rouge paradigm.

These findings provide relevant information for the understanding of those environmental variables – for example, the experience of early maltreatment by the primary care giver – that may interact with organismic and constitutional factors to influence development. The data for the maltreated infants suggest that early maltreatment may be such a potent variable as to alter or inhibit the demonstrated relationship between security of attachment and self-recognition. In addition, the results implicate the importance of qualitative differences in the attachment relationship for understanding and accounting for individual variation in the emerging capacity for self-recognition. There were no differences between the infants who did and those who did not recognize themselves in age or in level of performance on the object permanence subscale of the Uzgiris-Hunt scales. Thus, the results suggest that cognition is necessary, but not sufficient, for the emergence of the capacity for self-recognition, thereby providing compelling evidence for the relationship between affective and cognitive development of the infant.

Several investigators have studied representational development in Down syndrome toddlers. Even though most researchers consider symbolization to be within the purview of cognitive and language development, we think it may also reveal important information about the infant's affective life. In his discussion of affective schemas, Piaget (1954, 1973) argued that they appear to be more inaccessible to consciousness in part because they are exposed to less accommodation than are intellectual schemas. However, as Anthony (1976) has noted, affective assimilation takes place with less conscious awareness than does cognitive assimilation. Studying symbolic processes may help make us more aware of these affective assimilations, as their content is likely to become manifest in symbolic play. For example, just as infants repeat cognitive acts that they are on the verge of mastering, they may also "practice" novel affective schemes to which they may be adapting within symbolic play activity. Werner and Kaplan (1963) claimed that the ability to symbolize develops as the mother-child-object matrix becomes differentiated, thereby enabling the child to contemplate the object at a distance. Similarly, the capacity to represent emotional experiences symbolically enables the infant to think about and to recognize affective responses of the self as distinct from one another.

Wing, Gould, Yeates, and Brierly (1977) discovered in a survey of more than 100 retarded subjects between 5 and 14 years of age that no child with a mental age less than 20 months engaged in symbolic play. The Down syndrome children were the most likely group to develop the capacity for symbolic representation, whereas those with identifiable organic anomalies associated with mental retardation (such as childhood psychosis, encephalitis, and rubella) were not. Taken in tandem with the results of Hill and Tomlin's (1981) study, it appears that the chromosomal condition associated with Down syndrome does not have as deleterious an impact upon development as do the constraints imposed by brain damage.

Hill and McCune-Nicholich (1981) observed 30 Down syndrome toddlers between the ages of 20 and 53 months in a play session with their mothers conducted in the toddlers' homes. The mental ages of these children ranged from 12 to 26 months. Hill and McCune-Nicholich (1981) reported that symbolic play was significantly positively correlated with mental age ($r = +.75$). Furthermore, they found greater variability on stage attainment of symbolic play, with fewer than half the sample capable of performing combined pretend acts. Those toddlers who did not manifest combined pretend play also were incapable of producing utterances greater than one word. This latter finding is congruent with the suggestion of Piaget (1954) and Werner and Kaplan (1963) that a child must have the capacity to combine symbols in order to combine symbolic play and language.

In our laboratory, we, too, have found that symbolic play and mental age are highly intercorrelated ($r = +.71$) in Down syndrome toddlers. Moreover, early affect ratings – in particular, whether or not a toddler showed fear of looming objects at 16 months – predicted stage rankings of symbolic play at ages 4 and 5 years (Motti, Cicchetti, & Sroufe, in press).

What can these data tell us about the nature of the relationship between affect and cognition? Current theoretical conceptions of this relationship are based upon the sequence of emergence of new cognitive or affective qualities or characteristics (see Hesse & Cicchetti, 1982). Emotions may be regarded as developing ontogenetically earlier than cognition, thereby providing the context within which cognitive development may occur (*cognitive epiphenomenalism*). The emergence of new emotions may be dependent upon cognitive advances that must be made before various emotions may be expressed (*emotional epiphenomenalism*). Emotions may develop along a separate pathway from cognitive advances so that the sequence, rate, and quality of change must be considered distinctly within each domain (*parallelism*). Finally, emotions may emerge in interaction with cognitive advances, thereby suggesting a progression that necessitates a consideration of developmental changes that occur across domains and that exert a reciprocal influence upon each other (*interactionism*).

Based on extant empirical data from studies of infants with Down syndrome, the high intercorrelations obtained with this developmentally heterogeneous sample of infants indicate that cognitive and emotional development are inextricably intertwined. However, when the Down syndrome babies are matched on mental age with samples of normal infants (Sroufe & Wunsch, 1972), they show less affect, both positive and negative, than would be predicted based on a purely cognitive interpretation. We take these data, as well as the data from empirical work with other populations of atypical infants, to mean that affect and cognition are indeed separate developmental systems and that both the cognitive and the emotional epiphenomenalist position are thus refuted. However, it is difficult to decide between a parallelist and an interactionist viewpoint. Since affect and cognition predicted later cognitive and symbolic development (Motti, Cicchetti, & Sroufe, in press), we lean toward an interactionist explanation, although additional data are needed to resolve this question. Furthermore, although interactionism may characterize the nature of the affect-cognition relationship during infancy, it is conceivable that other results may be obtained at later stages of development.

The investigation of atypical patterns of development may provide an important contribution toward understanding the temporal relationship between advances in the affective and cognitive domains. It may allow for an understanding of the relative contribution of emotion and cognition for the development of particular competencies during the sensorimotor period. Because the development of normal infants is generally more rapid than is the case with infants with developmental deviations, the study of atypical infants will permit us to examine more closely the unfolding of various domains. Additionally, it will contribute to our current theoretical conceptions of the relationship between cognitive and affective development in both normal and atypical populations of infants.

Conclusion

When there are prominent and pervasive disturbances in the transaction between the infant and the care giver, the infant is at a greater risk for suffering the negative consequences of the "continuum of caretaking casualty" (Sameroff & Chandler, 1975). It is likely that consistent deviations in patterns of infant–care-giver interaction, such as those that may characterize the relationship between atypical infants and their parents, will manifest themselves in the form of difficulties in accomplishing the salient developmental tasks of infancy. Because affective and cognitive competence may be the most useful and important predictor of later adaptation of invulnerability to psychopathology, it is essential that an attempt be made to identify adequacies and strengths, as well as vulnerabilities and disturbances, in the developmentally salient capacities of atypical infants so that the quality of their adaptation or maladaptation may be better understood.

Accordingly, it is necessary for future work to be directed toward assessing the processes underlying the development of emotional and cognitive competence in atypical populations of infants. Consistent with the organizational perspective of development, efforts should be made not toward cataloguing specific capacities in the cognitive and affective domains but rather toward obtaining a more holistic picture of the infant in which the changing integration and organization of competencies becomes the central objective. Instead of describing the characteristics that comprise the clinical picture of infants with early deviations in developmental patterns, it is necessary to recognize the theoretically important goal of considering the *processes* by which developmental outcomes are achieved. If early cognitive or emotional deviations do have primary impact on later development, then it becomes important to employ assessment techniques in a manner that will maximize the chances of detecting important strengths, vulnerabilities, or disabilities. The specific measures used should represent central organizing constructs so as to tap developmentally salient issues in the acquisition of affective and cognitive competence. One would not expect to use the same measures, or even to focus on the same developmental issues, in infants or in toddlers of differing ages. Therefore, the methodology employed must be determined with regard to the particular age of the infant being studied and to the nature of the salient issues that are of vital importance in this developmental stage. Furthermore, the chosen measures must be capable of detecting covert vulnerabilities, which may only become apparent under some challenge or stress. It is necessary to use progressively more demanding and difficult tasks in an effort to test the infant "at the limits" and to detect vulnerabilities or strengths. Measures that are not demanding enough – those that do not test the limits of the infant's adaptation, those that tap developmentally inappropriate skills or competencies, or those that are not guided by any coherent, rational, theoretical framework – may miss the most crucial developmental disabilities.

Similarly, it is necessary to assess cognitive and affective competencies concurrently. Implicit in the infant's emerging affective capacities is an underlying cognitive component that guides the development and expression of these skills and regulates the processes by which these functions emerge; conversely, there is an interrelationship between emerging cognitive abilities and underlying affective capacities. Thus, the constructs that are selected to guide the measurement of these competencies, the techniques that are chosen to be most appropriate for their assessment, and the framework within which the results will be evaluated, all need to reflect the mutually influencing advances made by the infant in the affective and cognitive domains.

The investigation of atypical populations of infants provides a basis for examining claims of universality of a developmental sequence and for affirming and challenging developmental theory while simultaneously contributing precision to current theoretical formulations. By studying various samples of infants who manifest disorders with different etiologies, it will be possible to discover the processes and structures that are necessary and/or sufficient for achieving the same or different developmental outcomes. By examining the nature of these outcomes, it will be possible to understand the sequencing, structuring, organization of advances, and mechanisms of change in the affective and cognitive domains in atypical infants. In this way, a reformulation and extension of Zigler's (1969, 1973) developmental/difference argument may be made by illuminating the similarities and variations in the processes and outcomes of development in different clinical populations of infants. Longitudinal studies of these atypical infants will reveal whether there tends to be a correlation between affective and cognitive problems, or whether retardations or delays may occur in one domain but not in the other. The examination of similarities or variations in cognitive or affective deviations that may become manifest in infants with different etiologies underlying their early developmental problems will contribute to our current systems of diagnosing and classifying pathology in infancy and will facilitate the direction of therapeutic intervention. Furthermore, longitudinal investigations that depict development as a series of behavioral reorganizations reflecting the salient developmental tasks or issues at each stage will allow for an evaluation of continuities or discontinuities of early cognitive or emotional deviations. Finally, the analysis of the relationship between affective and cognitive growth in both normal and atypical populations of infants will provide a major advance toward the ultimate goal of formulating an integrative model of development.

References

Ainsworth, M. The development of infant–mother attachment. In B. Caldwell & H. Ricciutti (Eds.), *Review of child development research* (Vol. 3). Chicago: University of Chicago Press, 1973.

Ainsworth, M., Bell, S., & Stayton, D. Infant–mother attachment and social development: "Socialization" as a product of reciprocal responsiveness to signals. In M. P. Richards (Ed.), *The integration of a child into a social world*. Cambridge: Cambridge University Press, 1974.

Ainsworth, M., Blehar, M., Waters, E., & Wall, S. *Patterns of attachment*. Hillsdale, N.J.: Erlbaum, 1978.

Ainsworth, M., & Wittig, B. Attachment and exploratory behavior of one-year-olds in a strange situation. In B. M. Foss (Ed.), *Determinants of infant behavior* (Vol. 4). New York: Wiley, 1969.

Als, H., Tronick, E., & Brazelton, T. B. The achievement of affective reciprocity and the beginnings of the development of autonomy: The study of a blind infant. *Journal of the American Academy of Child Psychiatry*, 1980, *19*, 22–40.

Anthony, E. J. Emotions and intelligence. In V. P. Varma & P. Williams (Eds.), *Piaget psychology and education*. Itasca, Ill.: Peacock, 1976.

Arend, R., Gove, F., & Sroufe, L. A. Continuity of individual adaptation from infancy to kindergarten: A predictive study of ego resiliency and curiosity in preschoolers. *Child Development*, 1979, *50*, 950–959.

Arieti, S. *The intrapsychic self*. New York: Basic Books, 1967.

Bates, E. *Language and context: The acquisition of pragmatics*. New York: Academic Press, 1976.

Beck, A. *Depression: Causes and treatment*. Philadelphia: University of Pennsylvania Press, 1967.

Becker, J. *Affective disorders*. Morristown, N.J.: General Learning Press, 1977.

Bell, R. A reinterpretation of the direction of effects in studies of socialization. *Psychological Review*, 1968, *75*, 81–95.

Bell, R., & Harper, L. *Child effects on adults*. Hillsdale, N.J.: Erlbaum, 1977.

Berlyne, D. *Conflict, arousal, and curiosity*. New York: McGraw-Hill, 1960.

Berlyne, D. Laughter, humor, and play. In G. Lindzey & E. Aronson (Eds.), *Handbook of social psychology* (2nd ed., Vol. 3). Boston: Addison-Wesley, 1969.

Berlyne, D. Struktur und motivation. In G. Steiner (Ed.), *Die Psychologie des 20. Jahrhunderts* (Vol. 7). Piaget und die Folgen. Zurich: Kindler-Verlag, 1978.

Berry, P., Gunn, P., & Andrews, R. Behaviour of Down's syndrome infants in a strange situation. *American Journal of Mental Deficiency*, 1980, *85*, 213–218.

Bertenthal, B. I., & Fischer, K. W. Development of self-recognition in the infant. *Developmental Psychology*, 1978, *14*, 44–50.

Bleuler, E. *Naturegeschichte der Seele* (2nd ed.). Berlin: Springer, 1932.

Bleuler, E. *Dementia praecox or the group of schizophrenias*. New York: International Universities Press, 1950.

Bowlby, J. *Attachment and loss* (Vol. 1). New York: Basic Books, 1969.

Brachfeld, S., Goldberg, S., & Sloman, J. Parent–infant interaction in free play at 8 and 12 months: Effects of prematurity and immaturity. *Infant Behavior and Development*, 1980, *3*, 289–305.

Brazelton, T. B., Koslowski, B., & Main, M. The origins of reciprocity: The early mother–infant interaction. In M. Lewis & L. Rosenblum (Eds.), *The effect of the infant on its caregiver*. New York: Wiley, 1974.

Brentano, F. *Psychologie vom empirischen Standpunkt*. Leipzig: Meiner, 1924.

Bretherton, I., & Ainsworth, M. Response of 1-year-olds to a stranger in a strange situation. In M. Lewis & L. Rosenblum (Eds.), *The origins of fear*. New York: Wiley, 1974.

Bridges, F., & Cicchetti, D. Mothers' ratings of the temperament characteristics of Down's syndrome infants. *Developmental Psychology*, 1982, *18*, 238–244.

Bridges, K. Emotional development in early infancy. *Child Development*, 1932, *3*, 324–341.

Buckhalt, J., Rutherford, R., & Goldberg, K. Verbal and nonverbal interaction of mothers with their Down's syndrome and non-retarded infants. *American Journal of Mental Deficiency*, 1978, *82*, 337–343.

Buium, N. Early maternal linguistic environment of normal and Down's syndrome language learning children. *American Journal of Mental Deficiency*, 1974, *79*, 52–58.

Butterworth, G., & Cicchetti, D. Visual calibration of posture in normal and Down's syndrome infants. *Perception*, 1978, *1*, 513–525.

Campos, J. Heart rate: A sensitive tool for the study of emotional development in the infant. In L. Lipsitt (Ed.), *Psychobiology: The significance of infancy*. Hillsdale, N.J.: Erlbaum, 1976.

Campos, J., Hiatt, S., Ramsay, D., Henderson, C., & Svejda, M. The emergence of fear on the visual cliff. In M. Lewis & L. Rosenblum (Eds.), *The development of affect*. New York: Plenum, 1978.

Campos, J., & Stenberg, C. Perception, appraisal, and emotion: The onset of social referencing. In M. Lamb & L. Sherrod (Eds.), *Infant social cognition*. Hillsdale, N.J.: Erlbaum, 1981.

Carey, W. A simplified method for measuring infant temperament. *Journal of Pediatrics*, 1970, *77*, 188–194.

Charlesworth, W. Development of the object concept: A methodological study. Paper presented at the meeting of the American Psychological Association, New York, September 1966.

Charlesworth, W. R. The role of surprise in cognitive development. In D. Elkind & J. Flavell (Eds.), *Studies in cognitive development: Essays in honor of Jean Piaget*. New York: Oxford University Press, 1969.

Charlesworth, W. R. *Surprise reactions in congenitally blind and sighted children*. National Institute of Mental Health Progress Report, 1970.

Charlesworth, W., & Kreutzer, M. Facial expressions of infants and children. In P. Ekman (Ed.), *Darwin and facial expression*. New York: Academic Press, 1973.

Cicchetti, D., & Hesse, P. Affect and intellect: Piaget's contributions to the study of infant emotional development. In R. Plutchik & H. Kellerman (Eds.), *Emotion: Theory, research, and experience* (Vol. 2). New York: Academic Press, 1983.

Cicchetti, D., & Mans, L. Sequences, stages, and structures in the organization of cognitive development in Down's syndrome infants. In I. Uzgiris & J. McV. Hunt (Eds.), *Research with scales of psychological development in infancy*. Urbana, Ill.: University of Illinois press, in press.

Cicchetti, D., & Pogge-Hesse, P. The relation between emotion and cognition in infant development. In M. Lamb & L. Sherrod (Eds.), *Infant social cognition*. Hillsdale, N.J.: Erlbaum, 1981.

Cicchetti, D., & Pogge-Hesse, P. Possible contributions of the study of organically retarded persons to developmental theory. In E. Zigler & D. Balla (Eds.), *Mental retardation: The developmental-difference controversy*. Hillsdale, N.J.: Erlbaum, 1982.

Cicchetti, D., & Rizley, R. Developmental perspectives on the etiology, intergenerational transmission, and sequelae of child maltreatment. In R. Rizley & D. Cicchetti (Eds.), *Developmental perspectives on child maltreatment*. San Francisco: Jossey-Bass, 1981.

Cicchetti, D., & Serafica, F. The interplay among behavioral systems: Illustration from the study of attachment, affiliation, and wariness in young Down's syndrome children. *Developmental Psychology*, 1981, *17*, 36–49.

Cicchetti, D., & Sroufe, L. A. The relationship between affective and cognitive development in Down's syndrome infants. *Child Development*, 1976, *47*, 920–929.

Cicchetti, D., & Sroufe, L. A. An organizational view of affect: Illustration from the study of Down's syndrome infants. In M. Lewis & L. Rosenblum (Eds.), *The development of affect*. New York: Plenum, 1978.

Cummings, E. M., Zahn-Waxler, C., & Radke-Yarrow, M. Young children's responses to expressions of anger and affection by others in the family. *Child Development*, 1981, *52*, 1274–1282.

Cytryn, L. Studies of behavior in children with Down's syndrome. In E. J. Anthony (Ed.), *Explorations in child psychiatry*. New York: Plenum, 1975.

Darwin, C. *The expression of the emotions in man and animals*. London: Murray, 1872.

Decarie, T. *Intelligence and affectivity in early childhood*. New York: International Universities Press, 1965.

DesLauriers, A. Play, symbols, and the development of language. In M. Rutter & E. Schopler (Eds.), *Autism*. New York: Plenum, 1978.

DiVitto, B., & Goldberg, S. The development of parent–infant interaction as a function of newborn medical status. In T. Field, A. Sostek, S. Goldberg, & H. Shuman (Eds.), *Infants born at risk*. Jamaica, N.Y.: Spectrum, 1979.

Duffy, E. An explanation of "emotional" phenomena without the use of the concept "emotion." *Journal of General Psychology*, 1941, *25*, 283–293.

Egeland, B., & Sroufe, L. A. Developmental sequelae of maltreatment in infancy. *New Directions for Child Development*, 1981, *11*, 77–92.

Eibl-Eibesfeldt, I. Human ethology: Concepts and implications for the science of man. *Behavioral and Brain Sciences*, 1979, *2*, 1–57.

Ekman, P. Universals and cultural differences in facial expressions of emotion. *Nebraska symposium on motivation* (Vol. 19). Lincoln: University of Nebraska Press, 1972.

Ekman, P. Biological and cultural contributions to body and facial movement. In J. Blacking (Ed.), *The anthropology of the body*. London: Academic Press, 1977.

Ekman, P., & Friesen, W. *Manual for the facial action coding system*. Palo Alto, Calif.: Consulting Psychologists Press, 1978.

Ekman, P., Friesen, W., & Ellsworth, P. *Emotion in the human face: Guidelines for research and an integration of findings*. Elmsford, N.Y.: Pergamon Press, 1972.

Ekman, P., & Oster, H. Facial expressions of emotion. *Annual Review of Psychology*, 1979, *30*, 527–554.

Emde, R. Levels of meaning for infant emotions: A biosocial view. In W. A. Collins (Ed.), *Minnesota symposia on child psychology*. Hillsdale, N.J.: Erlbaum, 1980. (a)

Emde, R. Toward a psychoanalytic theory of affect. In S. Greenspan & G. Pollock (Eds.), *Psychoanalytic contributions toward understanding personality and development* (Vol. 1). Atlanta, Ga.: National Institute of Mental Health, 1980. (b)

Emde, R., & Brown, C. Adaptation to the birth of a Down's syndrome infant: Grieving and maternal attachment. *Journal of the American Academy of Child Psychiatry*, 1978, *17*, 299–323.

Emde, R., Gaensbauer, T., & Harmon, R. *Emotional expression in infancy: A biobehavioral study*. New York: International Universities Press, 1976.

Emde, R., Katz, E., & Thorpe, J. Emotional expression in infancy: II. Early deviations in Down's syndrome. In M. Lewis & L. Rosenblum (Eds.), *The development of affect*. New York: Plenum, 1978.

Engel, G. Attachment behavior, object relations and the dynamic-economic points of view: Critical review of Bowlby's *Attachment and Loss*. *International Journal of Psychoanalysis*, 1971, *52*, 183–196.

Erikson, E. *Childhood and society*. New York: Norton, 1950.

Fairbairn, W. Steps in the development of an object-relations theory of the personality. *British Journal of Medical Psychology*, 1949, *22*, 152–161.

Field, T. Effects of early separation, interactive deficits and experimental manipulation on mother–infant interaction. *Child Development*, 1977, *48*, 763–771.

Fraiberg, S. Blind infants and their mothers: An examination of the sign system. In M. Lewis & L. Rosenblum (Eds.), *The effect of the infant on its caregiver*. New York: Wiley, 1974.

Fraiberg, S. *Insights from the blind*. New York: International Universities Press, 1977.

Freedman, D. Smiling in blind infants and the issue of innate versus acquired. *Journal of Child Psychology and Psychiatry*, 1964, *5*, 171–184.

Freud, S. Analysis terminable and interminable. *Standard Edition* (Vol. 23). London: Hogarth Press, 1955. (Originally published, 1937.)

Freud, S. Studies on hysteria. *Standard Edition* (Vol. 2). London: Hogarth Press, 1955. (Originally published, 1895.)

Freud, S. Inhibitions, symptoms, and anxiety. *Standard Edition*, 20:75–175. London: Hogarth Press, 1959. (Originally published, 1926.)

Freud, S. The ego and the id. *Standard Edition*, 19:3–66. London: Hogarth Press, 1961. (Originally published, 1923–4.)

Freud, S. On the grounds for detaching a particular syndrome from neurasthenia under the description "Anxiety Neurosis." *Standard Edition*, 3:87–139. London: Hogarth Press, 1962. (Originally published, 1895.)

Freudenberg, R., Driscoll, J., & Stern, G. Reactions of adult humans to cries of normal and abnormal infants. *Journal of Infant Behavior and Development*, 1978, *1*, 224–227.

Frodi, A., & Lamb, M. Child abusers' responses to infant smiles and cries. *Child Development*, 1980, *51*, 238–241.

Gaensbauer, T., Mrazek, D., & Harmon, R. Affective behavior patterns in abused and/or neglected infants. In N. Frude (Ed.), *The understanding and prevention of child abuse: Psychological approaches*. London: Concord Press, 1980.

Gaensbauer, T., & Sands, S. Distorted affective communications in abused/neglected infants and their potential impact on caretakers. *Journal of the American Academy of Child Psychiatry*, 1979, *18*, 236–250.

Gallagher, R., Jens, K., & O'Donnell, K. The effect of physical status on the affective expression of handicapped infants. *Journal of Infant Behavior and Development*, in press.

Goldberg, S. Social competence in infancy: A model of parent-infant interactions. *Merrill-Palmer Quarterly*, 1977, *23*, 164–177.

Goldberg, S. Some biological aspects of early parent–infant interaction. In S. Moore & C. Cooper (Eds.), *The young child: Reviews of research*. Washington, D.C.: National Association for the Education of Young Children, in press.

Goldstein, K. *Human nature in the light of psychopathology*. Cambridge, Mass.: Harvard University Press, 1939.

Goldstein, K. *The organism: A holistic approach to biology derived from pathological data in man*. New York: American Book, 1940.

Green, A. Conceptions of affect. *International Journal of Psychoanalysis*, 1977, *58*, 129–156.

Greenspan, S. *Intelligence and adaptation*. New York: International Universities Press, 1979.

Greenspan, S., & Lourie, R. Developmental structuralist approach to the classification of adaptive and pathologic personality organizations: Infancy and early childhood. *American Journal of Psychiatry*, 1981, *138*, 725–735.

Gunn, P., Berry, P., & Andrews, R. The temperament of Down's syndrome infants: A research note. *Journal of Child Psychology and Psychiatry*, 1980, *21*, 1–6.

Gunn, P., Berry, P., & Andrews, R. The affective response of Down's syndrome infants to a repeated event. *Child Development*, 1981, *52*, 745–748.

Gunnar, M. Control, warning signals, and distress in infancy. *Developmental Psychology*, 1980, *16*, 281–289.

Haviland, J. Looking smart: The relationship between affect and intelligence in infancy. In M. Lewis (Ed.), *Origins of infant intelligence*. New York: Plenum, 1976.

Hesse, P., & Cicchetti, D. Perspectives on an integrated theory of emotional development. In D. Cicchetti & P. Hesse (Eds.), *Emotional development*. San Francisco: Jossey-Bass, 1982.

Hill, P., & McCune-Nicholich, L. Pretend play and patterns of cognition in Down's syndrome children. *Child Development*, 1981, *52*, 611–617.

Hill, P., & McCune-Nicholich, L. Pretend play and patterns of cognition in Down's syndrome children. *Child Development*, 1981, *52*, 611–617.

Hill, S., & Tomlin, C. Self recognition in retarded children. *Child Development*, 1981, *52*, 145–150.

Hoffman, M., Salapatek, P., Kuskowski, M., & Cicchetti, D. Evidence for visual memory in the evoked potential of human infants. Presented at the Society for Research in Child Development Meeting, San Francisco, April 1979.

Izard, C. *Human emotions*. New York: Plenum, 1977.

Izard, C. On the ontogenesis of emotions and emotion-cognition relationships in infancy. In M. Lewis & M. Rosenblum (Eds.), *The development of affect*. New York: Plenum, 1978.

Izard, C. Emotions as motivations: An evolutionary-developmental perspective. *Nebraska symposium on motivation* (Vol. 26). Lincoln: University of Nebraska Press, 1979. (a)

Izard, C. *The maximally discriminative facial movement coding system*. Newark, Del.: Instructional Resources Center, University of Delaware, 1979. (b)

Izard, C., & Buechler, S. Emotion expressions and personality integration in infancy. In C. Izard (Ed.), *Emotions in personality and psychopathology*. New York: Plenum, 1979.

James, W. *Memories and studies*. New York: Longmans, Green, 1917.

James, W. *Collected essays and reviews*. New York: Longmans, Green, 1920.

Jones, O. Mother–child communication with prelinguistic Down's syndrome and normal infants. In H. Schaffer (Ed.), *Studies in mother–infant interaction*. New York: Academic Press, 1977.

Kagan, J. *Change and continuity in infancy*. New York: Wiley, 1971.

Kagan, J. *The second year*. Cambridge, Mass.: Harvard University Press, 1981.

Kagan, J., Kearsley, R., & Zelazo, P. *Infancy*. Cambridge, Mass.: Harvard University Press, 1978.

Kanner, L. Autistic disturbances of affective contact. *Nervous Child*, 1943, *2*, 217–250.

Keogh, B., & Kopp, C. From assessment to intervention. In L. Lloyd and F. Minfie (Eds.), *Early communicative and behavioral assessment*. Baltimore: University Park Press, 1978.

Kessen, W. Early cognitive development: Hot or cold? In T. Mischel (Ed.), *Cognitive development and epistemology*. New York: Academic Press, 1971.

Kopp, C. Antecedents of self-regulation: A developmental perspective. *Developmental Psychology*, 1982, *18*, 199–214.

Lanzetta, J., Cartwright-Smith, J., & Kleck, R. Effects of nonverbal dissimulation on emotional experience and autonomic arousal. *Journal of Personality and Social Psychology*, 1976, *33*, 354–370.

Lewis, M., & Brooks, J. Self-knowledge and emotional development. In M. Lewis & L. Rosenblum (Eds.), *The development of affect*. New York: Plenum, 1978.

Lewis, M., & Brooks-Gunn, J. *Social cognition and the acquisition of self*. New York: Plenum, 1979.

Liben, L. (Ed.). *Deaf children: Developmental perspectives*. New York: Academic Press, 1978.

Ling, D., & Ling, A. Communication development in the first three years of life. *Journal of Speech and Hearing Research*, 1974, *17*, 146–159.

Loevinger, J. *Ego development*. San Francisco: Jossey-Bass, 1976.

Londerville, S., & Main, M. Security of attachment, compliance, and maternal training methods in the second year of life. *Developmental Psychology*, 1981, *17*, 289–299.

Main, M. Analysis of a peculiar form of reunion behavior seen in some daycare children: Its history and sequelae in children who are home-reared. In R. Webb (Ed.), *Social development in daycare*. Baltimore: Johns Hopkins University Press, 1977.

Main, M., Tomasini, L., & Tolan, W. Differences among mothers of infants judged to differ in security. *Developmental Psychology*, 1979, *15*, 472–473.

Malatesta, C., & Haviland, J. Learning display rules: The socialization of emotion expression in infancy. *Child Development*, 1982, *53*, 991–1003.

Mandler, G. The interruption of behavior. *Nebraska symposium on motivation* (Vol. 12). Lincoln: University of Nebraska Press, 1964.

Mandler, G. *Mind and emotion*. New York: Wiley, 1975.

Mans, L., Cicchetti, D., & Sroufe, L. A. Mirror reactions of Down's syndrome infants and toddlers: Cognitive underpinnings of self-recognition. *Child Development*, 1978, *49*, 1247–1250.

Matas, L., Arend, R., & Sroufe, L. A. Continuity of adaptation in the second year: The relationship between quality of attachment and later competence. *Child Development*, 1978, *49*, 547–556.

McCall, R., & McGhee, P. The discrepancy hypothesis of attention and affect. In F. Weizmann & I. Uzgiris (Eds.), *The structuring of experience*. New York: Plenum, 1977.

Meadow, K. The development of deaf children. In E. M. Hetherington (Ed.), *Review of child development research* (Vol. 5). Chicago: University of Chicago Press, 1975.

Motti, F., Cicchetti, D., & Sroufe, L. A. From infant affect expression to symbolic play: The coherence of development in Down's syndrome children. *Child Development*, in press.

Neuman, C., & Hill, S. Self-recognition and stimulus preference in autistic children. *Developmental Psychobiology*, 1978, *11*, 571–578.

Oster, H. Facial expression and affect development. In M. Lewis & L. Rosenblum (Eds.), *The development of affect*. New York: Plenum, 1978.

Peiper, A. *Cerebral function in infancy and childhood*. New York: Consultants Bureau, 1963.

Piaget, J. *The origins of intelligence in children*. New York: International Universities Press, 1952.

Piaget, J. *The construction of reality in the child*. New York: Basic Books, 1954.

Piaget, J. *Play, dreams and imitation in children*. New York: Norton, 1962.

Piaget, J. The affective and the cognitive unconscious. *Journal of the American Psychoanalytic Association*, 1973, *21*, 249–261.

Piaget, J. *Intelligence and affectivity: Their relationship during child development*. Palo Alto, Calif.: Annual Reviews, 1981. (Originally published, 1954.)

Pribram, K. The new neurology and the biology of emotion: A structural approach. *American Psychologist*, 1967, *22*, 830–838.

Pribram, K. The biology of emotions and other feelings. In R. Plutchik & H. Kellerman (Eds.), *Emotion: Theory, research and experience* (Vol. 1). New York: Academic Press, 1980.

Plutchik, R. *Emotion: A psychoevolutionary synthesis*. New York: Harper & Row, 1980.

Rapaport, D. *Emotions and memory*. New York: International Universities Press, 1950. (Originally published, 1942.)

Rapaport, D. On the psychoanalytic theory of affects. *International Journal of Psychoanalysis*, 1953, *34*, 177–198.

Rapaport, D. Psychoanalysis as a developmental psychology. In B. Kaplan & S. Wapner (Eds.), *Perspectives in psychological theory*. New York: International Universities Press, 1960.

Reese, H., & Overton, W. Models of development and theories of development. In L. R. Goulet & P. Baltes (Eds.), *Lifespan developmental psychology: Research and theory*. New York: Academic Press, 1970.

Robson, K. The role of eye-to-eye contact in maternal–infant attachment. *Journal of Child Psychology and Psychiatry*, 1967, *8*, 13–25.

Saarni, C. Cognitive and communicative features of emotional experience, or do you show what you think you feel? In M. Lewis & L. Rosenblum (Eds.), *The development of affect*. New York: Plenum, 1978.

Sagi, A., & Hoffman, M. L. Empathic distress in newborns. *Developmental Psychology*, 1976, *12*, 175–176.

Sameroff, A., & Chandler, M. Reproductive risk and the continuum of care-taking casualty. In F. Horowitz (Ed.), *Review of child development research* (Vol. 4). Chicago: University of Chicago Press, 1975.

Santostefano, S., & Baker, A. The contribution of developmental psychology. In B. Wolman (Ed.), *Manual of child psychopathology*. New York: Wiley, 1972.

Schlesinger, H. The hearing impaired preschooler. In N. Enzer (Ed.), *Social and emotional development: The preschooler*. New York: Walker, 1978.

Schlesinger, H., & Meadow, J. *Sound and sign: Childhood deafness and mental health*. Berkeley: University of California Press, 1972.

Schneider-Rosen, K. S., & Cicchetti, D. The relationship between affect and cognition in maltreated infants: Quality of attachment and the development of visual self-recognition. *Child Development*, in press.

Serafica, F., & Cicchetti, D. Down's syndrome children in a strange situation: Attachment and exploratory behaviors. *Merrill-Palmer Quarterly*, 1976, *22*, 137–150.

Shultz, T., & Zigler, E. Emotional concomitants of visual mastery in infants. *Journal of Experimental Child Psychology*, 1970, *10*, 390–402.

Simner, M. Newborn's response to the cry of another infant. *Developmental Psychology*, 1971, *5*, 136–150.

Skinner, B. F. *Science and human behavior*. New York: Macmillan, 1953.

Sorce, J., & Emde, R. The meaning of infant emotional expressions: Regularities in caregiving responses in normal and Down's syndrome infants. *Journal of Child Psychology and Psychiatry*, 1982, *23*, 145–158.

Spiker, D., & Ricks, M. Visual self-recognition in autistic children: Developmental relationships. *Child Development*, in press.

Spitz, R. *A genetic field theory of ego formation*. New York: International Universities Press, 1959.

Sroufe, L. A. The coherence of individual development. *American Psychologist*, 1979, *34*, 834–841. (a)

Sroufe, L. A. Socioemotional development. In J. Osofsky (Ed.), *Handbook of infant development*. New York: Wiley, 1979. (b)

Sroufe, L. A., & Waters, E. The ontogenesis of smiling and laughter: A perspective on the organization of development in infancy. *Psychological Review*, 1976, *83*, 173–189.

Sroufe, L. A., & Waters, E. Attachment as an organizational construct. *Child Development*, 1977, *48*, 1184–1199. (a)

Sroufe, L. A., & Waters, E. Heart rate as a convergent measure in clinical and developmental research. *Merrill-Palmer Quarterly*, 1977, *23*, 3–28. (b)

Sroufe, L. A., & Wunsch, J. The development of laughter in the first year of life. *Child Development*, 1972, *43*, 1326–1344.

Stechler, G., & Carpenter, G. A viewpoint on early affective development. In J. Hellmuth (Ed.), *Exceptional infant*. Seattle, Wash.: Special Child Publications, 1967.

Steiner, J. The gustofacial response: Observation on normal and anencephalic newborn infants. In J. Bosma (Ed.), *Fourth symposium on oral sensation and perception*. Bethesda, Md.: U.S. Department of Health, Education, and Welfare, 1973.

Stern, D. *The first relationship*. Cambridge, Mass.: Harvard University Press, 1977.

Thomas, A., & Chess, S. *Temperament and development*. New York: Brunner/Mazel, 1977.

Thomas, A., Chess, S., & Birch, H. *Temperament and behavior disorders in children*. New York: New York University Press, 1968.

Thomas, H. Discrepancy hypotheses: Methodological and theoretical considerations. *Psychological Review*, 1971, *78*, 249–259.

Tomkins, S. *Affect, imagery, consciousness* (Vol. 1). New York: Springer-Verlag, 1962.

Tomkins, S. *Affect, imagery, consciousness* (Vol. 2). New York: Springer-Verlag, 1963.

Tomkins, S. Affect as amplification: Some modifications in theory. In R. Plutchik & H. Kellerman (Eds.), *Emotion: Theory, research, and experience* (Vol. 1). New York: Academic Press, 1980.

Ulrich, S. *Elizabeth*. Ann Arbor: University of Michigan Press, 1972.

Vygotsky, L. *Thought and language*. Boston: MIT Press, 1962.

Waddington, C. H. *Principles of development and differentiation*. New York: Macmillan, 1966.

Waters, E., Wippman, J., & Sroufe, L. A. Attachment, positive affect, and competence in the peer group: Two studies in construct validation. *Child Development*, 1979, *50*, 821–829.

Wedell-Monning, J., & Lumley, J. Child deafness and mother-child interaction. *Child Development*, 1980, *51*, 766–774.

Weiss, P. Deformities as cues to understanding development of form. *Perspectives in Biology and Medicine*, 1961, *4*, 133–151.

Weiss, P. *Principles of development*. New York: Hafner, 1969.

Werner, H. *Comparative psychology of mental development*. Chicago: Follett, 1948.

Werner, H., & Kaplan, B. *Symbol formation*. New York: Wiley, 1963.

White, R. Motivation reconsidered: The concept of competence. *Psychological Review*, 1959, *66*, 297–333.

Wing, L., Gould, G., Yeates, S., & Brierly, L. Symbolic play in severely mentally retarded and in autistic children. *Journal of Child Psychology and Psychiatry*, 1977, *18*, 167–178.

Wundt, W. *An introduction to psychology*. London: G. Allen, 1912.

Zelazo, P., & Komer, M. Infant smiling to non-social stimuli and the recognition hypothesis. *Child Development*, 1971, *42*, 1327–1339.

Zigler, E. Developmental versus difference theories of mental retardation and the problem of motivation. *American Journal of Mental Deficiency*, 1969, *73*, 536–556.

Zigler, E. The retarded child as a whole person. In D. K. Routh (Ed.), *The experimental study of mental retardation*. Chicago: Aldine, 1973.

Zigler, E., & Trickett, P. I.Q., social competence, and evaluation of early childhood intervention programs. *American Psychologist*, 1978, *33*, 789–798.

Part III

Language, memory, and emotion

13   Children's understanding of emotions

Reid M. Schwartz and Tom Trabasso

What does it mean when we say that we understand an emotion? To illustrate our approach to how children (as well as adults) might show their understanding, consider the following protocols obtained on two 8-year-old children, John and Jane:

1. Interviewer: "One day, Mary gave her mother a present. How did Mary feel? Did she feel *care* or did she feel *safe*?"
   John: "Care."
   Interviewer: "Why did you say that Mary felt *care* instead of *safe*?"
   John: "Well, care is when you love someone. When you feel safe, you feel like no monsters are going to get you or no one is going to take away your bike."

2. Interviewer: "One day, Mary cried and cried. How was she feeling? Was she feeling *worried* or was she feeling *sad*?"
   Jane: "Sad."
   Interviewer: "Why did you pick *sad* instead of *worried*?"
   Jane: "Well, if I had to take a hard test and I knew I couldn't do it, I would feel worried. But if my cat died I would feel sad and cry."

In these interviews, the children were asked to select an emotion word that was appropriate as a description for how a story character felt when (1) something had happened to her and (2) she was expressing an emotional reaction. These causal antecedents and consequences were responded to by the respective children by selecting the appropriate term over a contrasting word. In the first example, the contrast is between two positive emotions on a dimension of whether the emotion is directed toward another or is an assessment of the self. In the second, the contrast is on whether things are *going* or *went* badly.

The choice between the contrasts is made possible by the child's knowledge about antecedent and consequences. In the first example, Mary did something socially desirable and is assumed to express an action that is a causal consequence of care (or love) toward her mother. In the second, Mary cried and is assumed to express an action that one shows when one feels sad, such as after experiencing a loss.

In answering the Why questions, both children justify their choices in mean-

The research reported in this chapter was supported by funds from the National Institute of Education Grant NIE-G-79-0125 and the Spencer Foundation to T. Trabasso.

ingful ways. John recognizes that care is equivalent to love. He further makes a distinction by illustrating what he means by safe, in contrast, namely, when there exists no threat. Jane, too, illustrates or instantiates her choice with contrasting causes. For her, anticipating a difficult test is a cause for worry over possible failure, while a loss of her cat is a cause for sadness and crying.

In our study of how children understand emotions, we took, as a fundamental part of our definition of meaning, a functional definition used by philosophers of language. For example, John Dewey provides a succinct definition of the type we have in mind: "To grasp the meaning of a thing, event or a situation is to see it in its relations to other things; to note how it operates or functions, what consequences follow it; what causes it; what uses it can be put to" (1963, p. 135).

This definition captures a major set of components of what, for us, constitutes an understanding of emotions. To understand an emotion is to know the situations in which it occurs, to know the states, events, and actions that relate to it, to know how it operates physiologically and how it functions motivationally, to know what actions and expressions follow as consequences from it, to know what states, state changes, events, and actions cause it, and to know what uses emotions can be put to. We shall, in the research reported here, operationalize this functional definition and use it to find out how children understand emotions. In addition to determining whether or not they can understand the antecedent, concurrent, and consequent aspects of emotion, we are also interested in knowing whether they can find similarities and differences among emotions in terms of semantic features or dimensions. These dimensional contrasts are yet another major aspect of meaning, common to a variety of theories on emotion.

Thus our study on the meaning of emotions deals with two levels of meaning: (1) a more concrete, instantiated level of contexts in which emotions occur and (2) an abstract level of semantic features or characterizing dimensions. Both levels and their interaction seem to be of use in answering the question of what we mean by understanding emotions.

Understanding emotions appears to require that children and adults have and use naïve theories about emotions. It may be the case that these naïve theories are not very different in their simplest forms from the sophisticated theories of those who study emotions. In fact, we shall use one such theory (Dahl, 1978) to construct our interview items in the belief that the difference between naïve and sophisticated theories is much less than one may normally assume. Our use of theory about emotion is out of a concern with providing a systematic rather than an intuitive approach to the study of children's understanding of emotion. Our definition of emotion in terms of the logical relations of cause and consequence is also in contrast to most developmental studies, which assume that young children lack such capabilities (Chandler & Greenspan, 1972; Harris & Olthof, 1982; Piaget, 1962, 1964, 1965).

Developmental studies

We shall now briefly review previous studies on what children know about emotions. For the most part, these studies are atheoretical and rely upon intuitive notions about emotions. However, an examination of the purposes and methods as well as findings and interpretations reveals implicit assumptions held by the investigators. For example, factor analytic or multidimensional scaling studies (Davitz, 1969; Russell, 1978, 1979, 1980) seek a set of basic dimensions that categorize the meanings that children attach to emotion words. On the other hand, open-ended or partially structured interviews (Demos, 1964; Harris & Olthof, 1982; Harter, 1980; Surbey, 1979; Wolman, Lewis, & King, 1971, 1972a, 1972b, 1972c, 1972d) try to assess the child's concept of emotions in terms of what *the child* can tell the interviewer about emotions. The child's answers are interpreted and categorized, however, in ways that either reflect implicit theories about emotion or are examined from a Piagetian perspective. The categorized data are most often presented in terms of age- and sex-related differences (or similarities). Prediction studies (Borke, 1971; Burns & Cavey, 1957; Gnepp, 1982) ask children to assign an emotional state term to pictured or story characters on the basis of their facial or situational cues. Here the interest is in whether the child prefers or uses one cue or the other and whether these preferences change with age. The data are frequently interpreted in terms of Piagetian issues concerning decentration, egocentrism, and empathy.

Farmer (1967) was among the first modern researchers to study children's understanding via answers to questions about personal feelings. Farmer found that older children could demonstrate greater knowledge about the physiological functioning, language, expression, control, arousal, and so on of emotions than could younger children. Using cluster analysis, Davitz (1969) reanalyzed Farmer's data and found that older children responded more like adults and that strong adult clusters appeared earlier in children's reports, whereas clusters that were least emphasized by adults appeared later in development. Thus children demonstrate knowledge about emotions similar to that of adults; when they begin to manifest this knowledge corresponds directly to the degree to which adults demonstrate such knowledge.

Other interview studies by Wolman and his colleagues and by Demos represent expanded versions of Farmer's (1967) work. In particular, questions concerning conditions of emotional arousal and intentions were included. For example, Wolman and his associates (1972a) found that children's attributions of emotional feelings to internal events increase as they become older; 5-year-olds make equal external–internal attributions, whereas 75% of young adolescents report antecedents of emotional states within themselves. Likewise, the youngest children showed a high understanding of intentions and actions in response to physical, but not emotional, states, whereas the older children demonstrated a clear knowledge of intentions related to emotions (see also Harris & Olthof, in press, who find increasing mentalistic explanations of emotions with age).

Demos (1974), in an unpublished Ph.D. thesis, has conducted perhaps the most comprehensive study of children's understanding of emotions, using interview methods and merging the clinical orientation of the previous work just cited with Piaget's and others' (e.g., Ericson's) notions of development. Demos studied conditions that arouse emotions, understanding emotion in others and in inanimate objects by children 6 to 12 years in age for ten affect terms.

Of interest here are Demos's questions and data concerning (1) conditions that arouse emotions, (2) experience of emotion, (3) consequences of emotional states, and (4) distinctions made between affects. First, as to antecedents, there emerged clear categories and consensus for the different emotions, with more variation resulting from the emotions than from age. Demos also replicated the finding of Wolman and his associates (1972a) that demonstrates a relationship between age and internal attribution and the Davitz (1969) finding that clusters most emphasized by adults appear earlier in the children's reports. Her data on consequences were less systematic, yielding no clear conclusions. Distinctions were assessed by having independent raters make general impressions of the child's ability to distinguish between pairs of emotions. The ability to make these distinctions increased with age, with the largest shift occurring between 6 and 9 years.

Surbey (1979; see also Trabasso, Stein, & Johnson, 1981), in a master's thesis directed by the second author, explored emotional state understanding in 3-year-old children (range: 3.0 to 4.6 years, mean = 3.10 years), using a generation paradigm. For six emotional states (the emotions, happy, surprised, excited, scared, angry, and sad, were taken from Izard's, 1971, list of basic emotions), each child was shown a picture and was told the beginning of a story, such as: "This is a picture of Jennifer. She was so *angry* that her mother and father could tell she was *angry*. And all of her friends could tell she was very *angry*." In one condition, causal antecedents were elicited by a question, for example, "Why do you think that Jennifer was so angry?" In another condition, consequences were elicited, for example, "And then what do you think Jennifer did?"

Surbey analyzed the answers generated to these questions in two ways. First, the answers were judged by independent judges as to whether they were plausible causes or consequences. The range of proportions of plausible judgments was from .56 to .94 and averaged .73 for these very young children. Second, to assess whether the children differentiated emotions as well as causes and consequences, their responses were sorted into content categories and the distributions of children over these categories were intercorrelated and subjected to a cluster analysis. Causes were highly differentiated from consequences, as the correlation between the distributions of the children's answers for causes and consequences was low ($r = -.25$). Further, positive and negative emotions were highly differentiated within causes and consequences ($r = -.19$ and .00, respectively). The negative emotion scared was highly differentiated from angry and sad. The latter as a group were more differentiated than were happy, excited, and surprised.

These data indicate that children as young as 3 years in age can communicate meanings and distinctions between emotions in terms of their causal antecedents and consequences. In addition, in comparing their distinctions with those made by adults (Davitz, 1969; Izard, 1977), the 3-year-olds' understanding bears a strong similarity to that of the adults. For example, Davitz (1969) had adults rate 50 emotional terms for the presence or absence of 556 descriptive terms (e.g., my head spins, there is a radiant glow). A factor analysis yielded two main dimensions, negative and positive, similar to that found by Surbey. A further analysis by Davitz yielded more detailed categories, the main ones being happy or cheerful terms, sad or depressed terms, and another set of negative terms, including angry and afraid. Apparently, children tend to combine sad and angry more than do adults. These data also support Borke's (1971) claim that young children are capable of complex, logical, cognitive tasks involving emotions.

Recent work by Russell (1978, 1979, 1980; Russell & Ridgeway, 1981), using factor analytic and multidimensional scaling on children, 8 years of age and older, as well as adults, shows that the positive–negative dimension is a strong semantic component of affect. Russell asked children such questions as, "Do you feel _____ today?" for each of 51 emotion words. Clusters and dimensions were determined for the resultant answers. In other experiments, 28 emotion words were sorted into different numbers of piles, the results of which were scaled. Both children and adults organized emotions around two bipolar dimensions: pleasure–unpleasure and degree of arousal.

As mentioned earlier, a third experimental paradigm involved cue-prediction studies. Burns and Cavey (1957), using a conflicting-cue technique, asked the child to decide how a protagonist feels given two cues, a specific situation and a facial expression. The conflict results from dissonance between each cue, that is, a happy face in a sad situation or sad face in a happy situation. They found that older children (5–6 years) gave significantly more responses consistent with the facial expression than did younger children (3–5 years). They concluded from this that younger children "project" their own feelings onto the situation, have difficulty comprehending the experimental task, use egocentric thinking, and have less social sensitivity than do older children (see also Chandler & Greenspan, 1972).

However, when Borke (1971) presented to children a series of stories depicting a protagonist in situations that evoked happiness, sadness, anger, and fear and asked the children to select one of four faces (happy, sad, angry, and afraid) to complete the stories, she found that 3-year-olds could differentiate happy and unhappy emotions in others and that by age 4 children could differentiate anger/fear/sadness at greater than chance expectations. This was taken as evidence that the very young child is not egocentric, that they are aware of others' emotions and can differentiate between emotions that another person is feeling.

Additional support for this conclusion comes in a cross-cultural study by Izard (1971). He administered both an emotion recognition and an emotion labeling task to American and French children 2 to 9 years old. In the emotion labeling task, the children were shown 18 photos of faces with different facial expressions (2 depicting each of the 9 categories of emotion defined by Izard) and asked, "How is this person feeling?" For the emotion recognition task the children were administered a forced comparison procedure in which they selected 1 of 3 facial expressions to illustrate "Show me who is feeling . . ." Izard found that children even as young as 2 years were able to recognize the emotions of joy, sadness, anger, fear, and surprise at greater than chance expectations. Although there were age-related differences, there was also significant variation in scores resulting from specific emotions. The emotion labeling task showed that young children have far more difficulty producing their own emotion labels than in recognizing different emotions. The author concluded that experimental procedures that depend upon the subjects' verbal production of emotion terms may "grossly underestimate the role of emotion in the child's life."

In an attempt to resolve the controversy, Gnepp (1982), in a Ph.D. thesis directed by the second author, presented 4-, 7-, and 12-year-olds with sets of conflicting and nonconflicting cues. For example, in the conflicting cue series children were shown a picture of a birthday party in which a protagonist had a sad face and asked, "Here is a boy at a birthday party. How do you think he feels?" Following the initial response, questions such as: "How can you tell how he feels? (turning picture over). What do you remember about the story and how the boy looked? Why does the boy look sad when he is at the birthday party?" In the nonconflicting series, emotion-evoking situations were paired with blank or corresponding facial expressions and a blank situation (a boy sitting in a chair) was paired with various facial expressions. Gnepp found that the youngest children prefer facial cues over situations and this preference decreases with age. In addition, there are developmental differences in how children integrate the conflicting cues; however, even 4-year-olds are capable of such integration. These findings run counter to Burns and Cavey (1957), and lead to the conclusion that 3- and 4-year-olds possess a capacity for social sensitivity and that developmental differences may be accounted for by the increased knowledge and experience of older children.

In sum, the studies on children's understanding of the language of emotions found evidence of developmental differences in regard to such comprehension. Primarily, these differences related to the type of language used by children to convey their comprehension. The number of responses increased with age, the types of answers most frequently given by adults appeared earlier, the types of responses least emphasized by adults appeared later, older children's responses were more specific and scorable, older children qualified their statements more, and older children were better able to describe their intentions to resolve emotional states.

The authors in general, with the exception of Surbey, argued that these findings suggest cognitive immaturity in children younger than 9 years. They felt that the reasoning of younger children was different from that of older children and adults.

Despite these interpretations, another pattern of findings also emerged. Scores varied from one emotion to the next. At times (e.g., in understanding the circumstances that arouse affect), more variation occurred in the scores as a result of the emotion than of the age of the subject. Although younger children did not give as many responses, at times, their responses were as complex as those of 12-year-olds and adults. Three-year-old children showed a causal understanding of emotions, which varied on a positive to negative dimension, and a discrimination among the causes and consequences of negative emotional states (Surbey, 1979). Further, the data from Farmer (1967), Davitz (1969), Izard (1971), and Russell (1980; Russell & Ridgeway, undated) show that children organize emotions along the same lines as do adults. The finding of interest here is in Davitz (1969), where the age at which distinctions emerge coincides with the ease with which adults make these distinctions. The age at which these dimensions appear to be discriminated is not clear.

As a consequence of these general findings, we sought a system for organizing our conception of meaning for emotions in order to generate systematic interviews with children. We found that our two-level definition, namely, the concrete, instantiated level of antecedent events or actions, concurrent states and consequential expressions or actions, and the more abstract, semantic feature level, was captured, in large part, by Dahl (1977, 1978, 1979). Therefore, we shall now briefly review Dahl's theory and its implications for the understanding of emotions by children.

Dahl's theory

Dahl's (1977, 1978, 1979) theory is based on a psychoanalytic framework that incorporates elements of other theories about emotions (Arnold, 1960; Darwin, 1872; Freud, 1915/1957; James, 1884; Tomkins, 1962/1963). The framework was designed to capture all emotion words, including those thought to be basic (Izard, 1977; McDougall, 1923; Roseman, 1979; Tomkins, 1962/1963) or those that identify facial expression (Emde, 1980; Emde, Gaensbauer, & Harmon, 1976; Ekman & Friesen, 1975). Dahl's system, however, is largely derived from the seminal work of De Rivera (1962, 1977).

Dahl's definition, which resembles Arnold's (1960) and Tomkins's (1962/ 1963), is that an emotion is "an integrated unit of experience consisting of (1) a distinctive perception; (2) an implicit wish and implied action (motive); and (3) a typical expression (facial and/or postural) that is species specific and in man is culturally adapted" (1979, p. 211).

Dahl's model is also based on three separate dimensions that closely resemble those examined by Emde (1976) and Izard (1977). Dahl makes a distinction between *Me* and *It* (corresponding to the internal–external dimension of Emde and his associates) emotions. We shall use the term *reference* to encompass this dimension. The *It* emotions are directed toward others as objects. The *Me* emotions are how one feels about oneself. A second distinction is between *Attraction* (positive) and *Repulsion* (negative) emotions. In the case of *It* emotions, one either wants to be involved with, or to distance oneself from, the object. For the *Me* emotions, the emotions are either pleasurable or un- pleasurable (Emde's "hedonic tone"). Third, Dahl makes the distinction between To/From and Active/Passive for *It* and *Me* emotions, respectively. We shall call the To/From and Active/Passive distinctions *direction*, after Dahl. The latter dimension for *Me* emotions appears to have in it some notion of arousal such as that espoused by Emde. However, this use of the term seems inappropriate here since there are many types of arousal besides activity. For positive *It* emotions, one may be attracted to (love, care, friendly) or stand away from (surprised, thrilled, amazed) objects or persons. For positive *Me* emotions, some states are active (brave, strong, powerful), while others are passive (glad, good, safe). For negative *Me* emotions, one finds parallel levels: active (tense, worried, nervous) and passive (sad, bad, alone).

Dahl attributes motivational properties to *It* emotions (consummatory acts), for example, taking care of, beholding, getting rid of, escaping. The *Me* emotions, on the other hand, serve as messages to the individual about the status of his goals (appetites). An interesting relation can be inferred between Dahl's arousal distinction and positive–negative (valence) emotions. If a person has not as yet attained his goal but there exists the possibility of attainment ("things are going well"), active, positive emotions ensue, whereas if there is the possibility of failure ("things are going badly"), active, negative emotions occur. If the person achieves his goal, things have gone well and he feels passive, positive affect. However, if he fails in his attempts to attain his goal, he experiences passive, negative affect.

Research plan

The purpose of our research was to study, in a systematic way, the two levels of meaning for emotions. To do so, we selected words that were known to children. The set of words provided all pairwise contrasts on the three dimensions of valence (positive vs. negative), direction (to/from and active/passive), and reference (*It/Me*).

In Experiment 1, a closed-interview procedure was used. Six-year-old children were asked to choose a word appropriate for an *antecedent* event. The choice pairs contrasted the dimensions of valence and direction such that mismatches could be assessed on the basis of one or the other or both dimensions. In effect, a mismatching choice indicates that the child did not make the intended distinction between the emotion words in the set of response alternatives.

In Experiment 2, one group of children, 6, 9, and 12 years in age, was asked to choose which one of two emotion words was most similar in meaning to a target word. These choices had no accompanying contexts. The no-context condition assessed the extent to which the children could find similarities and differences among meanings of the words when contrasted on the two dimensions of direction and reference. That is, how well do the children make discriminations in meaning between words on features involving *It* emotions, which move to or away from external objects, and *Me* emotions, which are active or passive? Likewise, how well do they discriminate between emotions directed externally, or toward others, and ones about the self when other features are held constant?

The next question of interest in our research was the role that the first level of meaning, that is, the concrete instantiation of component meanings of emotions or "contexts," play in the understanding of the words. Developmentally, one would expect instantiation of terms to aid children, but it also seems to be an aid to, and characteristic of, word knowledge in adults (Anderson et al., 1976). The question, however, is, given a system of emotional word meanings such as Dahl's, are some contexts more helpful than others? Dahl's system, at least with respect to the reference (*It/Me*) distinction, depends upon an assessment or knowledge of outcomes. Hence, antecedent conditions, while allowing prediction, may be incomplete or ambiguous as to which reference emotion one should select. In some cases, both kinds of emotion can co-occur (e.g., angry and sad when someone breaks a valued object). Antecedents could, however, aid in determining direction (e.g., the antecedent context provides sufficient information to infer potential harm; i.e., fear vs. intent to injure, i.e., anger). Wishes and thoughts would also help direction, as this dimension is included in the presuppositions of the definition of the wish, for example, to attack or to escape. They are, however, less likely to aid in making the reference distinction unless the object of the emotion is expressed in the wish or thought. Consequences are, however, helpful since an assessment of whether things are going well or badly or went badly can be made. We therefore expected the consequence context to be most facilitative of understanding distinctions between emotions.

Therefore, in Experiment 2, we added three context conditions that instantiated, respectively, an event antecedent to the emotion, a concurrent goal or wish state, or an actional or expressive outcome. Given these hypothetical story contexts, the child had to choose one of two emotions where the words contrasted on either the direction dimension or the reference (*It/Me*) dimension.

Experiment 1

Method

Subjects. In Experiment 1 the subjects included 11 children, 5 boys and 6 girls, ranging in age from 5.6 to 6.4 years (mean = 6.0 years), who attended kindergarten at the University of Chicago Laboratory School.

Words. The 24 emotion words were selected from Dahl and Stengel's (1978) classification of 371 words and were cited earlier in our introduction to Dahl's dimensional contrasts. Three words were selected from each of the eight categories in their system. The words selected in most cases also appeared in Wepman and Hass's (1969) spoken word count for children 5 to 7 years in age to assure that the children would know or use the words.

Procedure. Each child was presented with a set of 8 items (Appendix A). Each item contained an antecedent story context that was intended to elicit an emotional reaction that could be described by a word from one of the eight categories in Dahl's classification scheme. The questions following each story required the child to select one emotion from a set of three alternatives. One alternative matched the category of the item. The remaining alternatives were taken from adjacent categories in Dahl's system such that they matched the item's category on only one of the two possible dimensions. The contrasting dimensions were valence (positive vs. negative) and direction (either to/from or active/passive). In this experiment, the emotions did not contrast reference (*It/Me*). An example of an antecedent item is:

"One day, John's little brother took John's model airplane and wrecked it. How did John feel? Did he feel afraid or angry or friendly?"

In this example, the matching answer is angry (a negative, to, *It* emotion). The alternative afraid matches on the negative valence but contrasts on direction (away rather than toward). The alternative friendly matches on direction (toward) but not on valence (positive rather than negative). Thus, if the child chose angry, the answer was scored as matching on both dimensions of valence and direction. If the choice was afraid, it was scored as matching on valence. If the choice was friendly, it was scored as matching on direction. In this manner, matching on one or the other but not both dimensions was assumed to be a result of a failure to make a distinction between the terms or that the child used one dimension to find a similarity between terms.

Results

The proportion of choices that matched the context on *both* direction and valence was .78. For the remaining choices, .16 matched on direction and .06

matched on valence. Thus, a high level of choices matched on both dimensions and direction is *less* well differentiated than valence.

Statistical assessment of these data was done using a Rasch method (Rasch, 1980; Wright & Stone, 1979) of linear scaling. This method enables one to make comparisons between items and subjects on the same linear scale. The analysis (see Schwartz, 1981, for details) indicated that the children differentiated all emotion words. The lowest-scoring child had a higher scale value than the most difficult item. The analysis showed further that .64 of the children had 100% over the valence dimension, whereas only .18 did so on direction ($p <$ .05).

To compare the children's performance with that of adults, the data of Dahl and Stengel (1978) were reanalyzed. Dahl and Stengel (1978) asked adults to classify each of 371 emotion words along the three dimensions of their system. A subset of their data was used to calculate the proportions of adults who chose a particular dimension for the identical words used in the present study. We found that .97 of the adults agreed on valence, .90 agreed on direction. The disagreement proportions of .03 and .10 correspond, respectively, to the mismatch proportions of .06 and .16 for the present study. Thus, despite design differences, the adult and child patterns are alike. Of general interest, then, are the findings that valence is differentiated better than direction for both groups. In other terms, both young children and adults, as was also found by Surbey (1979) for 3-year-olds, distinguish positive from negative emotions better than they distinguish within either class on other dimensions.

Experiment 2

Method

Items. Each child was asked 32 questions, consisting of four sets of 8 questions each. Each question was answered by a choice from two possible answers. One set used only emotion words, one used antecedents, one used wishes concurrent with emotional states, and one used consequences of emotional states (Appendix B). Within each set, 8 items were included. Each item was based upon one of the eight categories drawn from Dahl's classification scheme.

All sets were used for two independent groups of children. One group was asked questions that required the children to make semantic distinctions between the reference (*It/Me*) emotions. The second group was asked to make distinctions on direction (to/from or active/passive) dimensions.

For the words-only set (no context), a child was presented with an emotion word and was asked to select one from two other emotion words. An example is:

1. Words only: "Is feeling *love* like feeling *care* or like feeling *good*?"

Table 13.1. *Proportion of matching choices: age and dimensional contrasts*

Dimensional contrast	6 years	8 years	12 years
Reference	.70	.82	.85
Direction	.88	.88	.90

For the context items, a child was presented with a brief story and asked to select one of two words:

2. Antecedent: "One day John's little brother took John's model airplane and wrecked it. How did John feel? Did he feel afraid or angry?"
3. Concurrent Wishes: "One day John wanted to run away from the mean dog. How did he feel? Did he feel afraid or hate?"
4. Consequence: "One day Mary smiled and laughed. How was she feeling? Was she feeling good or brave?"

For each child, a different random order of the sets of items was used and within each set the items were also randomized, as were the emotion word orders.

Subjects. The subjects, 30 boys and 30 girls from the University of Chicago Laboratory School, were from three age levels, with 20 children per level. The respective age level ranges (and means) were 6.3–7.2 (6.8), 8.4–9.5 (8.9), and 11.11–12.11 (12.5).

Results

The responses of each child on each item were scored according to whether the choice matched the target word or context on the appropriate dimension. When it was scored for reference (*It/Me*), either direction (to/from or active/passive) would be the mismatching choice. Likewise, for the direction, mismatching choices would be on the reference dimension.

Distinctions and age. The children showed a high rate, 84%, of selecting those responses that matched on the expected dimension. Table 13.1 summarizes the proportions of matching choices for the two experimental and the three age groups.

Dimension and age-related differences were found (Table 13.1). The number of children who selected appropriate dimensions increased with age, but the reference distinctions were more difficult to make than those having to do with direction. Finally, the direction distinctions appear to be mastered by age 6, whereas the reference distinction improves with age. Analyses of variance confirmed these conclusions. For age, the *F*-ratios were 11.21 and 0.20 (*df* =

Table 13.2. *Proportion of matching choices for words, contexts, and dimensional contrasts*

		Context		
Dimensional contrast	Words	Antecedents	Wishes	Consequences
Reference	.74	.74	.79	.89
Direction	.81	.90	.91	.93

2/27, $p < .01$) for the reference and direction contrasts, respectively. Individual comparisons showed that there was no statistically significant difference on age for the direction dimension, but there was for ages 6 and 8 on the reference dimension ($p < .01$).

Context effects. The effect of finding similarities and differences between emotion words in isolation and those in contexts was assessed by comparing the words-only condition with the other three context conditions. Table 13.2 summarizes the relevant findings for context and dimensions.

Children were able to make the appropriate matches on the words to a high degree and these distinctions were better made for the direction dimension than for the reference dimension (Table 13.2). Contexts aided in making these distinctions but not in all cases, as anticipated. The direction distinctions, already made to a high degree among words, were further facilitated by all three contexts ($F(1/27) = 7.07, 9.66, 14.94$, respectively). However, for the reference contrast, antecedents had no effect over words without context ($F < 1$); wishes had a small, nonsignificant effect ($F(1/27) = 1.26$); consequences clearly facilitated the distinction ($F(1/27) = 18.98, p < .01$).

Adult-child comparison. To compare the performance of children of the present study with those of adults, we analyzed the words of Dahl and Stengel (1978) that corresponded to the set used here and found the proportions of adults who chose the particular dimensional combination to classify the words. Further, we combined data from Experiment 1 with the average data (all conditions) of Experiment 2 (Table 13.3).

Those distinctions adults find easiest to make between emotion words are also the ones children can make at the earliest age (Table 13.3). The valence (positive vs. negative) distinction is most clearly made and is made at a high level by the young 6-year-olds of Experiment 1. The direction distinctions (to/from or active/passive) *within* each polar category are the next most easiest and show a small developmental increase (6% from age 6 to adulthood). The most difficult dimension for adults and children, given the emotions we studied,

Table 13.3. *Age and dimensional contrasts*

Dimensional contrasts	Proportion of matching choices				
	6.0[a] years	6.8 years	8.9 years	12.5 years	Adults[b]
Reference	—	.70	.82	.85	.78
Direction	.84	.88	.88	.90	.90
Valence	.94	—	—	—	.97

Note: Dash indicates absence of data.
[a] Data from Experiment 1.
[b] Data from Dahl and Stengel (1978).

is the reference (self/other or internal/external) distinction, but this distinction also shows the most improvement with age.

These generalizations hold when one compares the children with adults on *words alone*, without supporting contexts (Table 13.4).

Further, these relations held when we compared the *best* context (consequences) for the children with the Dahl–Stengel adult data (Table 13.5).

The 6-year-olds' data resemble those for adults (Table 13.5). That is, when the 6-year-olds had a supporting context that made clear whether things were going or went badly, they were able to make the requisite distinctions between emotions directed externally and those that are messages about one's motives to the same degree as do adults without such contexts. These data indicate that the young child *knows* the difference between such emotions but may not be able to instantiate the terms as easily as do adults.

Item analysis and context effects. The Rasch method (see earlier) was repeated in Experiment 2 to determine estimates of item and child abilities for each condition. In general, this analysis (see Figure 4 in Schwartz, 1981) showed that Dahl's categories were differentiated across age groups, dimensional contrasts, and experimental conditions. Children of all age groups have nearly complete mastery of all direction distinctions. The children had complete mastery (all children had the items correct) of 8 of the 32 direction items. Scaling with the remaining items showed no age differences in mean ability for direction distinctions, with the abilities of the children being significantly higher than even the most difficult items.

Although reference distinctions were also differentiated, they were significantly more difficult to make than were the direction distinctions for children of all three age groups, and significantly more difficult for 6-year-olds than for either 8- or 12-year-olds. Whereas children had obtained a total mastery of 25% of the direction items, only 3% of the reference items (one item) was completely mastered by the children. Of the 31 reference items upon which

Table 13.4. *Age and dimensional contrasts: words alone*

Dimensional contrasts	Proportion of matching choices			
	6.8 years	8.9 years	12.5 years	Adults[a]
Reference	.64	.76	.84	.78
Direction	.80	.80	.83	.90

[a] Data from Dahl and Stengel (1978).

scaling was based, 10 matched or surpassed the mean ability of the 6-year-olds. Although these same 10 items did not surpass the mean ability of the 8- and 12-year-olds, the items' difficulties did match, statistically, the older children's abilities.

To see how the context affected item difficulty, the 10 most difficult items identified by the Rasch analysis were examined for their distribution of the four conditions (Table 13.6).

The same *It/Me* items are among the most difficult for words alone and for antecedent conditions (Table 13.6). These results are consistent with our earlier conclusion, namely, that the antecedent contexts had no effect on the reference contrast. However, the wishes context removed two items from the most difficult set. Most strikingly, consequences removed all four items from the most difficult list. Emotions such as love are confused with glad and worried is confused with scared unless an outcome context is given.

Explanations. The inclusion of "why" questions for 6- and 8-year-olds allowed us to assess the child's ability to reflect on emotions and to determine if the choice made to the item was plausible. The child's reasons for each choice were scored as plausible or not by two independent judges. The percentage of agreement was 85% and differences were resolved by discussion (Table 13.7).

We then examined how plausible each justification was with respect to whether or not the choice matched its intended category. For *matching* choices, the respective proportions of plausible justifications were .62 and .88 for the 6- and 8-year-old groups ($p < .05$). Thus, the 8-year-olds were better than the 6-year-olds in justifying choices when judged by criteria consistent with Dahl's system. However, the 6-year-olds demonstrated high competence here, being able to justify more than half their matching choices.

When the choice selected mismatched the word or context, the proportions of plausible justifications decreased ($p < .05$) *but* was still high, signifying that the children picked up on ambiguities in the items as to which distinctions were to be made. The respective proportions here were .47 and .73 for the 6- and 8-year-olds.

Table 13.5. *Optimal performance adult-child comparisons: consequences context*

	Proportion of matching choices			
Dimensional contrast	6.8 years	8.9 years	12.5 years	Adults[a]
Reference	.80	.94	.94	.78
Direction	.96	.95	.96	.90

[a] Data from Dahl and Stengel (1978).

The plausible but mismatched justifications frequently involved selection of an aspect of the antecedent context that allowed an *It* emotion (Table 13.7), for example, liking housework (item 1), angry that one can't fight back (item 4), feeling good that one is loved (item 5), amazed that one could lift a heavy rock (item 6), sad over loss of bike (item 7), and afraid of a test (item 8). Note, too, that some justifications show that *It* and *Me* emotions can co-occur as in items 4, 5, 6, and 7. These dualistic interpretations both support the reference distinction and highlight the problem in constructing antecedent items that distinguish them.

Discussion

The main findings of these experiments are that children can make the same basic semantic distinctions among emotion words as do adults and that the age at which children show a high level of such ability is related to the ease with which adults make such distinctions. These findings mirror those of Davitz (1969), Demos (1974), and Wolman and his associates (1972a).

Why might the ease of distinction be related to development? One possibility is that the valence difference in experience is so highly distinct that there is little or no confusion between pleasant and unpleasant feelings even very early in life. These emotions are, in reality, mutually exclusive feelings, although they can co-occur as *It* emotions when one is ambivalent toward someone else or an object. The discrimination of direction depends upon the development of knowledge about objects, including knowing what to avoid and what to approach. The co-occurrence of reference emotions and the necessity to self-reflect or assess one's goal attainment or failure create complexities of interpretations for reference distinctions. Thus there seems to be, upon analysis, a complexity factor that underlies the correlation between age and ease of distinction. The development of emotional understanding, then, seems to be a result of increased experience and acquired knowledge about the contexts in which emotions occur. This increased experience and knowledge aids in

Table 13.6. *Distribution of ten most difficult items over conditions*

Item	Words	Antecedents	Wishes	Consequences
1. It, attraction, to (love, care)	1	1	1	—
5. Me, positive, passive (good, glad)	5	5	—	—
7. Me, negative, passive (sad, alone)	7	7	—	—
8. Me, negative, active (tense, worried)	8	8	8	—

Note: Dash indicates not in ten most difficult items.

the construction of links between emotions and between emotions, cognitions, and actions.

As far as interview methods and verbalization are concerned, our best guess is that at least by age 3 (Borke, 1971; Surbey, 1979) children have formed a basic understanding of the valence factor. Differentiation between emotions within these polarities is also apparent. For example, Surbey (1979) found little overlap for scared in either causes or consequences with anger or sadness. These data suggest that direction is already becoming differentiated, at least with *It* emotions; they also suggest the co-occurrence of the two other negative emotions, which may preclude showing understanding of the reference distinction.

In our data, all distinctions are made by age 6 to a high degree, although the reference distinction lags behind that for direction. By age 8, this distinction appears to be mastered.

Contexts, or the instantiating of components of emotion, facilitated the distinctions. This may be because children (as well as adults, Anderson et al., 1976) prefer to think of terms this way but the facilitation was also of theoretical reference. In Dahl's system, with respect to the reference analysis, the *Me* emotions depend upon knowledge of what happens to one's goals over time – whether things are going well or badly and whether things went well or badly. Indeed, we found that only such contexts helped the children make the *It/Me* distinction. In contrast, all sources helped the direction distinction, as anticipated.

"Why" questions revealed that 8-year-olds were better able to reflect upon and justify reasons for emotions, not a surprising phenomenon (cf. Harris & Olthof, 1982). However, 6-year-olds also showed this kind of logical ability by doing so for better than half the items. This is contrary to what has been argued to be the case, especially from a Piagetian perspective (e.g., Chandler

Table 13.7. *Examples of children's affect-response justification*

Item	Justification		
	Plausible/match	Plausible/mismatch	Not plausible
1. One day Mary's mother felt sick and asked Mary to clean the house. How did Mary feel? Did she feel care or safe?	It was more what the sentence sounded like. Care is when you care or love someone and safe feels like no monsters are going to get you or no one is going to take your bike.	She liked doing housework.	Because care is something gooder than love.
2. One day John saw a bear riding a bicycle. How did he feel? Did he feel care or surprised (thrilled)?	Not all bears can ride bikes. Surprised because he didn't know the bear could do it.	None	Don't know what thrilled means.
3. One day John's little brother wrecked John's model airplane. How did John feel? Did he feel angry (mad) or alone (sad)?	I get mad at my baby sister a lot for this; I know how John would feel.	None	Don't know.
4. One day Mary ran away from the mean boys who were chasing her. How was she feeling? Was she feeling tense (worried) or afraid (scared)?	Because worried is like bad boys caught her and were going to do something to her; scared is when they haven't caught her yet and she is trying to get away.	Well I picked mad because she wouldn't like boys that are chasing her and felt mad. Felt mad because she couldn't get back at them, this is how I feel when someone hurts me and I can't get back at them. I feel really mad. Would feel afraid, too, but mad more.	

426

5. On her birthday, Mary got nice presents from everyone in her family. How did Mary feel? Did she feel care (love) or good (glad)?

Because when you get birthday presents you feel really good because you like them and want to play, feel care about three days later, for a while you just want to play.

Because they cared for her on her birthday and felt love and knew they wanted her to have presents to feel good. Felt love and would feel good.

6. One day John tried to lift a heavy rock with one hand. How was he feeling? Was he feeling strong (brave) or amazed (surprised)?

Because brave is like feeling strong, think that you can do it; even if you can't you have pride in yourself that you can do it.

If rock was heavy he could have dropped it and hurt himself; if feeling amazed it would have been after he lifted the rock.

7. One day John's bike got stolen. How did John feel? Did he feel safe (alone) or mad (angry)?

Because if my friends would have their bikes and go riding around and I wouldn't be able to go with them because mine was stolen, I would feel sad.

Mad at people for stealing, but sad that lost bike.

8. One day John knew he would have to take a hard test. How did he feel? Did he feel worried (tense) or afraid (scared)?

Thought he might get the test wrong, he was nervous, might have never did a test before.

Because you know when you are going to take a hard test you feel afraid for a while, if you feel tense you are just sort of jumpy. If feeling afraid thinking, "What if I don't make it? What if I get bad grades?"

& Greenspan, 1972; Demos, 1964; Harris & Olthof, 1982; Piaget, 1962, 1964, 1965).

The justification data reveal more about the problem of making the distinctions than originally suspected, since co-occurrence of both *It* and *Me* emotions was acknowledged, and in some cases children selected one emotion to answer the question. Apparently, 6- and 8-year-olds can entertain ("coordinate") more than one emotion at a time but report only one emotion, even though they know both can occur (see Harter, 1980, for studies on coordination of emotion in children). The issues of coordination and co-occurrence would seem to be in need of conceptual clarification. First, which emotions are experientially mutually exclusive? It appears that positive and negative emotions are highly distinct as *Me* emotions but can co-occur in *It* emotions, for example, ambivalent feelings toward parents. It also appears that certain negative emotions can co-occur as *It/Me* emotions, for example, sad and angry. Likewise, positive *It/Me* emotions can co-occur, for example, love and good. If questions were worded in ways to elicit the external/internal distinctions, such coordination would perhaps be more readily seen. Coordination and/or co-occurrence knowledge might not be revealed when one asks How does one feel? because the respondent selects one emotion for report. The questions would have to require and explicitly ask something about the agent or object of the emotion or about the child's goals. For example, if the context is:

"One day, John's little brother took John's model airplane and wrecked it." Then, instead of asking How did John feel? one might ask:

1. (*It*-emotion): How does John feel toward his brother?
2. (*Me*-emotion): How does John feel about losing his airplane?

Although we did not ask these directed questions, one 8-year-old explained his choice, showing both emotions: "Sometimes little brothers do it because they don't know any better; big brothers get angry, but then make up. Angry is when someone does something to you. He'd also feel sad because he thought his airplane was nice and didn't want it to be wrecked. It was special to him."

We believe that an understanding of the conceptual basis for emotional terms is crucial for effective communication between adults and children as well as between researchers. Further, knowing how this understanding changes with development, as well as which aspects allow distinctions between emotions to be made in communication, helps us to understand, in turn, the nature of how humans conceptualize emotions. Theories and approaches to the study of emotion are frequently less than explicit and systematic about the *meaning* of emotion. Studies on how emotions are understood by children and adults deal directly with this semantic aspect. Here, we have adapted assumptions about causal thinking and semantic features to the concept of emotion. We have found that children, as well as adults, understand emotions in terms of their antecedent events, their concurrent internal states, thoughts, and feelings, and their consequent actions and expressions. Further, we found that they make semantic distinctions between emotion labels in terms of their polarity of affect – whether the state is pleasant or unpleasant – the direction of the emotion – whether it is toward or away from objects or reflects an assessment of whether things are going well or went well or are going or went badly for the person – and the reference of the emotion – whether it is directed externally or reflects an assessment of self. These findings indicate that the concept of emotion is context-dependent and that people use these contexts to infer emotional states in the self and others.

The extent to which labels for emotional states and the underlying meaning captures information contained in feelings per se remains unknown. We assert that the assessment or evaluation of feeling states into pleasant or unpleasant is a basic, highly discriminable, and coded semantic property of emotional feelings. This semantic feature emerges earliest in development and is the best differentiated. The distinctions between direction and reference depend less upon the feeling per se. Rather, they seem to require further reflection, taking into account antecedent and ongoing events, whether there is an outside agent who is the object of the feeling and whether or not things are going or went well or are going or went badly. The assessments could be reflected directly in the experience of the affect if one can discern differences in feeling states of depression versus anxiety or excitement versus calm. The dimension here is, as we noted, closely akin to arousal. Thus for polarity and direction, we can detect some direct relation to feelings, but for reference, less so. The latter, of course, may be experienced more in terms of goals and actions toward others or the self. This, however, broadens the definition of feeling into consequences expressed or experienced.

Dahl's (1977, 1978, 1919; Dahl & Stengel, 1978) system proved to be useful and revealing in constructing emotion word contrasts. Coupled with a two-level definition of meaning, the theory lent itself to operationalization of the feature contrasts in contexts. The data show that children can make the distinctions between emotion terms specified by Dahl and that the making of these distinctions is facilitated by certain contexts. In this sense, children show sophisticated distinctions in their naïve theories about emotion. They are able to define emotions in terms of logical relations. They demonstrated knowledge that people feel brave, strong, or powerful when they are succeeding in what they wanted to do and good, glad, or safe when they have succeeded. They also showed that they understood people to feel nervous, tense, or worried when they were failing to obtain what they wanted and sad, bad, and alone when they failed. These *Me* emotions were distinguished from, but not as well discriminated as, *It* emotions where the children knew that one loved, cared for, or was friendly toward parents and people in need and felt surprised, thrilled, and amazed about unexpected events. They also were aware of the negative feelings people have toward others, such as wanting to hurt someone when you feel anger, hatred, or mad. Finally, they understood that one tries to avoid things that make one afraid, scared, or frightened.

Conclusion

Two levels of the meaning of affect labels were studied on children 6 to 12 years in age. One level defined emotions in terms of the contexts in which they occur: their antecedents, their concurrent states, and their consequences. The second level contrasted the emotions on the semantic features of valence (positive or negative), direction (to/from an object and active/passive), and reference (other versus self). In Experiment 1, 6-year-olds chose words that were appropriate to antecedent events where the choice pairs contrasted the features of valence and direction. In Experiment 2, children 6, 9 and 12 years in age chose emotion words that were either (1) similar in meaning to another word without a context or (2) appropriate antecedent events, concurrent thoughts or wishes, or consequential actions or expressions of emotions. In all choices, the emotion words contrasted on direction or reference dimensions.

In Experiment 1 valence was differentiated better than direction (.94 vs. .84) by 6-year-olds, corresponding to similar patterns and degree of discrimination by adults. In Experiment 2, it was found that the direction dimension was mastered by age 6, whereas the reference dimension improved with age. Contexts aided in the making of direction distinctions but on consequences aided in the making of reference distinctions. The latter result indicates the necessity of knowing outcomes in order to decide whether things are going or went badly (or well).

Adult–child comparisons showed that those distinctions adults find the easiest to make are also the ones children master first in development. The valence (positive vs. negative) distinction is most clearly made by age 6. The direction distinctions (toward/away or active/passive) are next most easiest and show a small developmental increase. The most difficult dimension, for adults and children, is the reference distinction (self/other or internal/external), but this distinction also improves with age. However, when a supporting context made clear whether things were going or went badly (or well), 6-year-olds were able to make distinctions between emotions directed externally and those that assess motives to the same degree as do adults without contexts. Young children *know* the differences between emotions but may not be able to instantiate the terms as easily as do adults.

Appendix A: Items used in experiment 1

Antecedents of Emotional States

(1) One day Mary's mother lost her new hat. The next day Mary went to the store and bought her mother a new hat. How did Mary feel? Did she feel caring (love) or thrilled (amazed) or mad (angry)?

(2) One day John saw a bear riding a bicycle. How did he feel? Did he feel loving (caring) or frightened (scared) or amazed (surprised)?

(3) One day John's little brother took John's model airplane and wrecked it. How did John feel? Did he feel afraid (scared) or angry (mad) or friendly (loving)?

(4) One day there was a fire where Mary lived and she had to leave by the back door. How did she feel? Did she feel afraid (frightened) or surprised (thrilled) or angry (hateful)?

(5) On her birthday Mary got nice presents from everyone in her family. How did Mary feel? Did she feel sad (alone) or brave (strong) or glad (good)?

(6) One day Mary lifted a heavy chair up all by herself. How did she feel? Did she feel worried (tense) or strong (powerful) or good (glad)?

(7) One day John's new bike got stolen and he didn't get it back. How did he feel? Did he feel sad (helpless) or tense (worried) or good (secure)?

(8) One day John found out he had two cavities and would have to go to the dentist to get them fixed. How did he feel? Did he feel lonely (sad) or powerful (brave) or worried (nervous)?

Appendix B: Items used in experiment 2

Set 1 – Word Set with Direction Confusions

(1) Is feeling friendly (love) like feeling care (friendly) or like feeling surprised (thrilled)?

(2) Is feeling amazed (surprised) like feeling thrilled (amazed) or like feeling love (care)?

(3) Is feeling hate (angry) like feeling afraid (scared) or like feeling mad (hate)?

(4) Is feeling scared (afraid) like feeling fear (scared) or like feeling angry (mad)?

(5) Is feeling good (glad) like feeling brave (strong) or like feeling safe (good)?

(6) Is feeling strong (powerful) like feeling powerful (brave) or like feeling glad (good)?

(7) Is feeling alone (bad) like feeling worried (tense) or like feeling bad (sad)?

(8) Is feeling tense (worried) like feeling anxious (tense) or like feeling
     sad (alone)?

Set 1 - Word Set with It-Me Confusions

(1) Is feeling love (friendly) like feeling care (love) or like feeling
     good (safe)?

(2) Is feeling surprised (amazed) like feeling brave (powerful) or like
     feeling amazed (thrilled)?

(3) Is feeling mad (hate) like feeling hate (mad) or like feeling sad
     (alone)?

(4) Is feeling afraid (scared) like feeling tense (worried) or like
     feeling scared (fear)?

(5) Is feeling glad (good) like feeling safe (glad) or like feeling
     friendly (care)?

(6) Is feeling strong (powerful) like feeling powerful (strong) or like
     feeling thrilled (surprised)?

(7) Is feeling alone (bad) like feeling angry (mad) or like feeling bad
     (sad)?

(8) Is feeling worried (tense) like feeling fear (scared) or like feeling
     anxious (worried)?

Set 2 - Antecedents of Emotional States
(Direction Confusion)

(1) One day Mary's mother felt sick and asked Mary to clean the house.
     How did Mary feel? Did she feel love (care) or thrilled (amazed)?

(2) One day John saw a bear riding a bicycle. How did John feel? Did
     he feel surprised (thrilled) or care (love)?

(3) One day John's little brother took John's model airplane and wrecked
     it. How did John feel? Did he feel afraid (scared) or angry (mad)?

(4) One day there was a fire where Mary lived. How did she feel? Did
     she feel scared (afraid) or mad (angry)?

(5) On her birthday Mary got nice presents from everyone in her family.
     How did she feel? Did she feel glad (good) or brave (strong)?

(6) One day Mary rushed into a swimming pool to save a little boy who
     could not swim. How did Mary feel? Did she feel good (glad) or
     strong (brave)?

(7) One day John's new bike got stolen and he didn't get it back.
     How did he feel? Did he feel alone (sad) or tense (worried)?

(8) One day John knew he would have to take a hard test. How did he
     feel? Did he feel sad (alone) or worried (tense)?

Set 2 - Antecedents of Emotional States
(It-Me Confusion)

(1) One day Mary's mother felt sick and she asked Mary to clean the house.
How did Mary feel? Did she feel love (care) or glad (good)?

(2) One day John saw a bear riding a bicycle. How did he feel? Did he
feel strong (brave) or surprised (thrilled)?

(3) One day John's little brother wrecked John's model airplane. How
did John feel? Did he feel angry (mad) or alone (sad)?

(4) One day there was a fire where Mary lived and she had to leave by
the back door. How did Mary feel? Did she feel worried (tense) or
scared (afraid)?

(5) On her birthday Mary got nice presents from everyone in her family.
How did Mary feel? Did she feel care (love) or good (glad)?

(6) One day Mary rushed into a swimming pool to save a little boy who
could not swim. How did Mary feel? Did she feel brave (strong)
or thrilled (surprised)?

(7) One day John's bicycle got stolen and he did not get it back. How
did John feel? Did he feel mad (angry) or sad (alone)?

(8) One day John knew he would have to take a hard test. How did he
feel? Did he feel tense (worried) or afraid (scared)?

Set 3 - Wishes While Experiencing Emotional States
(Direction Confusion)

(1) One day Sue wanted to give her mother a Mother's Day present. How
was she feeling? Was she feeling friendly (thankful) or surprised
(amazed)?

(2) One day Jim wanted to stare at the elephant that could hop on one
leg. How was he feeling? Was he feeling thrilled (surprised) or
thankful (friendly)?

(3) One day Mary wanted to smash her pillow to pieces. How was she feeling?
Was she feeling angry (hate) or fear (afraid)?

(4) One day Jim wanted to run away from the mean dog. How was he feeling?
Was he feeling afraid (fear) or hate (angry)?

(5) One day Jim thought about how he got to go to the circus just like he
wanted. How was he feeling? Was he feeling good (glad) or strong
(powerful)?

(6) One day Sue thought about climbing a mountain by herself. How was she
feeling? Was she feeling glad (good) or powerful (strong)?

(7) One day Sue was thinking about how no one likes her. How was she feeling?
Was she feeling worried (anxious) or alone (sad)?

(8) One day Jim was thinking about having to go to the doctor to get a shot.
How was he feeling? Was he feeling sad (alone) or anxious (worried)?

Set 3 – Wishes While Experiencing Emotional States
(It–Me Confusion)

(1)   One day Sue wanted to give her mother a Mother's Day present. How
was she feeling? Was she feeling friendly (thankful) or good (glad)?

(2)   One day Jim wanted to stare at the elephant that could hop on one foot.
How was he feeling? Was he feeling powerful (strong) or thrilled
(surprised)?

(3)   One day Mary wanted to smash her pillow to pieces. How was she feeling?
Was she feeling angry (hate) or alone (sad)?

(4)   One day Jim wanted to run away from the mean dog. How was he feeling?
Was he feeling anxious (worried) or afraid (fear)?

(5)   One day Jim thought about how he got to go to the circus just like he
wanted. How was he feeling? Was he feeling glad (good) or friendly
(love)?

(6)   One day Sue thought about climbing a mountain by herself. How was she
feeling? Was she feeling hate (angry) or sad (alone)?

(7)   One day Sue was thinking about how no one likes her. How was she
feeling? Was she feeling hate (angry) or sad (alone)?

(8)   One day Jim was thinking about having to go to the doctor to get a
shot. How was he feeling? Was he feeling fear (afraid) or worried
(anxious)?

Set 4 – Consequences of Emotional States
(Direction Confusion)

(1)   One day Mary gave her father a present. How was she feeling? Was she
feeling love (care) or amazed (thrilled)?

(2)   One day John looked and looked at the man who was juggling ten Coke
bottles. How was he feeling? Was he feeling surprised (amazed) or
care (love)?

(3)   One day John yelled at his sister. How was he feeling? Was he feeling
scared (afraid) or hate (mad)?

(4)   One day Mary ran away from the mean boys who were chasing her. How
was she feeling? Was she feeling afraid (scared) or mad (hate)?

(5)   One day Mary smiled and laughed. How was she feeling? Was she feeling
good (safe) or brave (strong)?

(6)   One day John tried to lift a heavy rock with one hand. How was he
feeling? Was he feeling safe (good) or strong (powerful)?

(7)   One day Mary cried and cried. How was she feeling? Was she feeling
worried (tense) or sad (bad)?

(8)   One day John got a headache. How was he feeling? Was he feeling
alone (sad) or tense (worried)?

Set 4 - Consequences of Emotional States
(It-Me Confusion)

(1) One day Mary gave her father a present. How was she feeling? Was she feeling love (care) or good (safe)?

(2) One day John looked and looked at the man who was juggling ten Coke bottles. How was he feeling? Was he feeling brave (strong) or surprised (amazed)?

(3) One day John yelled at his sister. How was he feeling? Was he feeling hate (mad) or alone (bad)?

(4) One day Mary ran away from the mean boys who were chasing her. How was she feeling? Was she feeling tense (worried) or afraid (scared)?

(5) One day Mary smiled and laughed. How was she feeling? Was she feeling glad (good) or care (love)?

(6) One day John tried to lift a heavy rock with one hand. How was he feeling? Was he feeling strong (brave) or amazed (surprised)?

(7) One day Mary cried and cried. How was she feeling? Was she feeling mad (hate) or bad (sad)?

(8) One day John got a bad headache. How was he feeling? Was he feeling scared (afraid) or worried (tense)?

References

Anderson, R. C., Pichert, J. W., Goetz, E. T., Schallert, D. L., Stevens, K. V., & Trollip, S. R. Instantiation of general terms. *Journal of Verbal Learning and Verbal Behavior*, 1976, *15*, 667–679.

Arnold, M. B. *Emotion and personality*. New York: Columbia University Press, 1960.

Borke, H. Interpersonal perception of young children: Egocentrism or empathy? *Developmental Psychology*, 1971, *5*, 263–269.

Burns, N., & Cavey, L. Age differences in empathic ability among children. *Canadian Journal of Psychology*, 1957, *11*, 227–230.

Chandler, M. J., & Greenspan, S. Ersatz egocentrism: A reply to H. Borke. *Developmental Psychology*, 1972, *7*, 104–106.

Dahl, H. Considerations for a theory of emotions. In J. De Rivera (Ed.), *A structural theory of emotions. Psychological Issues*, Monograph 40, 1977.

Dahl, H. A new psychoanalytic model of motivation: Emotions as appetites and messages. *Psychoanalysis and Contemporary Thought*, 1978, *1*, 373–408.

Dahl, H. The appetite hypothesis of emotions: A new psychoanalytic model of motivation. In C. Izard (Ed.), *Emotions in personality and psychopathology*. New York: Plenum, 1979.

Dahl, H., & Stengel, B. A classification of emotion words: A modification and partial test of De Rivera's decision theory of emotions. *Psychoanalysis and Contemporary Thought*, 1978, *1*, 269–312.

Darwin, C. *The expression of emotions in man and animals*. London: Murray, 1872.

Davitz, J. *The language of emotion*. New York: Academic Press, 1969.

Demos, V. Children's understanding and use of affect terms (Doctoral dissertation, Harvard University, 1974). *Dissertation Abstracts International*. (University Microfilms No. 75-26, 902).

De Rivera, J. A decision theory of emotions (Doctoral dissertation, Stanford University, 1961). *Dissertation Abstracts International*, 1962. (University Microfilms No. 62-2356).

De Rivera, J. A structural theory of emotions. *Psychological Issues*, Monograph 40, 1977.

Dewey, J. *How we think*. Portions published in R. M. Hutchins & M. J. Adler (Eds.), *Gateway to great books* (Vol. 10). Chicago: Encyclopaedia Britannica, 1963.

Ekman, P., & Friesen, W. *Unmasking the face*. Englewood Cliffs, N.J.: Prentice-Hall, 1975.

Emde, R. N. Shaking the foundations: Changing models of infancy and the nature of early development. Unpublished manuscript, 1980.

Emde, R. N., Gaensbauer, T. J., & Harmon, J. R. *Emotional expression in infancy*. New York: International Universities Pres, 1976.

Farmer, C. Words and feelings: A developmental study of the language of emotion in children (Doctoral dissertation, Columbia University, 1967). *Dissertation Abstracts International*. (University Microfilms No. 67-14, 040).

Freud, S. Instincts and their vicissitudes. *Standard Edition* (Vol. 14). London: Hogarth Press, 1957. (Originally published, 1915.)

Gnepp, J. *Children's social sensitivity and ability to reconcile conflicting affective cues*. Unpublished doctoral dissertation, University of Minnesota, 1982.

Harris, P. L., & Olthof, T. The child's concept of emotions. In G. Butterworth & P. Light (Eds.), *Social cognition: Studies of the development of understanding*. Chicago: University of Chicago Press, 1982.

Harter, S. A cognitive-developmental approach to children's understanding of affect and trait labels. In F. Serafica (Ed.), *Social cognition in context*. New York: Guilford Press, 1980.

Izard, C. *The face of emotion*. New York: Appleton-Century-Crofts, 1971.

Izard, C. *Human emotions*. New York: Plenum, 1977.

James, W. What is an emotion? *Mind*, 1884, *9*, 188–205.

McDougall, W. *Outline of psychology*. New York: Scribner, 1923.

Piaget, J. *The origins of intelligence in children*. New York: International Universities Press, 1962.

Piaget, J. *Six psychological studies*. New York: Random House, 1964.

Piaget, J. *The moral judgment of the child*. New York: Free Press, 1965.

Rasch, G. *Probabilistic models for some intelligence and attainment tests*. Chicago: University of Chicago Press, 1980.

Roseman, I. *Cognitive aspects of emotion and emotional behavior*. Paper presented at the annual meeting of the American Psychological Association, New York, 1979.

Russell, J. A. Evidence of convergent validity on the dimensions of affect. *Journal of Personality and Social Psychology*, 1978, *36*, 1152–1168.

Russell, J. A. Affective space is bi-polar. *Journal of Personality and Social Psychology*, 1979, *37*, 345–356.

Russell, J. A. A circumplex model of affect. *Journal of Personality and Social Psychology*, 1980, *39*, 1161–1178.

Russell, J. A., & Ridgeway, D. *The structure of affect in children*. Unpublished manuscript, University of British Columbia, Vancouver, Canada, 1981.

Schwartz, R. *A developmental study of children's understanding of the language of emotions*. Unpublished doctoral dissertation, University of Chicago, 1981.

Surbey, P. *Preschool children's understanding of emotional states in terms of causes and consequences*. Unpublished master's thesis, University of Minnesota, 1979.

Tomkins, S. *Affect, imagery, and consciousness* (2 vols.). New York: Springer-Verlag, 1962/1963.

Trabasso, T., Stein, N. L., & Johnson, L. R. Children's knowledge of events: A causal analysis of story structure. In G. H. Bower (Ed.), *The psychology of learning and motivation* (Vol. 15). New York: Academic Press, 1981.

Wepman, J., & Hass, W. *A spoken word count (children ages 5, 6, 7)*. Chicago: Language Research, 1969.

Wolman, R., Lewis, W., & King, M. The development of the language of emotions: Conditions of emotional arousal. *Child Development*, 1971, *42*, 1288–1293.

Wolman, R., Lewis, W., & King, M. The development of the language of emotions: I. Theoretical and methodological introduction. *Journal of Genetic Psychology*, 1972, *120*, 167–176. (a)

Wolman, R., Lewis, W., & King, M. The development of the language of emotions: II. Intentionality in the experience of affect. *Journal of Genetic Psychology*, 1972, *120*, 303–316. (b)

Wolman, R., Lewis, W., & King, M. The development of the language of emotions: III. Type of anxiety in the experience of affect. *Journal of Genetic Psychology*, 1972, *120*, 325–342. (c)

Wolman, R., Lewis, W., & King, M. The development of the language of emotions: IV. Bodily referents and the experience of affect. *Journal of Genetic Psychology*, 1972, *120*, 372–385. (d)

Wright, B., & Stone, M. *Best test design*. Chicago: MESA Press, 1979.

14   Children's and adults' understanding of the causes and consequences of emotional states

John C. Masters and Charles R. Carlson

Research on emotion has always been an important area of inquiry, but there has been a distinct upsurge of interest within the past decade. The rapid growth in laboratory and naturalistic investigations of emotions has developed within several different theoretical orientations. In fact, it is somewhat remarkable that such sustained growth in interest can occur without having broad consensus regarding one or even several theories of emotion. The variety of theoretical foci is almost as great as the number of investigators reporting research findings (e.g., Izard, 1972; Lazarus, 1969; Plutchik, 1970; Schachter, 1959, 1972; Tomkins, 1962, 1963, 1981). It is perhaps because of this diversity of theories about emotion that there is an increasing volume of experimental data that chronicle the impact emotions have on the thoughts and actions of people. This growing pool of formal knowledge about emotion has opened the door to an allied domain of concern, the informal knowledge and beliefs[1] people develop about the cognitive and behavioral determinants and consequences of emotional states. It is this domain of "meta-emotion" on which the present review will focus.

Definition of emotion

To place the discussion of children's and adults' understanding of emotion in perspective, a working definition of emotion is needed. Initially, such a task appears monumental or at least rather arbitrary, given the extensive history of concern with emotion going back at least to the time of Aristotle and given the diversity of current theoretical conceptions. Numerous definitions of emotion have been forwarded in the ensuing years, and as might be expected, there has been little agreement. For example, Aristotle described emotion as a complex phenomenon primarily involving cognitions as the efficient cause, accompanied by bodily changes (Fortenbaugh, 1975). Centuries later, James (1884) suggested that emotion is a bodily sensation caused by some environmental event that is then consciously labeled. Within the last 100 years, definitions of emotion by a variety of scholars have been forwarded, but none has gained broad acceptance within the field of psychology (Cannon, 1932; Izard, 1972; Lazarus,

438

1969; Schachter & Singer, 1962; Tomkins, 1962, 1963, 1981; Watson, 1929, 1930). Lest this point be misunderstood as criticism, we should note that there has been an inherent heuristic in these definitions to the extent that they have provoked considerable research with infants, children, and adults in a broad variety of settings and focused upon a wide array of behaviors and other dependent variables.

Given the range of perspectives and productive research efforts concerning emotion, a unifying theoretical definition of emotion need not assume broad importance (Skinner, 1950). Elsewhere in this volume, specific definitions are embraced that are most pertinent for a given research question (see, e.g., Schwartz & Trabasso, Chapter 13). For our purposes, no formal definition of "emotion" is required other than an assertion that it is a shared concept among children and adults in a given society. Indeed, in one sense the definition of emotion *is* the variable under study, emotion as it is operationally defined (Bridgman, 1927) by the beliefs and expectancies of persons. Thus, the specific working definition of emotion in this review involves what persons who participated in the research studies subjectively defined it to be, as reflected in the data on their understanding of emotion, its causes and its consequences. Specific emotional states are thus defined merely in terms of common terminology (happy, sad, angry, etc.) and its contemporary use in this society.

In the present review we will address two dimensions of beliefs or knowledge about emotions: their causes and their consequences. We will also deal briefly (because there has been little research so far) with the potential relationships between knowledge/beliefs about emotion and patterns of behavior.

Knowledge and beliefs about the determinants of emotional reactions

In the last two decades the burgeoning experimental literature concerning emotions has dealt primarily with the consequences of emotion, not its determinants, and emotions have been found to influence a broad range of social behaviors and cognitive processes. There has been little systematic study of the antecedents of emotional states nor, until recently, of children's and adults' understanding of the causes of emotion. There are, of course, so many different experiences that tend to provoke some emotions that their exhaustive study would be laborious and generally trivial. It may even be the case that common emotional reactions to common experiences are considered to be so well understood that their ubiquity and common understanding makes them trivial scientifically. If this be so, it is particularly interesting that people's understanding of emotional reactivity and its place in their own implicit personality theories (Mischel, 1968, 1973) has received so little attention. This may be due in part to a long-standing reluctance among experimental psychologists to view subjects as experts. With an increased acceptability of introspective methods that acknowledge subjects to be experts concerning at least their understanding of their own behavior (Mischel, 1973), investigators have been more willing to inquire directly about subjects' ongoing mentations. This is most clearly illustrated by the recent work of Flavell and others (e.g., Kreutzer, Leonard & Flavell, 1975; Flavell & Wellman, 1977) concerning children's knowledge of memory processes (meta-memory). The recent increased legitimacy granted to the study of people's own knowledge or beliefs about their behavior, competencies, and the psychological processes that govern them clearly extends to the sphere of emotions.

Children's understanding of the determinants of emotion

According to classic Piagetian theory (1926), children below the age of 7 or 8 do not generally have a grasp of causal relationships. Broad characterizations of this sort, especially in terms of children's *in*capabilities, are coming to be viewed more and more as gross underestimates of children's competencies (e.g., Gelman, 1978). With respect to a causal understanding of emotion there is substantial evidence that children as young as 2½ years of age use emotion terms appropriately not only on a descriptive basis (to label their own states and those of others) but on a causal basis as well. Bretherton and Beeghly (in press) employed mothers to record their 28-month-old children's use of emotion terms. Not only did children use common emotion terms (happy, sad, mad, scared) appropriately from 60% to 100% of the time, they also used them causally with great frequency: Approximately 50% of all causal statements recorded referred to emotions! Bretherton and Beeghly report that a reanalysis they conducted on data from a study by Zahn-Waxler, Radke-Yarrow, and King (1979) revealed similar findings with respect to very young children's causal use of emotion terms.

Trabasso, Stein, and Johnson (1981) and Surbey (1979) examined slightly older (3 to 4½ years of age) children's understanding of antecedents by asking about the events that might have led a pictured child to feel a certain way. Children were asked about three positive emotions (happy, excited, surprised) and three negative emotions (sad, angry, afraid). While causal events were readily nominated, children better differentiated those events that might lead to the various negative emotions than they did those that were proposed for the positive ones.

Green (1977) devised a procedure whereby 6-year-old children could match pictures of other children experiencing a given emotional state (happiness, sadness, fear, or anger) to short movie episodes that showed the causal events for the emotions. The children were also asked to describe how the emotion had been produced by the event depicted in the movie episode. Green found that 6-year-olds were consistently able to identify appropriate causal events and to give acceptable reasons for the impact of those events on emotional experience. However, no information was given about the degree to which children may have varied in their accuracy for identifying appropriate causal events leading to different emotional states. Certainly some states are more common (frequently experienced) than others, and this commonality as well as the type of experience eliciting a given state may change with age. For these and other reasons it might be expected that children's understanding of the causes of emotion would be imperfect, would vary as a function of the emotion and the type of causal event, and would develop with age and experience.

To shed light on the development of children's understanding about specific determinants of common emotional states, Barden and his associates (1980) interviewed kindergarteners (4- and 5-year-olds), third graders (9- and 10-year-olds), and sixth graders (12- and 13-year-olds). Children were presented with 40 vignettes of potential emotion-inducing experiences that were divided into eight categories. The categories chosen for this study were not intended to be exhaustive but were meant to reflect a sample of common childhood experiences, including (1) success, (2) nurturance (being nurtured), (3) dishonesty that is detected or (4) that is not, (5) justified punishment, (6) unjustified punishment, (7) aggression (being aggressed against), and (8) failure. Children responded to five vignettes developed for each category by indicating the emotion they thought the experience would evoke (happiness, sadness, fear, anger, or no reaction).

There was significant agreement among children about the emotional consequences for all categories of experience, but the expected emotional consequence was not always the same for children of different ages. Nearly all children agreed that success ("If you played hide and seek so well no one found you") and nurturance ("If your friend told you what a nice person you are") led to happiness. In addition, older children showed a secondary tendency to expect nurturance to produce no emotional reaction, which could be interpreted as an indication of emerging motives for independence or a masking of the overt display of emotion in a nurturant context. In this same vein, older children also expected neutral reactions to failure, whereas younger children, surely more accurately, expected sadness. Children of all ages saw sadness as the likely reaction to justified punishment ("If you were playing with your mother's glass and you were not careful and broke it"). Younger children, perhaps with a candor not yet masked with socialization, expected *un*detected dishonesty to elicit happiness, whereas older children expected to be fearful. Older children may have been demonstrating their more accurate appraisal of the probabilities of encountering eventual detection, and they also nominated fear as the likely emotional consequence of dishonesty that was apprehended. The emerging picture is that children develop a shared understanding of the various emotional reactions likely to be produced by common experiences. Children's understanding also changes with age in ways that seem likely to reflect increasing experience, cognitive development, and changing socialization pressures.

More recently, Harris, Olthof, and Terwogt (1981) used an interview procedure to investigate children's understanding of how they could identify three
emotional states, happiness, fear, and anger, in themselves and others. Subjects
were Dutch 6-, 11-, and 15-year-olds. Although the investigators do not report
specific information regarding classes of experience children may have nominated as likely to induce emotional states, their results indicated that younger
children relied more on situational determinants to infer their own emotional
states ("it's my birthday"), whereas older children used internal cues such as
how their thoughts appeared to have been affected ("then you think everything
is just fine"). Harris and his colleagues also asked children about their own
strategies for influencing ongoing emotional states. All children (6-, 11-, and
15-year-olds) suggested that changing situations (e.g., call your friends up to
play) would result in changing one's ongoing emotional experience, but only
the older children (11- and 15-year-olds) suggested that refocusing thoughts
could have an impact on emotion. The investigators proposed that older children
were more able or willing to link inner thoughts and feelings with emotional
expression than were younger children.

Harter (1980) explored children's understanding of sources for emotions
their *parents* might feel. Using an interview procedure, children of three ages
(4–5, 6–8, and 9–11 years of age) were asked what sort of parent experiences
might lead their parents to feel various emotions (happy, sad, mad, and scared).
Three general categories were found for children's responses. First were antecedent experiences that were child-appropriate but not adult-appropriate
("Mommy would be scared if a monster came into her room"). Another category
concerned adult-appropriate antecedents that included the child as part of the
antecedent, generally as a target of the emotion ("Mom gets mad when I break
something"). The third category included antecedents that were totally adult-
appropriate and did not involve the child ("Mom was sad when her car got
wrecked in an accident").

Other investigators (Barden et al., 1980) have reported that children make
no differentiation between determinants of emotion that apply to themselves
and those that apply to other children. Harter found that the youngest children
in her sample appeared, inappropriately, to do the same in construing the
antecedents of parental emotions. Compatible with the cognitive developmental
concept of a progressive ability to decenter with age, children of increasing
age tended to move from providing antecedents of the first category to providing
ones from the second and then the third categories. It was also found, however,
that the type of antecedent was dependent as well upon the emotion in question.
For example, for the emotion of anger, fully 83% of the children, across all
ages, indicated that they were the cause of parental anger, whereas for the
emotion "scared," only 41% of the children indicated that they were the cause.

Another line of research that indirectly addresses children's understanding
of the causes of emotion involves the assessment of their accuracy in inferring

the emotional states of others when they have information about what has happened to them. In these studies, children are read short stories or shown short film segments that describe experiences or events likely to evoke particular emotional states. Children are then asked to assign appropriate emotional states to the vignettes. Sometimes children provide verbal labels of emotion to the vignettes (Deutsch, 1974; Farber & Moely, 1979; Feinman & Feldman, 1982; Greenspan, Barenboim, & Chandler, 1976; Reichenbach & Masters, 1983), and in other cases they may match photographs depicting various emotional states to the vignettes (Borke, 1971, 1972; Camras, 1980; Chandler & Greenspan, 1972; Odom & Lemond, 1972). Generally, children as young as 3 years of age appear to have an awareness of the determinants of common emotional states (happiness, sadness, anger, fear). For example, when a situation is described that is likely to produce happiness, children are quite accurate, generally more that 75% of the time. Accuracy in recognizing determinants of fear, anger, and sadness is generally lower but well above chance for all age groups considered (age range: 3–11 years). It is also generally found that accuracy in identifying the emotional consequences of various experiences increases with age except, of course, for those categories of experiences (e.g., success) or emotions (e.g., happiness) for which even very young children are quite accurate.

There are fewer investigations in which the multiple sources of information children may use to make inferences about emotion have been simultaneously examined. These studies compared children's use of contextual cues to their use of expressive (facial) cues for identifying the emotional states of others. Farber and Moely (1979) reported a study that investigated 4-, 5- and 6-year-old children's abilities to infer the emotions of others (happiness, sadness, fear, or anger) on the basis of facial cues, interpersonal/contextual cues, and vocal cues. As in earlier studies, it was found that all children were able to differentiate the emotions expressed in facial, situational, or verbal modes alone at levels well above chance, and the degree to which emotions were accurately inferred across all dimensions increased with age. Again, happiness was most easily recognized by all children across sources for inference, whereas sadness and anger were often confused, especially in the interpersonal context. No analyses were reported that would provide an indication of the relative importance for the various sources of expressive (facial, vocal) and contextual information for inferences about emotional experience.

Children's use of contextual information in inferring the emotional states of other children was also investigated by Kurdek and Rodgon (1975). As part of a broader study of perspective taking, these investigators developed an inquiry procedure similar to one used by Borke (1971) in which children (ages 5–12) were presented with eight drawings that depicted a boy or a girl in four situations that would typically induce happiness, sadness, fear, or anger. For half the drawings, the emotion expressed was consistent with the context.

After viewing each picture children were asked how the depicted child felt. When the situation and the emotional expressions in the pictures were consistent, it was found that children's accuracy increased with age, and by about the age of 10 children were essentially perfect in their performance. When there was a discrepancy between contextual and expressive cues, with increasing age children also tended to infer emotional states more on the basis of contextual cues than facial expressions. In this study the accuracy of children's inferences given multiple sources of consistent or discrepant information was not contrasted with their ability to infer states from expressive or contextual cues alone, so the interaction or integration of different types of information cannot be examined.

Most recently, Reichenbach and Masters (1983) showed children of two age groups (4 and 7 years) photographs of other children who were experiencing happiness, sadness, anger, or no emotional state. With each photograph, subjects were also presented with a story to provide contextual cues for the experiences leading to the emotional states of the children depicted in the photographs (e.g., for sadness: "Mary left her favorite toy at someone else's house. Mary couldn't get the toy for a long time"). In some cases the vignettes matched the facial expressions in the photographs and in other cases they were different. There were also groups of children who received only expressive (pictorial) or contextual cues.

For children of both ages, contextual cues led to greater accuracy than did expressive cues. Contextual information was appropriately identified as producing happiness, sadness, anger, or no specific emotion well over half the time (range: 64%–91%). The only instance when children were more accurate in inferring the emotional states of others was when both contextual and expressive cues were available and consistent with one another (e.g., happy context, happy face), suggesting a cognitive advantage of older children in processing more complex information. When there were inconsistencies between contextual and expressive cues, younger children relied more on expressive cues, whereas older children used contextual cues, indicating that even though contextual cues are truly more informative (leading to greater accuracy), the discovery of their advantage over expressive cues may come only with greater amounts of experience and the realization that some factors, such as display rules promoting the expressive disguising of some emotional reactions, impair the validity of expressive cues.

Gove and Keating (1979) proposed that even during the preschool years children may develop different skills to recognize the determinants of emotion. Specifically, they proposed that children first learn to infer emotional states others are likely to experience by reading situational cues and only later develop the skill of using subjective characteristics of the individual as a means to infer emotional states. In this study, one group of 4- and 5-year-old children were read short stories describing events likely to produce two divergent emotional states and then shown drawings of the two story characters that did not provide cues indicating the characters' emotional states. Another group of children were read stories and shown pictures of the story characters who displayed different emotional responses, even though the actual outcomes of the stories were the same for each character. Younger children were able to infer the emotions of others accurately from situational cues alone, but were not as accurate when required to make inferences based on situational cues in which two emotional responses apparently resulted from the same experiences. Older children not only were able to infer the emotions of others accurately from situational cues but also recognized that people can have differing emotional responses to the same situation and were able to provide sensible rationales for different reactions to the same experience.

Somewhat allied to children's integration of multiple sources of information to infer emotional states is their understanding of the experience and expression of two emotional states simultaneously. Harter (1980) examined children's understanding of multiple emotions using an interview procedure. Children between the ages of 3 and 13 were asked about both the temporal sequencing of two emotional states (e.g., "I was happy that I could watch television and then mad 'cause I had to go to bed") and the actual co-occurrence of two states ("I was excited about my first airplane ride but I was also a little scared"). She found that the youngest children were simply unable to comprehend that two different feelings could go together, but that with increasing age children began to recognize first the possibility of temporal sequencing (average minimum age: $= 6\frac{1}{2}$ to $7\frac{1}{2}$) and then coexistence (average minimum age: 9). Harter found further that in temporal sequence children were more likely to describe emotions with different valences expressed toward different objects, whereas co-occurring emotions were likely to be of similar valence (e.g., both positive) and toward the same person or object.

Studies that induced emotional states in children typically have used a procedure in which children generate thoughts that make them happy, sad, and so on (e.g., Barden et al., 1981; Masters, Barden, & Ford, 1979; Rosenhan, Underwood, & Moore, 1974). The mere fact that this procedure is effective (Masters et al., 1979) indicates that young children are aware of valid determinants of emotional states from which they identify thoughts that produce specific emotional states. Masters and his associates (1979), for example, presented the emotion-producing thoughts that preschool children had generated to adult raters and to other preschool children. Both children and adults were able to identify the emotional states supposedly characterizing the thoughts.

In summary, children as young as 3 years of age do have an understanding of the relationships between events that produce emotional reactions and the actual experiences of emotion. For a number of classes of common childhood experiences likely to lead to emotional responses, children show consensus for the emotional consequences they expect to follow. Finally, as children grow older, they show increasingly sophisticated skills for inferring emotional experiences, both in terms of integrating multiple sources of information and through an understanding of individual differences in emotional response.

Adults' understanding of the determinants of emotion

Few empirical investigations have been concerned directly with adults' knowledge or beliefs about the determinants of emotions. After a review of the literature on emotion, Ekman, Friesen, and Ellsworth wrote: "No one has provided a description of the social variables, or the individual differences which might clarify why and when certain classes of stimuli evoke emotional behavior" (1972, p. 11). Since that writing several research efforts have been aimed toward changing the situation as it existed in 1972, but these efforts do not appear to be conceptually linked together.

In an effort to categorize pleasant and unpleasant mood-related events, Lewisohn and Amenson (1978) administered a questionnaire to more than 850 adult volunteers. Subjects were asked to rate 640 events according to subjective enjoyability or aversiveness and frequency of occurrence. The responses were then factor analyzed. Positive experiences, rated as highly enjoyable, fell into the following categories: (1) social interaction (e.g., seeing old friends, complimenting or praising someone, or thinking about people I like), (2) sexually related actions (e.g., kissing, being with someone I love, expressing my love to someone), (3) positive feedback (e.g., being popular at a social event, amusing people), (4) experiences of comfort and competence (e.g., having peace and quiet, being relaxed, doing a job well), and (5) passive outdoor experiences (e.g., being in the country, seeing beautiful scenery, watching wild animals). Unpleasant, negative-mood-related experiences fell into the following categories: (1) interpersonal discord (e.g., realizing that someone I love and I are growing apart, being near unpleasant people), (2) physical discomfort (e.g., being physically uncomfortable, eating food I don't enjoy), (3) incompetence (e.g., realizing I can't do something I thought I could, having someone disagree with me), (4) work failure (e.g., failing at something, having a project or assignment overdue), and (5) work pressure (e.g., having too much to do, having someone evaluate or criticize me). Although these results have not been cross-validated, they probably capture many of the dimensions on which adults classify positive and negative experiences. Remaining for future exploration are more detailed issues, such as the derivation of a more discriminated conceptualization about the determinants of specific emotional states that may lie within larger categories of postive or negative experiences (e.g., serenity vs. delight, anger vs. fear vs. sadness).

Rippere (1977) asked a cross section of persons identified with psychology (undergraduates, graduates, and faculty members) about their beliefs concerning the everyday experiences of depression. It is important to note that her emphasis was not on information relating to clinical depression but rather on those experiences that occur on a daily basis among the population-at-large. There were three major classes of experience that were felt to produce feelings of depression: (1) letdown (when one has just accomplished an important, long-term goal); (2) boredom (when people haven't got enough to do); and (3) loss of control (when people lose control over important things that happened to them). Rippere also explored beliefs about the exacerbation of depression. Subjects felt that when individuals are *already* feeling depressed they are likely to feel even worse if they are (1) in situations in which one would have little control or choice (e.g., bad news, something breaks), (2) saying negative things to themselves, or (3) trying to engage in activities that have previously been known to be positive experiences (e.g., going to a party, working very hard).

Averill (1979) investigated adults' knowledge about determinants of anger. He integrated data from a survey of a cross section of a New England community with earlier data from studies of anger and aggression. The survey involved asking persons to evalutate their most recent incident of anger using a multiple-choice format. The events leading to anger in adults were categorized along two dimensions: justification and intrinsic characteristics of the situation. For example, more than half the subjects participating in the study indicated that anger would result from events that affected them negatively "in which the instigator knew what he was doing, but he had no right to do it" or when they experienced a "potentially avoidable accident or event which was the result of negligence, carelessness, or lack of foresight" (p. 51). With regard to intrinsic characteristics of the situation, more than 75% of the respondents indicated that anger was a natural and frequent consequence of incidents that led to frustration, to the disruption of ongoing or planned activities, or to the violation of expectations and wishes that were particularly important to them. In addition, subjects indicated that situations that damaged pride/self-esteem or involved socially inappropriate conduct would result in anger. Events that involved property damage or physical harm to the individual also would result in provocation of anger, but such events were not thought to be as frequent in occurrence.

Izard (1977) used a procedure proposed by Triandis (1972) in which subjects were shown photographs that displayed each of nine basic emotions. Subjects were then asked to write a brief statement about the feelings, thoughts, and actions that would precede and follow the particular emotional state in adults. The inventory was administered to more than 100 students at a large university. For most of the emotions studied there was at least one antecedent or consequence, often two, that was nominated by more than 25% of the subjects, although Izard did not present the statistical significance of these shared beliefs.

The determinants proposed by these adult subjects were generally compatible with findings described earlier for children (e.g., Barden et al., 1980), with adults nominating age-appropriate determinants that fell into expectable categories of experience. For instance, antecedents of distress/sadness commonly included thoughts about a specific, personal problem, actions involving something "stupid" or a mistake, and feelings of being lonely or isolated. In contrast to data obtained from young children who indicated that nurturant experiences led to happiness, adults, like older children (Barden et al., 1980), did not often state that nurturant experiences would lead to happiness. Izard also found that adults consistently nominated one or two categories of *feelings* that led to experiencing *other* feelings. Interestingly, investigations with children have not addressed whether children hold shared beliefs about experiencing feelings that lead to other emotional states, although research such as that by Harris and his colleagues (1981) has shown that internal factors (e.g., thoughts) are perceived as potential determinants, at least by older children. This would seem to be a fruitful area for future developmental research.

Little attention has been given (in either the adult or child literature) to the development of an understanding about ways that the characteristics of the person experiencing an emotion may influence the relationship between an emotion-inducing experience and the particular emotion that results. Do adults, for example, assume different emotional responsiveness, in general or to particular events, as a function of a person's age, or sex, or past history? Ekman (e.g., 1972) has nominated such individual characteristics as potential determinants of the *display* of emotion, but this begs the additional possibility that in some instances different personal characteristics lead to actual differences in emotional responsiveness that are recognized by others. In one relevant study, Zelko and his colleagues (1979) investigated adults' beliefs about the determinants of emotion in preschool children. The beliefs of adults were then contrasted with those of children (Barden et al., 1980). For some categories of emotion-producing experience, adults and children held similar beliefs about children's emotional reactions, e.g., success (happiness), nurturance (happiness), failure (sadness), and justified punishment (sadness). There were other categories of experience for which there were age differences in expectancies that may reflect a failure of perspective-taking by adults when they attempt to understand children's feelings. Some of these age differences indicated what may be examples of how adults' understanding of children is less accurate than that of the children themselves. For instance, children were more inclined than adults to expect other young children to feel angry as a result of being aggressed against. In other cases, it appeared that adults may impose their own likely response on children, failing to appreciate the contribution of socialization or maturity to their own reactivity. In response to unjustified punishment, children expected sadness, whereas adults expected anger. For dishonesty, adults (like older children) consistently expected children to be fearful, probably either of being caught or of the punishment that comes after being caught. Young children expected anger following dishonesty that is caught but happiness following dishonesty that is not caught.

It is apparent that adults are at once knowledgeable and ignorant about various aspects of children's emotional response (were there more work on children's understanding of adult emotional reactions we could at this point discuss possible points of mutual understanding and ignorance). At the present time, because there is little evidence about children's *actual* emotional responses to the sorts of experiences surveyed, it is difficult to determine whether children or adults tend to be accurate in their understanding. We suspect that in many cases of disagreement children may be more accurate than adults in the understanding of their own emotional responding. This may occur to the extent that adults share invalid beliefs based on (1) an incorrect assessment of developmental differences between children and adults (e.g., not expecting children to be angry over unjustified punishment) or (2) a tendency to project adult-appropriate responses onto young children ("adultomorphism").

The development and use of mood-induction statements (Velten, 1968) has provided additional, indirect information concerning adults' understanding of the determinants of emotion. An examination of self-referent statements (e.g., "I feel the future is hopeless" or "It's a perfect day for me to stroll in the park") that induce emotional states reveals the sorts of thoughts, perceptions, and experiences that evoke various classes of emotional responding. Carlson, Gantz, and Masters (1983) developed a series of self-referent statements patterned after Velten (1968) for each of three emotional states: happiness, sadness, and neutrality. There were 32 statements rated as likely to produce each emotional state, with the statements being validated for the specific emotional categories on the basis of unanimous and independent ratings by nine adult judges. Subjects were asked to read and ponder the statements according to procedures outlined by Velten (1968). On the basis of pre/post self-report measures of emotional state (Nunnally, 1979), it was found that the statements did induce the targeted emotional states.

Content analyses of the statements revealed a limited number of general categories characterizing them. Sadness inducing statements tended to focus on negative feeling states (e.g., "feel like crying", "don't seem to care," or "feel lonely most of the time"), future outcomes that reflect failure or hopelessness or a lack of social reinforcement (e.g., "no one seems to understand" or "my feelings are easily hurt"). For happiness, two categories of statements were especially prominent: (1) achieving or anticipating success, and (2) feeling states that reflected self-confidence, enthusiasm, or satisfaction (e.g., "it's great to be alive" or "I am full of energy"). The findings from this study are also of interest because they address the validity of adults' judgments (knowledge) of what will lead to a particular emotion: Such thoughts actually *do* induce the targeted emotion.

One basic tenet of attribution theory is that persons seek to determine why an event has occurred (Heider, 1958; Kelley, 1967). Within paradigms developed to investigate adults' understanding of the causal circumstances for emotional reactions, there is thus an additional source of information regarding adults' knowledge about determinants of emotion. Weiner, Russell, and Lerman (1978) gave adult subjects a brief vignette that described a particular situation and subjects were then asked to provide the likely emotional response of an individual. Generally, and not surprisingly, experiences of success resulted in positive moods (happiness) and experiences of failure resulted in negative moods ranging from unhappiness to disgust. When successful situations could be explained in terms of factors residing within the individual (internal attributions), more complex positive emotions (or at least ones with different labels from simple happiness) were expected, such as pride, self-esteem, and confidence. When failure could be explained internally, subjects expected emotions associated with depression, apathy, and resignation.

In a study investigating beliefs about emotional reactions to situations involving requests for help, Weiner (1980) provided subjects with stories of persons seeking help because of uncontrollable causes (illness) or controllable ones (drunkenness, partying). It was found that persons were more likely to say they would react with emotions akin to sympathy, pity, and concern when persons needed help because of uncontrollable, internal causes. However, when help was required because of controllable, internal causes, subjects said their emotional reactions would be anger-related.

Graham and Weiner (1981) asked subjects to describe incidents in which they had experienced emotions of pity, anger, and guilt. The perceived causes of the incidents were then evaluated on dimensions of locus (person-internal/ environment-external), stability (temporary-unstable/lasting-stable), and controllability (controllable/uncontrollable). In anger-related situations, the majority of subjects identified the cause of anger as being external to themselves, temporary, and controllable by someone else. Causes of guilt were seen to be internal/personal, temporary, and controllable by the individual. When the causes were rated as lasting and uncontrollable, the emotion experienced was pity. These studies provide further evidence that adults' understanding of emotional states is rather articulated and that qualifying factors beyond what might be termed the "essence" of an experience (e.g., success, failure) are taken into account. Although there is some indication that children do this too (e.g., dishonesty caught vs. not caught), it has not yet been determined whether or by what age children may come to have an understanding of emotional reactivity that integrates qualifying factors such as locus of causation with more essential aspects of a given experience.

Knowledge and beliefs about the consequences of emotional states

The research reviewed thus far indicates that both children and adults have clearly defined belief systems about the determinants of emotional states. As a natural extension, it might also be expected that children and adults would have beliefs about the consequences of emotional experiences, particularly the consequences for their own behavior, and it is to this that we now turn our attention. In contrast to the paucity of literature concerning the determinants of emotion, there is a more extensive body of literature reflecting the *actual* consequences of emotional states. Where available, this information will serve as a basis upon which to gauge the accuracy of people's understanding about the consequences of emotion.

Children's understanding of the consequences of emotion

The major findings concerning what the actual consequences of emotion are for young children can be summarized briefly. Positive mood states enhance both the speed and accuracy of learning (Barden et al., 1981; Masters et al., 1979) and negative states retard them. Positive mood states also enhance self-control and negative mood states decrease it (Fry, 1975; Mischel, Ebbesen, & Zeiss, 1972; Moore, Clyburn, & Underwood, 1976). Both happiness and sadness increase children's self-reward behavior (Barden et al., 1981; Rosenhan et al., 1974; Underwood, Moore, & Rosenhan, 1973).

The determinants of generosity are more complex and change developmentally. For younger children (4–5 years), positive (happy) moods produce greater generosity than do sad moods (Barden et al., 1981; Cialdini & Kenrick, 1976; Kenrick, Baumann, & Cialdini, 1979; Moore, Underwood, & Rosenhan, 1973; Rosenhan et al., 1974), but for older children (over 10 years) sad moods also increase generosity (Cialdini & Kenrick, 1976; Cialdini, Kenrick, & Baumann, 1981). It has also been found that sad thoughts involving others generate more generosity than sad experiences that are personal in nature (Barnett, King & Howard, 1979).

Felleman, Fischer, and Masters (1981) examined children's consensual knowledge concerning the behavioral consequences of emotion. Children of three ages (4–5 years, 8–9 years, 11–12 years) were asked to imagine that they were in a particular emotional state (happy, sad, angry, or neutral). They were then read a series of brief vignettes that described possible actions and were asked whether they would or would not behave in a particular fashion when they were in the given emotional state. The vignettes represented several broad categories of behaviors known to be influenced by children's emotional states, including aggression, generosity, self-control, self-gratification, and success. There were also subcategories of vignettes representing social and nonsocial aggression, verbal and physical aggression, public and private generosity, and academic and athletic success. For example, a vignette for (private) generosity was as follows: "If you were by yourself and you were feeling (happy/sad/mad/just OK), do you think that you might put some candy on another child's chair?" One for (physical, nonsocial) aggression was, "If you were by yourself and were feeling (happy/sad/mad/just OK), do you think you might throw a toy?"

Children did share a number of expectancies for the behavioral consequences of emotion, but these expectancies were not always accurate. For example, essentially *all* children believed that happy emotions would result in increased generosity, something that is consistent with the literature. Even the youngest children also believed that sadness would lead to more generous behavior as well, although current experimental data indicate that this is true only for older children (over 10 years of age). In general, there were relatively few age differences in children's shared understanding. Some age differences appeared to represent a growing realization that different emotions may have similar effects on some behaviors. For example, young children (4–5 years) expected to show decreased self-control when they were angry, whereas older children expected less self-control when they were angry or sad. For some behavior categories, children held both accurate and inaccurate expectancies. For example, all children expected less self-gratification when they were sad or angry but did not feel that happiness would have any systematic influence. Rather surprisingly, children did *not* indicate that they would expect anger to increase aggression! This finding, because it is rather unbelievable and contrary to available evidence (Harris & Siebel, 1975), suggests that even in a benign experimental setting children may not readily share their knowledge about the aspects of their behavior of negative social value. Regardless of the emotional state, children expected more physical than social aggression and expected to be more aggressive in nonsocial than in social situations. None of the other subcategories for the vignettes were found to make significant differences in children's expectations for outcomes.

The interview study of Harris and his associates also dealt with this issue. Among the questions asked of children was one dealing with the effects of emotion on children's impressions of others: "If you're happy/angry/afraid, what do you think about other people? Do you find them nice or not so nice or doesn't it make any difference?" (1981, p. 255). Older children (ages 11 and 15) believed that people would seem to be nicer when one is in a positive mood rather than in a negative one (angry/afraid), whereas younger children did not expect emotion to influence their judgments of others. The former findings are consistent with early work on projection dealing with 11-year-olds (Murray, 1933), and the latter are consistent with recent findings of

Carlson, Felleman, and Masters (1983) indicating that emotion does not exert a broad influence on young children's judgments of emotion in peers.

Children were also asked how their emotions would influence their abilities to make drawings at school. All children believed that making a drawing would be easier when one was happy than when one was angry or afraid. When asked to explain their reasoning for the effects of emotion on performance, the majority of 6-year-olds did not give any justification for the effects of a positive or a negative mood on subsequent behavior. Although some older children were also unable to provide justifications, those who did said positive effects from positive emotions were due mainly to an increase in the availability of thoughts and ideas needed to create the drawing (e.g., "You can come up with something quicker"), whereas negative emotions reduced the availability of thoughts or ideas relevant to the task and also distracted their attention (e.g., "Your thoughts are somewhere else"). These assessments match findings on children's latencies in problem solving during positive and negative emotional states (Masters et al, 1979).

In summary, there is variability in the accuracy of children's understanding of the consequences of emotional states for cognitive and social behavior. Children appear to be generally accurate in their understanding of the effects of emotion on cognitive functioning (Masters et al., 1979) and on generosity (Barden et al., 1981; Kenrick et al., 1979; Moore et al., 1973). They are also accurate in their assessment of the effects of emotion on judgments of others (Carlson et al., 1983; Murray, 1933). Only older children are accurate concerning their beliefs about the influence of emotion on self-control (Fry, 1975; Mischel et al., 1972; Moore et al., 1976). Finally, children are generally inaccurate regarding their beliefs about the effects of emotions on aggression (Harris & Siebel, 1975) and self-gratification (Barden et al., 1981; Rosenhan et al., 1974). Overall, these findings indicate that children do have expectancies about various likely behavioral outcomes from their emotional states but that these expectancies are not as pervasive as those for the determinants of emotion nor are they consistently accurate. One tentative conclusion is that children's understanding of their own emotional response (Barden et al., 1980) precedes or at least develops more rapidly than their understanding of how emotions may influence their behavior. This suggests that self-monitoring and -appraisal focus first on internal states and only later come to include behavior, perhaps because internal states are themselves salient experiences, whereas one's behavior is noteworthy primarily when it is drawn to one's attention by others (e.g., socialization agents in the act of socialization).

Adults' understanding of the consequences of emotion

The recent development of procedures to induce emotional states in experimental settings under controlled conditions (Bower, 1981; Rosenhan, Salovey, & Hargis, 1981; Thompson, Cowan, & Rosenhan, 1980; Velten, 1968) stimulated the growth of knowledge about the consequences of emotional states for adults as well as children, and the basic findings from this adult literature serve as a means to evaluate the accuracy of adults' understanding of the consequences of emotion. The three general categories of behavior studied involve altruism, cognitive and motor functioning, and social judgment. It is generally found that positive moods increase altruism, but the effects of negative states have been less predictable (Aderman, 1972; Cialdini & Kenrick, 1976). More recently, investigators have reported that factors such as focus of attention during the mood induction (Rosenhan et al., 1981; Thompson et al., 1980), costs or rewards for helping (Weyant, 1978), and the nature of the helping task (Forest et al., 1979) interact with negative emotional states in influencing altruistic behavior. In general, it has been found that positive moods enhance adults' cognitive and motor abilities, whereas negative states retard them (Hale & Strickland, 1976; Strickland, Hale, & Anderson, 1975; Velten, 1968; Williams, 1980). In addition, state-dependent effects on memory processes have been found that indicate improved recall when the emotional state during recall is the same as that when the information was learned (Bower, 1981; Teasdale & Fogarty, 1979). Finally, adults' judgments of emotion in other adults have been found to be influenced by emotional states in a projective fashion (Feshbach & Feshbach, 1963; Hornberger, 1960; Schiffenbauer, 1974). Interestingly, in the one study addressing adults' recognition of emotional states in children, emotional states did not have a pervasive influence (Carlson et al., 1983).

Investigations of adults' beliefs about the behavioral and cognitive consequences of emotional states are relatively sparse. The most extensive work in this domain is that of Izard (1977). It may be recalled that Izard asked college students to write a brief statement about the feelings, thoughts, and actions that would precede or follow various emotional states. The emotions employed in the research with adults have been more diverse than the more "elementary" or "simple" states (happiness, sadness, etc.) that children have been asked about. For example, representative emotional states included interest, enjoyment, surprise, shame or contempt, as well as fear or anger. Just as many of the emotions are more "sophisticated" (it is difficult to find a proper term to capture the parameter of the difference), so are the sorts of beliefs that adults share. These beliefs include cognitive consequences of emotion as well as consequences for overt motoric and social behavior. For example, Izard found that emotional states of fear are thought to create feelings of nervous tension, thoughts and actions of running away and protecting oneself, and/or plans and actions to cope with the situations. When fearful, persons are often believed to have thoughts about how to regain control but to think less frequently about how to talk to someone about the fears or to take action against the cause of the fearful state. Anger is believed to precipitate thoughts of revenge and ways to develop and maintain control of oneself and the situation. Adults in

Izard's sample also believed that angry states resulted in negative thoughts about self and others, and that persons who are angry would take steps toward establishing control in a situation including action, either physical or verbal, against the precipitator of the anger.

Unfortunately, there is little experimental evidence that can be cited to evaluate the accuracy of adults' shared beliefs about the consequences of fear or anger or many of the other more complex emotions that Izard has studied. Work with adults has focused primarily on two emotions, happiness and sadness. Izard did find that adults accurately expected happiness to foster maximum cognitive performances and sharing with others (Aderman, 1972; Cialdini & Kenrick, 1976; Hale & Strickland, 1976; Rosenhan et al., 1981; Strickland et al., 1975; Velten, 1968; Williams, 1980). For sadness, adults predicted (1) a slowing down and (2) withdrawal from social involvement. Research conducted within the laboratory has shown that both beliefs are accurate under certain conditions (Cialdini & Kenrick, 1976; Hale & Strickland, 1976; Strickland et al., 1975; Teasdale & Fogarty, 1979; Thompson et al., 1980; Velten, 1968), but that adults' beliefs did not tend to include the appropriate qualifiers (it may be that the assessment procedure did not encourage adults to give such particulars). For example, Thompson and his associates found that sadness induced by self-referent thoughts reduced helping behavior but that sadness induced by thoughts about others actually increased helping.

The relative paucity of laboratory findings involving the consequences of a range of emotions makes it difficult to give a broad appraisal of adults' accuracy in understanding the consequences of emotion. The general picture that adults draw of emotional response does have surface validity, at least to us, but then we are adults, too, from the same society, and could also be participating in a shared, but incorrect, belief system. Where it has been possible to estimate accuracy, adults' understanding has generally proved correct, although it is not clear that they have an awareness of all the factors that may mediate the effects of emotion on various categories of thought and action.

Since adults do have a common, shared understanding about many emotional states (or labels), a related question concerns the potential consequences of the *beliefs* themselves. Do adults direct their behavior toward others differently as a function of the states they perceive others to be in, in part because of spontaneously generated expectancies about how others think and may behave because of those emotional states? Do adults expressly teach children about the likely consequences of emotional states or do these beliefs constitute a distillation from self-observation or the observation of others? The description of elaborate beliefs about emotional states as determinants of cognition and behavior sets the stage for further inquiry into the functions and development of such beliefs. It is with a consideration of that question that we will now conclude this review.

Behavioral consequences of the understanding of emotion

The role that information and beliefs about emotion play in determining behavior is an important issue that emerges from the study of children's or adults' understanding of emotion even though our knowledge about that understanding is incomplete. In addressing this issue let us briefly consider factors that may mediate the relationships between social perceptions, beliefs, or knowledge and resulting patterns of behavior. In many instances, it is likely that several factors will be involved in determining behavior (Mischel, 1977), but for the purposes of discussion two key factors will be considered, internalized rules for social conduct and expectancies for personal outcomes.

One major factor linking cognitions, emotions, and behavior is the individual's set of rules that direct behavior when there are inadequate external guidelines or contingencies (Mischel, 1973). These internal rules provide a sense of what actions are appropriate in various contexts, the standards for those actions (criteria for adequate performance), and the consequences for achieving or not achieving those standards. Expectations concerning personal outcomes constitute a second potential mediator of the relationship between emotion knowledge or beliefs and behavior. An individual's learning history results in personalized expectations for the outcomes of his or her own behavior and those of others, and these expectations serve to direct personal and social behavior (Mischel, 1973). When outcomes are seen as valuable (rewarding), behaviors designed to elicit those outcomes will often be initiated, but when the potential outcomes are negative, it is likely that behaviors leading to those outcomes will be held in check.

These factors are particularly well illustrated in the development of display rules for emotion in children and adults. Display rules refer to the culturally learned understanding of the conditions under which various emotional states should or should not be expressed. For example, Ekman and his colleagues (e.g., Ekman, 1972; Ekman & Friesen, 1969a, 1969b) have detailed four management techniques for altering the voluntary display of emotion: (1) intensification, that is, increasing display of emotion according to the demands of a situation; (2) deintensification, that is, decreasing the display of emotion, as when victors subdue displays of happiness when in proximity to the defeated competition; (3) emotion neutralization, that is, attempting to maintain little or no display of emotion; and (4) emotion masking, that is, switching one emotional expression for another, as often occurs when one smiles when one is really angry. Ekman (1972) has also given attention to the sorts of factors that may define conditions for the operation of display rules. These include such things as personal characteristics (e.g., age or sex: big boys don't cry) or the particular social situation in which one finds oneself (e.g., a party vs. a funeral).

Saarni (1979a, 1979b, 1981) has studied children's understanding of the use of display rules extensively. In two studies (Saarni, 1979a, 1981), three groups of children (6-, 8-, and 10-year-olds) were asked to indicate the probable emotional states and emotional expressions for themselves and for other children after they or the other child had supposedly encountered situations that involved interpersonal conflict. Children did not always indicate emotional expressions that matched the emotional state they thought they or the target child would be in. When children were given opportunities to explain such discrepancies, Saarni found that even the youngest children gave some display rules (largely after some prompting), but the number of specific rules increased greatly with age. There were several general categories of reasons given for using display rules: (1) to avoid trouble, (2) to maintain self-esteem, (3) to avoid embarrassment and derision, (4) to support relationships, and (5) to express social norms. These data indicate that young children have developed some understanding of the social conventions for the appropriate display/control of emotional expression and that this understanding develops with age and, presumably, experience with outcomes for emotional displays in various situations.

Harris and his associates (1981) asked children about the use of display rules by inquiring about whether one might sometimes be unable to tell how someone else was feeling inside or how someone else might not be able to assess their (the children's) state. Six-year-old Dutch children showed little understanding of the possibility of a discrepancy between inner states and outward expressions, but 11- and 15-year-old children were quite aware of the possibility that display rules could come into play and produce such a discrepancy.

In a very recent study, Saarni (1979b) explored the degree to which children actually invoked display rules and controlled their emotional displays. For this investigation the experimenter posed as a textbook consultant and initially gave first- and fifth-grade children valuable rewards for participation in a workbook evaluation project. Children's facial responses were videotaped and served as a base line to gauge their responses during a second session. At this second session, after providing further evaluation assistance the children received disappointing rewards of little value to them (baby toys) and their facial expressions were again recorded. Younger children, especially boys, did not significantly use display rules and openly expressed their negative reactions. Older children, and in this case especially the girls, masked their likely emotions and in fact reacted (overtly) in a positive fashion.

Of course, display rules do not exhaust the behavioral consequences that may derive from one's understanding of emotion, but the research on display rules does constitute the primary body of systematic inquiry directed specifically at this domain. Other examples of theory and research that deal with the ways that one's understanding of emotion may influence behavior can be identified, but it is generally necessary to extract them from different literatures. For example, an individual's understanding of likely emotional reactions to certain experiences may influence behavior toward a person who has just undergone such an experience, and an understanding of display rules may promote the use of behavioral tactics based on an inferred emotional state even when that state is not apparent in expressive behavior.

On a formal level, theoretical training that deals with concepts such as unconscious or repressed emotional reactions, reaction formations, or projection clearly leads therapists and others so trained to behave (both therapeutically and socially) in ways dictated by their acquired understanding of emotion (Freud, 1896/1950; White, 1964). More informally, people may generate behavioral and emotional expectancies based on their personal theory (understanding) of emotion and, especially when these expectancies are incorrect, stigmatization may result.

Let us draw some illustrative findings from the literature on divorce. Santrock and Tracy (1978) showed 30 teachers a videotape of an 8-year-old boy's social behavior. Half the teachers were told that the boy was from a divorced family, and half were told that the boy was from an intact family. The teachers were then asked to rate the boy on 11 personality traits and to predict the boy's behavior in different school situations. Although the teachers watched the same videotape, teachers rated the divorced child more negatively on ratings of happiness, emotional adjustment, and the ability to cope with stress. In another study, Santrock (1977) found that teachers reported that father-absent boys were less advanced in moral development. Such stereotypic expectancies include both emotions and emotion-related behaviors.

Although these studies did not assess different behaviors directly, it seems a short inferential leap to propose that teachers may actually treat children from divorced families differently as a function of their implicit, stereotyped assumptions about their emotional states and proclivities for emotion-related behaviors. Within the divorce literature there are also common reports of marriages being held together because of anticipated emotional consequences of divorce for children (Tuckman & Regan, 1966).

There are clearly several dimensions to the relationship between an individual's understanding about emotional states and the behavior that may be influenced or directed by that understanding. In the case of display rules, understanding directs another facet of emotion, voluntarily controlled expression. In other instances, an understanding of emotional response may initiate expectancies about the behavior of others, modify how one chooses to interact with others, or even modify one's own behavior as when one decides not to enter a situation on the anticipation of its emotional consequences (e.g., the assessment of one's own transient or permanent vulnerability: "I don't think I could stand it if . . ."). The general point is that the understanding of emotion that an individual acquires does affect behavior. Questions of interest are not whether this is so but rather questions that address important classes of behavior that may relate to an individual's understanding of emotion. Examples of such behaviors include the use of display rules, the self-monitoring of vulnerability, and actions toward others that are modified by, or that are designed to modify, their emotional states.

Summary

It is difficult to summarize a review such as this, but there are a few points that bear brief mention once more. Children and adults share an understanding of the relationships between several classes of events that are likely to evoke emotional responses in peers and themselves. However, with age, there are systematic changes in such understanding that appear to reflect increasing experience, changing socialization pressures, and growing cognitive and social sophistication. For example, with increasing age more sophisticated skills to include multiple sources of information and an awareness of individual differences for emotional response are employed to infer the emotional states of others.

There is also evidence to suggest that adults generally nominate appropriate determinants of emotion in children, but data are not readily available that specifically address whether or not children have a broad understanding of the determinants of emotion in adults. Although laboratory inductions of mood states and studies of attribution processes provide cross-validation for the actual determinants of several specific emotional states, there remains within the larger categories of positive and negative experiences ample room for further inquiry to identify the dimensions on which experiences producing emotional reactions may be classified. Once such information is more readily available, it should be possible to refine still further theories about emotional response and expression.

Both children and adults also have expectancies, albeit not always accurate, concerning the likely consequences of ongoing emotional states. For children these expectancies are not as pervasive as those for the emotional consequences of experience, and their accuracy as judged by what has been found in laboratory studies is not particularly high. The consistency and accuracy of adults' understanding of the consequences of emotion, where data are available, appears to be greater than that of children. Even so, the extent to which adults have an awareness of the factors that mediate the effects of emotion on behavior and cognition remains unclear.

We gave only brief attention to the potential relationships between the understanding of emotion (meta-emotion), emotion-inducing experiences, and subsequent behavior. In particular, the use of self-control strategies with respect to emotional expression was presented within the context of display rule usage and emotion or emotional behavior stereotypes that one develops through common experience or formal training. This is surely one of the most important domains related to emotion and people's understanding of emotion, and one deserving of greater attention in future research.

Notes

1 We will generally attempt to draw a distinction between knowledge about emotion and beliefs about it. Knowledge will refer to beliefs about emotions for which there is confirming empirical evidence. The term *beliefs* will be reserved for those beliefs that are in contradiction to the evidence or for which there is no evidence, confirming or otherwise. To avoid excessive use of the cumbersome phrase "knowledge or beliefs," we will use the term *understanding* to embrace both knowledge and beliefs.

References

Aderman, D. Elation, depression and helping behavior. *Journal of Personality and Social Psychology*, 1972, *24*, 91–101.

Averill, J. R. Anger. In H. E. Howe, Jr. (Ed.), *Nebraska symposium on motivation* (Vol. 27). Lincoln: University of Nebraska Press, 1979.

Barden, R. C., Garber, J., Duncan, S. W., & Masters, J. C. Cumulative effects of induced affective states in children: Remediation, inoculation and accentuation. *Journal of Personality and Social Psychology*, 1981, *40*, 750–760.

Barden, R. C., Zelko, F. A., Duncan, S. W., & Masters, J. C. Children's consensual knowledge about the experiential determinants of emotion. *Journal of Personality and Social Psychology*, 1980, *39*, 968–976.

Barnett, M. A., King, L. M., & Howard, J. A. Inducing affect about self or other: Effects on generosity in children. *Developmental Psychology*, 1979, *15*, 164–167.

Borke, H. Interpersonal perception of young children: Egocentrism or empathy? *Developmental Psychology*, 1971, *5*, 262–269.

Borke, H. Chandler and Greenspan's "Ersatz egocentrism." *Developmental Psychology*, 1972, *7*, 107–109.

Bower, G. H. Mood and memory. *American Psychologist*, 1981, *36*, 129–148.

Bretherton, I., & Beeghly, M. Talking about internal states: The acquisition of an explicit theory of mind. *Developmental Psychology*, in press.

Bridgman, P. W. *The logic of modern physics*. New York: Macmillan, 1927.

Camras, L. A. Children's understanding of facial expressions used during conflict encounters. *Child Development*, 1980, *51*, 879–885.

Cannon, W. B. *The wisdom of the body*. New York: Norton, 1932.

Carlson, C. R., Felleman, E. S., & Masters, J. C. Influence of children's emotional states on the recognition of emotion in peers and social motives to change another's emotional state. *Motivation and Emotion*, 1983, *7*, 61–79.

Carlson, C. R., Gantz, F., & Masters, J. C. Adults' emotional states and recognition of emotion in young children. *Motivation and Emotion*, 1983, *7*, 81–101.

Chandler, M. J., & Greenspan, S. Ersatz egocentrism: A reply to H. Borke. *Developmental Psychology*, 1972, *7*, 104–106.

Cialdini, R. B., & Kenrick, D. T. Altruism as hedonism: A social developmental perspective on the relation of mood states and helping. *Journal of Personality and Social Psychology*, 1976, *34*, 907–914.

Cialdini, R. B., Kenrick, D. T., & Baumann, D. J. Effects of mood on prosocial behavior in children and adults. In N. Eisenberg-Berg (Ed.), *The development of prosocial behavior*. New York: Academic Press, 1981.

Deutsch, F. Female preschoolers' perceptions of affective responses and interpersonal behavior in videotaped episodes. *Developmental Psychology*, 1974, *10*, 733–740.

Ekman, P. Facial expressions of emotion. In J. K. Cole (Ed.), *Nebraska symposium on motivation* (Vol. 19). Lincoln: University of Nebraska Press, 1972.

Ekman, P., & Friesen, W. V. Nonverbal leakage and clues to deception. *Psychiatry*, 1969, *32*, 88–106. (a)

Ekman, P., & Friesen, W. V. The repertoire of nonverbal behavior. *Semiotica*, 1969, *1*, 49–98. (b)

Ekman, P., Friesen, W. V., & Ellsworth, P. *Emotion in the human face: Guidelines for research and integration of findings*. New York: Pergamon Press, 1972.

Farber, E. A., & Moely, B. F. *Inferring others' affective states: The use of interpersonal, vocal and facial cue by children of three age levels*. Paper presented at the biennial meetings of the Society for Research in Child Development, San Francisco, 1979.

Feinman, J. A., & Feldman, R. S. Decoding children's expressions of affect. *Child Development*, 1982, *53*, 710–716.

Felleman, E. S., Fischer, M. J., & Masters, J. C. *Children's expectancies about the behavioral consequences of their own emotional states*. Unpublished manuscript, Vanderbilt University, 1981.

Feshbach, S., & Feshbach, N. Influence of the stimulus object upon the complementary and supplementary projection of fear. *Journal of Abnormal and Social Psychology*, 1963, *66*, 498–502.

Flavell, J. H., & Wellman, H. M. Metamemory. In R. V. Kail, Jr., & J. W. Hagen (Eds.), *Perspectives on the development of memory and cognition*. Hillsdale, N.J.: Erlbaum, 1977.

Forest, D., Clark, M. S., Mills, J., & Isen, A. M. Helping as a function of feeling state and nature of the helping behavior. *Motivation and Emotion*, 1979, *3*, 161–169.

Fortenbaugh, W. W. *Aristotle on emotion*. New York: Harper & Row, 1975.

Freud, S. Further remarks on the defense neuropsychosis. In *Collected papers* (Vol. 1). London: Hogarth, 1950. (Originally published, 1896.)

Fry, P. S. Affect and resistance to temptation. *Developmental Psychology*, 1975, *2*, 466–472.

Gelman, R. Cognitive development. In M. R. Rosenzweig & L. W. Porter (Eds.), *Annual review of psychology* (Vol. 29). Palo Alto, Calif.: Annual Reviews, 1978.

Gove, F. L., & Keating, D. P. Empathic role-taking precursors. *Developmental Psychology*, 1979, *15*, 594–600.

Graham, S., & Weiner, B. *An attributional analysis of some commonly experienced emotional states*. Paper presented at the annual meeting of the American Psychological Association, Los Angeles, 1981.

Green, S. K. Causal attribution of emotion in kindergarten children. *Developmental Psychology*, 1977, *13*, 533–534.

Greenspan, S., Barenboim, C., & Chandler, M. J. Empathy and pseudo-empathy: The affective judgments of first- and third-graders. *Journal of Genetic Psychology*, 1976, *129*, 77–88.

Hale, W. P., & Strickland, B. R. Induction of mood states and their effect on cognitive and social behaviors. *Journal of Consulting and Clinical Psychology*, 1976, *14*, 155.

Harris, M. B., & Siebel, C. E. Affect, aggression and altruism. *Developmental Psychology*, 1975, *11*, 623–627.

Harris, P. L., Olthof, T., & Terwogt, M. M. Children's knowledge of emotion. *Journal of Child Psychiatry and Psychology*, 1981, *22*, 247–261.

Harter, S. A cognitive-developmental approach to children's understanding of affect and trait labels. In F. Serafica (Ed.), *Social cognition in context*. New York: Guilford Press, 1980.

Heider, F. *The psychology of interpersonal relations*. New York: Wiley, 1958.

Hornberger, R. H. The projective effects of fear and sexual arousal on the rating of pictures. *Journal of Clinical Psychology*, 1960, *16*, 328–331.

Izard, C. E. *The face of emotion*. New York: Appleton-Century-Crofts, 1972.

Izard, C. E. *Human emotions*. New York: Plenum, 1977.

James, W. What is an emotion? *Mind*, 1884, *9*, 188–205.

Kelley, H. H. Attribution theory in social psychology. In D. Levine (Ed.), *Nebraska symposium on motivation* (Vol. 15). Lincoln: University of Nebraska Press, 1967.

Kenrick, D. T., Baumann, D. J., & Cialdini, R. B. A step in the socialization of altruism as hedonism: Effects of negative mood on children's generosity under public and private conditions. *Journal of Personality and Social Psychology*, 1979, *37*, 747–755.

Kreutzer, M. A., Leonard, C., & Flavell, J. H. An interview study of children's knowledge about memory. *Monographs of the Society for Research in Child Development*, 1975, *40*, Ser. 159.

Kurdek, L. A., & Rodgon, M. M. Perceptual, cognitive and affective perspective taking in kindergarten through sixth-grade children. *Developmental Psychology*, 1975, *11*, 643–650.

Lazarus, R. S. Emotion and adaptation: Conceptual and empirical relations. In W. J. Arnold (Ed.), *Nebraska symposium on motivation* (Vol. 16). Lincoln: University of Nebraska Press, 1969.

Lewinsohn, P. M., & Amenson, C. S. Some relations between pleasant and unpleasant mood-related events and depression. *Journal of Abnormal Psychology*, 1978, *87*, 644–654.

Masters, J. C., Barden, R. C., & Ford, M. E. Affective states, expressive behavior and learning in children. *Journal of Personality and Social Psychology*, 1979, *37*, 380–390.

Mischel, W. *Personality and assessment*. New York: Wiley, 1968.

Mischel, W. Toward a cognitive social learning reconceptualization of personality. *Psychological Review*, 1973, *80*, 252–283.

Mischel, W. On the future of personality measurement. *American Psychologist*, 1977, *32*, 246–254.

Moore, B. S., Clyburn, A., & Underwood, B. The role of affect in delay of gratification. *Child Development*, 1976, *47*, 273–276.

Moore, B. S., Underwood, B., & Rosenhan, D. L. Affect and altruism. *Developmental Psychology*, 1973, *8*, 99–104.

Murray, H. A. The effect of fear upon estimates of the maliciousness of other personalities. *Journal of Social Psychology*, 1933, *4*, 310–329.

Nunnally, J. C. *The affect inventory*. Unpublished manuscript, Vanderbilt University, 1979.

Odom, R. D., & Lemond, C. M. Developmental differences in the perception and production of facial expressions. *Child Development*, 1972, *43*, 359–369.

Piaget, J. *The language and thought of the child*. New York: Harcourt, Brace & World, 1926.

Plutchik, R. Emotions, evolution and adaptive processes. In M. B. Arnold (Ed.), *Feelings and emotions*. New York: Academic Press, 1970.

Reichenbach, L., & Masters, J. C. Children's use of expressive and contextual cues in judgments of emotion. *Child Development*, 1983, *54*, 993–1004.

Rippere, V. Commonsense beliefs about depression and antidepressive behaviour: A study of social consensus. *Behaviour Research and Therapy*, 1977, *15*, 465–473.

Rosenhan, D. L., Salovey, P., & Hargis, K. The joys of helping: Focus of attention mediates the impact of positive affect on altruism. *Journal of Personality and Social Psychology*, 1981, *40*, 899–905.

Rosenhan, D. L., Underwood, B., & Moore, B. Affect moderates self-gratification and altruism. *Journal of Personality and Social Psychology*, 1974, *30*, 546–552.

Saarni, C. Children's understanding of display rules for expressive behavior. *Developmental Psychology*, 1979, *15*, 424–429. (a)

Saarni, C. *When not to show what you feel: Children's understanding of relations between emotional experience and expressive behavior*. Paper presented at the biennial meetings of the Society for Research in Child Development, San Francisco, 1979. (b)

Saarni, C. *Emotional experience and regulation of expressive behavior*. Paper presented at the biennial meetings of the Society for Research in Child Development, Boston, 1981.

Santrock, J. W. Effects of father absence on sex-typed behaviors in male children: Reasons for the absence and age of onset of the absence. *Journal of Genetic Psychology*, 1977, *130*, 3–10.

Santrock, J. W., & Tracy, R. L. The effects of children's family structure status on the development of stereotypes by teachers. *Journal of Educational Psychology*, 1978, *70*, 754–757.

Schachter, S. *The psychology of affiliation*. Stanford, Calif.: Stanford University Press, 1959.

Schachter, S. *Emotion, obesity and crime*. New York: Academic Press, 1972.

Schachter, S., & Singer, J. Cognitive, social and physiological determinants of emotional state. *Psychological Review*, 1962, *69*, 378–399.

Schiffenbauer, A. Effect of observer's emotional state on judgments of the emotional state of others. *Journal of Personality and Social Psychology*, 1974, *30*, 31–35.

Skinner, B. F. Are theories of learning necessary? *Psychological Review*, 1950, *57*, 193–216.

Strickland, B. R., Hale, W. D., & Anderson, L. K. Effect of induced mood states on activity and self-reported affect. *Journal of Consulting and Clinical Psychology*, 1975, *43*, 587.

Surbey, P. D. *Preschool children's understanding of emotional states in terms of causes and consequences*. Unpublished master's thesis, University of Minnesota, 1979.

Teasdale, J. D., & Fogarty, S. J. Differential effects of induced mood on retrieval of pleasant and unpleasant events from episodic memory. *Journal of Abnormal Psychology*, 1979, *88*, 248–257.

Thompson, W. C., Cowan, C. L., & Rosenhan, D. L. Focus of attention mediates the impact of negative affect on altruism. *Journal of Personality and Social Psychology*, 1980, *38*, 291–300.

Tomkins, S. S. *Affect, imagery, and consciousness*, Vol. 1: *The positive affects*. New York: Springer-Verlag, 1962.

Tomkins, S. S. *Affect, imagery, and consciousness*, Vol. 2: *The negative affects*. New York: Springer-Verlag, 1963.

Tomkins, S. S. The quest for primary motives: Biography and autobiography of an idea. *Journal of Personality and Social Psychology*, 1981, *41*, 306–329.

Trabasso, T., Stein, N. L., & Johnson, L. R. Children's knowledge of events: A causal analysis of story structure. In G. Bower (Ed.), *The psychology of learning and motivation* (Vol. 15). New York: Academic Press, 1981.

Triandis, H. *The analysis of subjective culture*. New York: Wiley, 1972.

Tuckman, J., & Regan, R. A. Intactness of the home and behavioral problems in chldren. *Journal of Child Psychology and Psychiatry*, 1966, *7*, 225–233.

Underwood, B., Moore, B. S., & Rosenhan, D. L. Affect and self-gratification. *Developmental Psychology*, 1973, *8*, 209–214.

Velten, E. A. A laboratory task for the induction of mood states. *Behaviour Research and Therapy*, 1968, *6*, 473–482.

Watson, J. B. *Psychology from the standpoint of a behaviorist* (3rd ed., rev.). Philadelphia: Lippincott, 1929.

Watson, J. B. *Behaviorism* (rev. ed.). Chicago: University of Chicago Press, 1930.

Weiner, B. A cognitive (attribution)-emotion-action model of motivated behavior: An analysis of judgments of help-giving. *Journal of Personality and Social Psychology*, 1980, *39*, 186–200.

Weiner, B., Russell, D., & Lerman, D. Affective consequences of causal ascriptions. In J. H. Harvey, W. J. Ickes, & R. F. Kidd (Eds.), *New directions in attribution research* (Vol. 2). Hillsdale, N.J.: Erlbaum, 1978.

Weyant, J. M. Effects of mood states, costs and benefits on helping. *Journal of Personality and Social Psychology*, 1978, *36*, 1169–1176.

White, R. W. *The abnormal personality*. New York: Ronald Press, 1964.

Williams, J. M. G. Generalization in the effects of a mood induction procedure. *Behaviour Research and Therapy*, 1980, *18*, 565–572.

Zahn-Waxler, C., Radke-Yarrow, M., & King, R. Child-rearing and children's prosocial initiations towards victims of distress. *Child Development*, 1979, *50*, 319–330.

Zelko, F. A., Duncan, S. W., Barden, R. C., Garber, J., & Masters, J. C. *Adults' understanding of children's understanding of emotional responding*. Paper presented at the annual meetings of the American Psychological Association, New York, 1979.

15 Emotion, self, and others

Bert Moore, Bill Underwood, and D. L. Rosenhan

Literature and life abound with evidence that our view of ourselves and our universe is profoundly colored by our moods. The last decade has seen an upsurge in investigations of the ways emotional states influence our responses to ourselves and others. This chapter reviews this emerging literature and derives some principles of how emotion moderates these processes. For our purposes emotion is seen as a sensory-feeling state that acts as a motivator, categorizer, and selector of perceptual and cognitive events and behaviors.

The literature that might support a coherent picture of the ways emotion influences reactions to the self and others has been scattered. Relevant elements exist in such work as the effects of success and failure on behavior; clinical literature on emotion; laboratory investigations of happiness, sadness, anxiety, and anger; and correlation work that relates mood to a variety of personality measures and day-to-day behavior. A comprehensive review of this literature is beyond our scope. Rather, this chapter is a selective review of areas that point to some important ways in which emotion influences reponses to the self and others. Examination of these complicated relationships is a step toward forming a general model of the role of emotions in self/other responses.

In this review, we focus on two emotions: happiness and sadness. We have chosen these over others because of the number and variety of studies of happiness and sadness, and because of the potential relevance of such studies for important clinical phenomena. Although our focus is on happiness/sadness at the expense of other affective states, it should be noted that many emotions are doubtlessly interrelated, perhaps even idiosyncratically so. It has been demonstrated recently that laboratory inductions designed to induce a single affective state, such as sadness, anger, or fear, can actually cause significant alterations in all those states simultaneously (Polivy, 1981; Underwood, Froming, & Moore, 1982). This possibility suggests that one must be cautious in attributing the results of a study to the operation of *an* affect and also argues for the inclusion of manipulation checks that assess multiple affective states.

This review will emphasize investigations that employ induced-mood states because of interpretational problems that arise when clinical moods, such as

This study was supported, in part, by a grant from the Kenneth and Harle Montgomery Fund to D. L. Rosenhan.

depression, are investigated. However, we will draw on the clinical literature to highlight comparable processes. Similar sorts of caveats must be stated regarding investigations that have employed success and failure as inducers of mood. Although such experiences undoubtedly influence affect, they also influence several different affective states, thus complicating the task of interpretation. Furthermore, success and failure also have been shown to influence such nonaffective states as self-rated competence (Kazdin & Bryan, 1971) and expectations for further success or failure (Feather, 1966), which further muddy the interpretive waters. For these reasons, the success-failure studies in this review are not a primary focus.

Emotion and reactions to self

Our moods are potent determiners of our responses to ourselves. The flush of buoyant self-approbation that accompanies a "high" and the self-abnegation and self-doubt that accompany depression are forms of self-reaction that are part of the defining characteristics of the emotions with which they are associated. The relationship between affect and self-reaction is undoubtedly bidirectional, with affect engendering certain cognitions and those cognitions leading to distinctive affective experiences. (For a comprehensive examination of these issues, examine Izard's *Human Emotions*, 1977, and Mandler's *Mind and Emotion*, 1975.) In this section we examine representative research on self-oriented cognitive and behavioral consequences of affect.

Availability and memory

Emotion alters attention and recall and, through them, cognitions about self. The power of emotion in this regard is seen in a study by Mischel, Ebbesen, and Zeiss (1976), who induced success and failure to explore the relationship between affect and memory for personality information. Their subjects were exposed to equal amounts of positive and negative personality information, which purportedly was derived from previous personality testing. They were subsequently tested for recall of the information. Those subjects who experienced success were better able to recall personality strengths than liabilities. Those who experienced failure, however, did not differ from controls. Similar findings were obtained by Isen (1970).

Although these findings suggest that only positive affect has potent effects on recall of personality-relevant information, later studies indicate that negative emotion has similar effects. Teasdale and Fogarty (1979) examined the personal memories that happy and sad moods evoke. On separate occasions, happy and sad moods were induced. On each occasion subjects were presented with a series of words. For each word they were asked to recall a past real-life experience, specified to be either pleasant or unpleasant, that they associated with the word. Using latency of retrieval for each experience, Teasdale and Fogarty found that happy subjects retrieved happy memories faster then sad ones and that sad subjects retrieved sad memories faster than happy ones.

Affect determines both the tone and the availability of memories. For example, people who are happy give more favorable evaluations of the performance and service records of their cars than do those who are not. Moreover, happy people recall more positive (but not more neutral or negative) words than do control subjects (Isen et al., 1978). Positive affect in particular may promote a "cognitive loop" that increases the salience and availability of positively toned memories.

Finally, the valence of an experienced emotion determines the valence of memories that are recalled. Subjects who had been maintaining daily diaries of "emotional events" were subsequently induced to experience emotion hypnotically. Those who were in a pleasant mood recalled more of their pleasant experiences than their unpleasant ones, whereas those who were in a negative mood recalled a higher proportion of their unpleasant memories (Bower, 1981).

Interestingly, some of these findings have been corroborated in clinical populations. An investigation by Lloyd and Lishman (1975) that used depressed patients closely parallels the findings of Teasdale and Fogarty (1979). Subjects were instructed to recall a happy or sad personal incident in response to neutral words. The more severe the depression, the longer it took to retrieve a pleasant, as opposed to an unpleasant, memory.

It appears then that mood, experimentally induced or existing endogenously, influences retrieval of self-relevant information in an affect-congruent fashion. The effect seems more clear-cut for positive than for negative memories.

In addition to information retrieval, the process of thinking about ongoing behavior has been investigated in relation to mood. One format for this investigation has been in the area of attribution research.

Emotion and self-attribution

Although a large literature exists on the manner in which people infer emotion (see Sherrod, 1982, for a discussion), fewer studies have explored the effects of emotion on attribution. This is an important area of investigation because self-attribution has potent effects on persistence and success at tasks, on expectancies regarding future performance, and on social comparison processes.

Emotion appears to influence attribution markedly. One investigation examined the effects of manipulated affect on self-attribution of causality. Subjects received false feedback about their performance on a person-perception task, with half the subjects told that they had done very well and half told that they had done badly. Subjects were then asked to generate either positive, neutral, or negative affective imagery. Finally, all subjects were asked to make causal attributions about their performance on the person-perception task. On three of the four measures of attribution there was a significant interaction between affective state and attributions for success and failure. Subjects who had generated sad thoughts took more personal responsibility for both failures and successes than did controls or positive-affect subjects (cf. Alloy & Abramson, 1979; Alloy, Abramson, & Viscusi, 1981). Clearly, sadness may predispose one toward negative self-referential information, as we have previously noted. At the same time, the tendency to take increased credit for success under negative affect serves to alleviate the sadness (Hoffman, 1978).

Although depressed people do not differ from the nondepressed in their initial estimates of how well they would perform on an ambiguous task, they are significantly more affected by failure feedback than are normals. Their estimates of performance are more profoundly affected by failure feedback and less affected by success feedback than are normals (Hammen & Krantz, 1976). Thus, depression does not merely produce global pessimism but rather predisposes toward attending to, and emphasizing, certain types of feedback.

This view is buttressed by the finding that depressives differ from normals in their retrospective causal ascriptions of performance on an achievement-related task. Depressives rate internal factors (ability and effort) as more important causal determinants of failure but less important determinants of success than do nondepressed subjects (Rizley, 1978).

Perception of control. Another issue relating to the self-cognition consequences of affective states is mood's effect on an individual's perception of control. Locus of control has been one of the heavily researched dimensions of the last fifteen years, and, in spite of its having been used in a broader fashion than was originally intended (Rotter, 1975), it has been found to be an important predictor of a number of behaviors. We would ordinarily expect that positive affect would be associated with greater expectations of the control of reinforcers being internal and that is precisely what was found by Natale (1978). Subjects completed Rotter's locus of control scale before and after an affect-induction procedure. Elation caused an increased sense of internality, whereas sadness caused an increased sense of externality. These findings are partially supported by Masters and Furman (1976), who found that positive affect generated greater expectations for noncontingent success on a task. (Masters and Furman, however, did not find a difference between neutral and sad conditions.)

Alloy and her associates (1981) examined the effects of mood on subjects' perceptions of personal control. Previous work by Alloy and Abramson (1979) had suggested that depressed people accurately judge their personal control, whereas nondepressed people may succumb to an "illusion of control" and overestimate their impact on objectively uncontrollable circumstances. Alloy and her colleagues (1981) induced sadness in nondepressed college women and elated mood in naturally depressed women and assessed the effects of these transient mood states on sense of personal control. They found that nondepressed women who were made transiently sad became more like chronically depressed women in that they gave *more* accurate assessments of contingencies. Correspondingly, naturally depressed women who experienced a positive-mood induction overestimated their control over contingencies.

Self-concept

One would not expect transient emotional states to markedly affect personality structure, and so far, no such effects have been found (Underwood, Froming, & Moore, 1980). But emotion might well influence transient self-concept – those aspects of self-concept that show high variability across relatively brief periods of time. The evidence suggests that that seems to be the case. When one examines daily mood ratings and compares them to self-descriptions and self-esteem questionnaires, one finds that self-concept varies with mood. Happy people describe themselves as productive and more able to excel than do unhappy ones. Moreover, mood ratings correlate significantly with self-esteem (Wessman & Ricks, 1966).

The effects of emotion on relatively transient, or "state," self-concept have now been demonstrated in a variety of studies, with some interesting implications. Underwood and his associates (1980) demonstrate that after the induction of happiness people feel more skillful, competent, proficient, and successful than they do after the induction of sadness. In a subsequent study, these investigators found negative affect generated by failure experiences made people feel less sociable. Finally, Amrhein, Salovey, and Rosenhan (1982) found that emotion has differential effects on men's and women's self-concept. When men are sad, they feel less sociable, intelligent, attractive, and even healthy than they do when they are happy. Women, in contrast, retain a relatively stable self-concept regardless of affective state. Conceivably, women have greater experience in dealing with emotion than do men, for whom emotional expression is considered the greater taboo. As a result, when men are overcome by strong emotion, the effects are relatively more powerful because they have less skill in handling such emotion.

Behavioral measures of self-reaction

We have described a variety of ways in which cognition about the self is influenced by affective state. We now turn to an examination of behavioral consequences of mood. Presumably these behavioral indexes have a variety of cognitive antecedents and consequences. However, for organizational purposes it is convenient to examine separately studies that have focused on affect-behavior relationships. We would expect that the self-relevant behaviors produced by affective states would reflect the operation of some of the cognitive mechanisms suggested thus far. Positive mood should be associated with behaviors reflecting optimistic, self-approving expectations. Negative mood may produce more complicated patterns of behavior, with examples of more pessimistic, self-denying behaviors in some situations and behaviors designed to ameliorate the negative affect in other contexts.

Task performance

One issue that relates to the question of how affective state influences self-reactions has to do with how actual task performance is affected for mood states. If moods influence achievement on tasks, they must perforce set conditions for positive or negative self-reactions, which in turn may well effect subsequent task performance. A comprehensive review of this issue goes well beyond the scope of this chapter, but some relevant examples of research on this issue are quite illuminating.

Emotion powerfully affects the task performance of very young children. Sadness increases the amount of time it takes for them to learn a discrimination task, as well as their response latencies and the number of errors they make. Happiness, on the other hand, reverses all of this, decreasing learning times, latencies, and numbers of errors (Masters, Barden, & Ford, 1979). These findings, however, have not yet been fully supported in studies of adults. Response latencies on anagram tasks, for example, are predictably influenced by sadness, since sadness slows down all responses. But performance accuracy is not differentially influenced by positive and negative emotion (Moore et al., 1982).

An early study by Gouaux and Gouaux (1971) also used adult subjects. They followed Velten's procedure for the induction of affective states but examined the consequences of induced states on adults' sensitivity to social and nonsocial reinforcers during the acquisition and maintenance of effortful behavior. They found that negative emotional states retarded the acquisition of the task and produced quicker extinction. These effects were accentuated when social reinforcers were involved, indicating not only that emotional states influence learning and persistence directly but also that the effectiveness of social incentives to learn is greater than that of tangible incentives.

To the extent that learning and recall can be considered tasks that mandate skill and effort, several studies find no direct mood effects. Bower (1981) and Gilligan and Bower (Chapter 18, this volume) discuss a number of experiments relating affective states to memory processes. We will not describe these studies in detail but do wish to note several points. The bulk of this research on affect and memory has focused on state-dependent memory, the facilitation of recall when it occurs in an affective state congruent with that which occurred during original learning. In general, Bower and others (Bartlett & Santrock, 1979; Moore, Underwood, & Terrazas, 1982) have not found main effects for mood on memory. There does not appear to be a general tendency for induced affect to produce either facilitative or debilitating effects on memory. It does appear that affect can serve as part of a contextual net by which material is retrieved. Additionally, Moore and his associates (1982) found that there was an interaction between affective state and affect-relevant stimulus materials.

One would expect that the associative strength of affective states would be greater for affect-relevant words than for affectively neutral words, because of the semantic connections that have been produced long before people come into a psychology laboratory. If this is true, then one should anticipate that the state-dependency effect would be stronger for affectively relevant words, as proved to be the case. One might also anticipate that a stronger associative value of affective states for affectively relevant words would produce a tendency for all affect induction groups to have relatively better memory for affectively relevant than for affectively neutral words, compared to the control group. This effect was also noted in the outcome of the experiment conducted by Moore and his associates (1982). Positive-affect subjects showed more efficient recall for both positive- and negative-affect words, whereas negative-affect subjects showed better recall for negative- but not positive-affect words. Compare this finding to the finding by Isen and her associates (1978) that positive-affect subjects recalled positive words more efficiently. It may be that there is a general affect congruence tendency in memory but that positive affect enables us to recall both positive- and negative-affect information, whereas negative affect acts more as a stringent filter, leading to selective focusing on negatively tinged memories.

Leight and Ellis (1981) used an interesting task to investigate the manner in which experimentally induced mood states influenced the recall and chunking of letter sequences. The task required the use of a chunking strategy to optimize performance, and Leight and Ellis included measures of both overall recall and the use of chunking strategy. They found that depressed mood hindered both recall and chunking. Interestingly, negative affect appeared to decrease the use of a facilitative strategy on not only a particular task but on the use of such strategy on a similar task 24 hours later. It appeared that sadness produced cognitive rigidity, which hindered task performance. Additionally, it may have reduced cognitive effort for task-specific demands.

Performance and attention

Isen (1970) investigated the effects of success and failure on memory for interpersonal information. She told subjects that they had performed very well or very poorly on a task related to creativity or gave no feedback. Subjects were then left to wait for the experimenter to return while an experimental confederate came into the room and performed a series of actions. When the experimenter returned, she questioned subjects about the confederate's actions. Subjects who had been told that they performed poorly, and were thus presumably in a negative affective state, remembered fewer of the confederate's actions than did control subjects or success (positive-affect) subjects.

Underwood, Froming, and Moore (1977), as part of a larger study, investigated the possible existence of attentional differences between positive- and negative-affect subjects. Using the reminiscence affect induction procedure, they had elementary-school children participate in an incidental learning task. They found no difference among affect and control conditions for their recall of items on a bulletin board. They concluded that, at least for these subjects under these manipulations, affect did not determine attention to extraneous environmental information.

However, another study by Moore and Underwood (1982), which used a measure of recall for behavior of a model, found that elementary-school children did differ in their ability to remember aspects of a behavior sequence depending on which affective state had been previously induced. Thus it appears that it is premature to draw firm conclusions regarding the influence of affect on memory. Based on the existing literature, it appears that the content of the material to be recalled may be a critical factor with affect-relevant words and interpersonal content showing effects of mood, whereas neutral stimuli do not necessarily show an effect.

Self-reward

A domain that has received a fair amount of investigation is the influence of emotions on the administration of rewards to oneself. This is an important domain for investigation in that self-reward would appear to be a major index of how one responds to oneself under different moods. Unfortunately, much of the research has used success and failure to create moods. Such procedures engender a variety of other processes, such as perceived competence or de-servingness, which may influence self-reward independent of emotional state.

To examine success and failure in relation to contingent and noncontingent self-reinforcement, Masters (1972) created a success or failure experience by having 7- and 8-year-old children play a bowling game in which feedback was predetermined. Masters found that success led to greater self-reinforcement regardless of whether rewards were contingent or noncontingent on performance. Oddly, there was no difference between failures and controls under contingent conditions. Under noncontingent conditions, failure subjects performed more like success subjects in that they self-rewarded more than controls.

Underwood, Moore, and Rosenhan (1973) used direct affect induction to investigate self-gratification in children. Third-grade children were brought to an experimental trailer and asked to help the experimenter test some new hearing equipment. After testing the equipment, the children were invited to help themselves freely and without limit to pennies from a "treasure chest." Pilot studies revealed that young children will help themselves very generously to such noncontingent rewards. Even so, Underwood and his associates found that the induction of affect had a potent effect on how many pennies children took. Both happy and sad children took more pennies than did control subjects. Although Underwood and his colleagues interpret these findings as illustrating that mood state does influence self-reward, they also hypothesize that different psychological processes may be involved for positive and negative affect. Positive affect may create a tendency to be kind to self and others, whereas negative affect may create an attempt to terminate the aversive affective state. In a situation that involves noncontingent self-gratification, such a tendency may lead to increased self-reward. But when gratification is contingent upon performance, as in Masters (1972), negative affect may lead one to devalue one's performance so that contingent self-reward does not increase compared to controls.

This view of self-reward finds support in a study by Jones and Thelen (1978) who used the Velten (1968) statements to generate elation, sadness, or a neutral mood. Subjects then evaluated their performance on an ambiguous word association task by marking a self-praise or self-critical point. Indexes of self-reinforcement indicated that subjects in the elation condition awarded themselves the highest rate of praise and the lowest rate of self-criticism, whereas those in the sadness condition administered the highest rate of self-criticism.

Research by Baumann, Cialdini, and Kenrick (1981) supports the notion that, at least under some conditions, self-gratification terminates the unpleasant experience of negative mood. They induced happy, sad, or neutral affect in college students using reminiscence procedures and then offered subjects an opportunity to self-gratify noncontingently by taking tokens that could later be turned in for a prize. Some subjects self-rewarded immediately after the affect condition, whereas others performed an interpolated task that assumedly produced positive affect. When there was no interpolated task, both positive and negative affect increased self-reward as compared to control subjects. However, when there was a positive-affect interpolated task, the tendency for sad subjects to increase self-reward disappeared. The interpolated task had no effect on the tendency of positive-affect subjects to self-reward.

The conclusions regarding sadness, however, must be tempered in light of a recent study by Sacco and Hokanson (1982) who examined depressed and nondepressed subjects on a task in which success was experimentally controlled and all subjects received either a high rate of success followed by a low rate of success or a low rate of success followed by a high rate. Subjects either self-reinforced publicly or privately. It was found that depression level interacted with sequence of feedback and public/private reward conditions. The most interesting result for our purposes was found among the depressed, private, high/low sequence subjects who rewarded themselves significantly more than did nondepressed subjects in the same condition. These results contrasted with previously obtained findings that depressives apply more stringent standards of self-reward. Sacco and Hokanson speculate that some of these earlier conclusions may have been produced by the public nature of the self-reinforcement. However, under private conditions (at least under conditions where some sense of deservingness has been created, as was the case here where subjects received initially high levels of success feedback), depressives may act in a "self-therapeutic" fashion. Clearly, these relationships are complicated and require further investigation.

Delay of gratification

If, as Underwood and his associates (1973) have argued, the tendency to self-reward under positive and negative affect is governed by different processes, then the delay of gratification paradigm may differentiate between those processes. Delay of gratification is a basic mechanism of self-control and has been found to be influenced by a number of situational and dispositional factors. In this particular instance, sad people, who presumably are acting to terminate an aversive emotional state, should show a preference for immediately available rewards. Happy people should show a preference for delayed larger rewards in that they are seen as not having as much felt need for immediate reward and therefore should opt for a reward-maximizing choice. Moore, Clyburn, and Underwood (1976) asked nursery-school children to think about happy, sad, or neutral events and then to choose between immediate and delayed rewards. They found the predicted relationships: happy children showed more delayed-reward choices than did controls and sad children made more immediate-reward choices.

These results are buttressed by a study in which success and failure were used as the affect-inducing procedure (Seeman & Schwarz, 1974). Children were told that their drawing had either been accepted or rejected for an art show and were then given a choice between small immediate and large delayed rewards. Happy children more often chose the delayed rewards than did unhappy ones.

Finally, Mischel, Ebbesen, and Zeiss (1973) investigated the role affect played in children's ability to successfully delay gratification once a choice has been made to wait for a larger, delayed reward. They found that nursery-school children who "thought happy thoughts" waited dramatically longer than those thinking sad thoughts. It would appear that focusing on events that evoke positive affect helps to bridge the aversive delay interval, whereas, not surprisingly, focusing on sad thoughts makes the delay interval more aversive and produces shorter waiting times.

The results of these studies appear consistent with an emerging picture of the relationship between affect and self-gratification which finds that affect differentiates patterns of contingent, not noncontingent, self-reward. However, findings from several areas suggest that the mechanisms underlying noncontingent self-reward differ for positive- and negative-affect subjects.

Reactions to others

We have described a number of studies that describe how emotion influences reactions to self. It is now time to examine the other side of the picture: how emotion influences response to others. As might be expected, the literature on this topic is much more limited. Since emotion is a private experience, the bulk of the behavioral correlates that have been investigated have been individual. However, it is intuitively persuasive that the manner in which we respond to other people is partially determined by mood.

Altruism

Research on prosocial behavior has provided a major vehicle for examining the influence of mood states. Altruism in particular provides an interesting setting for investigating the role of moods. Because there are no external, tangible rewards for altruistic behavior, the most parsimonious assumption is that it is sensitivity to the needs of others that promotes altruism. A number of studies have examined the role emotion plays in the maintenance of prosocial, and especially altruistic, behavior.

The earliest laboratory finding in this area is by Berkowitz and Connor (1966) who induced success in adults and found them more willing to help a supervisor make envelopes than were those who failed or controls. Subsequent studies (Isen, 1970; Isen, Horn, & Rosenhan, 1973) used less constrained tasks and found that adults and children would be more helpful and more charitable following a success induction. Both groups of investigators were struck by the emotional overtones of such experiences with success. Berkowitz and Connor explained their results in terms of the "glow of goodwill" generated by success, which makes people more tolerant of the costs of helping. Isen's "warm glow of success" similarly emphasizes the emotional aspects of a success experience.

The "feel good, do good" phenomenon is not limited to success, by any means. Competence produces similar effects. Subjects who believe themselves more competent are more willing to donate blood in an ongoing drive than those who feel less competent (Kazdin & Bryan, 1971; Midlarsky & Midlarsky, 1973).

Simple, even accidental, good fortune of the most trivial sort, apparently has effects that are similar to those of success and competence. Receiving a cookie for no apparent reason other than spontaneous kindness, finding a dime in a telephone booth (Isen & Levin, 1972), or being given free stationery (Isen, Clark, & Schwartz, 1976) predisposes people to help. Such helpfulness, it should be noted, is directed not toward the cookie or the stationery donor – that would be a simple quid pro quo – but toward third parties who were not involved, or even aware of, the gift giving.

Success, competence, and good luck are complex mixtures of cognition and emotion. The belief that the affective aspects of these experiences are those that are significant for altruism was confirmed in a study that attempted to examine directly the effects of affective state on children's prosocial behavior (Moore, Underwood, & Rosenhan, 1973). Second- and third-grade children were asked to recall events that had made them particularly happy or particularly sad. Children assigned to a control condition spent the same amount of time doing nothing or counting slowly while the experimenter listened. Immediately afterward, all children were given an opportunity to donate some of the 25 pennies that they had received for participating in the experiment to other children who would not have an opportunity to participate. The experimenter emphasized to the children that donating was entirely voluntary. The child was then left alone and allowed to make a donation.

The child's affective state had a potent effect on the child's tendency to donate. Children who had focused on happy thoughts gave significantly more than did children in the control or sad conditions. Children who had recalled unhappy events contributed significantly less than control subjects. Moore and his associates (1973) concluded that even the transient emotional states tapped in this experiment may influence the child's orientation toward others' needs. Positive affect may generate a general expansiveness to the external world, a feeling that one has more than adequate resources. Negative affect may generate the opposite sense, a turning inward emotionally, perhaps even perceptually, and a sense that one's resources are inadequate. A subsequent unpublished study by the same authors extended these findings by demonstrating the same relationship with a measure of helpfulness toward an anonymous other child.

One possibility that would account for the relative failure of negative affect to promote altruism is an attentional one: that negative affect diminishes attention to external cues and thus to the needs of others. This hypothesis was investigated in an experimental situation that was almost identical to that of Moore and his associates (1973), except that a bulletin board containing a number of pictures was included. If negative affect decreased attention to external information, the negative-affect subjects should be less able to report what was on the bulletin board. Whereas the previously obtained difference in donation between positive- and negative-affect subjects was replicated, there was no difference in subjects' ability to recall the items on the bulletin board. Thus attentional deficit does not produce reduced sharing under negative affect (Underwood et al., 1977).

The special effects of negative mood. Cialdini and Kenrick (1976) have raised a number of questions regarding the effects of negative mood on altruism.

They contend that as the child matures, he or she increasingly internalizes social norms regarding the desirability of exhibiting prosocial behavior. Because prosocial action is valued by society, we are able to feel good about ourselves when we help others. Thus one would expect people in a negative mood to be more helpful to others than people in a neutral mood, since the people in a negative mood should want to improve their mood by doing something as socially desirable and reinforcing as altruism. Cialdini and Kenrick therefore contend that the negative mood that inhibits prosocial action in young children prior to the internalization of norms regarding such behavior should reverse the relationship in older subjects.

To test their explanation, Cialdini and Kenrick replicated the procedures used by Moore and his colleagues but included subjects at three different age levels to determine whether negative affect had different consequences for altruistic behavior at different ages. They found that younger children tended to donate less money after reminiscing about sad experiences. However, with tenth- and twelfth-grade subjects, the manipulation led to increased rates of donation as compared to neutral controls. The authors interpreted these results as supporting their ideas regarding the developmentally acquired reinforcing value of prosocial action.

However, two studies using adult subjects (McMillen, Sanders, & Solomon, 1977; Underwood et al., 1977) point out the need for further clarification of this issue. Underwood and his associates, using movies prerated for affective content, and McMillen and his colleagues, using negative personality feedback, found lower donation rates and helping, respectively, under conditions of negative affect. So, while the general results are fairly consistent regarding the facilitative effects of positive moods on prosocial behavior, the role of negative affect is less certain and may involve counteracting tendencies.

This confusion may be partially reconciled by recent work that shows that negative mood can increase helping when the costs of helping are low and the potential benefits are high (Kenrick, Bauman, & Cialdini, 1979; Weyant, 1978). This suggests, however, that we must not perceive the costs of helping as too great if we are to help and that we need to expect to derive some benefits in terms of recognition and feeling good about ourselves (cf. Rosenhan et al., 1981).

Focus of attention

Another important issue that has grown out of research relating mood to altruism has to do with the focus of attention of the mood. As noted earlier, to speak of positive or negative mood is clearly too general a way to conceptualize the subtle shades of affect that may be experienced. Recent work has begun to explore the differences.

Rosenhan, Salovey, and Hargis (1981) induced joy in two groups of subjects. The first experienced joy for themselves, an egocentric joy. The second experienced empathic joy for a close friend. Those who experienced egocentric joy were markedly more altruistic toward a third party than those who experienced empathic joy. Indeed, the latter were less altruistic than a comparable control group that did not experience these affects. In a further exploration of this area, it was found that egocentric joy facilitates altruism toward the same- or higher-status persons. Empathic joy, however, promotes helpfulness toward lower-status people (Salovey & Rosenhan, 1982).

When sadness rather than joy is the dominant mood, findings are reversed. Subjects listened to a tape that solemnly described a friend's tragic death from cancer. They were directed to attend either to the worry, anxiety, and intense pain suffered by their friend or to their own pain and sorrow caused by their friend's death. Subjects in a control condition listened to a boring, emotionally "neutral" tape. Both other- and self-oriented subjects were much sadder than the controls (but did not differ from each other). However, subjects who attended to the thoughts and feelings of their friend were significantly more helpful than the self-focused or control subjects. Thus, "negative moods . . . facilitate altruism only among people who are attending to the problems of others, but not among people who attend to their own needs, concerns and losses" (Thompson, Cowan, & Rosenhan, 1980).

Barnett, King, and Howard (1979) also argued that the focus of the negative affect influences prosocial behavior. Barnett and his associates asked children to focus on happy, neutral, or sad events that had been experienced either by themselves or by another child. Following the affect induction, the children were given the opportunity to share their experimental earnings with some less fortunate children. It was found that children who focused on their own sad events were less likely to share their earnings than were neutral subjects but that children who focused on the sad events of others were more likely to share.

Distribution of rewards

Altruism involves contributing to others' welfare in the absence of a quid pro quo. Related to, but differing in significant ways from, the altruism situation is the issue of whether emotion influences how rewards are distributed to self and others. Consider the following study. Individual elementary-school children were asked to perform a simple task in a research trailer and were told that another child would be working on the same task elsewhere. Following completion of the task, the children were assigned randomly to one of three mood conditions: happy, sad, and control. Emotion was induced via the reminiscence procedure (Moore et al., 1973). Subsequently, the children were given 40 pennies to divide anonymously between themselves and the other child. The children were told either that they had performed better (positive social comparison) or worse than the other child (negative social comparison).

Not surprisingly, children who had been told they performed better than the other child kept more pennies for themselves than did children who had been told they performed worse. Within the positive social comparison condition, there was a significant linear increase from happy to neutral to sad in the number of pennies the children kept for themselves. The pattern was quite different for negative social comparison. There, control children kept significantly more pennies for themselves than did happy or sad children who did not differ significantly from each other.

Examining the data, one notes that five of the six conditions are very much in accord with the linear trend found in earlier research on altruism. The linear trend is not substantiated, however, by the sad mood in the negative social comparison condition, where children kept fewer pennies for themselves. One might speculate that sadness, while increasing children's motivation to keep more pennies for themselves, also sensitized them to negative information about their performance and therefore, their deservingness. Hence, they kept fewer pennies for themselves because of the enhanced impact of the negative social comparison. Thus it appears that happiness generates behavior that is consistent with the altruism findings of previous research. The effects of sadness, however, are more selective, depending on whether deservingness is involved.

Generally, these findings suggest the importance of examining how sadness influences the social comparison process. For instance, it would be illuminating to compare how depressives recall and evaluate others' performance in comparison with their own.

Finally, one study highlights the different processes that may be engendered by mood. Rosenhan, Underwood, & Moore (1974) examined donations and self-rewards under different affective states within the context of a single experiment. They found that happy children were generous to both themselves and others. Sad children, however, were generous only to themselves and niggardly with others. Thus, sadness appears to generate resource conservation both through self-gratification and lack of sharing with others. Happiness, however, encourages a generosity to self and others. Conceivably, different mechanisms promote responsiveness to self when people are happy or sad.

Attraction to others

In addition to our willingness to help and reward others, a number of researchers (e.g., Tomkins, 1962) have suggested that moods may influence more general social tendencies. Tomkins refers to the "sociophobia" of sadness and the "sociophilia" of joy. If, as has been suggested throughout this chapter, happiness promotes an outer orientation, a willingness to be generous to oneself and to others, and a generally positive self-orientation, then we might expect happy people to seek out others. The situation for sad people is probably more complex. On the one hand, negative self-evaluation and the inward focus that accompanies sadness might lead sad people to eschew social contact. Alternately, sad people may seek social contact as a means of alleviating the sadness.

One study by Mehrabian and Russell (1974) addresses these issues. They induced mood by exposing adults to slide-presented scenes that had been previously rated for their affective consequences and found that people had a greater desire to affiliate when they were watching the pleasurable than the unpleasurable slides. These tendencies were accentuated as the pleasurableness of the slide increased. Similar findings were obtained by Gouaux and Gouaux (1971).

Research by Bell (1978) found general support for these ideas but found that, as one might expect, aspects of the affiliation target moderated the tendency to affiliate. Specifically, Bell had subjects read happy, sad, or neutral prose passages and then provided them with a potential work partner who was in a happy, sad or neutral mood. Overall, happy subjects were more willing to have a work partner than were sad subjects, confirming the view that happiness generates sociophilia. However, there were interactions between the affective state of the subjects and the affective state of the target. Both happy and sad subjects were more willing to work with happy partners. But sad partners preferred sad, rather than happy partners, confirming the view that miserable company has a slight preference for misery!

Summary

We are still a long way from describing how, precisely, emotion influences reactions to self and others. That goal is remote for several reasons. In the first place, emotion is no unitary phenomenon: Different emotions likely influence these reactions differently, and the full panorama of emotion has not yet been explored. Second, the processes through which emotions exert their influences are not yet fully understood. Finally, perhaps as the result of these considerations, there is little by way of theory to guide these explorations. The horizon is dotted with studies that, separately, are both interesting and challenging but that, together, do not yet suggest the substantial fabric of theory.

Yet, for all these disclaimers, the literature on the relations between emotion, self, and others is not wholly without coherence. We begin with the assumption that the effects of emotion on self are mediated through perception and memory. We do not expect emotion to affect absolute memorial performance levels and know of no study in which that is the case. Rather, we expect that the *availability* of memories, the readiness with which they "come to mind," will be differentially affected. Here the data are rich, as will be seen elsewhere in this volume (Gilligan & Bower, Chapter 18). Happy people retrieve pleasant information – whether that information consists of personality descriptions, memories, or pleasant words – more readily than they do unpleasant information. For reasons that remain unclear, the situation regarding affect-retrieval relationships is less certain, and likely more complex, for unhappy people. It seems clear that unhappiness blocks the retrieval of happy memories in much the same way that happiness makes the retrieval of unhappy memories more difficult. But while happiness clearly facilitates the retrieval of happy memories, unhappy states may be less effective in making unhappy memories available because unhappy memories perpetuate an aversive emotional state. In short, it remains to be seen whether, and under what conditions, the cognitive loop that is facilitated by happy feelings will find its counterpart in negative feelings.

Emotion, it turns out, is a powerful and variable state that deeply affects reactions to self and others. Its power resides, in part, in its pervasiveness: There is hardly an area of self- or other-reaction that is not touched and altered by emotion. Happiness affects attribution, perception of control, self-reward, task performance and evaluation, self-concept and delay of gratification – all in the expected direction. Sadness affects these aspects of self too and again in the expected direction. Current evidence suggests that emotion seems *not* to influence the relatively stable and well-anchored aspects of personality, but the proposition has not yet been well tested. The more ephemeral aspects of personality, however, are clearly vulnerable to the vagaries of mood.

What holds for reactions to self seems also to hold regarding reactions to others, although explorations in this area have been restricted mainly to altruistic and other prosocial behaviors. In the main, happiness promotes altruism, helpfulness, sharing, and sociability, whereas sadness retards them. These findings hold only when the emotions are egocentric. When they are empathic, that is, when one is happy or sad for *others*, the findings reverse.

Generally, as others have observed, the findings regarding positive emotions are more consistent and stable than those regarding negative emotions, and our review of the effects of emotion on self and others provides no exception to that conclusion. Why that should be the case remains an interesting issue for a future agenda.

References

Alloy, L. B., & Abramson, L. Y. Judgment of contingency in depressed and nondepressed students: Sadder but wiser? *Journal of Experimental Psychology: General*, 1979, *108*, 441–485.

Alloy, L. B., Abramson, L. Y., & Viscusi, D. Induced mood and the illusion of control. *Journal of Personality and Social Psychology*, 1981, *41*, 1129–1140.

Amrhein, J., Salovey, P., & Rosenhan, D. L. *Joy and sadness generate attributional vulnerability in men.* Unpublished manuscript, Stanford University, 1982.

Barnett, M., King, L. M., & Howard, J. A. Inducing affect about self and other: Effects on generosity in children. *Developmental Psychology*, 1979, *15*, 164–167.

Bartlett, J. C., & Santrock, J. W. Affect-dependent episodic memory in young children. *Child Development*, 1979, *50*, 513–518.

Baumann, D. J., Cialdini, R., & Kenrick, D. Altruism as hedonism: Helping and self-gratification as equivalent processes. *Journal of Personality and Social Psychology*, 1981, *40*, 1039–1036.

Bell, B. A. Affective state, attraction and affiliation: Misery loves happy company, too. *Personality and Social Psychology Bulletin*, 1978, *4*, 141–145.

Berkowitz, L., & Connor, W. H. Success, failure and social responsibility. *Journal of Personality and Social Psychology*, 1966, *4*, 664–669.

Bower, G. Mood and memory. *American Psychologist*, 1981, *36*, 120–148.

Cialdini, R. B., & Kenrick, D. T. Altruism as hedonism: A social development perspective on the relationship of negative mood state and helping. *Journal of Personality and Social Psychology*, 1976, *34*, 907–914.

Feather, N. T. Effects of prior success and failure on expectations of success and subsequent performance. *Journal of Personality and Social Psychology*, 1966, *3*, 287–298.

Gouaux, C., & Gouaux, S. The influence of induced affective states on the effectiveness of social and nonsocial reinforcers in an instrumental learning task. *Psychonomic Science*, 1971, *22*, 341–343.

Hammen, C. L., & Krantz, S. Effects of success and failure on depressive cognitions. *Journal of Abnormal Psychology*, 1976, *85*, 577–586.

Hoffman, S. *Affect and attributions*. Unpublished manuscript, Stanford University, 1978.

Isen, A. M. Success, failure, attention and reaction to others: The warm glow of success. *Journal of Personality and Social Psychology*, 1970, *15*, 294–301.

Isen, A. M., Clark, M., & Schwartz, M. F. Duration of the effect of good mood on helping: Footprints on the sands of time. *Journal of Personality and Social Psychology*, 1976, *34*, 385–393.

Isen, A. M., Horn, N. C., & Rosenhan, D. L. Effects of success and failure on children's generosity. *Journal of Personality and Social Psychology*, 1973, *27*, 239–247.

Isen, A. M., & Levin, P. F. The effects of feeling good on helping: Cookies and kindness. *Journal of Personality and Social Psychology*, 1972, *21*, 384–388.

Isen, A. M., Shalker, T. E., Clark, M., & Karp, L. Affect, accessibility of material in memory and behavior: A cognitive loop. *Journal of Personality and Social Psychology*, 1978, *36*, 1–12.

Izard, C. *Human emotions*. New York: Plenum, 1977.

Jones, G. F., & Thelen, M. H. The effects of induced mood states on self-reinforcement behavior. *Journal of Psychology*, 1978, *98*, 249–252.

Kazdin, A. E., & Bryan, J. H. Competence and volunteering. *Journal of Experimental Social Psychology*, 1971, *7*, 87–97.

Kenrick, D. T., Bauman, D. J., & Cialdini, R. B. A step in the socialization of altruism as hedonism: Effect of negative mood on children's generosity under public and private conditions. *Journal of Personality and Social Psychology*, 1979, *37*, 747–755.

Leight, K. E., & Ellis, H. C. Emotional mood states, strategies, and state dependency in memory. *Journal of Verbal Learning and Verbal Behavior*, 1981, *20*, 251–266.

Lloyd, G. G., & Lishman, W. A. Effects of depression on the speed of recall of pleasant and unpleasant experiences. *Psychological Medicine*, 1975, *5*, 173–180.

Mandler, G. *Mind and emotion*. New York: Wiley, 1975.

Masters, John C. Effects of success, failure, and reward outcome upon contingent and noncontingent self-reinforcement. *Developmental Psychology*, 1972, *7*, 110–118.

Masters, J. C., Barden, R. C., & Ford, M. E. Affective states, expressive behavior, and learning in children. *Journal of Personality and Social Psychology*, 1979, *37*, 380–390.

Masters, J. C., & Furman, W. Effects of affect states on noncontingent outcome expectancies and beliefs in internal or external control. *Developmental Psychology*, 1976, *12*, 481–482.

McMillen, D. S., Sanders, D. Y., & Solomon, G. S. Self-esteem, attentiveness, and helping behavior. *Personality and Social Psychology Bulletin*, 1977, *3*, 257–262.

Mehrabian, A., & Russell, J. Environmental effects of affiliation among strangers. *Humanitas*, 1974, *11*, 219–230.

Midlarsky, E., & Midlarsky, M. Some determinants of aiding under experimentally induced stress. *Journal of Personality*, 1973, *41*, 305–327.

Mischel, W., Ebbesen, E., & Zeiss, A. Cognitive and attentional mechanisms in delay of gratification. *Journal of Personality and Social Psychology*, 1973, *21*, 204–218.

Mischel, W., Ebbesen, E. E., & Zeiss, A. Determinants of selective memory about the self. *Journal of Consulting and Clinical Psychology*, 1976, *44*, 92–103.

Moore, B. S., Clyburn, A., & Underwood, B. The role of affect in the delay of gratification. *Child Development*, 1976, *47*, 237–276.

Moore, B. S., & Underwood, B. *Affect and aggressive modeling*. Unpublished manuscript, University of Texas at Dallas, 1982.

Moore, B. S., Underwood, B., Doyle, L., Heberlein, P., & Litzie, K. Generalization of feedback about performance. *Cognitive Therapy and Research*, 1979, *3*, 371–380.

Moore, B. S., Underwood, B., Heberlein, P., Doyle, L. *Effects of induced mood on anagram solution*. Unpublished manuscript, University of Texas at Dallas, 1982.

Moore, B. S., Underwood, B., & Rosenhan, D. L. Affect and altruism. *Developmental Psychology*, 1973, *8*, 99–104.

Moore, B. S., Underwood, B., & Terrazas, D. *The affective-state dependency of memory*. Unpublished manuscript, University of Texas at Dallas, 1982.

Natale, M. Effect of induced elation and depression on internal external locus of control. *Journal of Psychology*, 1978, *100*, 315–321.

Nelson, R. E., & Craighead, W. E. Selective recall of positive and negative feedback, self control behaviors, and depression. *Journal of Abnormal Psychology*, 1977, *86*, 379–388.

Polivy, J. On the induction of emotion in the laboratory: Discrete moods or multiple affect states. *Journal of Personality and Social Psychology*, 1981, *41*, 803–817.

Rizley, R. Depression and distortion in the attribution of causality. *Journal of Abnormal Psychology*, 1978, *87*, 32–48.

Rosenhan, D. L., Karylowski, J., Salovey, P., & Hargis, K. Emotion and altruism. In J. P. Rushton & R. M. Sorrentino (Eds.), *Altruism and helping behavior*. Hillsdale, N.J.: Erlbaum, 1981.

Rosenhan, D. L., & Messick, S. Affect and expectation. *Journal of Personality and Social Psychology*, 1966, *3*, 38–44.

Rosenhan, D. L., Salovey, P., & Hargis, K. The joys of helping: Focus of attention mediates the impact of positive affect on altruism. *Journal of Personality and Social Psychology*, 1981, *40*, 899–905.

Rosenhan, D. L., Underwood, B., & Moore, B. S. Affect moderates self-gratification and altruism. *Journal of Personality and Social Psychology*, 1974, *30*, 546–552.

Rotter, J. Some problems and misconceptions related to the construct of internal versus external control of reinforcement. *Journal of Consulting and Clinical Psychology*, 1975, *43*, 55–67.

Sacco, W. P., & Hokanson, J. E. Depression and self-reinforcement in a public and private setting. *Journal of Personality and Social Psychology*, 1982, *42*, 377–385.

Salovey, P., & Rosenhan, D. L. *Effects of joy, attention, and recipient's status on helpfulness*. Unpublished manuscript, Stanford University, 1982.

Seeman, G., & Schwarz, J. C. Affective state and preference for immediate versus delayed reward. *Journal of Research in Personality*, 1974, *4*, 384–394.

Sherrod, D. R. *Social psychology*. New York: Random House, 1982.

Teasdale, J. D., & Fogarty, S. J. Differential effects of induced mood on retrieval of pleasant and unpleasant events from episodic memory. *Journal of Abnormal Psychology*, 1979, *88*, 248–257.

Thompson, W. C., Cowan, C. L., Rosenhan, D. L. Focus of attention mediates the impact of negative affect on altruism. *Journal of Personality and Social Psychology*, 1980, *48*, 291–300.

Tomkins, S. S. *Affect, imagery, consciousness* (Vol. 1). New York: Springer-Verlag, 1962.
Underwood, B., Berenson, J. F., Berenson, R. J., Cheng, K. K., Wilson, D., Kulik, J., Moore, B. S., & Wenzel, G. Attention, negative affect and altruism. An ecological validation. *Personality and Social Psychology Bulletin*, 1977, *13*, 541–542.
Underwood, B., Froming, W. J., & Moore, B. S. Mood, attention, and altruism: A search for mediating variables. *Developmental Psychology*, 1977, *13*, 541–542.
Underwood, B., Froming, W. J., & Moore, B. S. Mood and personality: A search for the causal relationship. *Journal of Personality*, 1980, *48*, 331–339.
Underwood, B., Froming, W., & Moore, B. S. *Dimensions of affect*. Unpublished manuscript, University of Texas, 1982.
Underwood, B., Moore, B. S., & Rosenhan, D. L. Affect and self-gratification. *Developmental Psychology*, 1973, *8*, 209–214.
Velten, E. A laboratory task for induction of mood states. *Behavior Research and Therapy*, 1968, *6*, 473–482.
Wessman, A. E., & Ricks, D. F. *Mood and personality*. New York: Holt, Rinehart and Winston, 1966.
Weyant, J. M. Effects of mood states, costs and benefits on helping. *Journal of Personality and Social Psychology*, 1978, *36*, 1169–1176.

Richard A. Dienstbier

The major aim of this chapter is to discuss a research program designed to assess emotion-cognition-behavior relationships in moral decision making. While pursuing that aim, I will discuss the relationship of that research to some of the more enduring theoretical issues in emotion.

Theories of emotion wax and wane across a more extended time frame than is typical for theoretical approaches in many other areas in psychology. Perhaps these extended cycles of emotion theory result from the relative difficulty in the recent past in doing definitive research within the area of human emotion. The field was thereby insulated from sudden shifts in focus precipitated by dramatic research relevant to basic theory.

One of those areas of enduring concern to philosophers and psychologists interested in human emotion has been whether to conceive of emotion as dimensional versus discrete in structure. Those on the discrete side of this controversy generally trace their theoretical lineage to Charles Darwin, whereas dimensional theorists often credit William James. Discrete theorists hold that there are eight or nine basic emotions, which are inborn syndromes of feeling and behavior (e.g., Izard, 1971, 1977; Tomkins, 1963). Although proponents of that view would usually acknowledge that general physiological arousal (cerebral, autonomic and/or endocrine) may affect some dimension of intensity or duration of experienced emotion, the role of general arousal is regarded as minor. On the dimensional side of the debate, several modern theorists argue that the physiological arousal underlying emotional experience combines with certain cognitive assessments of the meaning of that arousal to form a specific emotional experience, so that the number of different emotions one could experience would be limited only by one's ability to be cognizant of nuances of meaning in a situation that had stimulated general arousal (e.g., Mandler, 1975; Schachter & Singer, 1962). Similarly, the focus of the two approaches

The research and ideas of this chapter could not have progressed without the willing assistance and co-participation of many students and colleagues. In addition to those named as co-authors of the various papers mentioned in this chapter, thanks for research work with the children are due to Rod Cole, Ursela Fritsch, Dwight Heil, Julie Jorgensen, Charles S. Kaplan, Bob LaGuardia, Arlene and Max Lewis, Paula Mares, Kelly Martens, Jane McGinnis, Phil Nickel, Mischel and Terry Robacker, Shelley Stahl, Elinora Ward, Noreen Wilcox, Sharon Ziers, and Gail Zimmerman.

is on different response categories, with discrete theorists showing interest in the face and facial expression or voluntary muscle patterns and the dimensional theorists focusing on sympathetic nervous system arousal and hormonal changes or upon states of general cortical arousal. (For a review contrasting dimensional and discrete approaches, see Izard, 1971.)

Whatever the disposition of current theorists in this area, most acknowledge that for appropriate or inappropriate reasons, a major impetus toward the study of the interaction of emotion with cognition has been the attention given to the work of Schachter and Singer (1962), who attempted to support a radical dimensional viewpoint. The program of research reported in this chapter was stimulated by that dimensional work, now two decades old. Over the decade of this project, which is still ongoing, my students and I have had cause to modify our initial dimensional beliefs. Without dwelling on that personal progression, this chapter will discuss our theoretical evolution as our research developed. The final portion of the chapter will evaluate recent research designed to refute and to support the radical dimensional view with which we started and to evaluate our research in view of those observations.

A related theoretical concern is the interrelationship of emotion and cognition. Can emotion exist independently of cognition? While this is not a crucial issue for the discrete emotion theorists, for those who hold to strict post-Schachterian dimensional views, cognitions about the source and meaning of autonomic arousal are essential in the experience of emotion. "Pure" emotion without cognition is therefore not possible. (Such notions of the inseparability of emotion and cognition are consonant with the dominant view of attitude held during the 1950s and 1960s by most social psychologists.) Whereas the issue is sometimes couched in terms of whether cognitions precede and stimulate emotional states (e.g., Beck's, 1967, cognitive theory of depression) or whether emotional arousal precedes and stimulates consonant cognitive activities (e.g., various physiological approaches and pharmacological treatments of emotional disorders), Zajonc (1980) has recently refocused attention on the more basic question of whether emotion and cognition may exist independently of each other. The research reviewed in this chapter will be discussed in relation to this issue.

Emotion defined

Before discussing my research, let us consider establishing a definition of emotion. Each chapter author will undoubtedly confront this task differently, for differences in definition lie at the core of many theoretical disagreements. Like attempts to definitively establish *the* components of personality, the question of emotion definition should, at our present state of knowledge, be approached by first ascertaining which theoretical or practical questions will be pursued once the definition is established. Extending George Kelly's notions about theory in personality into the realm of emotion, each theoretical approach and, to a certain extent, each definition implies a set of constructs that may be most usefully applied toward a limited "point of focus"; similarly, there exists a range of convenience for the theory beyond which other theoretical structures and definitions need be sought.

Because of the nature of the research described in this chapter, my definition of emotion will stress aspects of motivation and arousal. Formally and simply put, *human emotion is conceived to be a motivation-laden feeling resulting jointly from shifts in arousal and from the meaning attached to those arousal shifts*.

To understand this definition, consider first the nature of arousal. Some arousal may be central nervous system arousal, and some may be peripheral, depending upon the emotional state elicited; certain of the arousal components may be general and common to many emotional states, and others may be unique to specific emotional states. The generation of the aroused state usually results from perceptions of external situations; those perceptions, together with later cognitions about the meaning of the external state, influence the nature of the experienced emotion and the direction and force of the experienced motivation.

Next, let us consider the motivational qualities of emotion. The motivational quality of the feeling of emotion is experienced as an increased tendency to avoid or pursue certain perceptual experiences (i.e., to attend to certain classes of stimuli), to remember and think about ideas and images with a similar affective tone, and to avoid or pursue certain behavioral options associated with changing our relationships with certain classes of goals (e.g., to fight with, run from, reject, avoid, or engage with). While following both Tomkins and Izard that the motivational quality of emotional experience is of paramount importance (e.g., see Izard & Tomkins, 1966), for me even low intensities of human emotion frequently stimulate far more effort than would be expected. That is, we may respond to the motivational quality of even slight emotion and to cognitions about the likelihood of emotional states as if we were experiencing a strong, current, emotion-instigated motivational force. While I will return to this theme at the chapter's end, it is time to consider the theoretical system that initially led to our research.

The development of modern peripheral-dimensional theory

Throughout the 1950s studies by a group of psychologists at the University of Rochester investigating the effects of various popular illicit drugs stimulated interest in the interaction of physiological states and cognitive information on the experience of mood and emotion (Vincent Nowlis, private communication).

Those researchers (including G. R. Wendt, Vincent and Helen Nowlis, Russel Green, and others) found, for example, that the impact on mood of a given drug varied dramatically as a function of whether other research subjects were simultaneously exposed to the same or to a different drug (e.g., whether an individual stimulated by an amphetamine remained with others similarly treated or with individuals who had taken barbiturates). Following those demonstrations, Schachter and Singer (1962) similarly demonstrated that following adrenaline injection, individuals appeared to act differently depending upon either the information they received through the social environment in which they were subsequently placed or through direct information about the impact of the adrenaline. Although the continuity between those two lines of research is easily apparent, the discontinuity is less obvious – whereas the drugs under study in the Rochester experiments were thought largely to affect mood as a result of the alteration of central nervous system conditions, the adrenaline used in the Schachter and Singer (1962) study was thought to impact emotion through feedback from peripheral body areas. Similarly, when Schachter and Wheeler (1962) demonstrated the impact of chlorpromazine in reducing laughter in response to a humorous movie, the peripheral impact was emphasized. Those interpretations led to a dramatic modification of previous dimensional approaches, which had emphasized cerebral arousal (e.g., Lindsley, 1970); instead, it was emphasized that feedback from peripheral areas and cognitive interpretations about the meaning of that feedback would be crucial in the experience of emotion. At the end of this chapter I will discuss research from other sources concerning the role of adrenaline (and noradrenaline) in the experience of emotion and those recently published studies that have challenged the Schachter and Singer findings and debated the role of autonomic (and facial) feedback in the experience of emotion. For the moment, the critical point concerning the early "emotion-attribution" interpretations by Schachter and his colleagues is that those interpretations stimulated a significant amount of research that could be (and was) interpreted as support for the importance of feedback from peripheral arousal in the experience of emotion and for the correctness of a dimensional approach with peripheral arousal as the central physiological dimension of importance.

The role of emotion in moral decisions

Schachter and Latané (1964) demonstrated that psychopathic criminals would learn to avoid punished errors much better if they were first aroused with an injection of adrenaline, and Schachter and Ono (reported in Schachter & Latané, 1964) demonstrated that college students tranquilized with chlorpromazine cheated more. Those demonstrations suggested that both the avoidance of punished errors and resistance to temptation were influenced by high levels of psychological arousal. Actually, it was inferred from that and other related research (which showed that psychopaths may be as physiologically reactive as nonpsychopaths) that the *experience* of inhibiting emotion, rather than physiological arousal per se, would reduce the probability of transgression.

Misattribution of peripheral arousal symptoms and cheating – the first study

Impressed by the coherence of those converging approaches to the role of emotion in resistance to temptation, and by the peripherally based dimensional theory of emotion, which underlay those approaches, I endeavored to ask the next logical question concerning the impact of peripheral arousal on resistance to temptation: Could it be demonstrated that one's interpretation of the meaning of the arousal modulated the effectiveness of that arousal in facilitating resistance to temptation?

Nisbett and Schachter (1966) had previously developed a technique that seemed to successfully influence the meaning of peripheral arousal and hence the experience of emotion. They had administered placebo pills with instructions that the pills would either contribute to four peripheral arousal symptoms (hand trembling, fast heart rate, face flushing, and stomach butterflies) or (for control subjects) would contribute to symptoms that were irrelevant to peripheral autonomic arousal. Those subjects who anticipated arousing side effects from their placebo pills subsequently withstood more electric shock (a graded series of mild shocks) before reaching the limit of their pain tolerance than did those subjects anticipating benign symptoms. It appeared that the misattribution of emotional arousal – stimulated by the electric shock and by fear of the shock – to the placebo pill lessened the avoidance-motivating quality of that emotional arousal.

We anticipated that this logic would hold equally well for our research subjects as they faced the temptation to cheat. That is, when facing such temptation in a natural environment, individuals would experience some emotional arousal – arousal that would signal their fear, shame, or guilt in anticipation of either the act of or the consequences of cheating. Whereas such emotional responses would motivate the avoidance of cheating in a natural setting, we anticipated that we could lessen that effect if we could induce misattribution of the emotional experience to a previously consumed placebo pill.

The first study with placebo pills in this series served as a prototype for the subsequent studies. Freshman introductory psychology students were recruited "in order to study the effects of a vitamin-related drug on vision." After being seated in individual booths, subjects were given a placebo and a form describing the pill's major effects on both vision and either the peripheral arousal side effects or the benign symptoms as described by Nisbett and Schachter. A vocabulary test was subsequently given to fill the interval "while the pill took effect" but that vocabulary test was to be taken seriously, because the "board of psychologists" developing that test was supposedly interested in interviewing college freshmen with particularly poor vocabularies. Following that test, subjects were exposed to the autokinetic illusion to substantiate the "visual effects" cover story and subtly reminded of the possible side effects. Subjects were then given the opportunity to cheat on their vocabulary test. The period during which subjects could cheat on their vocabulary tests was introduced as a delay period before rating any possible side effects (arousal-relevant or benign). Subjects were shown the correct vocabulary-test answers and told to "clean up" their machine-graded answer papers if needed (to provide an excuse for using their pencils and erasers) but warned "do not change any answers." Virtually all subjects "failed" the vocabulary test, which was designed to be deceptively difficult. Following the 7-minute period during which subjects could cheat by changing vocabulary test answers, a detailed post-experimental questionnaire concerning any suspicions was administered, followed by a complete debriefing.

With cheating defined as changing one or more answers, almost twice as many subjects anticipating arousal side effects from their placebos cheated (49% vs. 27%, $p < .02$). However, that effect was achieved almost entirely by the male subjects. (The procedure for detecting cheating using pressure-sensitive paper is described by Dienstbier & Munter, 1971.)

Before sex differences are discussed, let us consider some procedural questions and the meaning of the major findings. Did our suggestions about side effects lead to only the desired between-condition differences in the attribution of emotional arousal or were actual differences in arousal levels created between the experimental conditions? Once arousal-relevant side effects have been suggested to individuals in such research, there is no test free from very obvious demand characteristics, which could prove the null hypothesis that no arousal differences were actually created by direct suggestion. While we therefore have no definite answer to the question of between-condition arousal differences, we believe that such differences are unlikely, in part because of our technique for presenting side-effect information. We approached the induction of beliefs about placebo side effects in a low-key manner. That is, we suggested that we were not at all certain whether each individual would experience side effects and indicated that our reason for requesting feedback from each subject on whether such effects were experienced was a reflection of our uncertainty that such effects would occur. As observers of the experimental situation, it was our impression that the side-effects suggestions were among the least interesting and stimulating of the experimental maneuvers that our subjects experienced. A major reason for keeping our side-effect manipulation relatively tentative was to avoid the incredulity that frequently follows from overemphasizing such impacts. A recent review and analysis by Ross and Olson (1981) of both direct and "reverse" placebo effects substantiates these conclusions.

Assuming then that we did not induce differential arousal levels in our two subject groups, we are left with an emotion-attribution explanation for the cheating difference: That the attribution of arousal to a cause or source that is not relevant to the moral decision (the placebo, for the subjects in the experimental conditions) would attenuate the impact of that arousal in resisting temptation. Being neither hard determinists nor strict behaviorists, we were not aloof from speculation about the rational processes that might have intervened between our independent manipulations and altered cheating rates. The ideas that we then posited (and which have been subsequently modified by being placed in a more extensive context) were that individuals who face temptation think about their behavioral alternatives and, depending upon factors ranging from past punishment for options currently considered to the perception that certain actions would lead to value conflicts, experience emotional responses. We believed that we had demonstrated that if the peripheral symptoms of emotional arousal are experienced as irrelevant to the temptation dilemma (i.e., attribution to the placebo), then the emotional state would not be experienced as inhibitory – individuals would be as free to cheat is if they did not experience the emotions at all (as with the tranquilized students of the Schachter and Ono research described earlier). The research seemed to provide strong support for a dimensional emotion theory based upon peripheral feedback. More about that later.

Cheating and arousal misattribution – follow-up studies

Before we could progress with an understanding of the interaction of emotion and cognition in determining behavior in temptation situations, we had a conceptual cleanup chore required by the sex difference finding of our initial work; additionally, we wanted to be sure that an attributional explanation was necessary to account for our results rather than a simpler attentional one. (That is, would merely attending to the peripheral arousal side effects impact cheating or was the attribution of those symptoms to the placebo a necessary step.) With respect to the findings of sex differences, we reasoned that our female subjects may have been more upset by failing in the presence of the threat of the "board of psychologists" than were males. Subsequent research (Dienstbier, 1972) indicated that as threat intensity was systematically varied across four levels, at lower threat levels the placebo manipulation worked exactly as it had for males (with more cheating associated with the arousal side effects). Those results confirmed our suspicion that men and women use emotional cues similarly in making decisions about cheating and that the cause of our initial finding of sex differences was probably that our women subjects were more distracted by an intense social threat than were the men.

In a third study, using males, it was shown that when subjects focused attention on arousal-relevant (vs. benign) side effects it did not impact their cheating unless they could also attribute that arousal to a placebo. Half the subjects were given no pills at all but were instead told that they were a control condition to check for suggestion effects in a drug study. Thus they were to rate their (arousal or benign) side effects and do everything (except view the autokinetic illusion used to verify the effectiveness of the placebo) the "real" subjects did. Merely attending to whether they experienced the side effects had no impact on cheating, as contrasted to the replication (of Study 1) conditions where the arousal-condition subjects again cheated far more than did the controls. Apparently, the misattribution of emotional arousal to an irrelevant source is necessary before cheating rates increase.

Related emotion-attribution research

While our work progressed, other researchers were using similar independent manipulations to successfully test important variations of the peripheral dimensional approach. All these studies investigated and confirmed hypotheses that arousal would contribute *less* to a variety of emotional states when such arousal was misattributed to sources believed to be irrelevant to emotion (such as a placebo pill or a background noise). Younger and Doob (1978) found, for example, that administration of an "arousal" placebo reduced aggressive response. Ross, Rodin, and Zimbardo (1969) demonstrated that subjects who could attribute their arousal symptoms to a loud background noise worked less to avoid shocked punishment (contrasted with working to earn a positive reward) than did subjects who anticipated benign effects from the background noise; apparently the arousal from the anticipation of shock became attributed to the noise and hence was not experienced as fear. Rodin (1976) demonstrated that women who could attribute test anxiety to premenstrual symptomatology improved in test performance.

Emotion misattribution and the extinction of conditioned responses

Two related research programs were more directly important from the standpoint of our considerations of moral development. Loftis and Ross (1974) had subjects acquire a classically conditioned galvanic skin response to a light (having previously paired the light with shock) while an irrelevant tone sounded in the background. Following conditioning, some subjects were told that the tone was really responsible for their emotional response; others were not given such erroneous information. Those who attributed their conditioning to the tone extinguished more quickly (in a light-alone condition) than did subjects not given that misattribution-facilitating information. Thus, although previous research demonstrated that arousal misattributed to an emotion-irrelevant source would lose its impact on emotional experience, the Loftis and Ross study suggests that such misattribution will also lead to the quick extinction of acquired emotional responses.

Emotion misattribution and reduced attitude change in dissonance research

In a second research tradition, Zanna and Cooper (1974) showed arousal mis-attribution effects in the realm of dissonance research. In forced-compliance research, it is assumed that subjects induced to advocate attitudes that are quite different from their initial attitudes will experience some emotional tension. In turn, that tension will motivate attitude change, so that the subjects' attitudes shift in the direction of the position advocated. (Of course various parameters relevant to perceived coercion, payment, or lack of freedom attenuate this effect.) In a series of studies Zanna and Cooper demonstrated that postdissonance (following forced compliance) attitude change did not occur when arousal resulted from cognitive dissonance that was either misattributed to an irrelevant source or was the consequence of ingesting a tranquilizer (phenobarbital; Cooper, Zanna, & Taves, 1978); on the other hand, when subjects anticipated relaxation symptoms from an irrelevant source (but did not receive them) or were stimulated by an arousing amphetamine drug, postdissonance attitude change increased. Since those studies used both misattribution techniques and arousal-impacting drugs, they provide a powerful confirmation of arousal-misattribution working somewhat as suggested above. That is, the misattribution of arousal to an irrelevant source attenuates the impact of that arousal on subsequent decisions in a manner directly analogous to that obtained with a tranquilizer. The relaxation symptoms provided converging evidence; the misattribution of relaxation symptoms to an emotion-irrelevant source lead to behavioral outcomes similar to those caused by the administration of a stimulant drug. It should be noted, however, that in the case of this research both the arousing and the tranquilizing drugs used actually affect the central nervous system rather than peripheral processes. This observation has implications for a peripheral-dimensional theory of emotion. This issue will be discussed later.

Emotion misattribution and enhancement through the addition of naturally induced arousal

Another paradigm that was interpreted as supporting emotion-attribution theory involves inducing arousal in more natural ways than the adrenaline-injection technique used by Schachter and Singer and studying changes in a situation-appropriate emotional response. For example, Zillmann, Katcher, and Milavsky (1972) demonstrated that exercise-induced arousal facilitated aggression response; this facilitation was particularly strong (Zillmann, Johnson, & Day, 1974) when individuals mistakenly thought that they had returned to base line in their exercise-induced arousal. Similarly, Cantor, Zillmann, and Bryant (1975) found that exercise-induced arousal facilitated the judgment of aesthetic value of objects and the entertainment value of an erotic film, but only when subjects mistakenly believed that they had recovered from the exercise-induced arousal. Arousal induced by listening to complex (versus simple) tones delivered at loud volume (rather than mild) was found to increase aggression (Konecni, 1975).

A number of different approaches placed individuals in the company of attractive opposite-sexed others subsequent to arousal. Dutton and Aron (1974) found that more TAT story sexuality was elicited in males following passage over an arousal-inducing suspension bridge as contrasted to men who met the beautiful experimenter via a less-arousing bridge. Similarly, I have noted (Dienstbier, 1979a) that while attraction toward a beautiful (or handsome) opposite-sexed researcher is enhanced by startle-induced arousal (relative to nonstartled controls), attraction toward a same-sexed experimenter is reduced by that arousal-inducing startle.

With respect to the theoretical issue concerning a peripheral-dimensional theory, it should be apparent that the other placebo studies (including the Ross, Rodin, and Zimbardo study, 1969, in which arousal was attributed to sound) could be regarded as providing further supporting positive evidence. However, the conceptually similar second group of studies, in which naturally induced arousal apparently contributed to heightened emotional experience, could be more broadly interpreted. That is, while I have continued to use the term *arousal*, the operations inducing that arousal are not restricted to enhancing merely peripheral or autonomic arousal. Finally, as noted briefly earlier, the finding that *central* nervous system stimulants and tranquilizers lead to results similar to the misattribution of *peripheral* relaxation or arousal symptoms casts a pall over a radical peripheral-symptom dimensional emotion theory. This issue and the implications for theory will be reengaged later in this chapter.

Emotion attribution in self-control with children

Following the research with adult cheating, described earlier, I began to speculate with several colleagues and students about how normal socialization procedures with children might affect emotion-attribution processes in natural settings. Daryl Bem's work (1972), following that of the more traditional attribution theorists (such as Heider, 1959), had suggested that one reflected upon one's own previous behavior and searched for explanations of that behavior from among the possible internal motives and environmental forces. (Note here the similarity of that view to the traditional emotion-attribution view, which posits that following arousal one begins a search for explanations for the development of the arousal; both views have been challenged for their "cart before the horse" appearance.) These views were incorporated into thinking about the socialization of morality and self-control. Aronson and Carlsmith (1963) and Lepper and his colleagues (e.g., Lepper, Greene, & Nisbett, 1973) had demonstrated that whenever more force was used by a socialization agent than was needed to influence a desirable choice by a child, the child would attribute subsequent positive behavior to those external forces; no reduction in attraction toward the negative behavioral option would be experienced. On the other hand, if less pressure was applied to the child and especially if the child experienced some personal choice in adopting the positive behavior pattern, then the child would seek to justify his or her choice and, to achieve that justification, would value more the "chosen" positive behavior and devalue the "unchosen" negative option.

In our view, "overjustification" theory offered a substantial improvement over more traditional social learning conceptions of moral development, giving a clear prediction for the improved effectiveness of reduced coercion in socialization. (For an excellent recent review of attributional vs. social learning approaches to moral socialization, see Perry & Perry, in press.)

The major issue we took with the traditional attribution approach was simply that emotion had been left out of the process; we felt that the inclusion of consideration of attributions about emotion offered an important addition to the cool rational thinking proposed by the overjustification theorists (Dienstbier et al., 1975). Most traditional thinking about major moral socialization problems, from the development of psychopathy on the one hand to issues of oversocialization on the other had highlighted the central role of emotional processes. Indeed, the work just reviewed on cheating and emotion misattribution and the work of Schachter and Ono with chlorpromazine suggested to us that even in adulthood emotional processes were central in moral choices. We believed that they would be at least as important in childhood moral choices. In this regard the importance of emotional or affective processes in making judgments (as contrasted to "cool" cognition) parallels the recent thinking of Zajonc (1980), who has emphasized that when the balance between cool cognition and affect is assessed, "for most decisions, it is extremely difficult to demonstrate that there has actually been any prior cognitive processes whatsoever." Emotion plays a role of similar magnitude in our model.

As an illustration of emotion-attribution processes developing during a socialization encounter, consider two children confronting angry parents over some proscribed behavior. The confrontation and uncertainty would normally lead the children to experience a significant level of emotional arousal. If one of the children was subsequently physically punished, that child could arrive at quite different conclusions concerning the meaning (and cause) of continuing negative emotional states than would the child who was not given so salient a stimulus as physical punishment. Assuming some learning (similar to classical conditioning) of emotional responses following confrontation and/or punishment, it is likely that in subsequent temptation situations of a similar nature that the previously punished child would experience more emotional arousal than the child given an explanation of why such behavior was wrong. (See Hoffman, 1970, for an extensive discussion of "induction" techniques.) But emotional intensity may not be as crucial as the meaning of the emotional response. If the children were sure that detection of transgression was impossible, depending upon which of those previous treatments were received, the meaning of the emotional response would vary. The previously punished child might attribute arousal to the previous episodes of salient punishment, and, as in the experiment with an arousal-generating (placebo) pill, that emotional response would be assessed as irrelevant to the current detection-proof temptation dilemma. Having not experienced salient punishment in previous episodes, so that no alternative external explanation for emotional tension is available, the second child could believe that his or her tension is caused by the temptation to misbehave rather than to previous negative parental responses.

Early self-control studies

We attempted to abstract the emotion-attribution aspects of these socialization episodes into a laboratory procedure. Since that procedure is discussed extensively elsewhere (Dienstbier et al., 1975), it will be sketched here.

To effect as powerful a design as possible, identical or same-sex fraternal twins were used as research subjects. While the magnitude of the between-condition means are not affected by these special subjects, the use of such subjects allows the control of genetic and social background in a matched-pairs design. Individual subjects were left alone in a toy room with the assignment of watching a problematic slotcar (an electric toy car guided by a pin that slides through a slot in the track) in order to prevent an accident that could seriously affect the (very old) slotcar. After subjects abandoned their assigned task for a criterion time period, the accident was made to happen (by a hidden observer) and the experimenter was simultaneously signaled to return to the playroom. Subjects in the condition hereafter called internal (in which emotion-attribution was made relevant by association with the child's own behavior) were informed that they might feel unhappy because of what they had done and that children who do the right thing usually feel good *even if no one else ever knows* of that proper behavior. Subjects in the external condition (emotion-attribution to confrontation) were informed they might feel a bit bad because *the experimenter knew* what they had done and that children who can *show others* that they have done the right thing usually feel good. The emotional intensity of the two manipulations was carefully matched. The temptation situation was subsequently structured so that children believed that their watching of the slotcar was important but that now (with a new slotcar, the door locked from the inside, and with training in restarting the slotcar in case of accident) no detection by the experimenter of either good or poor behavior was possible. Twins in the internal condition (emotion attributed to own behavior) transgressed (failed to watch the slotcar) for an average of 177 sec out of 12 min, contrasted with 322 sec for their external-condition co-twins ($p < .001$). In a similar study with nontwins, transgression rates were 80 sec and 187 sec ($p < .07$), respectively. (The power of the twin design is seen in that whereas only 12 twins contributed to the first analysis, 24 subjects participated in the similar but marginally significant results of the nontwin study.) Subsequent research found almost identical results when the initial failure of the child was replaced by a story about another child who had "tried to help us out" but who had failed to watch the slotcar sufficiently to prevent the dreaded accident. The independent manipulation was couched in terms of how and why that other child responded emotionally to that failure.

Collectively, the research with twins and nontwins indicated that when a situation is perceived to be detection-free, emotional responses attributed to relevant sources (such as own behavior) play a large positive role in resistance to temptation, as contrasted to emotion attributions to irrelevant sources (such as previous confrontation). If these manipulations truly abstract important elements from real-life socialization episodes, they illustrate some of the reasons why more gentle and psychologically oriented socialization techniques may be more effective than harsh and punishment-oriented practices.

Integration of child and adult studies and theoretical reconceptualizations

Whereas the studies with placebo pills and cheating had at best only slight mundane realism, it being fairly unusual for one to ingest symptom-stimulating placebos prior to confrontation with moral dilemmas, the work with children provided a closer approximation to real life. We concluded that gentler socialization approaches have the dual virtues of being less likely to become the focus of emotion attribution and of providing a vehicle for specifically directing emotion attributions to the child's previous transgression.

Although at this point in our research most of our thinking was about the negative emotional response an individual would have while facing transgression, it was suggested by others (particularly Jerzy Karalowski, personal communication, 1978) that we should similarly focus upon the role of emotion attribution of positive emotions in prosocial choice situations. That is, if positive emotional responses are attributed to one's own choice to engage in altruistic behavior, then the likelihood of future similar altruistic behavior (in an anonymous situation) should be high relative to another person who believes that such positive feelings stem from recognition from others for one's positive accomplishments. In a variation on this thinking, Hoffman (1977) has discussed the efficacy of explaining to children how they impact upon the emotional states of those with whom they interact. The focus is not upon attributions about one's own emotional states but upon attributions about the other's states (e.g., "she will feel bad if you take that away from her"). Finally, similar approaches are used by Weiner (Chapter 6, this volume) in thinking about the emotional response of individuals to achievement situations.

The mundane realism of our independent manipulation and its application to children had been more than merely improved. The languge derived from the peripheral-dimensional approach to emotion had been replaced by language that simply discussed "feeling good" or "feeling bad" with no reference to specific symptoms of arousal or to peripheral or central locations of feelings. We wondered whether our peripheral-symptom messages of the college-student cheating research could have been replaced by far simpler messages about the experience of emotion resulting from the pill.

Adult cheating, schema activation, and emotion attribution

Although a complete answer is not available to that question, a partial one was provided by some subsequent research.. We launched a series of experiments in which our independent manipulations were presented to adults in the guise of reading-comprehension tests, with cheating on the vocabulary test the dependent measure (Dienstbier et al., 1980). Fortunately for our understanding of the interaction of emotion and cognition in temptation circumstances, our initial studies seemed to be complete failures; people who were sensitized to moral issues through their reading-comprehension test cheated more (on the vocabulary test) than did control-condition subjects who read nothing relevant to emotion or morality. We assumed that Study 1 was an example of the haunting reality that false positive results (or, as in this research, false negative) will strike once in 20 successful experiments when probability levels are set at $p < .05$. When, to our deep chagrin, we replicated the phenomenon (Study 2), we were forced to grow in our understanding of the interaction of emotion and cognition.

The intent of the five studies in this series was initially to ascertain whether a manipulation very much like that used with the children would similarly affect college students who were tempted to cheat. But whereas the children were presented with manipulations that directly addressed their future (dependent measure) behavior, in forms such as "you will feel bad if you do a poor job watching the slotcar, even if no one ever knows," adults were presented with messages in abstract form that were not directly related to the dependent-measure task. Passages were presented as reading-comprehension tests, which described the interaction of emotion and cognition in temptation situations using either internal or external emotion-attribution terms; a control group read about perception rather than morality. For example, in Study 2, the internal-condition subjects read that emotional tension develops when one contemplates or executes actions that are counter to one's own moral values. External-condition subjects read a matched passage that presented the idea that emotional tension signals that the contemplated or executed transgression is behavior that would have resulted in punishment in childhood, even though the real danger of punishment may no longer exist. The two messages we hoped to transmit to our subjects were that emotional tension experienced in the face of temptation is usually relevant to that decision (internal) or likely to be irrelevant to the decision (external). As in previous research, subjects were told that the "board of psychologists" developing the verbal tests was particularly interested in vocabulary test performance and would be interested in following the future grades and career of individuals who scored unusually low (defined as less than 18 of the 30 vocabulary items correct). When manipulation checks indicated that our subjects did not really understand the distinctions between internal and external manipulations, we knew that differences in cheating between the internal and external conditions would not be great; indeed they were not; but in Study 2, where control subjects read about long- and short-term memory, the finding of least cheating in the control group did replicate a similar finding from Study 1. (In both studies, 18% [14] of the 77 control-condition subjects cheated, as contrasted with 36% [51] of the 143 subjects in the combined internal and external conditions, $p < .01$.)

To explain our peculiar results, we began to speculate about the potentially elaborate roles of moral schemas in determining responses to temptation (Dienstbier et al., 1980); we temporarily suspended our thinking about emotion attribution. We defined a "schema" as a complex of values, attitudes, cognitions, and emotional responses that are either spontaneously made salient by internal thought processes or elicited by new relevant information; the interaction of new information with the elicited schema determines the resultant attributions, decisions, and behaviors.

We were sure that we had sensitized our subjects to moral issues by our internal and external emotion-attribution messages, since those manipulations contained detailed reference to various moral choices and how emotion plays a role in aiding people in the avoidance of lying, cheating, and stealing. Since those manipulations increased subsequent cheating on the vocabulary test, we reasoned that some other aspects of our experimental situation were providing information that interacted with heightened sensitivity to moral issues to increase cheating. We decided that the threat of embarrassment by an anonymous and powerful "board of psychologists" in the context of what should have been a simple one-hour experiment may have seemed unfair, particularly to those of our subjects who were stimulated to dwell on what is and is not moral;

potentially increased resentment could then have accounted for our peculiar results.

To test that hypothesis, we attempted to reduce such resentment in Study 3. We modified Study 3 to replicate Study 2 but with the research represented as the dissertation research of a graduate student (who acted as the experimenter in both studies). In addition, after the warning not to change any answers, the experimenter added that for his dissertation he needed accurate data or he might have to spend an extra semester gathering new data. As hypothesized, whereas few subjects in the internal and external conditions cheated, more subjects in the control condition did cheat (12% vs. 29%, $p < .05$). To be certain of our interpretation, we followed in Study 4 with a quasi-experiment in which both the Study 2 and 3 versions of the procedure were run, but with the experiment stopped just at the beginning of the period during which subjects could cheat. Questionnaire replies made at that moment indicated that the hypothesized resentment differences could account for the increase in cheating in Studies 1 and 2 in the moral schema activation conditions (internal and external) and a decrease in cheating in those conditions in Study 3.

Having apparently solved the problem of our initially surprising results, in Study 5 we carefully designed an internal and external emotion attribution manipulation with understandable and salient between-condition differences contrasted with a (long- and short-term memory) control condition for the last time. The hypothesized reduced cheating in only the internal emotion-attribution condition was achieved (with 15% cheating, differing from both the external condition rate of 30% and the control condition rate of 31%, $p < .05$).

As had been hoped at the inception of this series of five studies, the final study formed a conceptual bridge between the initial adult cheating studies, which employed the placebo-pill/misattribution manipulation, and the studies with children in which the misattribution information was provided at a conceptual level in a language that might be used in real socialization episodes. Additionally, this final study employed a significant methodological improvement over the work with children, for the independent manipulation was not related by the experimenter to the dependent-measure task. That is, in the work with children one salient alternative explanation for our results had haunted us: That the two emotion-attribution messages, by referring to the dependent-measure task ("you will feel bad if you don't watch the slotcar"), may have somehow increased the importance of that task in the internal condition relative to the external condition. This study achieved a conceptually similar result while effectively eliminating that alternative explanation.

The interaction of emotion attribution and schema activation

Following the research series just described, we concluded that whereas moral schema activation will enhance resistance to temptation (as in Study 3, given that no other information in the situation in interaction with the schema results in contrary analyses of what is moral), those increases in moral behavior will most likely occur when the appropriate emotion attributions are made. That is, in the external emotion attribution condition of Study 5 the elicitation of the relevant moral schema with an irrelevant emotion attribution resulted in *no* reduction in cheating (contrasted to the control group). Although a single study is far from definitive, those results, in combination with the placebo study results, allow the strong inference that, even for college-age adults, appropriate attributions about emotional tension in the face of temptation may be essential in determining the outcome of decision making when behavioral choices present a moral value conflict.

In the original presentation of the five studies we speculated about the inter-actions of emotion-attribution processes and schema activation in temptation situations; the following roughly parallels that speculation:

When an individual perceives the possibility of transgressing, schemas relevant to morality will typically become activated. In addition, emotional arousal will develop as a result of many processes, of which the following are examples:

1. Arousal may result from elements in the current temptation situation being perceived as like previous elements to which emotional responses have been conditioned (as through previous punishment for transgression in similar circumstances).
2. If aspects of the moral schema relate to self-concept ("I should be honest"), the consideration of behaviors that are contrary to those self-concepts may elicit emotional responses. In short, potential value conflicts from contemplating transgression may cause emotional arousal.
3. On the more external side, the individual may fear the potential shame or humiliation from others' knowing of the consideration, or the act, of transgression.

Even though the emotional tension in a single situation may have been elicited by several causes, the meaning of the emotional experience will be determined largely by the most salient cognitions about the meaning of the arousal. Those cognitions depend in turn on the nature of the schema elicited in interaction with elements in the current situation. Anxiety, fear, guilt, shame, or even excitement could result. As shown by the placebo-pill research and by Study 5 of the last series, the amount of arousal and the attributions made about its source and meaning will determine its impact on behavior in the temptation situation.

In addition, although this point is not illustrated by our research, it seems likely that the amount of emotional arousal elicited by elements of the immediate temptation situation would affect the degree to which the moral schema becomes salient and the specific components of the schema that are seen as relevant.

We are left with a complex interaction between elements of the situation that are salient and important because of relevance to either current or past socialization experience, the activation of some aspects of the moral schema by those elements, and the activation of emotional arousal by those elements. All these variables may have simple and interactive influences on all others; for example, both the initial intensity of the emotional response and the initial attributions concerning its source and meaning may influence, in turn, the search for either other relevant elements in the situation or aspects of the moral schema that bear on this situation. Out of this dramatic complexity one clear prediction remains: The meaning eventually accorded to the emotional experience in the temptation situation will play a major role in subsequent behavior.

Relating this research to dissonance and extinction research

It is useful to consider this model in the light of the similar work of Zanna and Cooper (1974) concerning the role of emotional tension in dissonance. They demonstrated that emotional arousal mediates attitude change when cognitions about attitude and about past behavior are dissonant unless that emotional arousal is misattributed to an irrelevant source. In our research, potentially similar dissonance was faced by our subjects before their behavioral decision. The "dissonance" centers around some aspect of the moral schema and the conflicting temptation to behave in a manner discrepant with that schema. As long as the resultant emotional arousal is experienced before the transgression, the emotional tension usually will be more easily resolved by resisting the behavior rather than by changing the moral schema. However, as with the dissonance research, where attributions of emotional arousal to an irrelevant source allow the dissonant elements to coexist without attitude change, emotion misattribution to irrelevant elements in the face of temptation apparently allows both the transgression and the contradictory moral schema to coexist.

But the coexistence of transgression and contradictory moral schemas will not be maintained indefinitely in the context of emotional tension thought to be irrelevant. The findings of Loftis and Ross (1974) suggested that the post-conditioning misattribution of emotional tension to an irrelevant source leads to the more rapid extinction of the conditioned emotional response. In moral dilemma situations, the repeated attribution to fear of punishment (when punishment is perceived as impossible) should lead to at least partial elimination of tension in the face of similar future temptations.

Further research on self-control with children

Our research program with children has led to some recent failures, which we hope will prove to be as heuristic as our initial "failures" in the adult series just described. That is, we have used a procedure similar to that used with

children just described, but have attempted to present emotion-attribution
messages in a form that does not relate directly to the temptation task in which
they will be engaged. We have been telling stories of temptation successfully
or unsuccessfully resisted, with the emotional response of the hero following
success or failure and the emotion-attribution messages emphasized (e.g., "he
felt very bad that he did not do what he was supposed to, even though no one
ever found out" as an internal message and, as an external message, "she felt
very good that her mother and father knew what a good job she had done").
To apply these messages to their own subsequent temptation, children must
translate them into abstract terms (we supply some help in this initial transition)
and apply them to the specific concrete situation in which they find themselves.
Children in grades two through seven have not been successful in doing this,
as no between-condition behavior differences have yet been demonstrated in
that research. However, some recent research by Rachel Karnoil (personal
communication) has led us to speculate about the potential source of our problems. Karnoil has demonstrated that the degree of post-transgression guilt
experienced by children (as assessed in fantasy projection) does not relate to
their actual resistance to temptation. She makes a strong and convincing case
that for young children there is not necessarily any relationship between post-
transgression emotions and emotional states experienced as inhibitory during
or prior to the contemplation of transgression. Although she did not measure
post-transgression guilt in response to exactly the same behavior as the subsequent temptation, this research does suggest that the automatic transition
from post-transgression arousal, induced initially by confrontation with socialization figures, to inhibiting arousal may be later in development than I
had previously believed. These ideas suggest that the most effective emotion-
attribution messages for parents to give in the context of confrontation over
transgression might involve describing the future feelings of children in similar
temptation situations in addition to labeling current emotional feelings.

A developmental perspective

In this section, I will discuss in a more speculative form how the changing
patterns of socialization of parents and the maturing symbolic capacity of the
child lead to changing patterns of emotional intensity and attributions as the
child develops.

   With very young children, the learning of prohibitions against injuring younger
siblings or animals is often an important concern. In such socialization encounters, the sheer intensity of the emotional response evoked by confrontation
with parents over transgression is crucial. That is, when the child with very
rudimentary symbolic capacity confronts a similar future "temptation," the
sheer volume of inhibiting emotional reaction in contrast to the positive desire
(as in a classic approach–avoidance conflict from animal research) determines

the outcome. As the child develops, just as the learning of language allows a cognitive symbolization of environmental (and behavioral) objects and events, a parallel symbolization of emotional response develops. That is, instead of the older child relying on the sheer intensity of inhibiting emotion to resist temptation, the symbolic representation of the transgression can lead to a similarly symbolic (or token) level of emotional arousal. At this point in development, even though the "approach gradient" toward a "sin of commission" may be very high, the child can understand the token inhibitory emotional response as a of sign the intensity of emotional response that would develop if the transgression were to be actually undertaken (and/or if detection were to result). Just as the purely cognitive representation of a delayed goal may allow the older child to delay immediate gratification (even without visualizing and reexperiencing all the wonders of the greater but delayed goal), the symbolism of small levels of emotional arousal allows the resistance of even mighty temptations without reexperiencing the horrors of a fully developed negative emotional response (depending upon the attributions made, as discussed in the earlier part of the chapter). No longer dependent upon the reactions of parents, the experienced levels of emotional tension are usually sufficiently small so that they are neither "aversive" as they develop nor particularly "reinforcing" as they decline but instead serve only to forecast symbolically the aversive emotional response that might develop with transgression.

Given that I am now invoking very small levels of emotional arousal, which may be experienced as shame (given external attributions) or as guilt (given internal attributions), would it not be more parsimonious and reasonable to abandon the emotion-as-symbol approach entirely in favor of verbal symbolic processes within the developing child? That question is quite close to the one with which I began this research program, hardly believing that people of college age would rely upon either token or large emotional responses in making judgments about such behaviors as cheating. Yet the research has provided an answer (as has the research of Schachter and Ono, who increased cheating rates through the tranquilizer chlorpromazine; reported in Schachter & Latané, 1964). Particularly for the placebo-pill research, it is difficult to pose an appealing alternative interpretation to the observation that emotion and emotion attributions play a major role.

The role of socialization intensity

Whereas in the foregoing sections of this chapter I considered the role of the *type* or quality of socialization procedure used in shaping the emotion attributions that developing children would make in the face of temptation, the intensity or quantity of socialization may also impact such attributions. Those forces impact the normal child's developing attributions in a way that may reinforce internal emotion attributions for intensely socialized dilemmas but stimulate external emotion attributions for temptations that have been weakly socialized. In this section, intense or strong socialization refers to pressures from social-ization agents that are neither more nor less internal or external in their focus than less rigorous or intense socialization but nevertheless evoke substantially more intense and enduring emotional responses.

Remember the logic of self-perception theory. The individual makes an analysis of those factors that apparently influenced his or her own behavior – an analysis based upon the same observations available to the onlooker. In my extension of that approach to emotional events, I propose that the emotional state itself will be attributed to internal causes when it is experienced for an extended period of time in the absence of obvious external causes. Consider the child who has been strongly socialized for episodes of lying. Following an apparently undetected subsequent lie, the child may experience an extended negative emotional response. The high intensity and long duration of the emo-tional response should motivate continued searches for understanding. But if no punishment or other salient external element is present in this episode, it is likely that the child may come to believe that the extended emotional response is due to internal causes – his or her revulsion for telling the lie.[1] On the other hand, when the child is weakly and infrequently socialized for a specific class of transgression, the emotional response subsequent to an episode of transgres-sion in that category will be weak and uncertain. The failure of a significant emotional response when the child is "getting away with it" provides further evidence to the child that the proper attribution for any emotional response in like episodes (when parents may have intervened) was indeed external. This approach would predict that many of the weakly taught moral lessons of our youth should be soon forgotten (because of the quick extinction of emotional responses with external attribution, as discussed above), but that the strong ones should go with us to the grave.

The role of temperament

This same logic leads to the view that individuals with different temperaments should similarly gravitate toward different emotion-attributional styles. That is, for the child who easily experiences high levels of emotional tension, a kind of attributional inevitability may foster internal attributions about transgression-inhibiting emotion, even in the absence of socialization agents specifically fostering such internal attribution. Such a child would experience his or her intense and lingering emotional tension following transgression as a result of his or her own sins, so that such individuals should frequently be guilt-ridden. The vast clinical literature on depression is, of course, supportive of this conclusion, since many chronically depressed individuals indicate high frequencies of guilt-laden thoughts.[2]

On the other hand, the child with only a slight tendency to experience any negative emotional responses will "condition" poorly even in the face of strong socialization practices and will often inspire harsh and repressive measures from parents. Such harsh punishment provides salient external stimuli to which the emotional responses may be attributed. But the failure of a significant emotional response to develop when the child is "getting away with it" provides further evidence to the child that the proper attribution for the emotional response in other episodes (when the socialization agent intervened) was indeed to the external cause. Thus, whereas the easily conditioned child may form increasingly internal emotion attributions, the unperturbable child may form increasingly external attributions, even in response to similar socialization techniques.

This logic would predict a population distribution of morality that would differ from the traditional bell-shaped curve. That is, with intensity of emotional experience and attributional tendencies not being additive but interactive, so that anxious individuals adopt internal emotion attributions and unperturbable people become external, a flattened curve, or even a trichotomous distribution, would be predicted, with (in the case of the trichotomous result) a major "bell" in the middle and two upturns on either end that would designate individuals who are either guilt-ridden, anxious, and depressed or psychopathic.[3]

Physiological dispositions and personality

If the foregoing speculations about the relationship of temperament to moral decision making have merit, there should be some research support. In fact, no research has been completed directly linking a tendency to form internal attributions about emotion in moral decision making with any aspect of temperament or personality. In the preceding section, I suggested that those with a more emotionally responsive temperament would become more internal. If we can assume that being more internal in emotion attributions (within the normal range) leads to the perception by others that one is better socially adjusted (by virtue of demonstrating appropriate levels of *self*-control), then indirect support for the basic relationship would be achieved by demonstrating a link between high emotional responsivity and positive social adjustment.

Relevant to this issue of psychological responsivity and positive personality (or adjustment) characteristics, three branches of research do exist. One branch of that research, undertaken largely in Europe, indicates that within individuals, increases in the catecholamines adrenaline and noradrenaline in the context of challenge or stress are correlated with many positive characteristics of temperament and personality. The second branch of relevant research demonstrates relationships between the physiological responsivity of the sympathetic nervous system and positive personality characteristics. Finally, work with psychopathic individuals suggests similar relationships.

Concerning the first branch of this research, high catecholamine levels during stress or high catecholaine level increases from control conditions to stress conditions have been associated with: high "ego strength" or greater "adaptive capacity or stress tolerance" in American male college students (Roessler, Burch, & Mefferd, 1967); low neuroticism and low experience of day-to-day stress for Swedish male college students (Forsman, 1980); more trust, less apprehension, and less anxiety (measured on Cattell's Sixteen Personality Factors Inventory) for Finnish male high school students, and low psychosomatic symptomatology for both male and female Finnish high school students (Rauste-von Wright, von Wright, & Frankenhaeuser, 1981); better ratings by teachers of social adjustment and emotional stability and more school satisfaction for 12-year-old Swedish girls and boys (Johansson, Frankenhaeuser, & Magnusson, 1973). Finally, in contrast to the substantial catecholamine increases of normal criminals as they experienced the approach of their trial dates, psychopathic criminals showed no such catecholamine increases (Frankenhaeuser, 1979).

The literature just cited is not an exhaustive review of the research showing positive relationships between catecholamine increases in stress or challenge and positive personality characteristics. Although it is compatible with major approaches to undersocialization and psychopathy to assume that catecholamine deficits may be associated with those states, finding that such deficits may be associated with anxiety and other forms of maladjustment is not as easily incorporated into most existing theories. However, to ease that problem, Johansson and Frankenhaeuser (1973) found that whereas improved performance accompanied catecholamine increases, neuroticism was identified with slow recovery (return to catecholamine base line) following stimulation.

Investigators of the second branch of research linking arousal indexes to temperament, who are largely American, have measured direct indices of the activity of the sympathetic branch of the autonomic nervous system and have come to similar conclusions about arousal and positive personality dimensions and/or socialization. J. Schachter and his associates (1965) found that for a sample of 46 college males, intimacy and involvement (a trait correlating .61 with tolerance for anxiety) was positively correlated with both heart-rate variability and skin-conductance levels under stress. They concluded that those subjects with calm temperaments showed the highest physiological reactivity to stress. Valins (1967) found similar results. The most important study for our purposes was that of Waid (1976), who found that skin-conductance responses to both signaled and unsignaled noxious stimuli were positively correlated with level of socialization as measured by the California Personality Inventory.

Concerning the third branch of research linking arousal to temperament, physiological response patterns have been related to psychopathy by Mednick (1977). Mednick was primarily interested in high-rate offenders and those diagnosed as psychopathic (in Denmark where extensive records are maintained, allowing this type of research). To assess autonomic activity recovery, Mednick focused on the electrodermal response and the speed of recovery from that response (EDRec). Having measured autonomic characteristics in a large population of Copenhagen males in a longitudinal study, Mednick noted that the EDRec was slower in those 36 men who subsequently violated the penal code and slowest of all for those 9 individuals who were diagnosed as psychopathic. Mednick also noted a high heritability component for EDRec, with the children of criminal fathers showing a pattern significantly like their criminal fathers (contrasted to noncriminal fathers and their children). (Similarly, the number of skin-conductance responses was almost double for the children of the non-criminals, indicating more orienting responses to the cues presented.) In studying maximum-security prisoners identified as psychopathic, Hare (cited in Mednick, 1977) has found similar correlations of EDRec and psychopathy.

Taken together, the three lines of research suggest the conclusion we had been looking for: That indices of increased physiological responsivity, suggesting greater ease in the learning of emotional responses, are positively related to positive personality dimensions and to level of socialization.

A return to basic issues in emotion theory

Let us return to the question of a dimensional theory of emotion emphasizing peripheral visceral feedback. Although the initial research using placebos suggested support for the peripheral feedback version of a dimensional theory of emotion, the independent manipulation in the research with children, which discussed "feeling good" or "feeling bad," allowed other interpretations. Subsequently, the final series of studies presented internal and external manipulations to college students in a textual format that described "emotional tension" rather than specific peripheral symptoms. The positive results of Study 5 in that series indicated that emotion attribution to an external source (previous punishment) facilitated cheating; that finding suggests strongly that the peripheral-dimensional language of the initial placebo studies was not essential. Of course, if that peripheral-symptom language was not essential in the early placebo cheating studies of our series, it probably was similarly nonessential in all the other noise-attribution and pill-attribution studies that appeared to support the peripheral-dimensional view. I now suspect that upon being told that peripheral arousal symptoms may be increased by a placebo, the research subject associated those systems (of muscle tension, pounding heart, face feeling flushed, and stomach "butterflies") with tension and/or anxiety and then understood the message to be that *feelings of emotional tension* would be pill-induced. Given this interpretation, I suspect it would have been as effective a technique for inducing emotion misattribution to have suggested symptoms relevant to muscle tension in facial areas ("you may begin to experience feelings of tension in your brow and jaw"). The findings in the dissonance literature, cited earlier, that a central tranquilizer was similar in effect to misattribution of "peripheral" arousal symptoms and that the misattribution of peripheral relaxation symptoms achieved effects similar to a central stimulant support this line of reasoning. Together, these observations suggest modifications of emotion-attribution theory away from the "classic" notion that one's understanding of the causes of one's peripheral arousal symptoms determines the quality of the emotion experienced. I would suggest instead that *one's ideas about the source and meaning of one's emotional experience determine* (to some extent, with caveats to be elaborated) *the quality of that experience and the impact of that experience on behavior.*

Necessary modifications to peripheral-dimensional theory have been prompted by recent experimental efforts that have identified increasing emotional arousal with more negative than neutral emotional tone (i.e., Marshall & Zimbardo, 1979; Maslach, 1979). Although those data suggest that one should not assume that an emotional state is merely "standard" undifferentiated arousal with a specific cognitive label, some of the research cited earlier shows that arousal induced by startle, exercise, and acrophobia can contribute to increased attraction toward others, increased sexuality in stories, and so on. These data strongly suggest that negative rather than neutral undifferentiated arousal can still contribute to a positive emotion if the environmental elements fostering that attribution are strong and salient. That is, in the context of those strong environmental cues, prior arousal from the sources described leads to increases on the dependent measure dimensions to a greater extent than if no prior arousal has been established. Elements within the individual similarly foster or inhibit such an emotional attribution. (For a detailed discussion of the parameters affecting emotion attribution, see Dienstbier, 1979b.)

Concerning studies favoring the facial-feedback hypothesis, usually attributed to discrete emotion theorists, several studies that bear on the issue have recently appeared. While Torangeau and Ellsworth (1979) were unable to show any impact of feedback from facial expressions when their subjects held a facial expression for an extended time period, Zuckerman and his colleagues (1981) found strong evidence that both the experience of emotion and various peripheral autonomic arousal indexes increased when subjects exaggerated their facial responses (in response to short films), as contrasted with either neutral instructions or instructions to minimize facial responses. Similarly, Laird and his associates (1982) have found that cognitions are influenced by facial expressions in the direction of emotional tone compatible with the expression assumed.

As I have discussed more extensively elsewhere (Dienstbier, 1979b), it is apparent that there are components of arousal similarity between the various emotional states characterized generally by sympathetic nervous system arousal, just as there are obviously components that are different (such as facial expression). Whether one focuses on the similarities and works with questions best answered from a theoretical stance, which emphasizes those similarities (such as has been my research approach), or whether one focuses on the differences and emphasizes compatible research and theoretical positions, the "opposing" theoretical position is not even addressed. I would suggest, however, that just as Laird and Crosby (1974) have suggested that individual differences may exist in sensitivity to facial feedback, similar between-individual differences probably exist for responsivity to more general forms of arousal.

Similarly, although no convincing data exist (to my knowledge) on this point, I strongly suspect that the degree to which facial or autonomic feedback plays a relatively larger role in the experience of emotion depends upon which emotional state we focus upon. Working within the framework of discrete theories for a moment, if one focuses upon the probable origins of certain emotional states in terms of the major adaptive functions they evolved to serve, some strong hints as to likely sites of important feedback emerge. (See Scott, 1980, or Plutchik, 1962, for theories emphasizing the adaptive utility of emotional states.) For example, I would expect that feedback from the region of the mouth, throat, and esophagus would be extremely important in the experience of disgust (thought to relate originally to the rejection of tainted food), whereas the importance of genital feedback in advanced states of sexual arousal (certainly more appropriately thought of as an emotion than a traditional "drive," since it is evoked more by external stimuli than by internal physiological needs) seems obvious.

On the other hand, the emotional states with which I have been most concerned in thinking about the inhibition of temptation are quite different. Anxiety is thought to arise in circumstances where neither a clearly definable cause nor an obvious response are available; predictably, the facial response is not generally emphasized, in contrast to the sympathetic and hormonal arousal character of anxiety. From an adaptive standpoint, this balance makes good sense, as the organism that feels vaguely uneasy has nothing to combat, nor an obvious direction available in which to flee, nor specifics about which to communicate with others of its kind. But an increase in general arousal, probably supported by long-term hormonal responses, will facilitate the long-term vigilance that may be necessary for safety and, in the context of a developed culture, the avoidance of temptation.

This research program has not specifically addressed the issue of arousal balance between cortical, peripheral autonomic and peripheral muscular facial locations. Despite our inability to know with precision what specific events in our brains and bodies contribute to our experiences of anxiety, fear, shame, and guilt, it is apparent that such emotional states profoundly influence our behavior in temptation situations and that those emotional states and their impact on behavior greatly depend upon the attributions made about their meaning and origin.

Summary

Following an introduction of some modern theoretical issues in the area of emotion and the development of peripheral-dimensional theory and research, a brief review of literature is presented showing the impact of the intensity of emotional arousal on moral decision making. Several studies are then presented that were designed to demonstrate that one's interpretation of the meaning of emotional arousal moderates the effectiveness of the arousal in facilitating resistance to temptation. Using a paradigm in which emotional symptoms were misattributed to a placebo pill (or not, in the control group), it was shown that cheating on a vocabulary test was significantly increased by the misattribution to the pill of symptoms of peripheral arousal.

Following another brief review of related emotion-attribution research based upon hypotheses derived from a peripheral-dimensional approach to emotion, some conflicts are highlighted in what seems at first to be a smooth progression of support for the peripheral-dimensional approach.

Presented next is a series of studies on self-control with children, in which the experience of emotion (feeling good or bad) was attributed to "internal" (the child's own behavior) or to "external" (others knowing about the child's behavior) causes. The attribution of emotional experience to internal causes was shown to have powerful self-control facilitating effects on difficult watching assignments in "detection-proof" situations. Those findings are discussed in relation to the larger literature on moral socialization.

A third research series is then presented that demonstrates that adult cheating rates too may be affected by giving adults different explanations of the meaning of emotional experiences in moral decision making. In the context of a reading-comprehension test, when adults read that the tension experienced during temptation is a sign that one may be about to violate one's own values, they cheated less on a subsequent vocabulary test than if they had read that emotional tension during temptation is related to past (often currently irrelevant) punishment. We concluded that, as with self-control in children, the meaning adults attribute to their emotional response (not peripheral-arousal symptoms) is crucial in self-control. This section concludes with a discussion of the interaction of moral schemas and emotion-attribution processes during moral decision making.

The role of emotion in resistance to temptation is then discussed from a developmental perspective. Explanations are advanced for how the progression from more intense emotional responses in younger children to the more symbolic and mild representations of emotional states in adults may still result in emotion-mediated self-control. Approaches to socialization that facilitate a more internal basis for conscience are discussed, and the role of inherited temperament differences in fostering internal and external emotion-attribution dispositions is discussed. Subsequently, some evidence from the research of others concerning the possible link between temperament and internality is presented and discussed.

Finally, the broad theoretical issues concerning the nature of emotion with which the chapter began are reengaged in light of the evidence from our research. The state of the evidence concerning the importance of arousal feedback from different body areas is discussed, and conclusions are discussed concerning the relative merit of dimensional and discrete approaches to emotion.

Notes

1 The research of Zillmann and his colleagues has suggested a similar process for exercise-induced arousal. When subjects mistakenly believed that they had recovered from that lingering arousal, they misattributed it to such "internal" sources as their valuing of aesthetic stimuli, the entertainment value they perceived in a film, and their own anger (Zillmann et al., 1974; Cantor et al., 1975).

2 It should be noted that this represents a causal emphasis between emotion and cognition in depression that is opposite to that popularized by Beck (1967). I am suggesting that the ongoing emotional state of depression can cause an increased frequency of emotion-compatible cognitions and that guilt (rather than shame), as an emotion compatible with internal emotion attributions, is a natural product of a lingering negative emotional state. Although this view is compatible with recent work on the impact of emotion and memory (e.g., Bower, 1981; Laird et al., 1982), it is not offered as a replacement for the causal direction emphasized by Beck but as an addition to that opposite causal view.

3 With respect to this prediction of psychopathic behavior, it should be noted that several recent studies of crime (e.g., Mednick, 1977; Yochelson & Samnow, 1976) have concluded that most crimes in civilized societies are committed by a very small number of individuals, representing 1% or 2% of the total population.

References

Aronson, E., & Carlsmith, J. M. Effect of the severity of threat on the devaluation of forbidden behavior. *Journal of Abnormal and Social Psychology*, 1963, *66*, 584–588.

Beck, A. T. *Depression: Clinical, experimental and theoretical aspects*. New York: Harper & Row, 1967.

Bem, D. J. Self-perception theory. In L. Berkowitz (Ed.), *Advances in experimental social psychology* (Vol. 6). New York: Academic Press, 1972.

Bower, G. H. Mood and memory. *American Psychologist*, 1981, *36*, 129–148.

Cantor, J. R., Zillmann, D., & Bryant, J. Enhancement of experienced sexual arousal in response to erotic stimuli through misattribution of unrelated residual excitation. *Journal of Personality and Social Psychology*, 1975, *32*, 69–75.

Cooper, J., Zanna, M. P., & Taves, P. A. Arousal as a necessary condition for attitude change following induced compliance. *Journal of Personality and Social Psychology*, 1978, *36*, 1101–1106.

Dienstbier, R. A. The role of anxiety and arousal attribution in cheating. *Journal of Experimental Social Psychology*, 1972, *8*, 168–179.

Dienstbier, R. A. Attraction increases and decreases as a function of emotion-attribution and appropriate social cues. *Motivation and Emotion*, 1979, *3*, 201–218. (a)

Dienstbier, R. A. Emotion-attribution theory: Establishing roots and exploring future perspectives. In H. E. Howe, Jr., & R. A. Dienstbier (Eds.), *Nebraska symposium on motivation* (Vol. 26), Lincoln: University of Nebraska Press, 1979. (b)

Dienstbier, R. A., Hillman, D., Lehnhoff, J., Hillman, J., & Valkenaar, M. C. An emotion-attribution approach to moral behavior: Interfacing cognitive and avoidance theories of moral development. *Psychological Review*, 1975, *82*, 299–315.

Dienstbier, R. A., Kahle, L. R., Willis, K. A., & Tunnell, G. B. The impact of moral theories on cheating: Studies of emotion attribution and schema activation. *Motivation and Emotion*, 1980, *4*, 193–216.

Dienstbier, R. A., & Munter, P. O. Cheating as a function of the labeling of natural arousal. *Journal of Personality and Social Psychology*, 1971, *17*, 208–213.

Dutton, D. G., & Aron, A. P. Some evidence for heightened sexual attraction under conditions of high anxiety. *Journal of Personality and Social Psychology*, 1974, *30*, 510–517.

Forsman, L. Habitual catecholamine excretion and its relation to habitual distress. *Biological Psychology*, 1980, *11*, 83–97.

Frankenhaeuser, M. Psychoneuroendocrine approaches to the study of emotion as related to stress and coping. In H. E. Howe, Jr., & R. A. Dienstbier (Eds.), *Nebraska Symposium on Motivation* (Vol. 26). Lincoln: University of Nebraska Press, 1979.

Heider, F. *The psychology of interpersonal relations*. New York: Wiley, 1958.

Hoffman, M. L. Moral development. In P. H. Mussen (Ed.), *Carmichael's manual of child development* (Vol. 2; 3rd ed.). New York: Wiley, 1970.

Hoffman, M. L. Moral internalization: Current theory and research. In L. Berkowitz (Ed.), *Advances in experimental social psychology* (Vol. 10). New York: Academic Press, 1977.

Izard, C. E. *The face of emotion*. New York: Appleton-Century-Crofts, 1971.

Izard, C. E. *Human emotions*. New York: Plenum, 1977.

Izard, C. E., & Tomkins, S. S. Affect and behavior: Anxiety as a negative affect. In C. D. Spielberger (Ed.), *Anxiety and behavior*. New York: Academic Press, 1966.

Johansson, G., & Frankenhaeuser, M. Temporal factors in sympatho-adrenomedullary activity following acute behavioral activation. *Biological Psychology*, 1973, *1*, 63–73.

Johansson, G., Frankenhaeuser, M., & Magnusson, D. Catecholamine output in school children as related to performance and adjustment. *Scandinavian Journal of Psychology*, 1973, *14*, 20–28.

Karalowski, J. Personal communication, 1978.

Karnoil, R. Personal communication regarding her work with children in Israel, 1982.

Konecni, V. J. The mediation of aggressive behavior: Arousal level versus anger and cognitive labeling. *Journal of Personality and Social Psychology*, 1975, *32*, 706–712.

Laird, J., & Crosby, M. Individual differences in self-attribution of emotion. In H. London & R. E. Nisbett (Eds.), *Thought and feeling*. Chicago: Aldine, 1974.

Laird, J. D., Wagener, J., Halal, M., & Szegda, M. Remembering what you feel: Effects of emotion on memory. *Journal of Personality and Social Psychology*, 1982, *42*, 646–657.

Lepper, M. R., Greene, D., & Nisbett, R. E. Undermining children's intrinsic interest with extrinsic reward: A test of the "overjustification" hypothesis. *Journal of Personality and Social Psychology*, 1973, *28*, 129–138.

Lindsley, D. B. The role of nonspecific reticulo-thalamo-cortical systems in emotion. In P. Black (Ed.), *Physiological correlates of emotion*. New York: Academic Press, 1970.

Loftis, J., & Ross, L. Retrospective misattribution of a conditioned emotional response. *Journal of Personality and Social Psychology*, 1974, *30*, 683–687.

Mandler, G. *Mind and emotion*. New York: Wiley, 1975.

Marshall, G., & Zimbardo, P. G. Affective consequences of inadequately explained physiological arousal. *Journal of Personality and Social Psychology*, 1979, *37*, 970–988.

Maslach, C. Negative emotional biasing of unexplained arousal. *Journal of Personality and Social Psychology*, 1979, *37*, 953–969.

Mednick, S. A. The biosocial theory of the learning of law-abiding behavior. In S. A. Mednick & K. O. Christiansen (Eds.), *Biosocial bases of criminal behavior*. New York: Gardner Press, 1977.

Nisbett, R. E., & Schachter, S. Cognitive manipulation of pain. *Journal of Experimental Social Psychology*, 1966, *2*, 227–236.

Nowlis, V. Personal communication regarding the Rochester drug studies, 1968.

Perry, D. G., & Perry, L. C. Social learning, causal attribution and moral internalization. In C. Brainerd (Ed.), *Advances in cognitive development*. New York: Springer-Verlag, in press.

Plutchik, R. *The emotions: Facts, theories, and a new model*. New York: Random House, 1962.

Rauste-von Wright, M., von Wright, J., & Frankenhaeuser, M. Relationships between sex-related psychological characteristics during adolescence and catecholamine excretion during achievement stress. *Psychophysiology*, 1981, *18*, 362–370.

Rodin, J. Menstruation, reattribution, and competence. *Journal of Personality and Social Psychology*, 1976, *33*, 345–353.

Roessler, R., Burch, N. R., & Mefferd, R. B. Personality correlates of catecholamine excretion under stress. *Journal of Psychosomatic Research*, 1967, *11*, 181–185.

Ross, L., Rodin, J., & Zimbardo, P. G. Toward an attribution therapy: The reduction of fear through induced cognitive emotional misattribution. *Journal of Personality and Social Psychology*, 1969, *12*, 279–288.

Ross, M., & Olson, J. M. An expectancy-attribution model of the effects of placebos. *Psychological Review*, 1981 *88*, 408–437.

Schachter, J., Williams, T. A., Rowe, R., Schachter, J. S., & Jameson, J. Personality correlates of physiological reactivity to stress: A study of forty-six college males. *American Journal of Psychiatry*, 1965, *121*, 12–24.

Schachter, S., & Latané, B. Crime, cognition, and the autonomic nervous system. In D. Levine (Ed.), *Nebraska symposium on Motivation* (Vol. 12). Lincoln: University of Nebraska Press, 1964.

Schachter, S., & Singer, J. E. Cognitive, social, and physiological determinants of emotional state. *Psychological Review*, 1962, *69*, 379–399.

Schachter, S., & Wheeler, L. Epinephrine, chlorpromazine, and amusement. *Journal of Abnormal and Social Psychology*, 1962, *65*, 121–128.

Scott, J. P. The function of emotions in behavioral systems: A systems theory analysis. In R. E. Plutchik & H. Kellerman (Eds.), *Emotion: Theory, research and experience*. New York: Academic Press, 1980.

Tomkins, S. S. *Affect, imagery, consciousness*, Vol. 2: *The negative affects*. New York: Springer-Verlag, 1963.

Tourangeau, R., & Ellsworth, P. C. The role of facial response in the experience of emotion. *Journal of Personality and Social Psychology*, 1979, *37*, 1519–1531.

Valins, S. Emotionality and autonomic reactivity. *Journal of Experimental Research in Personality*, 1967, *2*, 41–48.

Waid, W. M. Skin conductance response to both signaled and unsignaled noxious stimulation predicts levels of socialization. *Journal of Personality and Social Psychology*, 1976, *34*, 923–929.

Yochelson, S., & Samnow, S. E. *The criminal personality*, Vol. 1: *A profile for change*. New York: Aronson, 1976.

Younger, J. C., & Doob, A. N. Attribution and aggression: The misattribution of anger. *Journal of Research in Personality*, 1978, *12*, 164–171.

Zajonc, R. B. Feeling and thinking: Preferences need no inferences. *American Psychologist*, 1980, *35*, 151–175.

Zanna, M. P., & Cooper, J. Dissonance and the pill: An attribution approach to studying the arousal properties of dissonance. *Journal of Personality and Social Psychology*, 1974, *29*, 703–709.

Zillmann, D., Johnson, R. C., & Day, K. D. Attribution of apparent arousal and proficiency of recovery from sympathetic activation affecting excitation transfer to aggressive behavior. *Journal of Experimental Social Psychology*, 1974, *10*, 503–515.

Zillmann, D., Katcher, A. H., & Milavsky, B. Excitation transfer from physical exercise to subsequent aggressive behavior. *Journal of Experimental Social Psychology*, 1972, *8*, 247–259.

Zuckerman, M., Klorman, R., Larrence, D. T., & Speigel, N. H. Facial, autonomic, and subjective components of emotion: The facial feedback hypothesis versus the externalizer-internalizer distinction. *Journal of Personality and Social Psychology*, 1981, *41*, 929–944.

17 Thinking and feeling in Woolf's writing: from childhood to adulthood

Jeannette M. Haviland

There is a great mystery in the human mind arising from its desire to make singularities from multiplicities and vice versa. Is a life a series of moments largely connected by chance or wish, each moment a unique piece of existence, or is a life a unique but singular entity, each moment only a slightly varied reflection of other moments? When we see and know well one moment in a life, have we only learned to marvel more at the multiplicity captured by lives or, if very lucky, do we hold the kernel of that life, one moment of many reflections never essentially changing? These questions may seem to be only murmurings of an adolescent searching for identity, but they compose two metatheoretical positions in psychology, as in literature. Can one move sensibly from microanalysis to macroanalysis, from one category to another, from one age to another? In creating a literary character, can one make the character all pieces or must there be some centrality or at least predictability? Clearly, literary characters that achieve greatness may be complex, but they must be understandable as a singular entity. Continuity in literary character requires no explanation, but the psychological character may be less predictable.

Inasmuch as the psychological character may be conceived as containing subsystems of processing or operating, such as cognition and affect, it becomes relevant to inquire into the interrelationships of cognition and affect in the total functioning of a person. Heuristically, it is useful to consider separate systems, but it is rare that one can conceive of the mechanical information processor as other than a machine or the cognitively blank, affective responder as other than a state of being – nirvana or nightmare. As one changes cognitively, becoming more complex, more logical, more aware of self-processing, what happens to affective process? As one becomes compelled by life to experience certain affect states intensely or frequently, what happens to cognitive processes? At certain points it is likely that the questions will not be discriminable, but it is the task of this chapter to demonstrate certain interactive aspects of cognition and affect in a single individual growing from childhood through young adulthood.

This research was partially supported by a grant from the Rutgers Research Council for 1981–82. The assistance of Livingston College undergraduates in coding diaries and letters is acknowledged and appreciated.

515

In this chapter the developmental changes and similarities in affect and cognition as contained in a longitudinal study of the writings of Virginia Stephen Woolf are presented. Several basic descriptions precede the presentation of the analysis. First there is a brief defense of the use of a single case to suit the current purpose and a biographical description of Virginia Stephen Woolf. Second, there is a description of the codes to be used for affect and cognition with some attempt at general definition of the terms as used in the present context. Third, the procedure for coding and training in coding is described. The resultant developmental description follows these preparations.

The use of a case study for developmental research

The analysis of single cases or individual lives can be done either to substantiate a theoretical perspective or method of analysis or it can be used to create a theoretical perspective. There are many classic or nearly classic examples of this approach. Much psychoanalytic psychology is based on theories derived from the single cases (e.g., Freud's "Analysis of a Phobia in a Five-Year-Old Boy," 1953). New developments in psychoanalytic approaches have emerged from case studies also; for example, the psychobiographical approach of Erikson (e.g., *Young Man Luther*, 1958) led to a more thorough integration of individual and cultural "personalities."

A few personologists have also used the study of an individual to analyze a method. Allport's *Letters from Jenny* (1965) was used to compose theoretical approaches. Rosenberg and Jones's analysis of Theodore Dreiser (1972) was used to demonstrate implicit personality theory and to compare statistical methods. Some cases have been instrumental in establishing whole schools of psychology even outside the areas of personality; for example, Ebbinghaus's self-study was central to long-term memory hypotheses, Watson's "Little Albert" case, to behaviorism, and Piaget's own children as individual studies, to cognitive development.

In the abstract, analysis of a single case has an advantage for developmental studies that cannot be gained in other realms. In any kind of analysis that requires a sequential rule, one always has to derive the description or hypothesis for one case, in mathematics it is usually called "k"th case. Then, to establish the rule or complete the proof, one demonstrates that the same solution works for the "k + 1" case. One does not use aggregate cases in the proof unless the criteria specifically allow for aggregate cases. Changes in the shape of a function are distorted or masked when aggregates are used. For this reason, as well as for parsimony, new areas may be best explored using the case method. In some instances they may be the only method of study; for example, when a developmental "rule" or theorem is discovered using the case study, it may be masked when the contents of two or more cases are added (to use the easiest possibility). This seemingly simple rule of mathematics and psychology (e.g., Skinner, 1938) is particularly germane for a study of sequential events such as the present one.

Biographical background

Before beginning the developmental analysis of thematic content, a brief introduction to Woolf's family setting and major events is useful. Some situational cues become very clear from the biographical background, including her literary inclinations and concern with death and loss. The biographical material presented here is condensed from her biography by her nephew, Quentin Bell (1972). Even though the analysis is restricted to the first half of Woolf's life – childhood, adolescence, and young adulthood prior to her marriage – some items from her later life are interesting for interpretive reasons.

Virginia Stephen (Woolf) was born into a literary, upper-middle-class British home at the end of the nineteenth century. Her family was complicated by her mother's and father's previous marriages and children from those marriages. Both first spouses had died. Virginia had one surviving stepsister who was mentally "weak" (she spent most of her life in an institution) on her father's side and one stepsister and two stepbrothers on her mother's side. These step-siblings were already adolescents when Virginia and her brothers and sister were added to the family. Virginia was the second daughter and the third child of her parents, not counting the three older stepsiblings who lived at home. Virginia's parents had strong feelings about childrearing and education. They kept their children at home and educated them, themselves, until the boys went to the university.

Following the custom, daughters did not receive quite the same education as sons, since they were not being prepared for the university. Subjects such as mathematics, ancient languages, geography, and philosophy were not often taught girls, although the Stephen girls learned more than most. The Stephen girls received an extensive education in literature and a spotty but intensive one in the arts, according to most accounts. For the most part, the parents spurned tutors and taught the children themselves.

Before the age of 7, Virginia and her sister, Vanessa, had determined their career interests. Virginia was to be a writer and her sister, an artist. The family encouraged their pursuits and they did, indeed, become a writer and an artist. Virginia's earliest writings were letters and home newspapers to which most of the children in the family contributed. Family anecdotes relate that Virginia would leave her articles lying about, then hide to hear her parents' chance remarks upon "finding" the articles written by her. She seems to have doubted their praise but to have been dying to hear it from the very beginning.

Virginia's childhood had happy times in the nursery with her younger siblings and happiest times on vacation at their summer retreat where they were visited by well-known intellectuals and artists. These happy times were once interrupted when both Virginia and Vanessa had the measles and were sent away to the seaside to recover – at that time, Virginia was about 7. Then happiness came to an abrupt halt when Mrs. Stephen died during Virginia's early adolescence. The family never recovered from her death. Mr. Stephen mourned his wife dramatically, placing a great burden upon the children. He also died when Virginia was barely out of her teens. The children's stepsister, Sophie, took their mother's place in the household temporarily, but she married after a few years and then also died quite suddenly during Virginia's adolescence. Virginia's older brother died from typhoid when she was 21. By the time Virginia was a young woman, her large family was reduced to herself, Vanessa, her two stepbrothers, and one younger brother, Adrian.

After her mother died, Virginia had an extreme grief reaction, seems to have suffered hallucinations, and lost weight dangerously. During this time, she was nursed and cared for by professionals and relatives for a year or more. Somewhat similar episodes plagued her the rest of her life. She ended her life at the age of 60 by drowning, fearing the recurrence of the hallucinations, she said.

During her twenties, Virginia and her brothers and sister, bereaved of parents and guardians, set up housekeeping together and rented part of their house to other young people with scholarly or literary interests. At this time, Virginia began writing with the serious intent of publishing her novels and also began reviewing and critical writing for publication. Her reviews were accepted immediately, but her first novel would be many years in the writing.

Virginia was courted and she received four proposals, at least. Her beauty and wit were undeniable. She seems not to have taken her suitors very seriously until she met and married Leonard Woolf in what became an apparently happy marriage.

The Woolfs always lived rather quietly, partly because of Virginia's breakdowns, living either in an apartment in London or at their country house where both, but particularly Virginia, could indulge in long walks. Leonard founded Hogarth Press and both he and Virginia, as well as their many friends, worked on and for the press a good part of their lives. Leonard was frequently active in politics as well as in their literary ventures. During her late thirties, Virginia began to receive considerable acclaim for her novels and short stories and received a wider press both on the continent and in the United States.

Virginia Woolf is clearly an uncommon person; her personal themes will not be found in every man or every woman. However, much of her life is quite common. She grew up in a relatively happy family, had a disastrous adolescence, found a career compatible with her talents, married, helped run a business, visited with family and friends, gossiped, went for walks, went on vacation, kept house sporadically, loved her pets – in short, she grew up, was a young adult and then a middle-aged woman and she grew old. She did not have children, although she was a doting aunt. Her sexuality and mental health were difficult items in her life, but these may or may not have either impeded or prodded other aspects of her life. She is not typical, but she serves well for inquiry into the development of stability and change in life. She demonstrates both flexibility and the lack of it in various ways to personal disaster and personal success.

In one respect, Woolf may be an unusually good subject for the present inquiry because she was as interested as a psychologist in character and the clarity of life as meaning. Her studies of people, though literary, and her studies of herself in her diaries reveal a profound concern for discovering "the central transparency" of people and life events. Her inquiry may be an aid to our own because she presents the material we need although our methods of scrutiny diverge.

Allport (1965) was often moved to inquire whether we as psychologists could add to the analyses of character done by literary genius. His question cannot help but rise again when faced by a literary genius such as Woolf. What will one learn about character that could not be better learned by reading the novels of Woolf? In the novels and even the letters and diaries, there is much to envy and to emulate. The sure beauty and the splendor of the one clear, exact phrase is not lost upon the readers. No matter how distilled the psychologist's work, the words and life of the originator emerge. Perhaps the psychologist has nothing to add when faced only with Woolf's question. If there is one "central transparency," she is more likely to see it. However, if we inquire into the process that allows her to see her own particular centrality, we will be asking a question about becoming or developing that kind of clarity. Woolf, at least, was drawn by the sheer existence of a trait or ability or thought; we are drawn to known how the trait came to be identified.

Method of analysis: definitions

The approach used to discover how Woolf became herself and what that self might be is similar to that of Allport (1965) and Rosenberg and Jones (1972). The intent is different from theirs because they, a bit like Woolf, were concentrating on describing the static self, whereas we are concentrating on early development – childhood, adolescence, and young adulthood – presumably a less static self. The case to be used, as in previous case studies, must contain certain things. It should cover as long a span as possible, the closer to a lifetime, the better, and the material should be original. Although much can be inferred from secondary sources, analysis of cognitive level and style as well as elements of the personality would be best served by original materials. Since the requirement developmentally is for life-span material, one must settle on a person whose words are recorded, a recorded speaker or writer, and even here there are many limitations. Speeches are rarely recorded except during the middle or late years. Few novelists' writings are available during childhood or adolescence, although there are some exceptions. Diaries and letters seemed promising, since many people write letters and keep diaries continuously beginning in late childhood. Some diaries are of little interest in this pursuit of personality because they are primarily household records with little or no commentary, no recording of what one said or thought. Many diaries are fragmentary bits and pieces found in attics when much of the original history of the person is forgotten. There are a few exceptions, and Virginia Woolf is one. She was a novelist and critic; she kept a diary much of her life and her diaries were maintained by herself and her family. Letters are available from her early and mid-childhood, extending the usefulness of the written word backwards considerably. Unfortunately, some of the early material available in print is very fragmentary and difficult to date. Also, because of illness, some fairly long time periods in mid-adolescence are not recorded. However, from among published material by many writers hers is remarkably continuous.

Within this material we searched for key affect terms and then turned to a content-analysis type of approach for cognitive style. In a pragmatic sense to define the existence of an affect by the use of an affect term is obviously simple. If the writer claims to be "sad," then sadness is accepted as the affect. Similarly, if the writer describes someone else, or metaphorically, some object, as sad, then sadness is the stated affect. The assumption that the stated affect is a true statement of the writer's feeling is necessary for this approach and contains a wide range of error. For personal or social reasons one may omit certain affects or one may mask one with another to deceive oneself or others. Much of this verbal masking or distortion occurs regularly in discourse and in self-concept. A mildly depressed individual may claim to be bored, a shamed one may claim sadness, an angry one, excitement, and so on. The error may be deliberate or not, but it arises principally from the more cognitive tasks of verbalizing feelings and thinking about oneself. Because we are dealing here with what could be called "cognized" affect, we may well offend the clarity desired in affect research, where more direct bodily measures are ordinarily used such as facial or vocal cues. No one would assume that each of us has an accurate moment-to-moment picture of our affect, but the longer lasting feelings may be fairly accurately labeled. In the crudest sense, a depressed person knows she or he is depressed and looks it; similarly someone who "flies off the handle" in anger may be assumed to know it. How far this crude relationship may be relied upon is open for study. For present purposes it is assumed that there is generally an isomorphic relationship between the "cognized" affect as reported in a diary or letter and the original affect program.

There is yet another problem with "cognized" affect contained in a developmental study that must be acknowledged. It is possible that what is referred to as affect will change with social and cognitive development. Without additional information we will not be able to differentiate changes in affect states or experiences from changes in verbal and cognitive competence. For example, if a 6-year-old were to commonly use only the terms "happy" and "sad," but six years later to use a wide range of terms including "disgust," "shame," "fear," and so forth, would his potential for certain affects have changed or not? Since the current study uses only the verbal information, this question cannot be answered here in its subtle forms. However, the simple form of the question has well-documented answers. Izard (1971) and Demos (1974) have verified that children's affect vocabulary and ability to correctly identify basic affects is very similar to that of adults by late childhood at the latest.

In addition to pure affect terms, we coded a limited amount of material for cognitive style or complexity. A detailed account of the approach is described by Neimark and Stead (1981). We adapted their coding approach for analyzing "everyday" thinking occurring in textual material. The categories used are (a) *focus* – personal or impersonal, (b) *content* – everyday trivia, issues or broad concepts, and (c) *mode* of presenting content – observation, free association, concrete comparison, abstract comparison, or logical problem solving.

The purpose of coding everyday thinking for focus, content, and mode is to have a check on potential cognitive changes in affect expression. Although Neimark's system is not aimed at detecting developmental differences, but rather at cognitive style, it has some helpful features. For example, one would anticipate that young children would tend to be more personal in focus, more concerned with everyday trivia, and generally more concrete than older children or adults. Cognized affect may also then have a tendency to become less personal, more symbolic of issues, and to achieve the status of concepts or it may remain the focus of childlike cognitive approaches. That is, along with other thoughts and reports on oneself, reports on one's affect may change. Whether this "cognizing" affects the emotional state itself remains problematic.

Finally, it seemed that the interaction or even the parallel development of cognition and affect would produce coherences in the individual's story of her life similar to Tomkins's (1979) description of scripts. Tomkins argues that people experience their lives as scenes. Each scene is composed of at least one affect and an object of the affect. The suggestion contained here is that the experience of affect, even the cumulative experience, is psychologically predictable when one knows the object of the affect in addition to the affect. Very simply, if one knows that Woolf is ever happy, is her happiness associated with particular people or events or ideas? She may not be a consistently "happy person," but her happiness may be quite predictable.

There are several ways to begin a study of such scenes, and although the way chosen here may not yield the clearest sort of information for all individuals, it seemed suitable for Woolf. Woolf, especially as an adult, is not very concrete in descriptions of people or places in her diary, but she is fairly explicit about issues or themes. For this reason, we developed a list of themes to code as objects of affect in a general sense. The construction of the list will be presented in the procedural section.

Method of analysis: procedure

In beginning to study the Woolf material, a primary concern was with "reading into" her writing the perceptions of the coder. A second concern was with missing important issues. To avoid these problems, at least in part, the approach engaged multiple readers who were usually undergraduate students. To develop a list of themes, I and my students delved into common repertoires of personality themes and ended up by relying initially on those used for the Thematic Apperception Test (Murray, 1943). The next year, with a separate class, we began by developing our own themes. I vaguely defined a personality theme, assigned some secondary source readings on personality, and then asked the class to develop its own set of themes from the Woolf material and, for contrast, from several pages of statements by adolescents and college students about the "most important things that happened to me during the past year." The latter was included to make the list more inclusive of adolescent themes and to modernize the terminology. Fortunately, most of the vocabulary translated into Murray's (1943) original themes and into common affect terminology as one can see from the following list:

Affects	Themes
Joy, Distress, Anger, Shame, Contempt, Emotionality	Affiliation, Control, Ability, Sensuality, Death, Health, Beauty, Masc-femininity, Success, Insanity, Age

There are several differences in the themes and in the application of them for coding. First, we differentiated affective expressions. The list used here is similar to Tomkins's (1962) but is missing interest, fear, and surprise; it has gained "emotionality." Interest is missing because we could not reach agreement on coding; fear and surprise were too infrequent. Emotionality is included because Woolf often speaks of her feelings, her emotions and her tempers, without differentiating her feelings. "Emotionality" denotes these statements.

The themes listed often include both positive and negative aspects. For example, "affiliation" includes both statements about loving or liking someone in maintaining a relationship and statements about losing love or a relationship. "Control" includes statements about needing to have control – over feelings, for example – as well as demonstrations of control in ordering and listing and direct statements of having life under control. "Sensuality" includes references to one's body, sexual discussions, and sexual feelings. It does not include nonsexually specific statements about passionate or intense feelings. Health, death, and age are frequent Woolf references and refer to just that – one's health; death, dying, suicide, wishes to die, euthanasia; one's age – child, young, middle-aged, old, or aging, itself. In these two lists, affects and ideation themes, we have included at least two aspects of Tomkins's "scenes" in order to describe both the affective qualities of an individual's life and the ideas or objects of the affect. A further differentiation of objects will occur when letters to different people are compared. In the final analysis, affects, ideational themes, and people will be compared.

This list has served classes for two years in coding and we have had relatively few problems with it. A few items were added when we partially coded new works, including the diaries of Anaïs Nin and the autobiographies of Simone de Beauvoir and Margaret Mead. The inclusion of the additional items was useful because it highlighted the absence of what are apparently important themes for non-Virginia Woolf persons. That is, while the list presented here is moderately inclusive, one is quite likely to find it necessary to add themes when analyzing different persons. One might note that except for adolescent boys, all other persons coded have been female and the themes may reflect a "femininity" bias, if one exists. However, in retrospect, previous attempts to analyze individual personality themes omitted affective material and thus may have reflected a "masculinity" bias, if one exists.

As we progressed from listing the frequency of particular themes to examining the relationships among the traits, the importance of separating the poles of each theme became obvious, although it is often difficult. Currently, we code separately affiliation and lack of affiliation, control and lack of control. The debatable utility of this will be examined later.

In assessing the reliability of the coding schemas used, we adopted a rather stringent measure, a percentage agreement of 80% or better among undergraduates enrolled in a psychobiography class. These students went through the following training procedure. First, we defined the themes to ensure that common dictionary meanings and synonyms were known to everyone. Then, using the lists, each student attempted to code about two paragraphs from Woolf without further instruction. The ostensible purpose of this naïve coding was to match previous attempts or to demonstrate the need for new codes.

Generally, the students were told to code sentence by sentence, but not to code the same theme twice when there were overlapping themes within a paragraph. This happened frequently. Several sentences within a paragraph tend to reiterate or contribute to one or two distinct codeable themes. To identify a theme, the student must find a word or short phrase that is synonymous with the coding word. For example, "I hesitate to ride in elevators" cannot be coded as "fearful" although initially some students will wish to do interpretation of this nature. They were constrained to find the direct statement, such as "I was afraid to ride in elevators," in order to use it. Very little was left to interpretation using this format.

When each student had done his or her coding independently, the class discussed each code and item until complete agreement was reached among all members (class size varied from 11 to 23 from one semester to another). Because of the great variety in "interpretation," the quite restricted criterion just described was chosen. The procedure was repeated for about three weeks, during which each class member independently coded about 2,000 words of diary per week. When the procedure seemed to be becoming rather obvious to everyone, we switched to groups of two or three, depending on class size, and in-class discussion generally ceased while the coding proceeded as lab and homework assignments (leading to assigned paper topics). At this point, the diaries and letters were divided and each group was assigned different readings to code. Each group met together for several weeks to reach agreement on coding. After about three more weeks, individual group members began to code separately and turned their codings into the central scoring person for percentage agreement scores. If a group fell below 80% simple agreement of each theme, we would meet once more to discover the source of the problem. The usual sources were a lazy scorer who omitted themes, or a person who, for reasons apparently related to his or her own personality, omitted a particular theme (the person who never saw any statement about insanity was one, and several people consistently missed words relating to distress, sadness, or despair). Once the problem was identified, it was usually easy to correct. Twice during the remaining part of the semester, all groups were assigned the same readings, unknown to themselves. They knew it would happen at some point but were not told when. Of course, some of them could have discovered it, just as some people might have continued to score together; however, it is doubtful that there was any underhanded collaboration. This was done to ensure that groups did not become idiosyncratic in their scoring.

In fact, over the semester, each group developed an idiosyncratic "amount" of coding. For example, one group might score in paragraph one: affiliation, joy, and distress. They would then identify the same themes in paragraph two and one additional theme in paragraph three. A second group would develop a shorthand to delete "minor" themes, making a decision about how obvious or major a theme was. Nothing formal was done to correct for this as long as the rank order of themes across groups remained stable. For example, Group 1 might have found that distress was a top-ranked theme for five pages of diary entry with joy a second-ranked theme and so forth and found 16 examples of the first and 10 of the second; then Group 2 would find the same order for the themes but code 12 and 9 examples. I would suggest to the second group that they look more carefully, but did not require them to recode as long as the within-group agreement remained at 80% and the agreement across ranks between groups matched absolutely.

This approach to coding is very generous in the number of coders and generous with the amount of training and rechecking. Also, the time span is rather generous, as the coding has been done for four years by four separate seminar classes of undergraduates, both male and female, of all ages and several ethnic and economic groups. A more heterogeneous set of coders is unlikely in the psychological literature. On the other hand, the absolute amount of coding agreement is not particularly high; 80% simple agreement is not very stringent and the laxness I used in requiring rank orders to correspond across groups rather than in absolute numbers of themes is also a weakness. Overall, there should be relatively little error resulting from the coders' personal biases and a fair amount of error resulting from omission of subtle data.

Although the goal of the coding varied slightly from year to year and there is some analysis of Woolf's creative work and later life material, this chapter presents the synthesized data from only her first 30 years, arranged so as to demonstrate developmental trends established in affective and personal themes. There is the least amount of data for the period of early adolescence and nothing at all during the mid-adolescent years, then there is an increasing amount of material during Woolf's twenties. In each time period for which there are analyzed writings, I will present the synopsis of themes and affects along with some examples that will give the reader the direct experience of coding and thus broaden his or her understanding of the analysis.

Developmental issues: the analysis

In the following three sections, childhood, adolescence, and young adulthood, we will report the changes in the frequencies of particular themes. The purpose of this is to discover whether the major issues for Virginia Woolf changed dramatically during her early years, whether new issues emerge and, if so, when. In a later section, the question of how these thematic issues are related to each other will be discussed.

Childhood

Half the codes of Virginia's early writings concern her happiness and sadness (Table 17.1). Nearly every codeable entry included a reference to her feelings. Only a few sentences have some clear thematic material that all the coders could agree upon. Since the earliest excerpt comes from letters written, of course, to absent friends, it is not surprising to find reference to absent friends and demands that the friends return. But the same theme of affiliation or loss

Table 17.1. *Frequency and rank order of affect and theme material in Woolf's letters*

	Childhood (until 1897)[a]		Adolescence (1898–1902)[b]		Adulthood (1903–1909)[c]	
	Rank	(%)	Rank	(%)	Rank	(%)
Affects						
Joy	1	(30)	5	(10)	4.5	(8)
Distress	2	(20)	2.5	(13)	3	(10)
Anger	6	(7)		(3)		(2)
Shame	—			(1)		(4)
Contempt	4	(12)	6.5	(5)		(4)
Emotionality	3	(16)		(4)	7	(5)
Themes						
Affiliation	7	(4)	2.5	(13)	1	(14)
Control	8	(3)	1	(15)	2	(13)
Ability		(8)	6.5	(5)		(3)
Sensuality				(3)		(4)
Death			6	(7)	6	(7)
Health			4	(12)	4.5	(8)
Beauty				(4)		(2)
Masc-femininity						(4)
Success				(1)		(3)
Insanity				(2)		(2)
Age				(2)		(3)

[a] Based on 120 entries from Bell (1972).
[b] Based on 180 entries from Bell (1972) and Nicolson (1975).
[c] Based on 440 entries from Nicolson (1975) and Woolf (1953).

of affiliation appears in Virginia's stories for the children's newspaper. At age 6 Virginia wrote to her godfather:

My dear Godpapa have you been to the Adirondacks and have you seen lots of wild beasts and have you seen lots of birds in their nests you are a naughty man not to come here goodbye. (Nicolson, 1975, p. 2)

When Virginia was about 9, she and her siblings began the *Hyde Park Gate News*. Although there may have been some collaboration, Virginia's biographer, her nephew Quentin Bell, seems to feel that these two excerpts capture her writing:

So the boy turned him (a dog) lose [sic] to wander at his own sweet will like a *drop searching for it's* [sic] *fellow traveller* in the vast ocean. Nothing more has as yet been heard of him. (Emphasis added.) (Bell, 1972, p. 28)

And later yet in the *News*:

Miss Millicent Vaughan has honored the family of Stephen with her company. Miss Vaughan has like a dutiful sister been to Canada to see her *long absent sister* who is residing there. We hope that no pangs of jealousy crossed her mind when she saw her sister so comfortably *settled with a husband* when she herself is searching the wide world in *quest of matrimony*. But we are wandering from one point like so many *old people*. She came on Monday and is still at 22 Hyde Park Gate. (Emphasis added.) (Bell, 1972, p. 29)

These brief statements do deal with affiliative thematic content: "lose," "long absent," "searching for matrimony," "searching for a fellow traveller," "comfortably settled with a husband," "you are naughty not to come here"; but they have little direct affective content, such as "with eyes expressing worlds of joy" (Bell, 1972, p. 28), a phrase also out of Virginia's early writings. As notable as these themes are, certain ones that are apparent in other children's writings are missing; perhaps these are contained in unpublished material. There are no references to themes of independence or dependence, no descriptions of parents. Sibling jealousy is hinted at, as well as closeness among siblings in the excerpt presented here, as in a few others.

In childhood, Virginia began a lifelong stylistic habit of referring to herself and her friends as members of the animal kingdom. Virginia referred to herself as Goat, Goatus, Capra, Il Giotto, Goatus Esq, loving old goat and Billy goat. The rest of the family also called her "the Goat." She called her sister the Sheepdog, and her friends even in adulthood were the Barbary Ape, Bruin, Chipmonk, Toad, and so forth. In addition to the animal names, she used affectionate diminutives and other substitutions. In her twenties, Virginia wrote to a friend about "accounts from the zoo" in which she pointed out that animals were made "to balance human beings." However, animals had to "be taught habits." This contrast is characteristic of much of Woolf's letters and diary accounts in which polar distances are juxtaposed in single events.

The codings of the rather meager material available for the childhood period indicate that the most common themes refer to feelings of exhilaration, happiness, or gladness, followed very closely by depression, despair, and gloom; all of these are words used by Virginia. The next large category is also feelings, those that cannot be distinguished and are coded as "emotionality." The fourth- and fifth-ranked categories are also affective. Although the three themes of affiliation, control, and ability are fairly infrequent as concrete categories, they can be coded. A more subtle method of coding might indicate a higher prevalence of these themes. The major "personality" themes, however, occur only one-third as often as the major affect themes.

Thus, the major affects of Virginia as a child can be pulled out of her writings in letters and writings for the newspapers. They are principally the contrast of happiness and sadness, often following each other in quick succession. The themes of affiliation and loss, as well as their connection with control and order (in the wildness and domesticity issue, although that is not a concrete example), come out early. Concerns about her ability are expressed very early also.

Each of these issues is mirrored in family stories about Virginia, lending the analysis some degree of credibility. As a child she was known for her moods, both rages and despairs. Although she does not often mention her rages, they become apparent in later agitations but are seldom identified as rage. The family also tells about her concern over her writing, much of which was private during these years, with the exception of the *News*. She had a "fortress" in a corner chair where she wrote until her stepsister married and she got a room of her own. Writing seems to have served even in childhood as a retreat and as a strategy for maintaining control. Writing was a source of conflict, also, but apparently not directly tied into her joy and despair. The conflict was more one of pride or shame in herself and contempt for some others who also pursued her craft with less ability. For achievement or success, there is little need in the usual sense, but to be acknowledged as having ability, even genius – that was important.

A partial explanation for the ascendency of affective themes and lack of well-defined personal themes may be found in an analysis of the cognitive level of these early writings. Although there is not much material to use, Neimark's (1981) approach to coding "everyday" thinking reveals certain explanatory tendencies in the early writing. Nearly all of the early writings have a personal focus. Diligent searching revealed two excerpts with an impersonal focus, one of which is the "lost dog" episode presented earlier. Thirty others were personal. The content is "everyday trivia" and "issues." Issues include "matrimony," for example. Broader issues such as "What is life" or the "value" of feelings are not at all apparent until late adolescence. The mode of presenting content is primarily observational with a little free association and a little concrete comparison.

The categories of thinking demonstrate a concentration of everyday thinking on personal, trivial, everyday occurrences (Table 17.2). Her observations are acute, her descriptions worthy of much older people, but the facility with which she uses more abstract and impersonal modes of thinking is clearly limited. A relationship, a value, a general category of existence – these are not yet objects of thought or writing for Virginia. This may indicate that the issues she is aware of do not have much personal or motivating significance for her as yet, or it may indicate that the personality themes from their inception require a slightly more complex cognitive approach than the reporting of feelings.

Adolescence

The second set of entries begins rather arbitrarily in 1898 when Virginia was already 16. Her half-sister had died the summer before, her mother in 1895, almost three years before. Virginia continued her education and her writing. She had the free use of her father's library and his advice or opinion on literature and writers; she had tutors in Greek and Latin. The household was

Table 17.2. *Analysis of cognitive style dimensions, including focus, content, and mode of entries, in Woolf's letters*[a]

	Frequency of occurrence	
	Childhood (until 1897)	Late Adolescence (1898–1902)
Focus		
Personal	30	15
Impersonal	2	17
Content		
Everyday trivia	12	10
Issues	15	13
Broad concepts	0	8
Unclassifiable	5	1
Mode		
Observation	18	6
Free association	7	12
Concrete comparison	2	6
Abstract-logical	0	3
Unclassifiable	5	5

[a] Based on 30 letters in Nicolson (1975).

still active with six children. Her two older stepbrothers still lived at home and took an interest in society. Thoby, the older brother, began to introduce his Cambridge friends. Letters were written to Thoby at school, to the stepbrothers when they are away, and to her cousins, principally Emma Vaughan. There are enough letters available to present both a summary frequency table (Table 17.1) and a table (Table 17.3) comparing themes in letters written to men (her brothers) and women (her cousins).

Several prominent changes are clear in comparing the material from adolescence and childhood, although some care must be taken in interpretation because the sheer amount of material has increased and the purposes of the material are more varied. There is no more *News*, but there are many more letters and many diary entries. As indicated previously, the content changes in a way that suggests a much greater facility to consider issues and concepts, including introspective issues. She has conclusions and concepts even in her descriptive passages:

This is one observation that I have made from my observation of many sunsets – that no shape of cloud has one line that is the least sharp or hard . . . Everything is done by different shades and degrees of light – melting and mixing infinitely – Well may an Artist despair! (Bell, 1972, p. 65)

This passage demonstrates not only the change in cognitive grasp but also the somewhat indiscriminate prevalence of distress or despair. Even an artist faced

Table 17.3. *Frequency and rank order of affect and theme material in Woolf's letters to men or women during late adolescence (1898–1902)*[a]

	Men		Women	
	Rank	(%)	Rank	(%)
Affects				
Joy	3	(12)	3	(13)
Distress	6.5	(7)	2	(14)
Anger				
Shame				
Contempt			7.5	(7)
Emotionality	6.5	(7)		
Themes				
Affiliation	7	(6)	1	(22)
Control	1	(25)	4	(11)
Ability				
Sensuality			6	(8)
Death	4	(11)		
Health	2	(15)	5	(10)
Beauty			7.5	(7)
Masc-femininity				
Success				
Insanity				
Age				
Dependence	5	(9)		

[a] Based on 140 entries from Nicolson (1975).
Note: Top-ranked themes are common in all letters, but lesser ranked themes distinguish the recipients.

with a cloud might "despair." Why this "despair" is not quite clear; supposedly, the difficulty of shading rather than using straight lines brings about despair.

A reexamination of Table 17.1 shows that distress and the issues of affiliation and control, the top-ranked themes, are quite frequent in the adolescent period. Joy is not far behind and two major thematic-ideational concerns, health and death, follow closely. The three areas of thematic concern in childhood – affiliation, control, and ability – are still most important. The dominance of affective material has declined, although joy and distress are still high-ranked themes. "Joy" is now less prominent than distress and will remain dampened. Virginia's memories of a happier childhood are reflected in her writings from each period.

The discussions of health and death on first reflection may seem to be references to events in her family. Although a few are references to current problems, many are references to distant problems or fantasies or are metaphors. Virginia's family remarked that she saw all the accidents at this time. She certainly saw or wrote about a fair number. For example, she reports on the health of a dog when they go visiting:

Mrs. Hills has a horrible pet dog, which is always getting *ill* – it was *sick* all over the carpet. (Emphasis added.) (Nicolson, 1975, p. 10)

Likewise, a neighbor's dog died:

A cab slowly passed over its middle: we were watching. (Nicolson, 1975, p. 12)

Here is another report:

Pat has been almost *killed* on his bicycle by a wagon, Maive has *sprained* her thumb, Dorothy is almost *mad* with earache. (Emphasis added.) (Nicolson, 1975, p. 13)

And in a more fantastic vein:

Poor Sophie locks her door carefully and vows that she will *die* on top of the silver chest. (Emphasis added.) (Nicolson, 1975, p. 16)

The usage of these terms is not restricted to recent deaths and illnesses in the family but encompasses broad reaches of Virginia's experiences.

The primary affiliative themes include mention of both affiliation and loss of affiliation. Just as with issues of health and death, affiliative issues are sometimes concrete, sometimes abstract, but always pervasive. Mentions of other people's friendships and marriages and feelings of loneliness for the person being addressed or some other family member are most common. For example, on feeling lonely, she writes:

Heavens! What a long letter this is. But it is Sunday morning and *I am sitting solitary in my room with no dear sheep dog* [this a pet name for her sister, Vanessa] to talk to, and I can't help writing for the life of me, and you must be my receptacle. (Emphasis added.) (Nicolson, 1975, p. 34)

In another example, she chides her friend to write to her:

Marny insinuates that I have planted the green fiend in your heart which makes me exceedingly *glad*. I wish though that the green fiend or any other fiend would prompt you to write to me. I have had to make all the advances in this *friendship*, which is quite against my morals. (Emphasis added.) (Nicolson, 1975, p. 33)

Virginia appears to be a most affectionate friend, teasing, asking frequently for love and company, regretting the loss of friends when their visits are over. Friendship themes are probably common to most people and it should not come as a surprise that Virginia is no exception. The constant juxtaposition of feeling friendly and feeling lonely is probably less common. In fact, it is not a constant factor in Virginia's letters but is dominant in her letters to women. It is the greatest category of themes in her letters to women, but it appears very seldom in her letters to her brothers (Table 17.3). They do not receive all the news about friendships and marriages, nor do they hear much about Virginia's loneliness or her desire for them to write and return. The letters to her brothers are more businesslike entirely, full of directions and reports on her reading or studies. Though still affectionate, these letters are restrained and have less teasing affection. Writing to her brother, Thoby, she says, "We are *left to ourselves* this afternoon, and as some relief to my *feelings*, I will write to your highness" (Nicolson, 1975, p. 9). If one contrasts that with the closing cited earlier, a bit of the difference emerges. There is no reference to pet names, for example, no requests to write back immediately, nor does she scold men for not writing or not responding in any way. In fact, on at least one occasion, she relayed the news that her brother was not to come when someone was ill because he was not needed.

The second major theme concerns control or order and the lack of it. This aspect is revealed in many ways. Virginia had the habit of listing events or people, thus "putting them in order." The order, such as it is, usually has no sequential sense; it is a quick listing. On other occasions, Virginia mentions directly that things are out of control, that she has lost the sense of order in herself or in the household. For example, she writes to her stepbrother:

I suppose Nessa told you about our journey. It was successful on the whole and (1) my bicycle which was left behind arrived yesterday. (2) Father has begun work again; (3) and is making poor old Thobs cram all the morning. (4) Adrian had Macpherter here this morning and (5) Nessa and I went to High Street. (6) We met Kitty which was nice: she was just rushing off to stay with Margaret and Gunby. (Numbers are mine.) (Nicolson, 1975, p. 15)

It is more difficult to find these straightforward listed accounts in letters to women because she interrupts herself with descriptions, commentary, and references to the recipient of the letter. To her cousin Emma (nicknamed "Toad" by Virginia), she writes and begins to list:

Go on the Punt – feed the seagull – visit the stables – examine the photographs . . . I fear that Susan Lushington may in some way interrupt our afternoon, but she . . . can play the spinet to perfection. *Some* other people – toads I should say – nasty slimy crawling things – *think* they can play – ahem! (Woolf's italics.) (Nicolson, 1975, p. 15)

And all this in a letter "meant only to be short and businesslike."

The other differences between letters written to men and to women during adolescence further emphasize the empathy that Virginia felt with her female cousins. She tells them more about her loneliness and distress. To her brothers, she writes more vaguely about intense feelings. To her cousins, she writes about somewhat sensuous items – the time Vanessa's skirt fell off, the state of her own underclothes, how she felt when soaking wet, the appearance of her legs, a woman's body looking as if it were "doing business with infants," and so on. To her brothers, she writes more concretely about who is well and ill and dead.

The differences between letters to men and women may be considered to be naturally occurring situations that produce differences in the personal attributes of the individual. In fact, there are some situational differences. There is a different emphasis, at least in terms of the frequency of themes; the rank order is different. There are also differences in the minor themes used in each situation;

hence, the differences in sensuality, death, and beauty. Overall, the similarities remain striking. The domain of affects and the main personal themes do not change even though their order of frequent use changes. The repertoire of responses is changed just a little, but the dominant characteristics are not deleted. (The exception seems to be "ability," but during this time period references to ability are low in the letters and contained principally in diaries.)

In summarizing the published pieces that remain of Virginia's adolescent writings, one first notices that there is continuity in the main affective components of exhilaration and despair, which still are there but not as strongly as in her childhood writings. The relationship between the wild beast and the bird in its nest or common domesticity and creative wildness, control and lack of control, is still apparent but not dominant. The affiliative themes – need for affiliation and the experience of loneliness – are the dominant ones. There is only the barest hint of adolescent issues such as identity, life, success, goals (see Blos, 1979; Erikson, 1968). The concern is with maintaining some kind of balance between great opposites in her feelings. There is also a prominent concern with health and death, issues that are not under her control but which she attempts to control in writing by making them slight or humorous, a part of the day's report, in some cases, the postscript of the letter.

Additionally, there is an obvious sensitivity to the nature of the reader; the letters vary in style and content between those written to her brothers and those written to her women friends. Those written to her friends seem more like her later writing, more full of free association, more metaphoric, more prone to the teasing, scolding, and intimacies that characterize her adult letters. Practice in making friends and getting close to people seems to have occurred with women in adolescence.

One has a view at this point, as Virginia enters her twenties, of a person who experiences great swings in her moods and is struggling to keep them under control as well as to grasp the uncontrollable in her life. She wants to be lovable and to be the center of attraction for a small circle of friends, and she is willing to work at these relationships, willing enough to write long, amusing, affectionate letters that draw the interests of the other person into the letter. All feeling states are known and mentioned: anger – at illness or shortness with her father; fear, again of illness or other invasions such as burglars, but principally, she is sad and lonely or she is excited and happy and not lonely. When she is not lonely, it is not just because there are people around. They have to be people that she can feel close to and appreciate, such as her sister, Vanessa. Most people arouse her humorous contempt and lead her to feel more alone; that is, she feels that most people do not like her and, as she admitted later in describing herself, she felt awkward, lacking in beauty, and the proper behavior. So she built a shield of her humor, but it worked to maintain her loneliness as well as to increase the specialness of the people she felt belonged on her side of the barriers.

Young adulthood

Here we will finish the present illustration of the frequency of themes suggesting stability and change in personality and affect. By the end of her twenties, Virginia was married and had written her first novel as well as many short published reviews. She was launched, but not acclaimed. In most senses, she was an adult, had her own career and household and friends. What would be left by this time of the child and adolescent personality? How much differentiation has occurred? Is there evidence of an increasingly single or central identity forming or evidence of increasing differentiation of affects and themes or something quite different?

For this analysis, we turn once more to Table 17.1 to note any changes in the frequencies of different affect or ideational themes – any developmental trends. To continue the examination of naturally occurring situations, as an object of affect, the category of persons to whom letters are written is expanded in Table 17.4 from men (brothers) and women (cousins), as was the case in late adolescence, to Vanessa (her sister), Clive (her brother-in-law), and men (includes friends such as Lytton Strachey and Leonard Woolf) and women (includes cousins and more distant relatives). Virginia's world is expanding, but does the range of common categories for experience also expand? Different findings might emerge from these analyses. For example, if her writings were always somewhat contemptuous, distant, and well ordered when they were directed toward journal reviews but were warm and affiliative and free associative in personal letters and completely introspective when writing in a diary, then one could describe her various adult roles and note situational inconsistency. On the other hand, if there is less change and increasing unity of affect and trait emerging in ideals and use of symbols across the board, one would have to argue for continuity of self in terms of integration even if the cognitive mode or unity of presentation and self-concept were to change with age. If ideational themes vary but affective ones do not, still another approach to interpretation would be opened.

The first part of the analysis in both Tables 17.1 and 17.4 is devoted to the affects. Here, the earlier appearance of Virginia is continued, not changed according to the frequency of themes. However, the alternation and intensity of feelings becomes more than mere report of moods or emotional experiences. Virginia comes to consider her feelings a part of her character, a somewhat grandiose part, but completely essential. In writing about herself to Leonard Woolf when they are seriously considering marriage, she reported, "I am fearfully unstable. I pass from hot to cold in an instant, without any reason" (Nicolson, 1975, p. 496). This is more than a description, it is also an ideal: "We both of us want a marriage that is a tremendous living thing, always alive, always hot" (Nicolson, 1975, p. 497). In writing to a friend about

Table 17.4. *Frequency and rank order of affect and theme material in Woolf's young adult letters (1903–1909)*[a]

	Sister		Brother-in-law		Women		Men	
	Rank	(%)	Rank	(%)	Rank	(%)	Rank	(%)
Affects								
Joy	6	(7)	3	(9)	6	(7)		(7)
Distress	1	(15)	4.5	(8)	4	(8)		
Anger		(3)						(4)
Shame		(4)		(3)				(5)
Contempt		(5)		(5)		(4)		
Emotionality		(4)				(6)		(7)
Themes								
Affiliation	3	(10)	1	(14)	1	(16)		(7)
Control	5	(8)	2	(12)	2	(13)	1	(23)
Ability		(4)		(2)		(3)		(4)
Sensuality		(2)	4.5	(8)		(4)		(6)
Death	3	(10)			4	(8)		
Health	3	(10)		(5)	4	(8)		(5)
Beauty		(4)				(2)		(4)
Masc-femininity		(2)	6	(6)		(5)		(4)
Success		(2)		(3)		(3)		(4)
Insanity	7	(6)						
Age		(3)				(6)		
Dependence						(3)		(4)

Note: There is only small variation in material according to the recipient, demonstrating considerable stability across person situations.
[a] Based on Nicolson (1975): sister, 114 entries; brother-in-law, 93 entries; women, 176 entries; men, 57 entries.

marriage and about Woolf, she makes the same point, indicating that it is a central consideration in marrying:

I only ask for someone to make me vehement, and then I'll marry him . . . I feel oddly vehement and very exacting and difficult to live with and so very intemperate and changeable. (Nicolson, 1975, p. 492)

For warm pleasures and manners and commonplace achievement, life's less "hot" events, Virginia has little but contempt and occasional wistfulness when she sees the side of the commonplace that is peaceful, but that is a rare event.

Feelings of all sorts in all the writings are closely related to remarks about separation, loneliness, and demands for attention. This continues an emphasis on affiliation that increased in frequency from childhood to adolescence and is now top-ranked in nearly all situations (the low rank for the "men" category is likely due to too few entries). She only wants to be with people who increase her feelings and intensity of feelings. She does not treat lightly the family and friends with whom she corresponds but alternately despairs of them or their attention to her and raves about her love. Writing to a long-time friend from her adolescent days, part mother, part companion, she says:

I wish sometimes the unpremeditated desire to write to me would come over you. Every word I must earn before I have. And yet you are a good, generous, *woman* too; and would give me pounds of blood if I asked it. Where are you, how are you, and *do you love me* – or have you found some choicer specimen somewhere! O no – I won't believe it. (Emphasis added.) (Nicolson, 1975, p. 311)

A generally separate issue is her ability and genius in writing – also a theme of concern continued from adolescence, which is low ranked but persistent. Since she has been working on a novel during her twenties, this is a rather natural topic for her correspondence. The ability to write is something about which she has enormous qualms. What she writes has to measure up to genius standards and so does everyone else's writings, but she is quite self-conscious about these demands and how they define her. When writing in guest houses or inns, she covers her work so that others will not know she is doing it. She claims to be writing letters to lady cousins, not writing reviews of a novel. She makes fun of her writing and denies that her letters require work or that one should work on them. Yet she comments on the style and lack of it even in her letters as well as in public writing and gets upset when her letters are passed around and critiqued, sometimes demanding to have them back. The person she makes her chief confidante during her late twenties in critiques of her novel is her brother-in-law, Clive. For the most part, she does not seem to hold his writing in very high regard, nor does she seem to take his comments much to heart. Yet she is very appreciative of the attention he gives to her writing, and through it, to her. Although analysis of the affects inspired by her writing most frequently show a connection to shame and contempt (the auxiliary affects according to Tomkins, 1962), rather than the prominent joy and distress that accompany affiliative themes, the following excerpt also ties her thoughts to the ever-present distress (melancholy):

I dreamt last night that I was showing father the manuscript of my novel; and *he snorted*, and dropped it on to a table, and I was very *melancholy*, and read it this morning, and thought it bad. You don't realize the depth of *modesty* in to which I fall. (Emphasis added.) (Nicolson, 1975, p. 325)

Issues of order and control also remain very frequent as was previously seen in adolescence; furthermore, the ranking is high across all "situations." Just as the other themes, affiliative and ability themes seem to have become not only prevalent but to have taken on grandiose character themselves, as has control. In one letter she writes about control over not only herself but the world:

With regard to *happiness* – what an interesting topic that is! Walking about here with Jean for a companion, I feel a great *mastery* over the world. (Emphasis added.) (Nicolson, 1975, p. 434)

Once again, a few themes appear to be raised in letters to particular people or types of people. The previously strong themes of death and health are still very frequent in letters to women friends and her sister, but friends who are new since adolescence, including her brother-in-law and male friends, hear less about health and death. This is so even though a good many of her letters concern her father's health as he died from cancer and then her brother Thoby's health and final illness. Discussions of maleness and femaleness, including the ability of the female mind or the feminine sensibility, are largely contained in letters to her brother-in-law. Finally, discussion of the bouts of "insanity" are scattered throughout her letters but principally in letters to Vanessa.

During her twenties, Virginia had several episodes of "insanity" during which she was put in mental nursing homes and had rest cures. Judging from the diagnosis of the time as well as from her letters, she had some sort of depressive or manic-depressive episodes. She would lose the ability to sleep, develop severe headaches, and then apparently lose control of her thoughts and do things that were considered insane for her day, such as walking barefoot, and insane for our days as well, such as jumping through a window. Generally, the manic phase occurred after a traumatic event, such as a death in the family (four in her immediate family before she was 24), and then also after her own marriage. Following each family event, including death, the family members would take a voyage or vacation during which or shortly after which Virginia would develop these "flight of mind" symptoms. Of course, they were of great concern to Virginia and to her family. Any depression or headaches brought concerned attention from her sister, friends, brothers, and family physician. Virginia herself had unresolved conflicting statements to make about her "insanity," as she herself called it. Writing to a friend after a short rest cure, she was quite offhand about it.

I've been ill, but I'm practically all right again now. It was a touch of my usual disease, in the head, you know. I spent a week in bed, but now that's all over, except for miraculous dreams at night. (Nicolson, 1975, p. 489)

Her mention of the "miraculous dreams" gives the impression that Virginia romanticized her insanity and often she did. In writing about another "lunatic" at the rest home where she stayed for several weeks, she wrote:

One of Miss Thomas's most excitable *lunatics*, the one who leapt when she saw me, has been almost *dying*, but is now better again. Miss Thomas says that these *excitements* are the wine of life. This bears out my theory, based on Aunt Fisher, and all the other *sepulchral* women, that what people like is *feeling*, it doesn't matter what. (Emphasis added.) (Nicolson, 1975, p. 441)

When she was nearer "recovery," she put a slightly different emphasis upon her illness. She was writing to Vanessa about the nursing home and wondering when she would be leaving and complaining about the staff, in particular, about their religious canting. She ends one paragraph on their religious peculiarities with "The religious mind is quite amazing" and begins another without preamble:

However, what I mean is that I shall soon have to jump out of a window. The *ugliness* of the house is almost inexplicable, having white, and mottled green and red. Then there is all the eating and drinking and being shut up in the dark. My God. What a mercy to be done with it. (Emphasis added.) (Nicolson, 1975, p. 431)

Any reader who has doubts whether Virginia in fact had manic "flights of the mind" has only to read the following excerpt from a letter to a woman friend:

At the same time poor Aunt Minna, who has been brooding constantly over her disappointment with Marny in the summer, set out for Fickmansworth, to find the Bluebell Walk. She got to Richmond and asked "have you any bluebottles? Is this the Star and Barter? Then I must be at Greenwich after all." But why did naughty Margaret Vaughan tell me B stood for bug? Well, well: I could run on, you could call it running, when every sentence draws a tear. So poor Will has followed John Bailey's example after all. With the exception of the bedroom poker, I hope. We call it poker, though it has another name. It's worse, though when the Quakers run amok. Happily though the earth spins round me, and it is rumored in Hoxton that Marny had a hand in the last butchers bill at the hospital . . . I keep calm and virtuous here by the sea shore. (Nicolson, 1975, p. 359)

Generally, in her writings Virginia's thoughts about insanity are linked to issues of control and lack of control; frequently, they are linked to dying and depression. In general, the issue is not a happy one. Although Virginia pokes fun at herself and others who express concern about her and she makes light of her cures, every now and then a note of despair creeps into the description. It is most notable when she speaks of others who are insane or lunatics – she views them as hopeless. The notion that one might really cure her seems to have never crossed her mind. She was constructing a theory about her bouts of depression and lunacy during her twenties that would be concretized in later years. She would write later that she feared a real cure would take away her genius. Yet in the end, the depressing aspects of her condition led her to drown herself, so it was not true that she was able to handle her feelings through such a theory. Frequently, she would turn from justifying the excitement and intensity of her insanity to writing of the birds who spoke to her or the dark and hairy devils who usurped her and were entirely unbearable.

Let us return to the issues addressed with reference to the frequency tables and pick up the pieces of evidence from childhood and adolescence before moving to a new level of analysis. Certain things seem abundantly clear from the analysis. First, it is evident that the affective traits of the individual in this case have been quite dominant and have characterized her from childhood throughout young adulthood. Virginia's intense exhilaration and despair of childhood were maintained in adolescence and were absolutely characteristic of her in adulthood not only as a descriptor but as a self-identified value. On the other hand, there are some changes with age in the frequency of certain terms, particularly personal themes.

During late adolescence, personal themes used both concretely and metaphorically across diverse situations are easily identified. In young adulthood, there is maintenance of adolescent themes and an increasing number of identifiable themes. There is also an increase in self-generated theories or values built around the themes. Not only are feelings valued; she writes thoughtfully also about the types of relationships she values, the necessity of mastery, order, and control. She even constructs self-theories about her "insane" episodes, about feminine traits and the effect of age on personality.

In adulthood, one sees the emergence of "broad problems" or "major conceptual issues," all of which are centered about, and explanations for, her previously identified traits. Similarly to psychologists, her "theories" of personality are constructed from her own experiences but are then generalized as rules and values (see Stolorow & Atwood, 1978). Even broader cognitive schema are anticipated in her more formal or "scholarly" writings – the newspaper reviews of books and literary events that are not included in this analysis. Presumably, they would reveal an even greater use of impersonal focus and more theoretical contexts. However, the point here was to demonstrate a change in the type of thinking about herself and her relationships that could be demonstrated even in writings of letters and diaries, a more informal everyday context.

What this analysis tends to show is that the maturing individual comes to think about the everyday interactions and objects more abstractly and more elaborately. There is a gradual change throughout childhood, adolescence, and young adulthood (and presumably later in adulthood as well). The result of this change is that conceptions of the self and relationships become more abstract and more elaborated; Tomkins's "scenes" are enunciated (Carlson, 1982).

Integrative analysis and hypotheses

In this section four hypotheses that delineate the development of affective and cognitive systems will be presented. These hypotheses are derived from the Woolf data already presented and lead to general rules that may be tested with additional research in the future.

1. *All thematic content that seems to have developed in childhood remains salient in adolescence and young adulthood.* This hypothesis is extrapolated directly from the Woolf data presentation. It is quite clear that the late childhood themes, both the affective and ideational, remain prominent in Woolf's young adulthood. Presumably, the origins of these themes are contained in undocumented childhood events or may even be so socially common as to be nearly universal.

The earliest detectable themes include all the affective experiences. In Woolf's case, joy-distress-affiliation combinations loom large in childhood and are predictive of both the core adult thematic content and the bipolar character of later themes. Even in childhood, and clearly in adulthood, neither joy nor distress had unidirectional relationships with other themes. If an event, idea, or person was important or "hot" in Woolf's terms, it usually had strong positive and negative affective ties.

The possibility that the major ideational themes may be relatively universal is heightened by the analogy between Woolf's primary ideational themes of affiliation, control, and ability to McClelland's three primary motives (1951) or to elements of developmental personality theories. For example, Erikson's (1968) "basic trust" may be analogous to affiliative ideation, "industry" to ability ideation, and "autonomy" to control ideation. These analogies do suggest a certain universality to the core ideational themes; however, the role of affect in unifying, polarizing, or splintering the ideational themes is unexplored as yet in developmental theories.

The potential impact of demonstrating the nature of continuity in character or personality development through analyses such as that presented here is substantial. Although philosophers and novelists as well as psychologists have logically assumed a developmental continuity, its existence in affective content and certain ideational themes has been obscure.

2. *New adolescent and adult ideational themes may arise and are tied to recurring events in later life.* In Woolf's case these themes include ideas related to health, death, femininity, insanity, and sensuality. These themes were not visible in late childhood but become the object of consciousness in adolescence or adulthood. The development of these ideational themes cannot be traced to any single event, since they gradually increase in frequency, and the number of events that might influence each theme also continues to rise. There is not a single death, nor a single bout of insanity, nor a single sensuous incident that could be said to be *the* setting event since there are many deaths, many bouts of insanity, many opportunities to deal with sensuous or sexual incidents and all were salient. Further, when an ideational theme becomes very frequent it begins to occur solely as an idea, not just as a description of an event. As the analysis demonstrated, frequently occurring themes, such as death, appear as descriptions of situations, as when the dog was run over, as metaphors, as when the maid claimed she would die on the silver chest, and finally as an abstract concept, as when Woolf discusses euthanasia or suicide as an ethical event. For Woolf, at least, a prominent theme is recurrent as an organizer of many events or thoughts.

3. *Affects have multiple functions in personality formation.* Not only does affect color ideas and experiences; it may become an idea and it may become the goal of experience. In Woolf's case, affect provides a directional or motivational quality to many experiences, functioning to unite different ideational content and helping to prevent a proliferation of subselves. In a different context, Bower (1980) has made a similar proposal about the use of affect as

a category in recalling any type of material. For Woolf, affect themes become abstract ideational themes as well as conjuncts of events or ideas. Woolf came to view her self as an emotional self, and she came to value that aspect of her self-concept, as when writing about the "vehemence" necessary for her marriage. Thus, the result of her reifying affect is that she begins to consciously organize her life situations, as well as her thoughts, so as to experience certain kinds of feelings. Very likely there are unconscious processes at work, but the conscious ones alone provide enough material to support the point.

Generally, it is not clear that everyone will reify affect; however, it is likely that at some level affect will unify and partially organize experience. This hypothesis is quite different from most conceptions of affects as disorganizers, as the opposite of a cognition system with a process and a logic. What is now proposed is that affect experience is an organizer in a different way. In providing for a self-generated sense of continuity, one uses affect to identify salient events and to classify them; also, particular affect experiences may become sought after for their own qualities. Because of their role in providing self-continuity, affects may lose apparent positive or negative qualities. A common example is provided by so-called thrill seekers, people who desire intensely exciting or frightening experiences almost regardless of the particulars of the thrilling situation. A less common example is provided by Woolf, who desires to experience life intensely and even includes intense depression as a natural aspect of her desire, though it produces insurmountable conflict.

Although there is little evidence, one should consider another possibility, namely, that certain cognitive styles are developed from or reflective of affects. As a simple example, there is an analogy between Woolf's emotional shifts from despair to exhilaration and her style of thinking in opposites. For Woolf to think of a reunion is to think of separation, to imagine desire is to contemplate revulsion, to sorrow at death is to rejoice in the well-completed life and so on. More generally, particular affective temperaments or experiences may be related to proclivities for impulsive or reflective cognitive styles. This approach to the interaction of cognition and affect is too speculative for present evidence, but it may be worthwhile to gather information on this topic.

4. *Ideational and affect themes are organized so that (a) certain affects are predictive of certain ideational themes and (b) there are very few frequently recurring affect-ideation combinations defining an individual.* This hypothesis is similar to Tomkins's (1979) statement that personality scenes contain affect and an object for the affect and that scripts are reiterations of certain salient scenes.

Although this last hypothesis cannot be "tested" in any statistical sense with the available information, it does require a stricter examination of the relationships between affect themes and ideational themes than has been provided. To make such an examination, the previously coded material was cross-coded to examine the co-occurrence of events. Each occurrence of a codeable

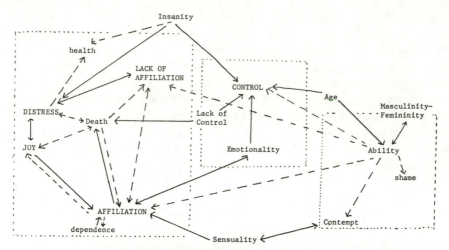

Figure 17.1. A map of co-occurring themes, showing three overlapping thematic spaces: affiliation, control, and ability with corresponding affective connections of joy/distress, emotionality, and shame and contempt.

Key: CAPITALIZED: 44-70 entries; Capitalized 16-28 entries: not capitalized: 10–14 entries; x → y: y follows x 20%–63% of all entries for x; x ----→ y: y follows x 8%–19% of all entries for x.

theme or trait was cross-coded with the theme following it. There was one restriction: Both had to occur within the same paragraph. A paragraph shift was treated as a legitimate shift in thought. For example:

Also I had a compliment on my *beauty*, this was a little dashed by hearing that Gumbo had felt a distinct *emotion* of *love* upon seeing Nessa. (Emphasis added.) (Nicolson, 1975, p. 450)

Here one codes *emotion* as following *beauty* and *affiliation* (love) as following *emotionality*. One will immediately wish to code all three as conjunctive, but the problems posed by this are too troublesome for the level of analysis proposed. The method used assumes a directionality to the thoughts; that is, it does not presuppose that *love* is likely to precede *emotion* as often as *emotion* will precede *love*. This is the same as saying – in multivariate analysis terms – that we do not assume that it is the same "distance" from *emotion* to *love* as it is from *love* to *emotion*. Generally, one must presuppose equal "distance" for multivariate analyses. Naturally, one decreases the total amount of codeable material to be used because it sometimes happens that there is one theme in a paragraph; it would be eliminated from this analysis. The only category markedly affected by this strategy was the "control" category, of which 13% is missing. For all other categories, less than 6% is lost. One could say that "control" predicts itself quite often.

Figure 17.1 is a spatial representation of the relationships among categories that have been derived in this way. The arrows indicate the simple percentage of time that one category follows another. For example, there are 52 "distress" codes and 47 "joy" codes in this analysis. Of the "distress" codes, 12 follow "joy," and of the "joy" codes, 11 follow "distress." In this one case, the distance between themes is reciprocal – one is just as likely to find "joy" following "distress" as to find "distress" following "joy," about one of four times in each case. On the other hand, there are 53 "control" codes and only 17 "insanity" codes. "Control" follows 24% (4) of the "insanity" codes, but "insanity" follows "control" only once in the material coded, so it is not the same "distance" each direction.

The figure demonstrates, as predicted, that each of the major themes of affiliation, control, and ability has a closely allied affective component. Affiliative themes are closely tied to joy and distress. Joy and lack of affiliation are not paired, but every other pairing occurs. Thoughts of joy are paired with thoughts of distress and affiliation, affiliation with joy, distress, and lack of affiliation, and so forth. Control themes are tied to emotionality and also to joy, but the ties are not reciprocal. Ability themes are linked to shame, contempt, and emotionality. There is overlap among affective components but each also has a separable thematic link. Minor themes can be closely related to many themes or restricted to one. Dependence and masculinity–femininity have single ties. Insanity, death, age, and sensuality have multiple ties that cut across major themes.

If one were to speak of Woolf as having three or so factors or trait clusters to her personality, one would be partially correct but would miss an essential characteristic; there are overlapping configurations. Although clusters such as affiliation-joy-distress do form, a major cluster such as this is also tied, usually through affects, to every other major cluster. It seems true, at least in Woolf's case, that affects and ideational themes do cluster and that a very few overlapping clusters account for almost all the codeable material. Minor or infrequently occurring clusters are also clearly defined. "Shame," for example, frequently follows thoughts about ability (usually grandiose thoughts). "Shame" and ability are not, however, central themes that receive consideration across situations; they are important minor issues. On the other hand, "emotionality" is tied to every major thematic area and receives attention as a conceptual issue, as well. "Joy" and "distress" form a strong category, nearly strong enough to be a single category. They also receive consideration as conceptual issues. So there is some additional evidence for the hypothesized dual functioning of affective experience as both ideational and expressive.

The developmental aspects of the "scene" clustering remain problematic because there is not sufficient information to present a separate analysis. However, a few comments may give helpful direction to future searches. An examination of the frequency tables may persuade the reader that the core of the themes is essentially the same throughout. The earliest detectable themes are the core themes; all the affective experiences are available in all the material. The joy-distress-affiliative combinations may have been connected to more or to other themes. The mix of joy and distress, with neither in clear ascendency and with neither having unidirectional relationships with other traits, is clearly characteristic of Woolf throughout this whole period.

The growth of satellite themes is apparent as a developmental trend, but these are not split off into separate "scripts" or "roles," nor do they draw randomly from all thematic characteristics. Each satellite theme, such as sensuality or age or insanity, ties into two thematic areas and has a principal affective content. "Death" may have been a similar satellite at one time but clearly has achieved a central position in Woolf's young adult life, having logically contradictory connections to control, lack of control, joy, distress, affiliation, and lack of affiliation. It is what Tomkins would probably call a problematic script in that it is polarized. This script is so polarized that one might prefer to call it fractionated. To relate such contradictory thematic content biographically, one has only to remember Woolf's suicide attempts and her desire to have everything in life and to live intensely. Her life behavior in relation to death is equally contradictory.

Summary

The analysis of the development of personality using affective themes, larger personality themes, and situational/trait themes from a single case has revealed previously unsuspected relationships among these elements. In going from the single case to the general case, several points developed from the Woolf material should be considered: (1) affective material is prominent and easily retrieved from childhood writings, much more so than ideational themes, (2) childhood affective material remains prominent in adult material, and (3) affect themes find a position in adult personal descriptions of self and become part of the metatheory of self.

The data from the Woolf case indicate that coherent personal ideational themes, ideas about personality and values attached to one's own themes, do not clearly exist in childhood writings. The central personal characteristics that give coherence to character in childhood seem to be primarily affective. Themes are elaborated both cognitively and experientially, and the first notable effect of this elaboration is seen in Woolf during late adolescence, although she does not have an obvious personality "theory" for herself until her twenties, a theory of self akin to Erikson's (1968) notion of identity.

The hypothesis that childhood affective themes are the primary organizers of early personal experience and that they are likely to remain prominent in adult personality organization is a novel hypothesis open to a variety of interpretations. We are unable to select a best interpretation because our ability to generate specific examples is seriously hampered by a general neglect of developmental studies of the self. The complexity of affective material is too great to yield to simple analysis based on simple data; the meaning of children's affect statements remains obscure. Continued observations lead to ever more complex rules. For example, one might predict, based on the Woolf material, that the early and persistent experience of extreme distress may lead to adult episodes of acute depression. On the other hand, it may lead to avoidance of depression or to competence in handling depression. Additional case information is needed to make such pragmatic predictions.

To make predictions about adult personality from childhood traits would be possible in the general sense primarily if one had rules for predicting from affective traits. For example, the affective polarity in Woolf's childhood made her vulnerable to thematic polarities; the high frequency of distress even before traumatic losses occurred in her family probably contributed to her vulnerability to depression. The continued loss and the juxtaposition of distress and joy in traumatic situations no doubt contributed to her losing control of her already polarized affects. The extent to which such statements can be true is the degree to which childhood or adolescent themes, both those that are affective and ideational, can be predictive of later vulnerability to traumatic situations in adulthood and of resistance to change in therapies. The resistance of depressives such as Woolf to therapy is legendary. One clear reason illustrated here for this resistance is that the distress is central to the personality, clarifies the meaning of various life situations, provides continuity, and, at least in Woolf's case, is as closely tied to life's pleasures as to its despair. Working within Woolf's own personality themes, one could only hope to make her less vulnerable by strengthening bonds between other affects and life themes. Taking the distress out of her life space would probably leave too large a gap in her experiences.

Thus this schematic method of discovering the continuity of affect and ideational themes and the emergence of themes and the relationships among them can be used developmentally to construct theories that describe the impact of affective experience on development and the interaction of cognition and affect in defining the self.

References

Allport, G. W. *Letters from Jenny*. New York: Harcourt, Brace and World, 1965.

Bell, Q. *Virginia Woolf: A biography*. New York: Harcourt, Brace, Jovanovich. 1972.

Blos, P. *The adolescent passage: Developmental issues*. New York: International Universities Press, 1979.

Bower, G. H. Mood and memory. *American Psychologist*, 1981, *36*, 129–148.

Carlson, R. Studies in script theory: II. Altruistic nuclear scripts. *Perceptual and motor skills*, 1982, *55*, 595–610.

Demos, E. V. *Children's understanding and use of affect terms*. Unpublished doctoral dissertation, Harvard University, 1974.

Erikson, E. H. *Young man Luther*. New York: Norton, 1958.

Erikson, E. H. *Identity: Youth and crisis*. New York: Norton, 1968.

Freud, S. Analysis of a phobia in a five-year-old boy. In *Collected Papers* (Vol. 3), pp. 243–287. New York: Basic Books, 1953.

Izard, C. E. *The face of emotion*. New York: Appleton-Century-Crofts, 1971.

McClelland, D. C. *Personality*. New York: Sloane, 1951.

Murray, H. A. *Thematic apperception test manual*. Cambridge, Mass.: Harvard University Press, 1943.

Neimark, E. D., & Stead, C. Everyday thinking by college women: Analysis of journal entries. *Merrill-Palmer Quarterly*, 1981, *27*, 471–488.

Nicolson, N. (Ed.). *The flight of the mind: The letters of Virginia Woolf, Vol. 1: 1888–1912*. London: Hogarth Press, 1975.

Rosenberg, S., & Jones, R. A method for investigating and representing a person's implicit theory of personality: Theodore Dreiser's view of people. *Journal of Personality and Social Psychology*, 1972, *22*, 372–386.

Skinner, B. F. *The behavior of organisms: An experimental analysis*. New York: Appleton-Century-Crofts, 1938.

Stolorow, R. D., & Atwood, G. E. *Faces in a cloud: The subjective world in personality theory*. New York: Aronson, 1978.

Tomkins, S. S. *Affect, imagery and consciousness* (Vol. 1). New York: Springer-Verlag, 1962.

Tomkins, S. S. Script theory: Differential magnification of affects. In H. E. Howe & R. A. Dienstbier (Eds.), *Nebraska symposium on motivation* (Vol. 26). Lincoln: University of Nebraska Press, 1979.

Woolf, V. S. *A writer's diary*. London: Hogarth Press, 1953.

18   Cognitive consequences of emotional arousal

Stephen G. Gilligan and Gordon H. Bower

Does the cheerful person really view the world through rose-colored glasses? Does the depressed person act and think in ways that sustain his misery? Does the pessimist describe as "half empty" the same beer bottle that the optimist calls "half full"? These familiar emotional stereotypes crystallize several important assumptions, specifically, that our perceptions, thoughts, and actions are strongly biased by our emotional feelings.

We have been interested in experimentally testing these assumptions and have thus examined how emotional mood states might influence such cognitive processes as learning, memory, perception, and judgments. The following discussion of our research in this area is divided into four sections. First, we describe our general procedure of using hypnosis to induce and sustain emotional states in experimental subjects. We then summarize our experiments according to four major results: (1) mood selectively biases the recall of affectively toned material; (2) mood enhances the learning of mood-congruent material; (3) the intensity of a mood affects learning differently, depending on the particular mood and the type of materials used; and (4) emotional states can bias many cognitive processes, such as interpretations, fantasies, projections, free associations, personal forecasts, and social judgments.

The second section marshals arguments against a "compliance with demand" explanation of the obtained findings. The third section then explains the results in terms of a semantic network theory of affect. This theory conceptualizes memory for an event in terms of an associative network of descriptive propositions and concepts. As central units in a network, emotions are proposed that have strong associative linkages to other aspects of the network – for example, to autonomic response patterns, expressive behaviors, beliefs, events, and themes. These associative connections are used to explain how activation of a mood influences cognitive processes in multiple ways.

The final section addresses some problems with the network model and offers speculations about how the theory might be extended to deal with various affect-related phenomena. Among the topics addressed are the interaction of

This research was supported by National Institute of Mental Health Grant MH-13905 to the second author.

cognition, behavior, and emotion; the development of affective structures; and the use of control processes to regulate emotional responses.

Empirical investigations

The general procedure

The experiments were conducted by the authors and a few colleagues over a five-year period. The general procedure shared by most of the experiments involved recruiting highly hypnotizable subjects, defined by their high scores (top 15% of population) on the Stanford Hypnotic Susceptibility Scale, Form C (Weitzenhoffer & Hilgard, 1962) or the Harvard Group Scale of Hypnotic Susceptibility, Form A (Shor & Orne, 1962). Approximately 60% to 70% of the subjects were Stanford undergraduate students; the rest were mental-health professionals who had attended hypnosis workshops given by the first author. Most subjects were run in groups of 1 to 4.

To experimentally induce the desired mood state, subjects were first hypnotized via a 10–15-minute general eye-closure induction (Weitzenhoffer & Hilgard, 1962). They were then asked to begin to develop a specific mood (e.g., happiness or sadness) by remembering and revivifying a personal experience in which that mood was prominent. Thus, a subject who was asked to feel happy would often recall an enjoyable vacation or an exuberant success; subjects who were requested to feel sad would remember funerals or crushing disappointments. When, as instructed, a subject signaled that an emotional incident had been accessed and replayed in imagination – usually within a minute or two – instructions were given to forget about the specific content of the revivified memory and instead simply concentrate on intensifying the accessed emotional state. These instructions were repeated for about 5 minutes until subjects were totally immersed in the suggested mood. They were told to maintain the mood until the experimenter asked them to do otherwise and then given further instructions regarding the specific tasks of the experiment. (Amnesia suggestions for the mood induction were usually also given to decrease possible compliance effects.) Following the experimental tasks, the experimenter would rehypnotize subjects, shift them back to a neutral mood, remove all other suggestions (e.g., posthypnotic cues), and then reorient them to their waking states. Subjects would then be thoroughly questioned and debriefed, usually paid or given credit for their participation, and then dismissed after ascertaining that they were suffering no ill effects from the mood induction.

The issue of demand compliance will be addressed later; here, however, preliminary comments about the use of hypnosis are in order. The sensational folklore and myths surrounding hypnosis have led many lay people to overestimate its value, with the result that skeptical academicians have reacted by rejecting its authenticity outright. We would emphasize that the scientific validity of hypnosis has been established by many reputable investigators (e.g., Hilgard, 1965; Hull, 1933; Orne, 1959). We have used it as a methodological tool because we have found it to be a highly reliable and effective way to experimentally induce and maintain mood states. The hypnotic alteration of physiological states is well documented (e.g., Crasilneck & Hall, 1959; Gottlieb, Gleser, & Gottschalk, 1967; Sarbin, 1956), as is the hypnotic production of emotional states (Blum, 1967; Damaser, Shor, & Orne, 1963; Gidro-Frank & Bull, 1950; Hepps & Brady, 1967; Zimbardo, Maslach, & Marshall, 1972). These findings are consistent with our general understanding of hypnosis as a naturalistic state in which the suggested development of relaxation enables complete absorption in suggested images to the extent that actual physiological changes may result (cf. Hilgard, 1965; Zimbardo et al., 1972). We therefore expected that our highly hypnotizable subjects would easily develop the suggested moods, and their success was confirmed by experimenter observations, subject reports, mood checklists, and experimental results.

The remainder of this section describes how the induced moods were used to test four general hypotheses: the *state-dependent recall hypothesis*, which postulates that superior memory occurs when the recall "state" (e.g., mood) matches the learning state; the *mood-congruity hypothesis*, which states that material agreeing in emotional tone with the subject's mood is learned best; the *mood-intensity hypothesis*, which predicts that learning is positively correlated with the intensity of a mood; and the *thought-congruity hypothesis*, which states generally that subjects' thoughts – free associations, fantasies, interpretations, and judgments – will be thematically congruent with their mood state.

State-dependent recall

General theories of memory proposed by Anderson and Bower (1973) and Tulving and Thomson (1973) share the premise that memory retrieval is positively correlated with the overlap of cues available during retrieval and those present at the time of learning; in other words, the more "learning context" cues present at recall, the better the memory. Because the "learning context" includes many variables – other items on a list, testing room, the subject's posture, his mood – there have been many tests relevant to this claim. In an early study by Abernathy (1940), for example, students taking a final exam in a room different from the regular classroom remembered less and performed worse than students tested in the regular room. More recently, Godden and Baddeley (1975) had deep-sea divers learn word lists while either on a boat or 20 feet underwater. When later tested in either the same or the different environment, subjects recalling in the same environment remembered significantly more words. Similarly, Smith, Glenberg, and Bjork (1978) had subjects learn a word list one day in one environment (a windowless, clean room with a well-groomed experimenter) and then another list the next day in a different environment (a sloppy basement room with a "hippie-type" experimenter). When on the third day subjects recalled *both* lists in either the first or second learning environment, they recalled more words (59% vs. 46%) that were learned in the same environment. State-dependent effects have also been found when subjects' internal states were manipulated. An early experiment by Nagge (1935) showed that interference caused by learning multiple word lists could be reduced by having subjects learn one list in a waking state and another while hypnotized. Eich and his colleagues (1975, 1980) independently varied whether a subject was drugged ("stoned") with marijuana or nondrugged when learning and later recalling a word list; the best memory prevailed when the recall state matched the learning state. Parker, Birnbaum, and Noble (1976) obtained a similar effect using alcohol.

Mood/state-dependency with multiple lists. These and other findings of state-dependent recall suggested to us that mood might also be a powerful context in this regard. In an initial study (Bower, Monteiro, & Gilligan, 1978), we first tried the straightforward approach of having subjects learn a word list composed of half happy words and half sad words (abstract nouns) while in a hypnotically induced happy or sad mood and then recall them in either the same or opposite mood. We were somewhat surprised and discouraged that the groups did not differ in recall during either learning or retention testing. Noting Nagge's (1935) results suggesting the list-differentiating properties of internal states, we modified the experimental design to include two word lists. Subjects first learned a list while happy or sad, learned another list while happy or sad, then recalled the first list twenty minutes later while happy or sad. Thus, mood was induced three times in each subject, with the type of mood (happy or sad) independently varied each time.

This design yields three relevant conditions. Subjects in a control condition learned and recalled both lists in the same mood, thereby providing base-line data against which to compare the other groups. Subjects in a facilitation condition learned the first list in one mood, switched moods to learn the second list, then shifted back to the original mood to recall the first list. Our prediction was that this group would show the best memory for the first list because (1) interference would be decreased because the second list had been isolated by having been learned under a different mood and (2) the matching mood at first-list recall would enhance its retrieval. Subjects in an interference condition learned the first list in one mood, then the second list in the opposite mood, then recalled the first list in that (opposite) mood. We expected this condition to have the poorest recall because (1) interference would arise from the second list, which had been learned in the retrieval mood and (2) retrieval problems would arise because the recall state differed from the learning mood of the first list.

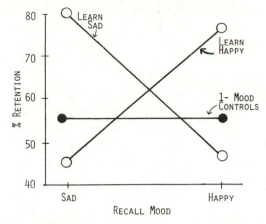

Figure 18.1. Percentage retention scores depending on the match between learning mood and recall mood. The sloping lines refer to subjects who learned the two lists under different moods. (From G. H. Bower, "Mood & Memory," *American Psychologist*, 1981, *36*(2), 129–148. Copyright 1981 by the American Psychological Association. Reprinted by permission.)

The results were scored in terms of the percentage of items recalled during an original learning phase and those that were recalled on the (later) critical test. Although mood had no influence on the type of word learned or recalled within a list, it did affect overall recall of a list (Figure 18.1). The flat line in Figure 18.1 indicates that recall percentages for the two control groups were about the same (56% for the always-sad subjects vs. 53% for the always-happy group). However, subjects in the other conditions performed remarkably differently. As shown by the crossing lines, recall was far better in the facilitation groups than in the interference groups (70% and 63% vs. 43% and 48%, respectively). In short, memory for a list was best when (1) its recall mood matched its learning mood and (2) the interfering list was isolated by being learned under a different mood. Memory was poorest when the opposite conditions held.

This state-dependent finding was replicated and extended in an undergraduate honors thesis carried out by Brett Thompson under Bower's direction (see Bower, 1981). Briefly stated, Thompson and Bower wondered if different degrees of mood/state-dependency could be produced. Using Plutchik's (1980) analysis of basic emotions, they selected the emotions of joy, sadness, anger, and fear. In Plutchik's scheme, the first two emotions are diametrically opposed to each other, as are the latter two. The main prediction was that a recall mood similar to the learning mood would result in a better memory. To test this, subjects were asked to learn a different word list in each of the four basic mood states and then to recall each list while either in the same mood (in which it was learned), a different but not opposite mood, or the opposite mood. The major finding was that emotional proximity affected recall: when learning and recall moods matched, recall averaged 85%; when moods were different but not opposite, 70% of the words on a list were remembered; but with opposite moods, recall averaged only 54%.

These generalization scores, predicted by Plutchik's theory, could also be interpreted in terms of the differential emotions theory of Izard (1972). That theory would claim that the nominal "emotional states" in this experiment are patterns or mixtures of elements from several primary emotions, for example, that sad situations may also evoke some elements of anger and/or fear. This theory would further claim that the coefficients of overlap in emotional elements among our experimental conditions follow the gradients predicted by Plutchik's model. These claims could be tested simply by asking subjects to fill out Izard's (1972) Differential Emotions Scale while in our four different emotional states and then checking for the overlap coefficients in the patterns of emotions checked off.

State-dependent recall of autobiographical events. To determine whether these results would obtain for more naturalistic situations involving the retrieval of autobiographical memories, we modified a methodology developed by Holmes (1970). Diaries were given to 26 highly hypnotizable subjects (Bower & Gilligan, 1980), in which they were to record the time, place, and gist of each emotionally laden event, along with a rating of its intensity on a 10-point scale, for a week. Thus, entries might read: "Monday 7:30 p.m.: just got angry at my mother on the phone; a −8 rating" or "Wednesday noon . . . got word that my vacation request has been granted . . . +6."

A week later, most subjects returned at their scheduled times. Not surprisingly, a number of them had been remiss in maintaining accurate diary recordings. Using the criterion of 15 or more adequately recorded incidents, only 14 of the 26 diaries were judged usable. The 14 subjects were asked to return a week later for some hypnotic experiments, ostensibly unrelated to the diaries. Upon their return they were hypnotized (in groups of 1−4), induced into a pleasant or unpleasant state (7 subjects in each condition), and then asked to recall as many incidents recorded in the diary as they could. Subjects later rated each recalled incident according to its *present* intensity value.

The major results, in terms of the average number of pleasant and unpleasant incidents as recorded in the diary and the corresponding numbers recalled (Table 18.1), indicate that more pleasant than unpleasant experiences were recorded by subjects, replicating a finding by Holmes (1970) and Matlin and Stang (1979). This may be due to a variety of factors, including a reporting bias, a greater frequency of happy events, or different forgetting rates for happy and sad events. Accordingly, more pleasant experiences were recalled by most subjects. The major data of interest, however, are the relative percentages of pleasant and unpleasant incidents recalled by subjects in the different moods. As indicated in the right column, the expected interaction occurred

Table 18.1. *Average number of pleasant and unpleasant incidents recorded in diary and later recalled by subjects in pleasant or unpleasant emotional state*

Recall mood	Pleasant incidents recorded	Pleasant incidents recalled	Unpleasant incidents recorded	Unpleasant incidents recalled
Pleasant	20.8	6.43 (31)	11.3	2.57 (23)
Unpleasant	20.0	6.57 (33)	14.1	5.29 (38)

Note: Figures in parentheses indicate percentages.

between mood state and type of incident recalled: subjects in a pleasant mood recalled more pleasant than unpleasant experiences (31% vs. 23%), whereas subjects in an unpleasant mood showed the reverse pattern (33% vs. 38%).

Another finding was that the original intensity ratings given to incidents were somewhat predictive of recall. Dividing each subject's ratings at the median, the more intense experiences were later recalled better than the less intense ones (37% vs. 25%). The second round of ratings, made at the time of recall, were largely influenced by the experimentally induced mood: happy subjects tended to rate happy incidents as more pleasant and unhappy events as less unpleasant than before, whereas sad subjects showed the opposite tendency. Thus, the current mood seemed to shift the evaluation scale for memories.

To ensure that the selective recall effect was not a design artifact, Monteiro and Bower (see Bower & Gilligan, 1980) ran a similar experiment in which hypnotized subjects made happy or sad were asked to recall for 10 minutes a succession of unrelated childhood incidents. They were also instructed to write down the gist, time, and place of each remembered event (e.g., "my party in fifth grade; we went to the fun house"). When subjects returned the next day for a different experiment, they rated (while in a neutral mood) each recalled event as being either pleasant, unpleasant, or neutral. The ratings indicated that 92% of the memories recalled by "happy" subjects were happy, whereas only 45% retrieved by "sad" subjects were happy and slightly more than 50% were sad. Thus, the overall bias toward recalling happy memories was again found, as was the more important effect of mood/state-dependent recall.

Supporting evidence. These experiments show that mood can bias recall, a finding consistent with those reported by others. For example, Isen and her associates (1978) found that positive moods induced by winning a game enhanced recall of positively toned experimental materials. Bartlett and Santrock (1979) used a design similar to the two-list state-dependency experiment described earlier (see Figure 18.1) – except that no hypnosis was used – and found that kindergarten children showed a similar state-dependent memory. Henry, Weingartner, and Murphy (1973) found that word associations learned by manic-depressives were remembered best when patients learned and recalled in the same mood (mania or depression). Similarly, both Teasdale and Fogarty (1979) and Lloyd and Lishman (1975) reported that a mood quickened access to mood-congruent memories. Given the differences in mood inductions, designs, and subject populations across these studies, it appears that our state-dependency results were not due simply to demand characteristics or design artifacts.

Recognition memory uninfluenced by mood. An interesting aspect of these experiments – including ours – is that none examined the possible effects of mood on recognition memory. Our intuition was that little if any mood effects would obtain under such testing conditions. This was based partly on Eich's (1980) report that drug/state-dependency did not occur with recognition memory tests and partly on our explanation of our recall results in terms of an associative network theory. A central assumption of this theory, to be described later, is that a learning mood constitutes a contextual cue that becomes encoded in an associative network representation of the event. Because of its associative links to other parts of the memory representation, reactivating the learning mood could boost recall by enhancing access to the rest of the memory. In this view, however, a recognition test would not be much influenced by mood mismatching, because the direct access that recognition provides to the memory minimizes such retrieval cues.

Despite these negative expectations, Gellerman and Bower (see Bower & Gilligan, 1980) decided to run an experiment involving recognition memory, partly because positive results would suggest the serious consideration of alternative explanations of our results. Pictures of human faces were chosen as the experimental stimuli, as they might be subject to emotional biases at encoding (e.g., Schiffenbauer, 1974). Slides of pictures from high-school yearbooks of Caucasian male high-school seniors with average physical features were made. Subjects studied some slides while in a hypnotically induced angry or happy state and then studied different slides in the opposite mood. Following an interval, they took one recognition test in one mood and a second test in the alternate mood. Each recognition test contained some distractor items not previously presented, some pictures that had been presented during the "angry" learning state, and some that had been presented during the "happy" learning state. This counterbalanced 2- × -2 design ensured that subjects saw half the "old" slides while in the same mood and half in the opposite mood, thus testing for state-dependent effects.

The results showed absolutely no differences in recognition memory stemming from input mood or test mood. More important, no interaction (state-dependent) effects were obtained. Old faces were recognized about 60% of the time in all input-by-output conditions, and about 84% of the distractor faces were correctly

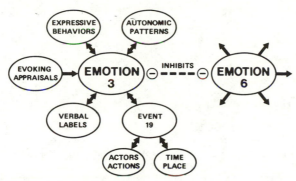

Figure 18.2. Small fragment of the connections surrounding a specific emotion node or unit. Bidirectional arrows refer to mutual exchange of activation between nodes. An inhibitory pathway from Emotion 3 to Emotion 6 is also shown. (From G. H. Bower, "Mood & Memory," *American Psychologist*, 1981, *36*(2), 129–148. Copyright 1981 by the American Psychological Association. Reprinted by permission.)

rejected. These results indicate that subjects could clearly discriminate old from new faces but were not affected in any way by their mood states. Thus, the generalization that state-dependent effects are minimized with recognition tests appears to pertain to mood states as well as to drug states.

Summary. To summarize, our experiments yielded several interesting findings. Mood biased memory when multiple word lists or autobiographical events were the recall targets. It did not affect memory for mood-related words within a list or when only a single list was used; nor did it influence recognition memory in any way. Other findings included that (1) mood shaded the subjective evaluation of a past event (in the diary experiment); (2) mood intensity correlated with the memorability of an event (in the diary experiment); and (3) pleasant experiences tended to be recalled more than unpleasant ones, an interesting finding but of no special relevance to our concerns.

Explaining mood/state-dependent recall

Our results are explained in the third section in terms of a theory of affect. A part of the theory will be introduced here to explain the state-dependent results. Network theories (e.g., Anderson & Bower, 1973; Collins & Loftus, 1975; Collins & Quillian, 1969) conceptualize memory as an associative network of nodes representing, among other things, numerous concepts, schemata, and events. Bower (1981) proposed that emotions might be considered as units in such a network, with each emotion "node" having strong associative links to other units in the network (Figure 18.2). An event becomes encoded in the network as a cluster of propositions with strong associative links to concepts and other units (e.g., emotions) and schemata to which they are related. These propositions might refer to individual words learned on a word list, actions in

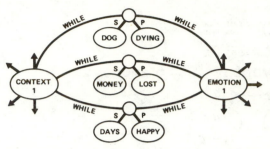

Figure 18.3. The crucial connections for explaining mood/state-dependent retrieval. The subject has studied many adjective-noun phrases (dying dog, lost money, happy days, etc.) in Context 1 while feeling Emotion 1. The associations indicated (and many others) are weakly formed. (From G. H. Bower, "Mood & Memory," *American Psychologist*, 1981, *36*(2), 129–148. Copyright 1981 by the American Psychological Association. Reprinted by permission.)

a story, autobiographical experiences, and so on. The propositions constitute the basic units of thought, and the activation of them or their related concepts is the basic process of thought. Activation can occur directly or indirectly. Direct activation occurs by presentation of a corresponding stimulus pattern: for example, stimulation of an emotion would activate the corresponding emotion node; presentation of a word on a recognition test would access its network representative. Indirect activation occurs when "energy" spreads from associated nodes that are activated, for example, the mood could be "turned on" via activation spreading to it from associated concepts or propositions.

The state-dependent results can be explained straightforwardly by this model. Figure 18.3 illustrates in a highly simplified fashion how two-word phrases like "happy days" or "dying dog" learned under different moods in one of our multiple-list experiments would be represented in a memory network. Each memory is represented as a subject-predicate (S-P) proposition, which was experienced and learned while (note the name on the association) the subject was in Mood 1 and List Context 1. At recall, reinstating the learning mood for, say, List 1 would reactivate that mood unit (Emotion 1) and spread activation down its associative links, thereby priming List 1 words. At the same time, asking the subject to recall the first list would activate the List 1 node, which would also spread activation. Thus, the target items (i.e., the List 1 words) would receive the summation of activation emanating from the two activated sources, thereby making them more highly accessible than alternative contents. Intersection of activation from the List 1 node helps to discriminate the target items from the many other associations to Emotion 1; it also provides the additional energy needed to push activation of target items over threshold, thererby bringing them into consciousness. Conversely, mismatching learning and recall moods would depress accessibility, because the recall mood not only would fail to activate the target items but would also activate interfering associations. As discussed in the third section, this inter-ference is especially pronounced when the recall mood is diametrically opposed to the learning mood.

The mood-congruity effect

The character identification experiment. In addition to the question of how mood biases memory, we have also been interested in whether mood might cause selective learning of affective material (see Bower, Gilligan, & Monteiro, 1981). Our first experiment in this area developed from an earlier interest in the role of character identification in the reading and recall of narratives (Bower, 1978). The basic question was whether a subject made happy or sad would identify more with, and thus learn and recall more about, a story character expressing the same mood. To test this idea, we composed a short third-person narrative about two students playing tennis on a Saturday afternoon. One character, André, is very happy – he sings, jokes, enjoys the sunshine, wins the game, and so on. The other character, Jack, is just the opposite – he is morose, worries about exams, feels scorched by the sun, loses the game, and so on. The number of (mostly happy) statements about André equaled the number of (mostly sad) statements about Jack.

Subjects were induced into a happy or a sad mood via a posthypnotic cue (see Bower et al., 1981) and then asked to read the narrative. Afterward, they filled out questionnaires regarding which character they identified with and attended to more. A written free-recall test of the story was given the next day while subjects were in a neutral mood. Of the facts recalled by "happy" readers, 55% were about Happy André, whereas of the propositions recalled by "sad" readers, 80% were about Sad Jack. In addition, all subjects reported identifying more with the character whose mood matched theirs at the time of reading. This is not a state-dependent effect, as a neutral mood prevailed at the time of recall; rather, the results suggest selective learning.

The single character experiment. The hypothesis attributing the recall differences to "character identification" was not uniquely tested in the André-Jack ex-periment because that story confounded the type of fact with the character. That is, all happy facts involved Happy André and all sad facts pertained to Sad Jack. Thus, the observed effect may have reflected selective learning of mood-congruent materials, unmediated by character identification. To test this possibility, we constructed a short narrative about a single character, a psychiatric patient, recounting a mixture of happy and sad memories uncovered during hypnotherapeutic age regressions. As before, subjects read the story while in hypnotically induced happy or sad moods. This time, though, they were also in an induced mood while recalling the story some 20 minutes later. By in-dependently manipulating learning and recall moods, we could isolate possible

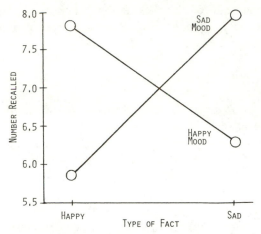

Figure 18.4. Number of happy versus sad story incidents recalled by readers who were happy or sad. (One character in the story described both types of personal incidents.) (From G. H. Bower, "Mood & Memory," *American Psychologist*, 1981, *36*(2), 129– 148. Copyright 1981 by the American Psychological Association. Reprinted by permission.)

learning, recall, and state-dependent (interaction) effects. The results indicate that learning mood does affect the type of facts recalled, with happy learners later recalling more happy incidents and sad learners more sad ones (Figure 18.4).However, there was no reliable state-dependent effect, that is, overall recall by subjects whose learning and recall moods matched was not significantly greater than that of subjects in different moods. Also, recall mood did not influence which type of material – happy or sad – was remembered.

The absence of a mood-matching effect here is consistent with our earlier failings using single lists. Remember, we had to use two interfering lists before the facilitation provided by mood-matching was shown clearly. The important result here is that mood during learning influenced selective learning, whereas mood during recall of a single list had little or no selective influence on recall.

The absence of a simple effect of recall mood surprised us, so we conducted two experiments that varied mood only at recall following neutral-mood learning. Subjects read either the two-character (André and Jack) or the single-character (the psychiatric patient) story while in a neutral mood, then returned six hours later to recall the story twice, first while happy or sad and then in the opposite mood. Results showed that recall mood had no selective influence on memory for pleasant versus unpleasant events in either story, thus replicating the null effects of the earlier experiment.

Character identification versus mood-episode congruity. The major positive finding, then, was that subjects' moods while reading a narrative caused superior learning of mood-congruent episodes. Whereas our first experiment assumed that selectivity was caused by mood-mediated character identification, the single-character study suggested that it could have resulted from congruity (agreement) between subjects' moods and the pleasant or unpleasant episodes. These two hypotheses are not mutually exclusive and could both be correct. To compare these hypotheses, a narrative was constructed that opposed the character-identification factor against the mood-congruity factor. The story was about two patients about to leave therapy. Joe was introduced as a happy-go-lucky manic type, and Mike was described as a gloomy depressive. In a final interview with their mutual therapist, the young men alternated in describing some of the key memories uncovered during their therapies, with an equal number of happy and sad incidents recited by each character. (Each incident was described in about two statements.) Thus the mood of the character and the type of episode he related were independently manipulated. Subjects were made to feel happy or sad as they read this narrative.

Subjects recalled the story 20 minutes later while in a neutral mood. The recall data revealed that readers learned more mood-congruent than mood-incongruent incidents but did not learn more incidents related by the mood-congruent character. (That characters were actually perceived as being happy or sad was confirmed by questionnaire data and by the fact that all subjects recalled more happy facts about Happy Joe and more sad facts about Sad Mike.) These results suggest that the mood-congruity of the episode outweighed the character-mood factor in determining the moody reader's selection of material for greater learning.

Explaining the mood-congruity effect. Four possible explanations of the mood-congruity effect might be briefly noted here. Three of the explanations assume generally that mood-congruent material receives *greater elaboration* and is thus better learned (see Anderson, 1976; Anderson & Reder, 1979). The first specifies a *greater ease of elaboration* for mood-congruent items. That is, the reader's mood primes affectively congruent cognitions and associations that facilitate various types of elaborations on mood-similar episodes, for example, thinking about their antecedents and consequents or imaging the character or one's self involved in the described actions. This hypothesis is supported by experiments reported later showing that associative thinking – interpretations, judgments, free associations – is biased toward the subject's mood.

A second hypothesis – one that is really a special case of the first – is *selective reminding*. This hypothesis suggests that subjects are more likely to access related memories while reading about a mood-congruent episode than a mood-incongruent episode. For example, a storybook character who fails an exam might more often remind a sad (than a happy) reader of a similar depressing incident; in contrast, a fantastic victory for that character would be more likely to trigger related memories in a happy (than a sad) reader. This state-dependent reminding, strongly suggested by subject reports and by other experiments (e.g., Lloyd & Lishman, 1975; Teasdale & Fogarty, 1979), would result in more elaboration on mood-congruent material. And as Bower and Gilligan (1979) have found in other work, memory is enhanced substantially by associating personal memories to the to-be-learned material. Thus selective reminding as a plausible explanation of the mood-congruity effect merits further investigation.

A third hypothesis is *selective attention* to mood-congruent material. A good case for this can be made via attribution theory. Specifically, our subjects were typically given amnesia for the mood suggestions and thus may have wondered why they were feeling so intensely happy or sad while reading the story. If so, they could have attributed their feelings to the story material; then, to justify their attribution, they might have spent more time attending to mood-congruent items.

However, this attribution hypothesis was not supported by further experiments, which showed that the mood-congruity effect obtained even when no amnesia was given for subjects' moods, so that subjects knew that their mood stemmed from the suggestion. Of course, a case could be made for selective attention independent of attribution processes; for example, more time might be spent on mood-congruent items because of ease of elaboration or selective reminding processes. This could be tested by controlling reading times for congruent versus incongruent items and checking whether the mood-congruity effect still obtained. Another possibility would be to let the mood-induced subjects pace their reading of the stories line by line, with reading time recorded for each line. Subjects should spend more time on the mood-congruent statements.

A fourth explanation of mood-congruent learning involves *mood intensity*. This explanation assumes that (1) the intensity of subjects' mood states increases while reading mood-congruent episodes but decreases while reading mood-incongruent episodes and (2) an episode's memorability increases with the intensity of the subject's emotional reaction to it at the time of learning. The first assumption was suggested by subjects' frequent postexperimental mentioning of mood fluctuations in response to happy or sad episodes in the story they were reading. Specifically, "sad" subjects often reported that their sadness intensified when reading sad events but lessened when reading about happy events; similarly, "happy" subjects noted that their emotional intensity was augmented by happy events but dampened by sad ones. That this intensity difference could have produced the mood-congruity effect is suggested by a number of sources, including (1) our finding in the "mood diary" experiment (described earlier) that emotional intensity ratings of events correlated with their recall, and (2) Kanungo and Dutta's (1966; Dutta & Kanungo, 1975) findings that emotionally provocative material was remembered better than neutral material.

Mood intensity and learning

The experiments just cited, showing results supportive of the mood-intensity hypothesis, systematically confound the nature of the material with the normal emotional reaction to it. Theoretical inferences would be simpler if we could disentangle the influence of emotional intensity per se from the stimulus materials. To rectify this, we conducted experiments in which mood intensity was manipulated hypnotically, with the materials presented at each intensity level randomized for each subject. We used a procedure adapted from Blum (1967) in which highly hypnotizable subjects were first trained to experience various intensity levels of a mood and then given various learning tasks at each intensity level.

Experiment 1. In the first experiment, subjects were trained to experience three intensity levels of happiness: low (calm and content), medium (joy), and high (ecstatic bliss). Once subjects could reliably shift (on cue from the hypnotist-experimenter) among the three intensity levels, they received an experimental learning task in which both mood-relevant and mood-irrelevant episodes were presented at the different intensity levels. Specifically, subjects were hypnotized, shifted to a randomly determined mood-intensity level, and asked to imagine themselves personally involved in twelve short episodes (vignettes) that were read to them. They were also asked after each reading to rate on a scale of 1 to 7 how imaginatively absorbed or involved they had become in that vignette. Following this, subjects were shifted to a different intensity level and asked to repeat the procedure with twelve additional vignettes. They were then shifted to the third intensity level and presented with more vignettes.

Half the vignettes presented at each intensity level were affectively neutral (e.g., "reading a newspaper and passing the time while doing your laundry"); the other half described happy incidents ("walking along the street and finding a five-dollar bill"). Aside from this constraint, presentation of the materials was randomized across subjects. Recall occurred in a neutral state following a 20-minute retention interval.

Both mood-congruent and mood-irrelevant vignettes were included because an earlier pilot study had shown that, contrary to the simple intensity hypothesis, increasing the intensity of a happy mood significantly *decreased* learning rates for neutral words (e.g., names of American cities, kitchen utensils). Extensive subject interviews suggested that the ease of relating the learning material to the mood might be critical in determining how intensity level influenced learning. Subjects commonly reported being unwilling or unable to attend to "kitchen utensils" and the like while feeling intense euphoria. The present experiment was designed in part to test this possible interaction between materials and intensity level.

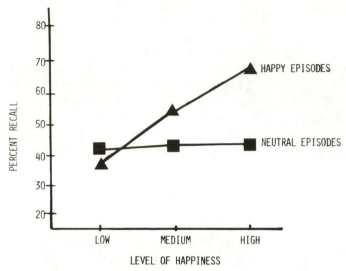

Figure 18.5. Free recall of happy and neutral episodes experienced when the subject was feeling mildly, moderately, or extremely happy.

We predicted that increasing intensity would enhance learning of mood-related materials but not of mood-irrelevant materials. The recall results generally confirm this prediction (Figure 18.5). As indicated by the sloping line, learning of happy incidents increased with intensity level. As illustrated by the relatively flat line, however, learning of affectively neutral incidents was not influenced significantly by mood intensity (recall percentages were 40%, 43%, and 47%). The imagery ratings were also interesting. While ratings were higher for happy than for neutral vignettes (4.99 vs. 4.08), ratings for both types of vignettes increased with intensity level (lower: 4.27; medium: 4.52; high: 4.83). Thus, overall imagery ratings are somewhat predictive of recallability.

The results suggest an interesting interaction between mood intensity and the type of materials. When the material was irrelevant to the happy mood, intensifying the mood had relatively little impact on learning; but when the material was relatable to the subject's happiness, increasing intensity enhanced learning. This pattern is quite consistent with Easterbrook's (1959) hypothesis that increasing arousal narrows attention so that "relevant" stimuli become more salient and attended. This hypothesis has been supported by several other investigations (Bahrick, Fitts, & Rankin, 1952; Bursill, 1958; Callaway & Stone, 1960; Cornsweet, 1969; McNamara & Fisch, 1964).

Experiment 2. The preceding experiment used only happy moods, and thus permitted no conclusions about learning and emotional intensity in general.

To see if the results would generalize to other moods, we conducted a second experiment in which the between-subjects factor of type of mood (happy or sad) was added to the within-subject factors of mood intensity (high or low) and type of materials (happy, sad, or neutral vignettes). Subjects were randomly assigned to the "happy" or "sad" group, and then trained as before to experience two intensity levels of the mood. In the experimental session subjects were shifted back and forth (twice) between these intensity levels. At each intensity level (two high and two low), they imagined themselves in 12 different vignettes (4 happy, 4 sad, and 4 neutral) that were read to them. They also gave a "degree of absorption" rating after imagining each vignette. Free recall of the 48 vignettes occurred in a neutral-mood waking state after a 20-minute retention interval.

Figure 18.6 shows an intriguing pattern of results for the happy and sad subjects for the happy and sad items. (Neutral items were recalled equally by both groups and thus for ease of understanding are not represented in the figure.)First, the sloping lines indicate the expected mood-congruity effect, with happy subjects learning happy vignettes better than sad ones, and sad subjects learning sad vignettes better than happy ones. Second, the highly intense happy state (Figure 18.6 top) produced better learning than the mild happy state (overall recall percentages were 43% vs. 29%); rather surprisingly, however, the exact opposite occurred for sad subjects (Figure 18.6 bottom), with vignettes learned in the mildly sad state being recalled better than those learned in the profoundly sad mood (overall scores of 44% vs. 26%). It thus appears that extreme sadness produces low motivation for learning or demanding tasks. Later, we will offer an explanation of this finding.

Interestingly, subjects' absorption and imagery ratings conformed to this general pattern of findings. Happy subjects gave higher ratings to happy vignettes than to sad ones (5.60 vs. 4.15), and sad subjects gave higher ratings for sad than for happy vignettes (4.19 vs. 3.85); this pattern is exactly as expected by the mood-congruity hypothesis. In addition, happy subjects gave higher imaginal absorption ratings when intensely happy than when mildly happy (5.09 vs. 4.52), whereas sad subjects showed more imaginal absorption in the vignettes when mildly sad than when intensely sad (4.72 vs. 3.76). These absorption ratings were completely consistent with the recall interaction between mood intensity and mood type. Thus, the recallability of an item could have been mediated by the degree to which the subject could become imaginally absorbed in it.

Summary and general explanation. The results of these several experiments on mood intensity suggest a state of affairs more complicated than predicted by our original hypothesis. Intensifying a happy state had little influence on learning of mood-irrelevant items, whereas it improved the learning of happy

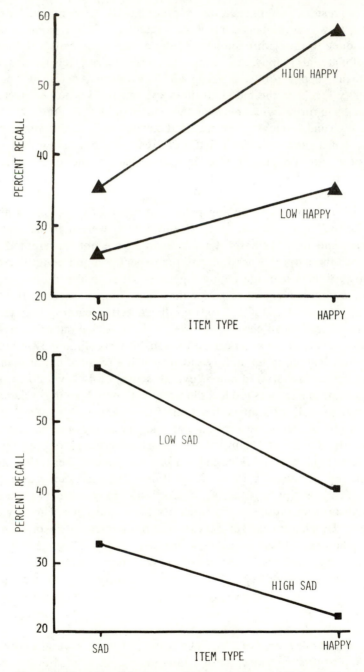

Figure 18.6(top) Recall by happy subjects under low and high mood intensities.
Figure 18.6(bottom) Recall by sad subjects under low and high mood intensities.

vignettes; intensifying a sad mood hampered the learning of even mood-relevant vignettes. Thus, both the mood and the relatedness of the learning materials are important variables in determining the effect of mood intensity on learning. Further experiments are currently under way to determine if these results can be replicated and generalized.

A preliminary explanation of the findings can be offered here in terms of the network theory of affect. As noted earlier (Figure 18.1), this theory assumes that emotions can be represented by central units in an associative network encoding memories, with each emotion node bearing associative connections to specific autonomic patterns, beliefs, events, response patterns, and inter-pretation schemata. The development of a mood state activates the corresponding emotion unit in the network; by virtue of spreading activation, its surrounding nodes (e.g., the specific autonomic patterns, event instances) are also brought into play. Roughly speaking, the activated components of the network become the "contents of consciousness."

Emotional intensity can be represented as the degree to which an emotion unit has been activated. Low-intensity emotion results in only minor spreading activation to nearby associative nodes; high-intensity emotion causes a large amount of activation to spread along many associated links as well as to distant parts of the network. The amount of emotional activation affects the contents of consciousness because the theory supposes that only those ideas that receive activation above their threshold will become conscious. Thus a stronger emotion will cause more ideas linked to that emotion to "flood into" short-term memory. This is true for both irrelevant, preexperimental associations and the associations specifically trained in the experiment.

This differential flooding of short-term memory by emotion-related material has several implications. First, the impact of the mood on processes of perceptual interpretation, learning, and memory will generally increase insofar as newly arriving stimuli are interpreted according to currently active categories in short-term memory. Second, the filling of consciousness by emotionally related ideas results in the phenomenon described as the "narrowing of attention" to mood-related material (Easterbrook, 1959). In certain cases, if the internally generated scenario is sufficiently compelling, the emotional flooding of short-term memory can lead to "lack of attention" to external stimuli. This may have happened with our high-sad subjects in the last experiment. In addition, the content of the mood-related ideas and their helpfulness for learning may differ for happy versus extremely sad moods. Thus, the very sad mood may evoke a preexperimental depressional syndrome of withdrawal, ruminating over failure, crying, predicting failures, feeling fatigued, and helplessness. In extreme form, these negative factors could lead to poor learning and poor performance by our very sad subjects. This implication agrees with the claims of differential-emotions theory, as well as the clinical observations of depressed people.

Mood effects on other cognitive processes

Associations, interpretations, and depictions. The multiple effects of mood on learning and memory processes led us and our colleagues to investigate whether other cognitive processes would be similarly affected. In one study, hypnotized subjects were induced into happy, angry, or sad moods and then given a series of tasks, including (1) generating chains of free associations to abstract affectively neutral words like *life, mind,* and *future*; (2) composing stories in response to pictures of the Thematic Apperception Test (TAT); and (3) giving "thumbnail personality sketches" of people familiar in their lives (e.g., first-grade teacher, uncle, best friend). Independent judges then blindly rated subjects' productions in terms of their mood content. The results showed that mood dramatically biased thought productions: Judges could reliably determine the mood of the subjects during the task. All subjects gave free associations, composed TAT stories, and retrieved selective sketches of their acquaintances in a manner congruent with their mood at the moment. Such results are consistent with the network theory. For example, in the TAT study, the theory implies that the person's emotional state will evoke a theme congruent with that of the story (e.g., *anger* will evoke themes of conflict of war).

Predicting the future. In another experiment, Wright and Bower (1981) investigated the influence of moods on probability estimates of future events. Two lists were constructed, each specifying 12 possible future events. One list referred to personal events, the other to national or global incidents; half the items on each list were happy, half were depressing and catastrophic. Thus, the 24 items were of four different types: Happy Personal Events (e.g., "You will take a European vacation in the next three years"), Happy National or Global Events (e.g., "There will be a cure for most cancers discovered within ten years"), Catastrophic Personal Events (e.g., "You will be involved in a serious auto accident within the next five years"), and Catastrophic National or Global Events (e.g., "World war will occur within the next ten years"). Subjects were made happy or depressed by hypnosis and asked to use a 1– 100 scale to estimate the probability of half the events, then shifted into the opposite mood and requested to estimate the probabilities of the other events. Special emphasis was placed on providing "objective" estimates, and subjects later stated that they felt their estimates were not influenced by their moods.

However, a mood bias was in fact revealed by the estimates (Table 18.2). The happy mood boosted estimates for blessed events and lowered them for tragic events, and the sad mood had the opposite effect. The influences are nearly symmetrical around the neutral-mood estimates.

That a transient mood could exert such a powerful effect was somewhat surprising but is nevertheless quite consistent with Tversky and Kahneman's (1973) heuristic principles of availability and representativeness. Three types

Table 18.2. *Probability of "blessed" and "catastrophic" future events as predicted by happy, neutral, and sad subjects*

Mood	Blessed events	Catastrophic events
Happy	.52	.37
Neutral	.44	.43
Sad	.38	.52

of strategies might have been used by our subjects in judging the likelihood of an event: (1) recalling related autobiographical episodes involving one's self or friends and using a representativeness judgment of the available sample to estimate the likelihood of a similar event in the future; (2) retrieving memories of news reports and using them in a similar way; and (3) constructing a "causal scenario" leading to the event and generating an estimate based on the ease with which such a scenario could be formed. Mood would have biased the first two strategies via state-dependent retrieval processes, that is, the availability of relevant episodes would be either lowered (for mood-incongruent material) or raised (for mood-congruent material) by the estimator's emotional state. Similarly, the third strategy could have been influenced by the mood-mediated "ease of elaboration," as discussed earlier. Further investigations of these possibilities are warranted. For now, we merely note that we have produced in the laboratory the fabled optimism of the happy person and pessimism of the depressed person.

Mood and social judgments

The network theory suggests than an emotional state may influence the interpretation of ambiguous stimuli because the emotion primes into readiness congruent concepts and categories. An especially interesting class of ambiguous stimuli are social behaviors of others directed toward us. Judgments of social actions are heavily tinged with subjectivism, because we must rely upon inferences about the actor's intention; and those inferences may differ, depending on the "emotional premise" from which the perceiver begins. Is someone who continues to disagree with you being admirably persistent or unreasonably stubborn and pigheaded? Is a student who disagrees with a professor's work assignment being assertive or lazy or aggressive? The interpretation will vary with how the perceiver feels in general, and how he feels about the actor in particular. Thus, happy people tend to be friendly, charitable, and merciful in their judgments of others; angry people tend to be the opposite.

Just as our emotional state influences our perceptions of others' social actions, so should it also influence perceptions of our own behaviors. This influence has clinical relevance. For example, depressed people are notoriously disparaging and castigating about their own behavior. Indeed, Roth and Rehm (1980) found that when clinically depressed patients rated videotapes of themselves for socially negative and socially positive behaviors, they "saw" twice as many negative as positive behaviors, even though neutral judges scored equivalent numbers of these behaviors. Forgas, Bower, and Krantz (1983) performed a similar experiment using hypnotically induced moods with undergraduate students. On Day 1 of their two-day experiment, 20-minute interviews with pairs of subjects about personal topics were videotaped (with the subjects' consent). When subjects returned the next day, they were first trained to score interview behaviors as either prosocial and positive (e.g., a friendly smile, a kind remark) or antisocial and negative (e.g., looking away, frowning). Subjects were then hypnotized and asked to develop either a feeling of social well-being and success or a feeling of social failure and rejection. They were told to maintain this feeling while viewing a videotape of their interview from the previous day and to mark down every 10 seconds (on cue) at least one positive or negative behavior displayed by themselves or their partner.

The results were as predicted. Subjects in the pleasant mood "saw" far more socially positive than negative behaviors for both themselves and others. In contrast, subjects who were feeling rejected and downcast "saw" mostly negative behaviors in themselves but a roughly equal number of positive and negative behaviors in their partners. The scoring was clearly subjective, as neutral judges rated the two groups as having roughly the same proportions of negative and positive behaviors. Thus, the results suggest that people who are feeling socially successful will tend to see the good points in themselves and others, whereas people who are feeling like social failures will see themselves as socially inept and ineffectual. These results are as expected by the network theory, because the emotional mood primes and brings into readiness perceptual categories and interpretive schemata that guide what people attend to as well as how they interpret it.

Summary. The experiments reviewed indicate that an emotion can have a surprisingly strong influence on how someone thinks and acts in his social world. In one study, mood was shown to bias free association, thematic storytelling, and personality descriptions of familiar people. In another, subjects seemed to be optimistic or pessimistic about the future – whether it involved personal or national affairs – according to their transient mood state. In a third study, whether a person felt socially successful or rejected biased self-observations of his or her socially positive or negative behaviors. Emotion thus seems to be inextricably related to how we perceive and think, influencing them at every turn. Indeed, results reported throughout this chapter suggest that emotion is often a central component of cognitive processes in general, and thus that a comprehensive theory of cognition should address it. The final sections of this chapter offer several initial steps in this direction.

The "compliance with demand" explanation

The results of our experiments indicate that mood can bias cognition in a wide assortment of ways. Both the learning and recall of mood-congruent memories – whether they be word lists, story events, or autobiographical events – are apparently enhanced by a mood's presence. Similarly, the evaluation of emotionally toned memories can be shaded by emotion, with more memories rated as pleasant under a happy mood and more as unpleasant under a sad mood. The intensity of an emotional reaction has variable effects on learning, depending on the specific mood and the type of learning materials. Specifically, intensifying a happy mood enhanced the learning of mood-related materials, whereas intensifying a sad mood decreased the learning of such materials. The implications of this intriguing finding are still under investigation. Finally, subjects' affective states slanted the emotional tone of their free associations, storytelling, personality descriptions, predictions about the future, and social perceptions of themselves and others.

The network theory supposes that these cognitive influences of emotional states follow "automatically" as a result of activation spreading from the emotion unit to related words, concepts, and themes. However, an alternative interpretation, applying specifically to those results obtained from hypnotic subjects, is that our suggestible subjects figure out what behaviors the experimenter is implicitly demanding by means of his mood-induction instructions. According to this hypothesis, having decided that the experimenter wants them to play the role of, say, a sad person, the subjects comply by behaving in all respects according to their conception of the "sad person" role. Thus, they report sad associations, sad memories, sad fantasies, and give pessimistic estimates of the future. Similarly, subjects told to be happy or angry comply by behaving according to their beliefs about the happy or angry role.

Clearly, if subjects are simply complying with experimental demands, our results are considerably less interesting. So the issue definitely must be confronted.

Ruling out the compliance hypothesis is relatively easy for the memory experiments; in those the explicit "demand" from the experimenter was for subjects to remember everything they could about the target material, regardless of its content. Nonetheless, the mood-matching effect on retrieval came through clearly in free recall. If the compliance hypothesis were to argue that our mood-dependent recall results show that subjects figured out what outcomes were wanted, the hypothesis would be strained beyond reason to explain why these prescient subjects did not show mood-dependency in memory tests involving recognition. Nor does the hypothesis explain why manipulations of mood only at recall (following neutral input of mixed items) caused no selective recall. The network theory explains both these anomalies, so it is the more parsimonious as well as the more fruitful theory.

In contrast to the memory studies, our results showing the influence of emotion on free associations, fantasies, social judgments, and probability estimates are more vulnerable to the charge of demand compliance. Ruling out the demand hypothesis has proven more challenging for such cases. Nonetheless, we believe several arguments can be marshaled against the demand-compliance hypothesis as a consistent explanation of the results, and we will review four such arguments here.

First, the emotions induced seem real and have little of the phenomenal character of a faked pretense. For example, measures of autonomic arousal such as changes in GSR and heart rate reveal changes during the suggested emotion similar to those during the actual emotional experience (e.g., Gidro-Frank & Bull, 1950; Zimbardo et al., 1972). Furthermore, our subjects looked, sounded, and acted as though they were really in the throes of their emotions: Sad subjects appeared morose, sometimes tearful, and happy subjects beamed, laughed, and exuded a sense of well-being. The authenticity of these moods was confirmed by subjects during postexperimental interviews that urged honest reporting.

Second, similar results have been obtained when the mood manipulation was not hypnotic in nature. We replicated the free-association and TAT results using disguised "mood music" (see Bower, 1981). Laird and his associates (1982) observed a mood-congruity effect in learning in a study where mood was induced by having subjects pose their face into unwitting frowning, smiling, or sorrowful expressions. Isen and her colleagues (1978) have obtained similar results when moods were induced in unobtrusive ways, including having subjects win or lose a computer game, find a dime in a phone booth, or receive a small gift (e.g., nail clippers, cookies). Bartlett and his associates (in press) induced moods in their kindergarten subjects by simply having them revivify and describe an emotional memory. Teasdale and Fogarty (1979) used the Velten procedure, in which subjects read a series of self-referent mood statements to access a particular mood. Thus, our results agree with those obtained when moods were induced by diverse means.

Third, the mood effects on performance often appear as predicted despite running counter to the experimenter's demand. A good example is the experiment by Teasdale and Fogarty (1979) in which happy or sad subjects were instructed to retrieve as fast as possible a stipulated pleasant or unpleasant incident from memory in response to neutral cue words. They found that happy subjects retrieved pleasant memories faster and sad subjects retrieved unpleasant memories faster, despite the experimenter's demand for fast retrieval in all cases.

Fourth, in some studies we have misled subjects about the experimenter's "demand." In one study, subjects wrote free-associations and TAT stories after being told that the experimenter's interest was in whether hypnosis would affect physical properties of handwriting. Whereas post-experimental interviews indicated that subjects believed the handwriting deception, the results showed that mood nonetheless biased the emotional content of subjects' associations and stories. Thus, systematically misleading subjects did not alter the general results.

We will tentatively conclude, therefore, that the mood effects we have observed are "automatic" and not the result of the subjects' compliance with a demanded role. Thus we believe that our use of hypnosis should be recognized as a minor and incidental aspect of our research. Of central importance is that mood can influence cognition in diverse ways. We will now consider an explanatory theory for these findings.

The network theory of affect

Basic assumptions

The results obtained in the preceding experiments can be accounted for by a network theory of affect, which represents memory as a rich associative network of concepts, schemata, and events. We will begin by stating some basic assumptions of the theory. First, emotions will be treated as central units in this network, with multiple associations to related schemata, concepts, and events. How these connections might include autonomic arousal patterns, action patterns, attitudes, beliefs, facial expressions, and interpretative schemata was illustrated in Figure 18.2. The contents of these general aspects of experience may be different for each mood.

To comment briefly on the "emotion node" hypothesis, a node in memory is defined primarily in terms of the other elements to which it is connected. An emotion node like "anger" differs from a concept node in only a few respects. First, at least some emotion nodes are liable to be inborn, with some innate connections to the facial musculature and autonomic nervous system. Second, once activated, emotion nodes receive reverberatory feedback from the autonomic response pattern they initiate, and this feedback cycle causes the activated emotion unit to persist for some time after its arousal. The activation eventually dies out (after removal from the evocative situation) by a natural dampening process. Such persistence of activation is unusual for a simple concept or idea, which typically disappears from working memory as soon as, say, the topic of conversation is changed. Third, the emotion nodes may be distinguished by the absolute amount of excitation that they transmit into the associative network once they pass threshold and are turned on. One might think of nodes in the network as small voltage sources (or signal boosters),

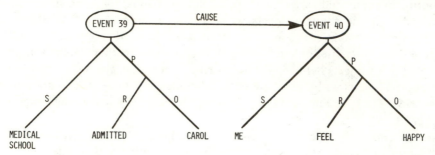

Figure 18.7. A semantic network encoding of a proposition ("medical school admitted Carol") and an emotion it causes. Lower nodes represent preexisting concepts, and lines represent new associations. S = subject; P = predicate; R = relation; and O = object.

and that, once aroused, emotion nodes simply send more "voltage" than concept nodes. This would cause an emotion to gain greater control than a thought over the direction and content of subsequent thoughts. Although we believe that "emotion nodes" in our theory have these unique properties, we should also note that none of these unique properties is needed to explain the results we have presented. We have listed these properties of emotion nodes in response to persistent requests to somehow distinguish emotion nodes from concept nodes within the framework of associative network theory.

Second, to continue our description of the theory, events become encoded within the network in terms of a set of propositions. For example, Figure 18.7 offers a simplified representation of how a person's joy at his friend's acceptance into medical school might be propositionally encoded.

Third, the process of thought is modeled by the activation (or excitation) of specific nodes in this network. Concept nodes that are activated above a threshold become available to consciousness and may issue into a response. Activation can spread among nodes (concepts, emotions, and propositions) according to their associative connections. An analogy is an electrical (or neuronal) network in which terminal junctures represent nodes, wires represent associative connections, a voltage imposed at specific junctures corresponds to activation of a pattern of nodes, and electrical current flowing from a voltage source to a remote juncture corresponds to the spread of activation. Spreading activation has become a standard retrieval theory in cognitive psychology (e.g., Anderson, 1976; Collins & Loftus, 1975); it also is suggestive of an analog for neural nets in the central nervous system.

Fourth, a concept or event can be activated directly by various means, including verbal symbols or physiological stimuli. For example, asking the person how he felt about his friend's medical school acceptance would activate the corresponding nodes in the network; similarly, inducing a mood in a subject (as in our experiments) corresponds to activating that emotion node.

Fifth, activation spreads from an activated node to varying degrees, thus providing a way to indirectly access associated nodes. For instance, activation of the "medical school" node in Figure 18.7 would likely spread to the "happy" node; similarly, activation of an emotion unit might activate neighboring nodes (e.g., mood-related autobiographical experiences).

Sixth, a propositionally encoded event becomes associated with other cognitive elements active at the time of learning. For example, Figure 18.3 illustrated how list words learned in a mood state might develop associative links to the node representing that mood. Finally, the "contents of consciousness" consist of those network nodes whose activation exceeds a threshold at a given time; the flow of activation is supposed to model the *process* of thought.

Explaining the mood-congruity effect. Subjects in the congruity experiments were placed in a happy or sad mood before reading a story consisting of a mixture of happy and sad episodes. According to the network theory, the induction of the mood activates the corresponding emotion node and (some of) its associates, thereby creating a mental context dominated by mood-related themata. Because of hypnotic suggestions to maintain the mood for the duration of the learning task, this mood-biased context is used by the subject to understand and elaborate upon the story materials. Mood-congruent material is easily elaborated because of its similarity to, and consistency with, the context themata, whereas mood-incongruent material is difficult to elaborate because it is inconsistent with such themata. The greater elaboration of mood-congruent material results in a network representation of it which has more interconnections with other memory structures than does mood-incongruent material. This greater number of connections results in better memory for the congruent items, because each link provides a potential retrieval path to the items during recall.

This "ease of elaboration" hypothesis may also explain why mood had no learning effect on mood-related items in our word-list experiment. Specifically, the nature of the learning task – a two-second presentation rate of relatively abstract words – did not encourage or permit elaboration of the words. This suggests, of course, that a mood-selective learning effect for single words could be produced if extensive elaboration were encouraged and enabled.

Explaining state-dependent recall. The network theory of affect provides a similar account of our results showing state-dependent recall of autobiographical events. An event becomes propositionally encoded in the network, with connections to its corresponding emotion node and other mood-related concepts (Figures 18.3 and 18.7). The induced mood activates these nodes, thus biasing the subject to initiate from them searches for mood-related memories. This biased search, in addition to the priming of mood-congruent memories via spreading activation from the excited emotion node, biases recall toward mood-congruent incidents.

This general explanation can be extended to the state-dependent recall study involving word lists. Figure 18.3 depicted the basic explanation of why mood provided a discriminating cue that enhanced or inhibited memory, depending on whether a list's learning and recall moods matched or mismatched. When lists are learned in opposite moods, each list would become associated to a different emotion node. At the time of recall, a mood would activate the corresponding emotion node and spread activation to its associates. Reinstating a target list's learning mood would result in superior recall because of the enhanced accessibility of *only* that list, as the other list would have been associated to a different emotion node. However, recalling while in a different mood – for example, trying to remember List 1 while in Mood 2 – would result in poor memory because the activated emotion node would (1) provide no retrieval paths to the target list and (2) make the alternate list more accessible (and thus augment its interference effect). As noted earlier, this explanation of state-dependent recall in terms of retrieval paths is consistent with the finding that the effect did not obtain when recognition tests were used, as the direct access to target items provided by recognition tests minimizes the need for retrieval cues.

Explaining the mood-intensity results. The network theory of affect explains the "mood-intensity" findings in terms of varying activation levels of an emotion concept. Specifically, intensifying a mood results in increased activation of its corresponding unit in the network and its associates. This causes consciousness to be flooded with mood-congruent associates, which narrows the subject's attention to mood-congruent cues (Easterbrook, 1959). This makes it difficult for the subject to respond to mood-irrelevant tasks or stimuli. The increased activation of a mood also amplifies the influence on behavior of an emotion's associated ideas and roles. As was illustrated in Figure 18.2, the nature of these concepts differs for each basic emotion. For example, "happiness" may be associated with high expectations of successful performances, optimism, confidence, and self-esteem; conversely, "sadness" probably calls forth expectancies of failures, exhaustion, and inwardly directed rumination, resulting in poor motivation for active performances. Each set of associates would have a different impact on a learning task. This may explain why the learning of mood-relevant items increased when a happy mood was intensified but decreased when a sad mood was intensified. Other theories such as Izard's (1972) differential-emotions theory do not derive such implications from first principles but rather simply assume that different emotions differ in their motivational properties.

Explaining the thought and judgment results. The network theory can also be applied to the research showing mood effects on other cognitive processes.

The mood biases in free associations follow by supposing that a person in a specific mood (say, sadness) will associate to a neutral word like *life* those words in the associative hierarchy to *life* that also receive activation from the mood. Thus, sad associations to *life*, such as *death* and *suffering*, will be chosen over more pleasant associations.

The mood bias in TAT stories is explained by supposing that the subject's mood activates and makes available certain themes such as success and romance (for happiness), or conflict and war (for anger), or failure and loss (for sadness). These themes are then elaborated using the characters shown in the TAT pictures.

The mood bias in personality sketches of acquaintances is viewed as a form of state-dependent memory. People probably have a heterogeneous collection of positive and negative opinions, facts, observations, and episodes about anyone they know well. When placed in, say, an angry mood and asked about an acquaintance, the person's memory selectively retrieves the negative (or unflattering) facts and opinions. Since these negative facts are highly available, the subject gives his "snap judgment" of the acquaintance based on them (see Tversky & Kahneman, 1973).

The mood bias in probability estimates of future events is explained as a form of state-dependent retrieval of past relevant events or opinions. For any given future event, whether a blessing or catastrophe, any well-educated person can usually think up some facts (or opinions) that argue for or against the likelihood of that event. The theory supposes that ideas that support positive ("happy") events and discourage negative events will be more available to the happy person, whereas the reverse will be true for the sad person. Introspections of happy and sad subjects during the event-estimation task provided some anecdotal support for this availability hypothesis.

Finally, the mood biasing of social perception of others or of oneself is predicted by the network theory, since social judgments are so heavily determined by the trait categories and schemata used by the observer. If the observer is happy, he tends to look for evidence of "positive" social behaviors in his target; if he is angry, he is biased to look for "negative" antisocial behaviors. Social behavior is sufficiently ambiguous and unconstrained that the perceiver will usually be able to find evidence for whatever trait category or schema he wishes to impose on the behaving target. This top-down determination of social impressions works just as strongly when people judge their own behavior as when they judge that of others.

Summary. The network theory of affect proposes that emotion plays a central role in a unified representation of mind. Basic emotions are viewed as innate elements or units that through experience become connected with various event memories, actions, roles, interpretation schemata, and themes. Activation of a mood is postulated to automatically activate varying numbers of these associates, depending on the intensity of the mood. This basic model provides an account of how mood affects cognitive processes of memory, learning, free association, interpretation, judgment, and prediction. It also explains how the influence of intensifying a mood can vary depending on the specific mood. The remaining section addresses some of the important questions that have not been discussed.

General comments

The network theory of affect suffices to explain reasonably well our experimental results. However, the theory has several flaws. In this final section we will identify some problems with the theory, and then discuss some issues central to theories of emotion. Because of space limitations, our discussion will be selective; the reader may consult Bower and Cohen (1982) for a fuller discussion of some of these ideas.

Retrieval cue overload. One of our major arguments has been that mood-congruent memories are recalled best because they are associated to the emotion node and are thus primed via spreading activation from that node. In other words, every event in a person's life involving, say, happiness is alleged to become linked to the "happy" emotion node in the network. An obvious problem with this assumption is that, without some means for separating different contexts, an astronomical number of experiences would become linked to each basic emotion node. With this many links, the small amount of activation spreading from that node distributed among its millions of outgoing branches would become extremely dissipated, to the extent that any specific targeted mood-related memory would receive insufficient activation to make its retrieval easier.

We must admit that this objection poses problems for our theory. Briefly stated, our best response is to assert that any retrieval within the network involves searches emanating from at least two cues, with the target items found at intersections of the retrieval paths. Thus the memory search process emanates not just from the happiness node but also from a node corresponding to other stimulus cues (e.g., "my friend" or "List 1" or "third grade"). By restricting the search domain in this manner, the "dissipation of activation" problem is a bit more manageable.

Representation of emotional intensity. Another potential problem is that our network model represents a basic emotion as a single unit that is qualitatively the same across different situations and different intensity levels. We noted earlier that intensity shifts, for example, could be conceived as involving quantitative (and not qualitative) changes in the activation of an emotion, perhaps indexed by autonomic arousal. However, certain problems are en-

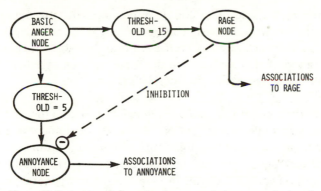

Figure 18.8. A network for activating one node (*annoyance*) when the system experiences a low level of anger and a different node (*rage*) when it experiences a high level of anger. Thresholds are indicated, as is an inhibitory connection (dashed line) from the higher-level to the lower-level node.

countered in an associative network when different emotional intensities are to be represented by the degree of activation of the same node.

An immediate problem is that people (and animals) can learn to make different responses to low versus high intensities of an emotion or drive. For example, we learn to label our mild angers as *annoyances*, moderate angers as *angers*, and extreme angers as *rages*. But to represent this in an associative network requires either special connections or something like an analog-to-digital converter that monitors the activation level of the node. The "special connections" are easily designed in networks using inhibitory links and different threshold elements. Figure 18.8 illustrates a simple network that will activate different nodes (*annoyance* or *rage*), depending on the activation level of the basic emotion node (of *anger*). The lower-intensity node requires a lower threshold for its activation, and the higher-intensity node must have inhibitory connections to all lower-intensity nodes, so that when the high-intensity node fires it shuts off the firing of any lower-intensity nodes connected to that basic emotion node. Whenever the *annoyance* or *rage* node fires, it sends activation to whatever actions and memories have been associated with the firing of that node (such as the label of *annoyance* or *rage*).

A similar complication caused by the assumption of a single unit for primitive emotions is that the theory should differentiate among subtle shadings of a given emotion, depending on its context of arousal and its object. Thus, the feeling of tender love will probably differ greatly between, say, a woman's tender love for her infant, husband, father, kitten, and old flame. Anger at one's failings probably differs from anger at an aggressive stranger or at a governmental policy. The theory handles all such cases by supposing that the anger (or love) node activated is the same in all cases; but that the context or object of the emotion are two other cognitive elements that, by intersection searches in conjunction with the basic emotion, cause different scripts, roles, and action patterns to be activated and retrieved into short-term memory. The subjective feeling reported is a mixture of the basic emotion together with the script appropriate to the target and the social situation.

Interaction of emotion, cognition, and behavior. Our research focused mainly on how emotional states influence cognitions. However, reciprocal interactions are to be expected; our cognitions obviously affect our emotions in many ways. Indeed, standard techniques for manipulating moods experimentally require the subject to dwell on certain thoughts or memories. Our hypnotic procedure is clearly of this kind. Another mood-induction method is that devised by Velten (1968), which suggests elation or depression in subjects by having them read a series of self-referential mood statements (e.g., "Things are going badly for me today") and imagine that these describe their feelings. Another procedure, used by Thompson, Cowan, and Rosenhan (1980), induces sadness by having subjects listen to a tape asking them to project themselves into a story about a close friend dying of cancer.

Almost all emotion theorists accord a central role to cognitions in emotional responses. Many theorists relate emotions to cognitive appraisals of actual, imagined, or anticipated transactions in terms of their meaning to the person's goals, self-image, beliefs, and well-being. The well-known "two-factor" theory of Schachter (1966; Schachter & Singer, 1962) suggested that emotion developed from a cognitive interpretation of physiological arousal; Mandler (1975) and Lazarus, Kanner, and Folkman (1980) present similar views about the complex interaction between autonomic arousal, cognitive interpretations, and actions.

The network theory is one representation of these interactions, as the theory conceives of the emotion node as being connected to patterns of autonomic arousal and to expressive behaviors (Figure 18.2). Importantly, these connections are reciprocal and two-way, that is, general autonomic arousal intensifies (amplifies) the activation of whatever emotional unit has already been selected by the cognitive system. This leads to the expectation that a background of excitement from irrelevant stimulation (such as physical exercise or a roller-coaster ride) will intensify any emotion (like anger or romantic love) elicited by a coincident provocation. Zillmann (1978) reviews much positive evidence for this "excitation transfer" hypothesis.

Another reciprocal influence on emotions comes from the face and bodily expressions. Cross-cultural research has shown that each of a limited set of basic emotions is associated with a characteristic facial expression (Ekman, Friesen, & Ellsworth, 1972). Facial expressions similar to those of real emotion occur even when the person simply produces imagery of a certain affective quality (e.g., Schwartz, Brown, & Ahern, 1980; Sirota & Schwartz, 1982). Evidence also suggests that the setting of the facial musculature and bodily postures will feed back activation to specific emotional units commonly associated with these poses. Laird and his colleagues (1982) found that subjects who configured their facial muscles unwittingly into a specific pose produced some of the corresponding emotional state. One could also expect competition among cognitive and facial determinants of emotion; thus, the time to retrieve and image clearly an anger scene should be slowed by having the subject's face posed in a smile; conversely, the image latency for a happy scene should be slowed by an angry facial pose. Such reciprocal influences are consistent with the network model, which posits two-way linkages.

The development of affective structures

Although the network model is a convenient summary of emotion-cognition interactions, it gives us no clue about how many emotions there are or how they are developed. We feel these issues are outside our area of research and expertise, but as a theory should address these issues, we will hazard a few comments.

An associative (or semantic) network is a kind of formal "language" in which to transcribe theoretical guesses about the internal representation of concepts and events. This is done at the functional level of those elements that are connected to other units. Every language needs a base set of primitive elements in its "vocabulary" to build up higher-level ideas of structures. Thus, semantic-memory theories (such as HAM of Anderson & Bower, 1973, or the conceptual-dependency theory of Schank, 1975) assume that each infant begins with a base set of neural elements that are genetically prespecified to become sensory elements, action elements, and perhaps conceptual elements under appropriate environmental stimulation. For example, given appropriate stimulation, certain neurons along the visual pathways and in the visual cortex would be prespecified to become sensitive, say, to red light. Thus, we would say that "red light" would be a primitive element in the base set of percepts of most infants.

Second, associative theories stipulate a set of relations (among elements) and rules for building up more complex descriptions of objects and events out of relations among primitive elements. For example, a visual square would be characterized by the visual cortex as an object formed by parallel vertical and horizontal lines connected at right angles. From the base set of elements and relations, the brain can then build up arbitrarily complex descriptions of physical or conceptual objects; and it is the internal representations of these structural descriptions that are stored in memory. There is nothing esoteric or mysterious about this: A familiar analogy is that natural languages like English build up an unlimited number of arbitrarily complex words from a vocabulary of 26 letters plus a space and the relation of "successor."

From such logical necessities, the network theory of emotions is led to postulate a beginning set of basic emotions that are genetically prespecified for each human infant. We do not know how to decide how many primitive emotions an infant has or what they are, but other scientists such as Izard (1972; Izard & Buechler, 1980) have come to reasonable conjectures of six to nine primitive emotions. Typical basic emotions are interest-excitement, enjoyment-joy, surprise-startle, distress-anguish, anger-rage, disgust-revulsion, contempt-scorn, fear-terror, and shame-humiliation.

The existence of such innate emotions is suggested by several lines of evidence: (1) the sharing across species of common emotional responses such as distress, startle, interest, revulsion, and aggression (see Strongman, 1978, chap. 7); (2) the cross-cultural similarities of facial expressions in various emotions (Izard, 1971; Ekman, Friesen, & Ellsworth, 1972); and (3) the emotional expressions of very young infants (e.g., Izard, 1971; Izard & Buechler, 1980).

The network theory would suppose that these primitive emotions exist as innate units in the network, each with innate connections to a cortical and autonomic arousal pattern and to its pattern of facial-bodily expression. Also a few innate "productions" (S-R connections) would be needed to recognize stimulus situations in which the indicated emotional unit should be fired. From these rudimentary beginnings, the infant enters into a lifetime of learning through acculturation. The associative network model is capable of representing most of this learning and differentiation.

This cultural learning is extensive and goes on at several different levels. One type of learning involves increasing "stimulus learning and differentiation," with the infant learning to recognize more and more subtle situations that call for a particular emotion. Included would be the infant's learning of specific emotional reactions to specific persons, events, and topics. A second type of learning involves increasing "response learning." Each culture teaches its members certain social "scripts" (see Abelson, 1981; Schank & Abelson, 1977) for conventional displays of specific emotions. These emotional scripts are lengthy action routines, which are modeled for the child repeatedly by his social community. Thus, he learns the accepted cultural scripts for showing romantic love, for grief, shame, loneliness, and so on. These scripts are elaborated around the core of innate behaviors associated with the emotion; thus, the shamed person may put on the same face across cultures, although what he does with his shame – retribution, public breast-beating, or quiet isolation – will vary across cultures. Of course, idiosyncratic variations on these emotional scripts are frequent.

A third form of learning involves increasing differentiations of the primitive emotions. This is accomplished by subcategorizing situations and appropriate behavioral scripts that formerly fell under a given primitive emotion. One subcategorization is according to the intensity of the appropriate emotional reaction. As mentioned earlier (in Figure 18.8), the network model can represent the experience of different intensities of an emotion by "turning on" different nodes in the network, and these will call forth different response repertoires. Another type of differentiation involves setting up a cognitive unit to represent subtle shadings in subjective feelings attendant upon arousal of different thoughts when a common core emotion is aroused. For example, the core emotion of *interest* will be differentiated and labeled *intellectual curiosity* in one evoking situation, *romantic pursuit* in another, and *thrill-seeking* in still another. Although arousal of the emotion of *interest* is common, these feelings are differentiated not only by their evoking situations and the scripts followed but also by the other emotions and thoughts aroused during prototypical occasions.

This differentiation process is both creative and unbounded, which explains why the English language has nearly 18,000 words referring roughly to shades of emotional feelings or character traits (reported in Allport & Odbert, 1936). Our emotion vocabulary is a motley collection of words that differ in describing the quality of a feeling, its cause, goal, intensity, and its duration; the vocabulary even includes enduring character traits. Such a vocabulary is neither well ordered, logically constructed, nor taught with any precision to language users. Consequently, psychologists cannot hope to discover much about the primitive emotions by factor analyses of adults' judgments about the similarities of emotion words, any more than we learned anything about the physiology of color vision by analyzing our color vocabulary. However, such analyses may tell us something about cultural commonalities in the teaching of emotional terms.

Automatic versus controlled processes in emotion

We have interpreted our results as indicative of automatic (or spontaneous) influences of emotion on cognition rather than as a result of conscious intention to play a role. We may follow Posner and Snyder (1975) in defining *automatic processes* as those that occur without awareness (attention), without intention, and without interfering with other mental processes. Posner and Snyder contrast automatic with *controlled processes*, which require awareness (attentional resources), intention, time and effort to implement, and interfere with other ongoing mental processes.

Following Clark and Isen (1982), we feel that this distinction is useful for emotions, too. Clearly, people have learned diverse methods for controlling their moods and emotional reactions – for prolonging or terminating a mood, for blunting or augmenting an emotional reaction, for even transforming the affective significance of emotional stimuli (e.g., the ecstasy of the religious martyr).

The control strategies for moods involve some purposive manipulation of either our physical state, our environment, or our thoughts, images, and memories. People learn to alter their physical state through the use of psychoactive drugs, muscle relaxation (with or without biofeedback), deep-breathing exercises, and physical exercise. People try to control their mood by environmental alterations, as when they go to parties, amusement parks, vacation resorts, entertainments (dramas, plays, movies, music), or when they call a friend or engage in absorbing activities to distract themselves from dwelling on their mood.

People also control their emotions by their cognitions about the event in question, by the way they categorize the event initially, by the evaluation and significance they assign to it, and by the persistent rehearsal of self-talk associated with the event. Thus, if someone publicly says that your hairstyle looks silly, you are likely to interpret that as a belittling insult that arouses anger. If you recycle the insult in short-term memory and repeat self-sentences about the event and the target ("What right does he have to embarrass me?"), such repeated thoughts will sustain the anger. Conversely, the anger could be circumvented by interpreting the remark differently in the first place. For example, you might regard it as simple information, or as reflecting good intentions of the observer, or as involving an unimportant issue for you. Alternatively, you can stop the angry self-sentences by counting to ten or by filling consciousness with well-rehearsed distracting or anger-coping thoughts such as "Don't lose your temper. Keep calm." The learning of such emotional self-control procedures is of major concern in psychotherapy with neurotic patients, especially in cognitive behavior therapy (e.g., Meichenbaum, 1977). In such therapy, patients are taught cognitive strategies ("thinking habits") for coping with emotional problems such as anxiety, stress, pain, anger provocations, and depression.

In the network theory, we would represent these cognitive coping responses as "implicit habits" that become associated with (and triggered by) the activation of the relevant emotion node. These coping responses are able to fill short-term memory with distracting or countervailing thoughts and thus prevent the emotional reaction from facilitating itself (via its activated thoughts). In the absence of self-facilitation, the emotion dies out within a few seconds. Thus, the functions of "counting to ten" when a person is provoked to anger are (1) to fill short-term memory with innocuous material, (2) to prevent thinking about angry ideas primed by the provocation, and (3) with the passage of time to allow the initial emotional arousal to dissipate to zero.

Interestingly, people also deliberately use emotional events as modulators of other behaviors they must perform. These sorts of strategies were noted by Lazarus and his colleagues (1980). Thus, to persist in a taxing goal-directed effort (e.g., writing a book), people may use *sustainers*, which rekindle the motivation for completing the task (e.g., imagining the rewards at the end); they may take *breathers* (a rest), which temporarily disengage them from the fatiguing or stressful task, allowing the stress system to recover; or they may use *restorers* (vacations), which allow recuperation from the long, exhausting tasks that overstressed them. These restorative measures are often useful in everyday stress management, and problems such as "job burnout" may result from their neglect.

Of course, emotional controls are not always socially appropriate or available. When they are not, psychological problems may result. For example, the person may overuse certain control strategies and thereby obstruct the natural "flow" of emotional experience. This is exemplified by the overly "inhibited" person who so rarely expresses his feelings that he loses the ability to feel much of anything. Furthermore, attempts at emotional control may backfire, as when a high-strung insomniac tries to command himself to relax and fall asleep and in this way exacerbates his tension. Strategies can also be socially inappropriate and dysfunctional, such as the drug addict who tries desperately to re-create a "high" through chemical means, or the person who habitually dulls the impact of negative emotions with tranquilizers. Finally, as noted earlier, many clinical problems arise from the absence of emotional controls: Examples include the depressive whose spiraling cycle of pessimistic cognitions and negative mood go unchecked; the premature ejaculator who cannot control the intensity of his sexual arousal; and the aggressive person who is easily provoked to outbursts.

In short, control processes can powerfully affect emotional experience. They may be overused, applied inappropriately, or not available. The vast number of them and their ability to enhance or limit the quality of one's experience suggest that it would be useful to gain a more thorough understanding of them. This knowledge could be used not only for furthering a theoretical understanding of emotion but also for therapeutic applications and perhaps the development of educational programs to enhance people's abilities to use control processes beneficially.

Appraisals of emotional events

In this chapter we have examined the cognitive consequences of arousing an emotion, but we have not discussed how emotional reactions are triggered in the first place. Bower and Cohen's (1982) work extends the network model to deal with the elicitation of emotional reactions. In principle, recognizing situations in which one should feel frightened, angry, or sad should not differ greatly from recognizing objects, scenes, and social situations that would be categorized in non-emotional terms. The same issues of stimulus-pattern recognition arise, and complex decision rules will be needed to characterize a person's social discriminations for evoking different emotions.

Bower and Cohen suggested that the initiation of emotional reactions could be modeled in terms of generalized habits, which they called "emotional interpretation rules" or "productions." A production is like an S-R habit designed to recognize a configuration or pattern of relevant variables (the S) that describe a situation; when its pattern is matched (recognized), the production is fired, causing the appropriate emotional units (the R) to become activated and to thus enter consciousness. An example of such an emotional interpretation rule is: IF someone harms you and he could have prevented it, THEN feel anger at that person. The stimulus conditions for such productions are presumed to exist in an abstraction hierarchy, so that diverse events can come to be categorized, say, as "harmful to you." Furthermore, a given situation or social remark might be recognized by several productions; for example, a sarcastic quip can be interpreted either as merely funny or as a personal attack. Which interpretation is selected depends on the current strength of the different productions. Bower and Cohen handled this issue by supposing that emotional interpretation rules are themselves connected to the emotions they turn on; thus, for example, when someone is feeling angry, productions that result in, or sustain, anger will be temporarily strengthened. Their greater strength implies that these rules will most likely be selected to control the interpretation of ambiguous situations. This means that people will interpret ambiguous emotional signals in a way congruent with their current emotion. These are exactly the sort of emotion-driven interpretive biases that one wants a theory to have.

Reappraisals of events from memory

Bower and Cohen also proposed that an episode causing an emotional reaction would be stored in memory as a triad: the description of the episode, the emotions it aroused, and the emotional interpretation rule by which that episode called forth those emotions. Bower and Cohen noted several reasons for storing the interpretative rule with the episode-emotion connection. One reason is that the rule enables the person later to explain why he had the emotional reaction that he did. A second important reason is that memory of the rule used in the original interpretation is often used in reinterpreting or changing one's appraisal of an earlier event. By replaying the remembered experience and reappraising it according to an altered rule or in an altered context, a different emotional reaction may be assigned to the event.

Some reasons for altering an emotional appraisal can be cited briefly. First, the person may receive *new information*. For example, the anger associated to the event of a friend not showing up for a date might be replaced with guilt when you hear that the friend had been seriously injured in an auto accident on the way to the date. Second, a *change in attitudes or values* may occur between the event and its reappraisal. For example, a teen-ager's contempt for his parents' physical weakness may be replaced later by tolerance and compassion for the infirmities of the aged. Third, a reinterpretation might be prompted by a *shift in evaluation mood*. For instance, a husband who is exhausted and cranky may be very upset with his wife's tardiness in preparing dinner; when feeling rested on the following day, he may reappraise that scene and now feel guilty about his insensitivity. Fourth, an event may *change in im-*

portance because of consequent events. For example, the sadness associated with being rejected from one job would dissipate quickly if soon afterward an offer of a better job was received. Finally, there may be a *change in goals or interests*. Thus, the excitement once associated with a honeymoon experience may be replaced with anger and sadness following a bitter divorce.

To summarize, control processes are used in many ways to alter emotional responses to past, present, and future (anticipated) events. The obvious therapeutic value of such controls is reflected by the many psychotherapies that emphasize methods for altering or coping with emotional associations; for example, aversive conditioning (e.g., McGuire & Vallance, 1964; Thorpe et al., 1964), systematic desensitization (e.g., Wolpe, 1958), and hypnotherapy (e.g., Kroger & Fezler, 1976). Many forms of psychotherapy strive for periodic reappraisals of critical life events and memories of them. Such reappraisals often lie at the heart of insight and growth toward psychological maturity.

References

Abelson, R. P. Psychological status of the script concept. *American Psychologist*, 1981, *36*, 715–729

Abernathy, E. M. The effect of changed environmental conditions upon the results of college examinations. *Journal of Psychology*, 1940, *10*, 293–301.

Allport, G. W., & Odbert, H. S. Trait-names: A psycho-lexical study. *Psychological Monographs*, 1936, *47* (1, Whole No. 211).

Anderson, J. R. *Language, memory and thought*. Hillsdale, N.J.: Erlbaum, 1976.

Anderson, J., & Bower, G. H. *Human associative memory*. Washington, D.C.: Winston, 1973.

Anderson, J. R., & Reder, L. M. An elaborative processing explanation of depth of processing. In L. S. Cermak & F. I. M. Craik (Eds.), *Levels of processing in human memory*. Hillsdale, N.J.: Erlbaum, 1979.

Bahrick, H. P., Fitts, P. M., & Rankin, R. E. Effect of incentives upon reactions to peripheral stimuli. *Journal of Experimental Psychology*, 1952, *44*, 400–406.

Bartlett, J. C., & Santrock, J. W. Affect-dependent episodic memory in young children. *Child Development*, 1979, *50*, 513–518.

Blum, G. S. Hypnosis in psychodynamic research. In J. E. Gordon (Ed.), *Handbook of clinical and experimental hypnosis*. New York: Macmillan, 1967.

Bower, G. H. Experiments on story comprehension and recall. *Discourse Processes*, 1978, *1*, 211–231.

Bower, G. H. Mood & memory. *American Psychologist*, 1981, *36*, 129–148.

Bower, G. H., & Cohen, P. R. Emotional influences in memory and thinking: Data and theory. In S. Fiske & M. Clark (Eds.), *Affect and social cognition*. Hillsdale, N.J.: Erlbaum, 1982.

Bower, G. H., & Gilligan, S. C. Remembering information related to one's self. *Journal of Research in Personality*, 1979, *13*, 420–432.

Bower, G. H., & Gilligan, S. G. *Emotional mood and remembering one's autobiography*. Unpublished manuscript, Stanford University, 1980.

Bower, G. H., Gilligan, S. G., & Monteiro, K. P. Selectivity of learning caused by affective states. *Journal of Experimental Psychology: General*, 1981, *110*, 451–473.

Bower, G. H., Monteiro, K. P., & Gilligan, S. G. Emotional mood as a context for learning and recall. *Journal of Verbal Learning and Verbal Behavior*, 1978, *17*, 573–587.

Bursill, A. E. The restriction of peripheral vision during exposure to hot and humid conditions. *Quarterly Journal of Experimental Psychology*, 1958, *10*, 123–129.

Callaway, E., & Stone, G. Re-evaluating the focus of attention. In L. Uhr & J. G. Miller (Eds.), *Drugs and behavior*. New York: Wiley, 1960.

Clark, M. S., & Isen, A. M. The relationship between feeling states and social behavior. In A. H. Hastorf & A. M. Isen (Eds.), *Cognitive social psychology*. New York: Elsevier North-Holland, 1982.

Collins, A. M., & Loftus, E. F. A spreading-activation theory of semantic processing. *Psychological Review*, 1975, *82*, 407–428.

Collins, A. M., & Quillian, M. R. Retrieval time from semantic memory. *Journal of Verbal Learning and Verbal Behavior*, 1969, *8*, 240–247.

Cornsweet, D. J. Use of cues in the visual periphery under conditions of arousal. *Journal of Experimental Psychology*, 1969, *80*, 14–18.

Crasilneck, H. B., & Hall, J. A. Physiological changes associated with hypnosis: A review of the literature since 1948. *International Journal of Clinical and Experimental Hypnosis*, 1959, *7*, 9–50.

Damaser, E. C., Shor, R. E., & Orne, M. T. Physiological effects during hypnotically requested emotions. *Psychosomatic Medicine*, 1963, *25*, 334–343.

Dutta, S., & Kanungo, R. N. *Affect and memory: A reformulation*. Oxford: Pergamon Press, 1975.

Easterbrook, J. A. The effect of emotion on cue utilization and the organization of behavior. *Psychological Review*, 1959, *66*, 183–201.

Ekman, P., Friesen, W. V., & Ellsworth, P. *Emotion in the human face*. New York: Pergamon Press, 1972.

Eich, J. E. The cue-dependent nature of state-dependent retrieval. *Memory and Cognition*, 1980, *8*, 157–173.

Eich, J., Weingartner, H., Stillman, R. C., & Gillin, J. C. State-dependent accessibility of retrieval cues in the retention of a categorized list. *Journal of Verbal Learning and Verbal Behavior*, 1975, *14*, 408–417.

Forgas, J. P., Bower, G. H., & Krantz, S. E. *Mood and self-perception in formal and informal settings*. Manuscript in preparation, 1983.

Gidro-Frank, L., & Bull, N. Emotions induced and studied in hypnotic subjects, Part I: The method. *Journal of Nervous and Mental Disease*, 1950, *111*, 91–100.

Godden, D. R., & Baddeley, A. D. Context-dependent memory in two natural environments: On land and under water. *British Journal of Psychology*, 1975, *66*, 325–331.

Gottlieb, A. A., Gleser, G. C., & Gottschalk, L. A. Verbal and physiological responses to hypnotic suggestion of attitudes. *Psychosomatic Medicine*, 1967, *29*, 172–183.

Henry, G., Weingartner, H., & Murphy, D. Influence of affective states and psychoactive drugs on verbal learning and memory. *American Journal of Psychiatry*, 1973, *130*, 966–971.

Hepps, R. B., & Brady, J. P. Hypnotically induced tachycardia: An experiment with stimulating controls. *Journal of Nervous and Mental Disease*, 1967, *145*, 131–137.

Hilgard, E. R. *Hypnotic susceptibility*. New York: Harcourt, Brace & World, 1965.

Holmes, T. S. Differential change in affective intensity and the forgetting of unpleasant personal experiences. *Journal of Personality and Social Psychology*, 1970, *15*, 234–239.

Hull, C. L. *Hypnosis and suggestibility: An experimental approach*. New York: Appleton-Century-Crofts, 1933.

Isen, A. M., Shalker, T., Clark, M., & Karp, L. Affect, accessibility of material in memory and behavior: A cognitive loop? *Journal of Personality and Social Psychology*, 1978, *36*, 1–12.

Izard, C. E. *The face of emotion*. New York: Appleton-Century-Crofts, 1971.

Izard, C. E. *Patterns of emotions: A new analysis of anxiety and depression*. New York: Academic Press, 1972.

Izard, C. E., & Buechler, S. Aspects of consciousness and reality. In R. Plutchik & H. Kellerman (Eds.), *Emotion: Theory, research, and experience*. New York: Academic Press, 1980.

Kanungo, R. N., & Dutta, S. Retention of affective material: Frame of reference or intensity? *Journal of Personality and Social Psychology*, 1966, *4*, 27–35.

Kroger, W. S., & Fezler, W. D. *Hypnosis and behavior modification: Imagery conditioning.* Philadelphia: Lippincott, 1976.

Laird, J. D., Wagener, J. J., Halal, M., & Szegda, M. Remembering what you feel: The effects of emotion on memory. *Journal of Personality and Social Psychology*, 1982, *42*, 646–657.

Lazarus, R. S., Kanner, A. D., & Folkman, I. Emotions: A cognitive-phenomenological analysis. In R. Plutchik & H. Kellerman (Eds.), *Emotion: Theory, research, and experience* (Vol. 1). New York: Academic Press, 1980.

Lloyd, G. C., & Lishman, W. A. Effect of depression on the speed of recall of pleasant and unpleasant experiences. *Psychological Medicine*, 1975, *5*, 173–180.

Mandler, G. *Mind and emotion.* New York: Wiley, 1975.

Matlin, M., & Stang, D. *The Pollyanna principle: Selectivity in language, memory, and thought.* Cambridge, Mass.: Schenkman, 1979.

McGuire, R. J., & Vallance, M. Aversion therapy by electric shock: A simple technique. *British Medical Journal*, 1964, *1*, 151–160.

McNamara, H., & Fisch, R. Effect of high and low motivation on two aspects of attention. *Perceptual and Motor Skills*, 1964, *19*, 571–578.

Meichenbaum, D. *Cognitive-behavior modification: An integrative approach.* New York: Plenum, 1977.

Nagge, J. W. An experimental test of the theory of associative interference. *Journal of Experimental Psychology*, 1935, *18*, 663–682.

Orne, M. T. The nature of hypnosis: Artifact and essence. *Journal of Abnormal and Social Psychology*, 1959, *58*, 277–299.

Parker, E. S., Birnbaum, I. M., & Noble, E. P. Alcohol and memory: Storage and state-dependency. *Journal of Verbal Learning and Verbal Behavior*, 1976, *15*, 691–702.

Plutchik, R. A general psychoevolutionary theory of emotion. In R. Plutchik & H. Kellerman (Eds.), *Emotion: Theory, research and experience* (Vol. 1). New York: Academic Press, 1980.

Posner, M. I., & Snyder, C. R. Attention and cognitive control. In R. L. Solso (Ed.), *Information processing and cognition: The Loyola symposium.*. Hillsdale, N.J.: Erlbaum, 1975.

Roth, D., & Rehm, L. P. Relationships among self-monitoring processes, memory, and depression. *Cognitive Therapy and Research.* 1980, *2*, 149–157.

Sarbin, T. R. Physiological effects of hypnotic stimulation. In R. M. Dorcus (Ed.), *Hypnosis and its therapeutic applications*, pp. 1–57. New York: McGraw-Hill, 1956.

Schachter, S. The interaction of cognitive and physiological determinants of emotional state. In C. D.. Spielberger (Ed.), *Anxiety and behavior.* New York: Academic Press, 1966.

Schachter, S., & Singer, J. E. Cognitive, social, and physiological determinants of emotional state. *Psychological Review*, 1962, *69*, 379–399.

Schank, R. C. *Conceptual information processing.* Amsterdam: North-Holland, 1975.

Schank, R. C., & Abelson, R. P. *Scripts, plans, goals, and understanding.* Hillsdale, N.J.: Erlbaum, 1977.

Schiffenbauer, A. Effect of observer's emotional state on judgments of the emotional state of others. *Journal of Personality and Social Psychology*, 1974, *30*(1), 31–35.

Schwartz, G. E., Brown, S. L., & Ahern, G. L. Facial muscle patterning and subjective experience during affective imagery: Sex differences. *Psychophysiology*, 1980, *17*, 75–82.

Sirota, A. D., & Schwartz, G. E. Facial muscle patterning and lateralization during elation and depression imagery. *Journal of Abnormal Psychology*, 1982, *91*, 25–34.

Shor, R. E., & Orne, E. C. *The Harvard Group Scale of Hypnotic Susceptibility, Form A.* Palo Alto, Calif.: Consulting Psychologists Press, 1962.

Smith, S. M., Glenberg, A., & Bjork, R. A. Environmental context and human memory. *Memory and Cognition*, 1978, *6*, 342–353.

Strongman, K. T. *The psychology of emotion.* New York: Wiley, 1978.

Teasdale, J. D., & Fogarty, S. J. Differential effects of induced mood on retrieval of pleasant and unpleasant events from episodic memory. *Journal of Abnormal Psychology*, 1979, *88*, 248–257.

Thompson, W. C., Cowan, C. L., & Rosenhan, D. L. Focus of attention mediates the impact of negative affect on altruism. *Journal of Personality and Social Psychology*, 1980, *2*, 291–300.

Thorpe, J. G., Schmidt, F., Brown, P. T., & Castell, D. Aversion-relief therapy: A new method for general application. *Behavioral Research and Therapy*, 1964, *2*, 71–84.

Tulving, F., & Thomson, D. M. Encoding specificity and retrieval processes in episodic memory. *Psychological Review*, 1973, *80*, 352, 373.

Tversky, A., & Kahneman, D. Availability: A heuristic for judging frequency and probability. *Cognitive Psychology*, 1973, *5*, 207–232.

Velten, E. A laboratory task for induction of mood states. *Behaviour Research and Therapy*, 1968, *6*, 473–482.

Weitzenhoffer, A. M., & Hilgard, E. R. *Stanford Hypnotic Susceptibility Scale, Form C*. Palo Alto, Calif.: Consulting Psychologists Press, 1962.

Wolpe, J. *Psychotherapy by reciprocal inhibition*. Stanford, Calif.: Stanford University Press, 1958.

Wright, W. F., & Bower, G. H. *Mood effects on subjective probability assessment*. Unpublished manuscript, Stanford University, 1981.

Zillmann, D. Attribution and misattribution of excitatory reactions. In J. H. Harvey, W. Ickes, & R. F. Kidd (Eds.), *New directions in attribution research* (Vol. 2). Hillsdale, N.J.: Erlbaum, 1978.

Zimbardo, P. G., Maslach, C., & Marshall, G. Hypnosis and the psychology of cognitive and behavioral control. In E. Fromm & R. E. Shor (Eds.), *Hypnosis: Research developments and perspectives*. Chicago: Aldine, 1972.

Author index

Abelson, R. P., 82, 580
Abernathy, E. M., 549
Abrams, R., 330
Abramson, L. Y., 467
Adamec, R. E., 30
Adams, J. A., 78
Aderman, D., 454, 455
Adrian, E., 141
Ahern, G. L., 578
Ainsworth, M., 237, 293, 295, 371, 385, 386, 394
Ajuriaguerra, J. D., 327
Akert, K., 329
Alford, L. B., 327
Alloy, L. B., 467
Allport, F., 234
Allport, G. W., 516, 519, 581
Als, H., 380, 382
Amenson, C. S., 446
Amrhein, J., 468
Anderson, J., 549, 555, 579
Anderson, J. R., 94, 196, 559, 572
Anderson, L. K., 454
Anderson, P. J., 329
Anderson, R. C., 417, 425
Andrew, R. J., 323
Andrews, R., 383, 386, 391
Anisman, H., 146
Anson, J. M., 323
Anthony, E. J., 395
Appel, M., 254
Archibald, Y., 354
Arend, R., 290, 291, 293, 367, 384
Arieti, S., 371, 374
Arnold, M., 234, 311
Arnold, M. B., 266, 415, 416
Aron, A. P., 493
Aronfreed, J., 104, 152
Aronson, E., 494
Asher, S. R., 298
Ashton-Jones, G., 135
Atkinson, J. W., 183
Atwood, G. E., 539
Averill, J. R., 46, 266, 447
Ax, A. F., 193

Baddeley, A., 83, 84
Baddeley, A. D., 549
Bahrick, H. P., 562
Baker, A., 367
Ballif, B., 22
Bandura, A., 244
Baranovskaya, Q. P., 329
Bard, P., 79
Barden, R. C., 441, 442, 445, 448, 451, 453, 469
Barenboim, C., 443
Bargh, J., 87
Barnett, M., 477
Barnett, M. A., 451
Barrera, M., 254
Barrett, K., 244
Barrett, K. C., 11
Bartlett, J. C., 469, 553, 570
Bashore, T. R., 352
Bates, E., 380
Baumann, D. J., 451, 472, 476
Bear, D. N., 327
Beck, A., 370
Beck, A. T., 330, 485, 511n2
Becker, J., 370
Beebe-Center, J., 230
Beeghly, M., 440
Bell, B. A., 479
Bell, P. A., 149
Bell, Q., 517, 526, 527, 529
Bell, R., 382, 383
Bell, S., 385
Bell, S. M., 108
Bem, D., 23
Bem, D. J., 75, 493
Benesh-Weiner, M., 174, 175
Bennett, J., 343, 344
Benson, D. F., 328, 355
Bergman, T., 254
Berkowitz, L., 474
Berlin, B., 45
Berlyne, D., 247, 369, 371, 378
Berlyne, D. E., 267
Berry, P., 383, 386, 387, 391
Berscheid, E., 252

Bertenthal, B., 244
Bertenthal, B. I., 394
Betts, G. H., 208
Bills, A. G., 83
Birch, H., 382
Birnbaum, I. M., 550
Birns, B., 290
Birthnell, J., 334
Bjork, R. A., 549
Bleuler, E., 370
Blevings, G., 83
Block, H., 83
Bloom, F. E., 135, 142
Blos, P., 533
Blum, G. S., 549, 561
Boccia, M., 243
Bolan, R., 89
Bolles, R. C., 187
Borke, H., 110, 411, 413, 425, 443
Bottenberg, E. H., 167
Boucher, J., 229, 239
Bower, G. H., 14, 22, 23, 33, 73, 80, 88, 139,
    140, 196, 210, 245, 274, 453, 454, 466, 469,
    480, 511n2, 540, 549, 550, 551, 552, 553,
    554, 555, 556, 557, 558, 560, 566, 568, 570,
    576, 579, 583, 584
Bower, T., 255
Bower, T. G. R., 145
Bowlby, J., 24, 231, 244, 371
Brachfeld, S., 382
Brady, J. P., 201, 549
Brazelton, T., 232, 293
Brazelton, T. B., 370, 379, 380, 382
Breedlove, D. E., 45
Brehm, J. W., 169
Brentano, F., 369
Bretherton, I., 386, 440
Breuer, J., 230
Bridges, F., 380, 383
Bridges, K., 374
Bridges, K. M. B., 173, 174
Bridgman, P. W., 439
Brierly, L., 395
Briggs, J. L., 39, 46
Brinker, R. P., 268
Broadbent, D. E., 139, 141
Brodal, K. A., 135
Bronson, G. W., 145, 147, 148, 150, 232, 247,
    303
Brooks, J., 377
Brooks-Gunn, J., 270, 392, 393, 394
Brophy, J. E., 179
Brossard, M., 232
Brown, B. B., 201
Brown, C., 375, 380, 382
Brown, S. L., 578
Brucken, L., 64
Bruder, G. E., 333
Bruner, J., 233, 246, 255

Bruner, J. S., 146
Bryan, J. H., 465, 474
Bryant, J., 493
Bryden, M., 337
Buck, R., 236, 271
Buckhalt, J., 380
Buddin, B., 255
Buechler, S., 151, 290, 370, 374, 580
Buhler, C., 252, 254, 255
Buium, N., 380
Bull, N., 76, 78, 89, 91, 549, 570
Bullowa, M., 233
Burch, N. R., 506
Burger, J. M., 168
Burns, N., 411, 413, 414
Bursill, A. E., 562
Burton, M. J., 135
Bush, L. E., 194
Bushnell, M. C., 141
Buss, A. H., 142
Butterworth, G., 380
Byrne, E., 149

Cacioppo, J. T., 85
Callaway, E., 562
Campbell, B. A., 146
Campbell, H., 283
Campos, J. J., 11, 25, 28, 30, 57, 142, 151,
    235, 237, 239, 240, 241, 242, 243, 244, 251,
    254, 270, 348, 350, 370, 372, 374, 387
Camras, L. A., 443
Cannon, W., 234
Cannon, W. B., 79, 195, 438
Canon, L. K., 77
Cantor, J. R., 493, 511n1
Carey, W., 383
Carlsmith, J. M., 494
Carlson, C. R., 13, 449, 453, 454
Carlson, G., 229, 239
Carlson, R., 539
Carpenter, G., 370, 371
Carstens, A. A., 268
Cartwright-Smith, J., 21, 376
Cavey, L., 411, 413, 414
Chance, J. E., 88
Chandler, C., 179
Chandler, M., 367, 397
Chandler, M. J., 410, 413, 425, 443
Charlesworth, W. R., 148, 233, 252, 254, 255,
    372, 374, 375, 376
Chess, S., 142, 382
Christoff, N., 329
Chute, D. L., 88
Cialdini, R., 472
Cialdini, R. B., 451, 454, 455, 475, 476
Cicchetti, D., 12, 311, 367, 369, 370, 372,
    373, 375, 377, 378, 379, 380, 382, 383, 386,
    387, 390, 391, 392, 393, 396
Clark, M., 474

Clark, M. S., 581
Clarke, S., 232
Clavier, R. M., 137
Clyburn, A., 451, 473
Cohen, B. D., 334
Cohen, P. R., 576, 583, 584
Cohn, J., 232, 254
Colby, C. Z., 89
Collins, A. M., 80, 555, 572
Comer, R., 21, 89
Connor, W. H., 474
Conrad, R., 83
Cook, E. W., III, 209, 214
Cooper, H. M., 168
Cooper, J., 492, 501
Corbitt, J. D., 283
Cornsweet, D. J., 562
Courts, F. A., 83
Cowan, C. L., 453, 477, 578
Coyle, J. T., 323
Crasilneck, H. B., 549
Cronin, D., 334
Crosby, M., 89, 509
Crowne, D. P., 331
Cummings, M., 387
Cytryn, L., 380

Dahl, H., 410, 415, 416, 417, 418, 419, 421, 422, 423, 424, 425, 429
Damaser, E. C., 549
Darwin, C. R., 21, 30, 44, 57, 90, 269, 272, 273, 366, 415
Davidson, R., 234
Davidson, R. J., 12, 89, 327, 330, 331, 332, 333, 336, 338, 339, 340, 341, 342, 343, 344, 345, 346, 347, 349, 350, 351, 352, 353, 354, 355, 357n1
Davison, C., 327
Davitz, J., 411, 412, 413, 415, 424
Davitz, J. R., 194
Dawson, M. E., 139
Day, K. D., 493
Day, R., 348
De Rivera, J., 415
Decarie, T., 232, 240, 367
DeCasper, A., 237
DeCasper, A. J., 268
deCharms, R., 169
Deci, E. L., 169
Decina, P., 334
Deckert, G. H., 201
Deglin, V. L., 334
d'Elia, G., 335
Demos, V., 411, 412, 424, 428, 521
Denenberg, V. H., 29, 322, 323, 324, 325
Dennett, B., 220
Dennis, W., 230
Denny-Brown, D., 327

Derryberry, D., 10, 29, 132, 135, 143, 153, 160, 161
DesLauriers, A., 371
Deutsch, F., 443
Dewey, J., 410
Dewson, J. H., III, 326
Diamond, S. R., 271
Dienstbier, R. A., 13, 489, 490, 493, 494, 495, 497, 498, 508
Dimberg, U., 341
Dimond, S., 338
DiVitto, B., 382
Dixon, N. F., 139, 141
Doi, T., 39
Doob, A. N., 491
Doty, R. W., 325
Doubleday, C., 179, 180
Dougherty, L. M., 278
Douglas, V. I., 149
Driscoll, J., 380
Driver, M. V., 329
Dru, D., 84
Duffy, E., 230, 369
Duncan, J., 21
Duncan, J. W., 89
Dutta, S., 560
Dutton, D. G., 493

Easterbrook, J., 246
Easterbrook, J. A., 562, 565, 574
Ebbesen, E., 451, 465, 473
Edinger, H., 141
Egeland, B., 293, 294, 295, 387
Ehrlichman, H., 330, 335, 336
Eibl-Eibesfeldt, I., 30, 371, 374
Eich, J., 550
Eich, J. E., 554
Ekman, P., 25, 30, 31, 75, 77, 87, 130n2, 229, 233, 234, 236, 238, 239, 251, 269, 321, 322, 337, 350, 357n1, 369, 371, 375, 376, 384, 415, 446, 448, 456, 578, 580
Eldridge, M., 83, 84
Elias, P. K., 54
Ellis, A., 218
Ellis, H. C., 470
Ellis, H. D., 88
Ellsworth, P., 25, 238, 269, 384, 446, 578, 580
Ellsworth, P. C., 508
Emde, R., 151, 232, 233, 235, 239, 240, 241, 243, 249, 251, 254, 367, 370, 371, 375, 380, 382, 383
Emde, R. N., 25, 28, 32, 51, 145, 150, 270, 346, 415, 416
Engel, G., 371
Epstein, S., 172, 176
Erdelyi, M., 139, 246
Erikson, E., 374
Erikson, E. H., 110, 516, 533, 540, 544

Escalona, S. K., 142
Evarts, E. V., 42
Ewy, R., 254
Exline, R., 234
Eysenck, H., 236
Eysenck, H. J., 133, 134, 135, 136, 157

Fairbairn, W., 371
Farber, E., 443
Farmer, C., 411, 415
Farrell, W. S., 325
Farrington, L., 338
Feather, B. W., 201
Feather, N. T., 465
Fedio, P., 327
Feinman, J. A., 443
Feinman, S., 242, 243, 270
Feldman, R. S., 443
Felleman, E. S., 451, 453
Fenichel, O., 93
Feshbach, N., 454
Feshbach, N. D., 113
Feshbach, S., 233, 454
Festinger, L., 77, 272
Fezler, W. D., 585
Field, J., 145
Field, T., 233, 255, 382
Field, T. M., 346
Fields, J., 348
Fifer, W., 237
Fisch, R., 562
Fischer, K. W., 394
Fischer, M. J., 451
Fiske, M., 232
Fiske, S. T., 311
Fitts, P. M., 562
Fitts, W. H., 21
Flavell, J. H., 31, 440
Fleming, D., 90
Flor-Henry, P., 330, 333, 344
Fogarty, S. J., 454, 455, 465, 466, 554, 560, 570
Folkes, V. S., 167, 168, 181
Folkman, I., 578
Folstein, M. F., 328
Foote, S. L., 135
Ford, M. E., 445, 469
Forest, D., 454
Forgas, J. P., 568
Forsman, L., 506
Fortenbaugh, W. W., 438
Fox, J., 22
Fox, N., 234, 347
Fox, N. A., 345, 346, 349, 350
Fraiberg, S., 379, 380, 382, 383
Frank, M., 243
Frankenhaeuser, M., 506
Freedman, D., 243, 379
Freud, S., 97n1, 230, 272, 366, 368, 371, 415, 458, 516

Freudenberg, R., 380
Friesen, W., 229, 233, 238, 239, 369, 384, 415, 446
Friesen, W. V., 25, 75, 130n2, 269, 357n1, 456, 578, 580
Frodi, A., 213, 217, 382
Froming, W., 471
Froming, W. J., 464, 468
Fry, P. S., 451, 453
Fryer, D. H., 84
Fuchs, A. F., 336
Furman, W., 467

Gaensbauer, T., 29, 232, 233, 367, 381
Gaensbauer, T. J., 28, 415
Gainotti, G., 327
Galin, D., 351
Gallagher, R., 375, 391
Gallistel, C. R., 135, 136, 138, 141, 142, 145, 146, 151
Galton, F., 91
Gantz, F., 449
Garbanati, J. A., 325
Garcia, J., 324
Garcia Coll, C., 49
Gardner, H., 328
Garner, W. R., 38, 54
Gazzaniga, M. S., 139, 325
Gelman, R., 109, 440
Gerbing, D., 241
Geschwind, N., 141, 354, 355
Giacoman, S., 235
Gibson, J., 233
Gibson, J. J., 83, 97n3
Gidro-Frank, L., 549, 570
Gilligan, S. G., 14, 22, 469, 480, 550, 552, 553, 554, 557, 560
Glenberg, A., 549
Gleser, G. C., 549
Glick, S. D., 323
Gnepp, J., 411, 414
Godden, D. R., 549
Goldberg, K., 380
Goldberg, M. E., 141
Goldberg, S., 264, 267, 268, 283, 382, 383
Golden, M., 290
Goldman-Rakic, P., 229
Goldsmith, H. H., 142
Goldstein, A., 88
Goldstein, K., 327, 366
Goldstein, M., 169
Goldstein, S. G., 333
Goleman, D. J., 343, 344
Goleman, J., 89
Goodman, G., 232
Gordon, P. G., 87
Gottlieb, A. A., 549
Gottschalk, L. A., 549
Gouaux, C., 469, 479
Gouaux, S., 469, 479

Gould, G., 395
Gove, F., 291, 293, 367, 384
Gove, F. L., 444
Graham, F., 240
Graham, F. K., 145, 146
Graham, S., 10, 13, 176, 177, 178, 179, 180, 182, 450
Gray, J. A., 134, 136, 137, 142, 143, 159, 195
Green, A., 368
Green, S. K., 440
Greene, D., 494
Greenson, R. R., 292
Greenspan, S., 367, 371, 410, 413, 428, 443
Grill, J. H., 26
Grossberg, J. M., 201
Grossman, S., 230
Guarino, P. A., 179, 180
Gunn, P., 383, 386, 391
Gunnar, M., 251, 377
Gunnar, M. R., 268, 269
Gunnar-Von Gnechten, M., 251
Gur, R. C., 335, 337
Gur, R. E., 335

Hainline, L., 254
Haith, M., 229, 232, 254
Haith, M. M., 148
Hale, W. D., 454
Hale, W. P., 455
Hall, G. C., 328
Hall, J. A., 549
Hall, M. M., 328
Halliday, A. M., 334
Hamilton, C. R., 325
Hamilton, V. L., 169
Hammen, C. L., 467
Hankin, W. G., 324
Hargis, K., 453, 477
Harmon, D. W., 344
Harmon, J. R., 415
Harmon, R., 232, 233, 251, 346, 367, 381
Harmon, R. J., 28
Harper, L., 383
Harris, M. B., 452, 453
Harris, P. L., 410, 411, 425, 428, 442, 448, 457
Harrison, A. A., 91
Hart, J. D., 201
Harter, S., 255, 411, 428, 442, 445
Hartmann, H., 272
Hass, W., 418
Hasset, J., 336
Hastrup, J. L., 49
Haviland, J., 14, 251, 311, 372, 384
Hayes, L., 255
Hebb, D., 247
Hebb, D. O., 133, 195, 267
Hécaen, H., 327
Heider, F., 169, 450, 493
Heider, K., 239

Heilman, K. W., 328
Hein, A., 83
Hein, P. L., 201
Held, R., 83
Hembree, E. A., 31
Henry, G., 554
Hepps, R. B., 549
Hesse, P., 369, 370, 396
Hettena, C., 22
Hetzer, M., 252
Hiatt, S., 151, 239, 241
Hiatt, S. W., 25
Hilgard, E. R., 202, 548, 549
Hill, P., 395
Hill, S., 229, 392, 393, 395
Hinde, R., 237, 238
Hintzman, D. L., 83
Ho, B. T., 88
Hoare, R. D., 329
Hochberg, J., 88
Hodgson, R. O., 193
Hoffman, M., 122, 233, 248, 380
Hoffman, M. L., 10, 24, 33, 103, 104, 105, 107, 111, 115, 123, 124, 125, 129, 184, 377, 495, 497
Hoffman, S., 467
Hofstadter, D., 264, 285
Hokanson, J. E., 472, 473
Holmes, T. S., 552
Hommes, O. R., 329
Homskaya, E. B., 329
Horenstein, S., 327
Horn, N. C., 474
Hornberger, R. H., 454
Horner, T., 236
Horowitz, F., 254
Howard, J. A., 451, 477
Huebner, R. R., 31, 32
Hull, C. L., 202, 549
Humphrey, G., 105
Huson, J., 201

Imamoglu, E. O., 109
Impastato, D. J., 334
Inhelder, B., 290, 311
Isen, A. M., 73, 80, 465, 466, 470, 474, 553, 570, 581
Izard, C. E., 9, 11, 17, 18, 21, 22, 25, 27, 28, 29, 30, 31, 32, 33, 57, 75, 76, 87, 96, 97, 115, 137, 138, 143, 150, 151, 159, 184, 233, 235, 238, 239, 249, 251, 252, 269, 270, 278, 290, 291, 292, 321, 346, 369, 370, 371, 374, 376, 377, 412, 413, 414, 415, 416, 438, 447, 448, 454, 455, 465, 484, 485, 486, 521, 552, 574, 580

Jackson, J., 240
Jackson, J. C., 145
Jackson, J. H., 144
Jacobson, E., 83, 85, 97, 201

Jaffe, R. H., 89
James, W., 21, 38, 39, 234, 270, 366, 415, 438
Jeffrey, W. E., 149
Jennings, J. R., 21, 22
Jens, K., 375
Jerussi, T. P., 323
Johansson, G., 506
Johnson, L. R., 412, 440
Johnson, P., 338
Johnson, R. C., 493
Johnson, W., 235
Jones, E. E., 123
Jones, G. F., 472
Jones, H., 236
Jones, O., 380
Jones, R., 516, 519
Jousse, M., 90, 97
Jouvet, M., 161

Kagan, J., 9, 25, 27, 40, 51, 52, 59, 60, 150, 231, 232, 240, 242, 264, 267, 371, 372, 374
Kahneman, D., 566, 575
Kandel, E. R., 135
Kanner, A. D., 578
Kanner, L., 370
Kanungo, R. N., 560
Kaplan, B., 367, 395
Kaplan, L. J., 112
Karalowski, J., 496
Karlin, R., 330, 343, 344
Karnoil, R., 181, 502
Katcher, A. H., 493
Katz, E., 375
Kazdin, A. E., 465, 474
Kearsley, R., 59, 232, 372
Keating, D. P., 444
Kelley, H. H., 450
Kelly, A. E., 329
Kelman, H., 327
Kenney, M., 229
Kenrick, D. T., 451, 453, 454, 455, 472, 475, 476
Kent, E. W., 138
Keogh, B., 371
Kessen, W., 369
Kestenbaum, C. J., 333
Kieras, D., 196
Kimura, D., 354
King, L. M., 451, 477
King, M., 411
King, R., 440
King, R. A., 112
Kingdon, J. W., 168
Kinsbourne, M., 335, 345
Kintsch, W., 198
Kleck, R., 376
Kleck, R. E., 21, 89
Klein, D. F., 193

Kling, L., 231
Klinnert, M., 235, 242, 243, 252, 254, 255
Klinnert, M. D., 70
Kocel, K., 335
Koenig, K. L., 270
Kohli, D., 89
Koivumaki, J., 81
Kolb, B., 329
Kolers, P. A., 74, 94
Komer, M., 372
Konecni, V. J., 493
Kopp, C., 371, 377
Koslowski, B., 246, 293, 370
Kosslyn, S. M., 82, 94
Kotsch, W., 241
Kozak, M. J., 213
Krantz, S., 467
Krantz, S. E., 568
Kremenitzer, J. P., 145
Kreutzer, M., 252, 254, 255, 376
Kreutzer, M. A., 440
Krogler, W. S., 585
Kronfol, Z., 333
Kuhn, D., 64
Kun, A., 174, 175, 181
Kunst-Wilson, W. R., 91, 245
Kurdek, L. A., 443
Kuskowski, M., 380

LaBarbera, J., 254
Lacey, B. C., 194
Lacey, J. I., 135, 143, 193, 194, 217
LaFreniere, P., 291
Laird, J., 251, 509
Laird, J. D., 21, 23, 31, 33, 34, 89, 271, 508, 511–2, 570, 579
Lamb, M., 254, 382
Lamb, M. E., 149
Lang, P. J., 11, 73, 82, 85, 97, 192, 193, 195, 196, 197, 201, 202, 203, 204, 205, 206, 207, 209, 213, 214, 221, 223n2
Langsdorf, P., 56
Lanzetta, J., 376
Lanzetta, J. T., 21, 89
Latané, B., 487, 503
Latz, E., 148
Lau, R. R., 167, 168
LaVoie, P., 328
Lawson, M. E., 176, 177, 178
Lazarus, R., 234
Lazarus, R. S., 73, 75, 266, 438, 578, 582
Lecours, A., 351
LeDoux, J. E., 139
Leight, K. E., 470
Leitenberg, H., 193
Lemond, C. M., 443
Leonard, C., 440
Lepper, M. R., 494
Lerman, D., 171, 172, 450

Lerner, M. J., 123
Levenson, R. W., 357n1
Leventhal, H., 75, 97
Levin, D. N., 202, 209, 210, 214, 223n2
Levin, P. F., 474
Levitt, E. E., 201
Levy, B. A., 83
Levy, R. I., 24
Lewis, M., 11, 264, 265, 267, 268, 269, 270, 283, 377, 392, 393, 394
Lewis, V., 83, 84
Lewis, W., 411
Lewisohn, P. M., 446
Ley, R., 337
Liben, L., 381
Liberman, A. M., 87, 338
Lidov, H. G. W., 146
Lifton, R. J., 92
Light, K. C., 49
Lindsley, D. B., 487
Ling, A., 381
Ling, D., 381
Lipps, T., 105
Lishman, W. A., 328, 466, 554, 560
Litman-Adizes, T., 169
Littlepage, G. E., 130n2
Livsey, W., 21, 22
Lloyd, G. C., 554, 560
Lloyd, G. G., 466
Loevinger, J., 371
Loftis, J., 491, 492, 501
Loftus, E. G., 80, 555, 572
Londerville, S., 367
Lorenz, K. Z., 195
Lourie, R., 367
Lumley, J., 383
Lund, J. S., 325
Luria, A. R., 329, 336, 341, 354
Lutz, C., 39, 45, 46
Lyons, W., 41

Mabry, P., 146
McArthur, L. Z., 89
Macauley, J., 213
McCall, R., 232, 247, 371
McCall, R. B., 264
McClelland, D. C., 540
McCune-Nicholich, L., 395
McDougall, W., 234, 415
McGhee, P., 247, 372
McGuigan, F. J., 83
McGuire, R. J., 585
McGuire, W. J., 64
McKeever, W. F., 337, 340, 341, 345
McKenzie, B., 348
McLean, A., Jr., 211, 212, 213
MacLean, P. D., 79
McMillen, D. S., 476
McNamara, H., 562

Maer, F., 327
Magnusson, D., 506
Maiberger, R., 328
Main, M., 293, 367, 370, 385, 387
Malatesta, C. Z., 32, 251, 384
Mandler, G., 40, 59, 73, 75, 95, 134, 135, 142, 186, 187, 195, 271, 310, 371, 465, 484, 578
Manning, E., 323
Mans, L., 383, 392, 393
Marks, I. M., 201
Markus, H., 9
Marlowe, D., 331
Marshall, G. D., 186, 508, 549
Maslach, C., 186, 508, 549
Mason, J. W., 135, 143
Mason, W., 229
Massonet, J., 327
Masters, J. C., 13, 443, 444, 445, 449, 451, 453, 467, 469, 471, 472
Matas, L., 244, 290, 293, 297, 384
Matlin, M., 552
Matlin, M. W., 91
Matthysse, S., 143
Maurer, D., 254
Max, L. W., 85
Mayer, D. J., 142
Mayr, E., 40, 44, 70
Meadow, K., 381
Mednick, S. A., 506, 507, 511n3
Mefferd, R. B., 506
Mehrabian, A., 194, 479
Meichenbaum, D., 218, 582
Melamed, B. G., 201
Meltzoff, A., 255
Mench, J., 323
Mendelson, M., 229
Meng, Z., 246
Mesulam, M., 141, 147
Mesulam, M. M., 328
Meutsch, P. R., 328
Meyer, D. E., 87
Meyer, M., 230
Meyer, S. T., 327
Michalson, L., 11, 265, 269, 270
Midlarsky, E., 474
Midlarsky, M., 474
Milavsky, B., 493
Miller, G. A., 208, 209
Miller, M., 89
Miller, N., 236, 238
Miller, R., 244
Milmoe, S., 244
Milner, B., 329
Mischel, T., 188n1
Mischel, W., 272, 439, 440, 451, 453, 456, 465, 473
Mishkin, M., 140
Moely, B. F., 443

Molliver, M. E., 146
Monakhov, K., 330
Monrad-Krohn, G. H., 81
Monteiro, K. P., 550, 557
Moore, B. S., 13, 445, 451, 453, 464, 468,
    469, 470, 471, 473, 475, 476, 477, 478
Moore, M., 254, 255
Mora, F., 135
Moreland, R. L., 91
Morris, L., 134
Moscovitch, M., 334
Moss, E., 339
Motti, F., 396
Mrazek, D., 381
Muensterberg, H., 83
Muir, D., 145
Munter, P. O., 489
Murdock, B. B., 83
Murphy, D., 554
Murphy, L., 290, 292, 293
Murray, A., 239
Murray, D. J., 83
Murray, H. A., 452, 453, 522
Mussen, P., 231

Nadel, L., 19
Nagge, J. W., 550
Nagler, S., 22
Nash, S. C., 64
Natale, M., 89, 467
Nauta, W. J. H., 320, 329, 336, 354
Negrao, N., 325
Neimark, E. D., 521, 528
Neisser, U., 81, 233
Neuman, C., 393
Newman, P. L., 46
Nicholls, J. G., 178, 181
Nicholson, N., 526, 529, 530, 531, 532, 534,
    535, 536, 537, 538, 542
Nierenberg, R., 169
Nikolaenko, N. N., 334
Nisbett, R. E., 123, 488, 494
Noble, E. P., 550
Nonneman, A. J., 322
Norgren, R., 26
Norman, D., 232
Norman, D. A., 18, 19, 82, 274
Nottebohm, F., 322, 323
Nottebohm, M. E., 323
Nowlis, V., 486
Nunnally, J. C., 449

Obrist, P., 240
Obrist, P. A., 49
Odbert, H. S., 581
Odom, R. D., 443
O'Donnell, K., 375
O'Keefe, J., 19

Oldfield, R. C., 332
Olds, J., 334
Olson, J. M., 490
Olthof, T., 410, 411, 425, 428, 442
Optin, E. M., Jr., 266
Orne, E. C., 548
Orne, M. T., 549
Orr, S. P., 21
Osgood, C. E., 91, 194
Oshinsky, J., 239
Oster, H., 87, 145, 254, 369, 370, 376
Overman, W. H., 325
Overton, W., 367

Padawer-Singer, A., 64
Pandya, D. N., 141
Panhuysen, L. H. H. M., 329
Pankey, W., 148, 150
Panksepp, J., 27, 137, 141, 144
Parcella, B. L., 334
Paris, S. G., 174, 175, 181
Parker, E. S., 550
Parsons, J. F., 181
Paskal, V., 104
Pazer, S., 122
Pearlson, G. D., 324, 326
Pearson, K., 91
Peiper, A., 376
Penick, S. D., 334
Perl, J., 352, 353
Perria, L., 329
Perris, C., 330
Perry, D. G., 494
Perry, L. C., 494
Peters, K. G., 149
Petersen, M. R., 326
Pettit, P., 167
Petty, R. E., 85, 91
Pfaff, D. W., 138, 142
Phillips, R. J., 88
Piaget, J., 73, 84, 108, 109, 138, 188n1, 268,
    290, 311, 369, 374, 395, 410, 412, 428, 440
Pien, D., 148, 152
Pietromonaco, P., 87
Pineault, M. H., 130n2
Plomin, R., 142
Plutchik, R., 371, 438, 509, 551
Plutchik, R. A., 273, 274, 552
Pogge-Hesse, P., 311, 367, 373
Polivy, J., 56, 464
Porges, S. W., 143
Posner, M. I., 144, 148, 581
Postman, L., 246
Pradhan, S., 146
Pradhan, S. N., 146
Prechte, H. F. R., 145
Pribram, K., 378
Pribram, K. H., 79, 329, 336

Price, D. D., 142
Provost, M., 240
Pylyshyn, Z. W., 81, 94

Quillian, M. R., 196, 555

Rachman, S. J., II, 193
Radke-Yarrow, M., 112, 233, 387, 440
Rainey, C., 323
Rakic, P., 346
Randall, D., 22
Rankin, R. E., 562
Raotma, H., 335
Rapacz, J., 181
Rapaport, D., 245, 368, 371
Rasch, G., 419
Rasmussen, T., 329
Rauste-von Wright, M., 506
Raven, P. H., 45
Rawles, R. E., 88
Ray, W. J., 344
Rayner, R., 266
Reder, L. M., 559
Reed, M. A., 152
Reese, H., 367
Regan, D., 252
Regan, R. A., 458
Rehm, L. P., 568
Reich, J., 240
Reichenbach, L., 443, 444
Reisenzein, R., 186, 187
Reuter-Lorenz, P., 339, 340
Reznick, J. S., 50, 51
Rhodewalt, F., 21, 89
Rice, D. G., 192
Rich, A. R., 202
Richard, D. W., 88
Ricks, D., 468
Ricks, M., 393
Ridgeway, D., 413, 415
Riggs, E., 231
Rioch, D., 79
Rippere, V., 446, 447
Rizley, R., 382, 467
Robinson, D. A., 336
Robinson, D. L., 141
Robinson, R. G., 323, 324, 326, 328, 355
Robson, K., 379
Rodgon, M. M., 443
Rodin, J., 491, 493
Roe, K., 113
Roessler, R., 506
Rogers, L. J., 323
Rohrkemper, M. M., 179
Rolls, E. T., 135, 137, 140
Rorty, A. O., 38
Rorty, R., 39
Rosadini, G., 329

Roseman, I., 234, 248, 415
Rosenbaum, R. M., 169
Rosenberg, S., 516, 519
Rosenblum, L., 265
Rosenfeld, H., 254
Rosenhan, D. L., 13, 445, 451, 453, 454, 455,
    468, 471, 474, 475, 476, 477, 478, 578
Rosenthal, R., 81
Ross, E. D., 328, 335
Ross, J., 181
Ross, L., 491, 492, 493, 501
Ross, M., 490
Rossi, G. F., 329
Roth, D., 568
Rothbart, M. K., 10, 29, 132, 143, 144, 148,
    152, 153, 160, 161
Rothenberg, B., 290
Rotter, J., 467
Rotter, J. B., 169
Routtenberg, A., 137
Rovee-Collier, C. K., 268
Royce, J. R., 271
Ruble, D. N., 181, 182
Rumelhart, D. F., 274
Rush, A. J., 328, 335
Rusiniak, K., 324
Russell, D., 167, 168, 171, 172, 450
Russell, J., 479
Russell, J. A., 194, 411, 413, 415
Rutherford, R., 380
Rychlak, J. F., 168
Ryle, G., 242

Saarni, C., 270, 384, 457
Sacco, W. P., 472, 473
Sackeim, H. A., 327, 328, 334, 337
Sackett, G., 229
Sagi, A., 104, 377
Salapatek, P., 254, 380
Salovey, P., 453, 468, 477
Sameroff, A. J., 54, 367, 397
Samnow, S. E., 511n3
Sander, L., 293
Sanders, D. Y., 476
Sandman, C. A., 78, 79
Sands, S., 381
Santostefano, S., 149, 367
Santrock, J. W., 458, 469, 553
Sarbin, T. R., 549
Saron, C., 330, 331, 332, 333, 339, 343, 344,
    352, 353, 355
Satinoff, E., 151
Saucy, M. C., 337
Scaife, M., 255
Schachter, J., 193, 506
Schachter, S., 73, 75, 115, 134, 135, 186, 199,
    217, 231, 232, 271, 357n1, 438, 439, 484,
    485, 487, 488, 492, 503, 578

Schaffer, C. E., 330, 331, 332, 333, 339, 355
Schaffer, H., 232
Schaffer, H. R., 267
Schank, R. C., 82, 579, 580
Schell, A. M., 139
Scherer, K., 234, 239
Scherer, K. R., 32, 81
Schiffenbauer, A., 454, 554
Schlesinger, H., 381
Schlosberg, H., 230
Schlumpf, M., 323
Schmidt, R. A., 78
Schneider-Rosen, K., 12, 387, 393
Schneirla, T. C., 195
Scholes, R., 328
Schork, E. J., 313, 317n3
Schroeder, H. E., 202
Schwartz, G., 233, 251
Schwartz, G. E., 25, 42, 55, 85, 89, 135, 143,
    201, 327, 335, 336, 341, 342, 343, 344, 351,
    354, 578
Schwartz, L., 241
Schwartz, M. F., 474
Schwartz, R. A., 419, 422
Schwartz, R. M., 12, 439
Schwarz, J. C., 473
Scott, J. P., 509
Scott, T. R., 26
Scripture, E. W., 84
Seeman, G., 473
Seifer, R., 54
Seligman, M. E. P., 68, 195
Serafetinides, E. A., 329
Seraficia, F., 379, 383, 386, 387
Shagass, C., 330
Shatz, M., 109
Shaw, W. A., 201
Sheehan, P. Q., 208
Shepherd, J. W., 88
Sherman, L. W., 292
Sherman, M., 230
Sherrrington, C. C., 90
Sherrod, D. R., 466
Sherrod, L. R., 149
Shields, S. A., 44
Shiller, V. M., 28
Shoemaker, W. J., 323
Shor, R. E., 548, 549
Shultz, T., 372
Siebel, C. E., 452, 453
Siegel, A., 141
Simernitskaya, E. G., 329, 354
Simmons, C., 123
Simner, M., 377
Simner, M. L., 104
Simon, H. A., 82
Simonov, P. V., 19, 267
Singer, J., 73, 75, 115, 186, 231, 232, 271,
    357n1, 439, 484, 485, 487, 492, 578

Sirota, A. D., 578
Skarin, K., 240
Skinner, B. F., 230, 369, 439, 517
Slackman, E., 122
Sloman, J., 382
Smith, M. O., 81
Smith, S. M., 549
Smith, T. L., 83
Smith, W. G., 83
Smythe, W. E., 74, 94
Snyder, C. R., 581
Sokolov, A. N., 83, 85
Sokolov, E. N., 283
Sokolov, Y., 247
Sokolov, Y. N., 198
Solomon, G. S., 476
Solomon, M. R., 89
Solomon, R. L., 283
Sorce, J., 242, 243, 254, 383
Sorenson, E., 229, 238, 239
Sparling, S., 252
Sperry, R. V., 217
Spiker, D., 393
Spitz, R., 231, 237, 367
Sroufe, L. A., 11, 24, 28, 32, 150, 151, 174,
    232, 233, 237, 240, 244, 290, 291, 293, 294,
    295, 297, 300, 301, 311, 313, 346, 348, 349,
    351, 367, 370, 371, 372, 374, 375, 376, 377,
    378, 379, 380, 383, 384, 387, 390, 391, 392,
    396
Stang, D., 552
Stang, D. J., 91
Stayton, D., 385
Stead, C., 521
Stechler, G., 148, 370, 371
Stein, L., 137
Stein, N. L., 412, 440
Steiner, I. D., 169
Steiner, J., 229, 378
Steiner, J. E., 26
Stenberg, C., 28, 80, 235, 239, 241, 242, 243,
    251, 374, 387
Stenberg, C. R., 57, 270, 348, 350
Stengel, B., 418, 419, 421, 422, 423, 424, 429
Stern, D., 152, 232, 292, 293, 370, 379, 380
Stern, G., 380
Stern, P., 176, 177, 178
Stern, R. M., 44
Sternbach, R. A., 192
Stevens, K., 234
Stinus, L., 329
Stolorow, R. D., 539
Stone, G., 562
Stone, M., 419
Stotland, E., 106, 119, 123
Strauss, E., 334
Strayer, J., 113
Strickland, B. R., 454, 455
Strock, B. D., 146

Stromgren, L. S., 335
Strongman, K. T., 272, 580
Suberi, M., 337, 340, 341, 345
Suci, G. J., 194
Sullivan, M. W., 11, 268
Surbey, P., 411, 412, 413, 415, 419, 425
Surbey, P. D., 440
Svejda, M., 243
Szetela, B., 328

Tanji, J., 42
Tannenbaum, P. H., 194
Tarter, R. I., 334
Taub, E., 78
Taves, P. A., 492
Taylor, M. A., 330
Teasdale, J. D., 454, 455, 465, 466, 554, 560, 570
Teitelbaum, P., 146
Tennes, K., 151
Terrazas, D., 469
Terwogt, M. M., 442
Terzian, H., 329
Thelen, M. H., 472
Thomas, A., 142, 284, 382
Thomas, H., 372
Thome, P. R., 213
Thompson, R. A., 174, 175, 181
Thompson, W. C., 453, 454, 455, 477, 578
Thomson, D. M., 549
Thorpe, J., 375
Thorpe, J. G., 585
Tieman, S. B., 325
Tinbergen, N., 138, 195
Titchener, E., 230
Tolan, W., 385
Tomasini, L., 385
Tomkins, S. S., 75, 87, 137, 269, 270, 321, 371, 375, 415, 416, 438, 439, 478, 484, 486, 521, 522, 523, 536, 539, 541
Tomlin, C., 392, 393, 395
Torangeau, R., 508
Trabasso, T., 12, 412, 439, 440
Tracy, R. L., 458
Triandis, H., 447
Trickett, P., 367
Trivers, R. L., 185
Tronick, E., 32, 232, 254, 380, 382
Tubylevich, D., 354
Tucker, D., 234
Tucker, D. M., 19, 328, 336, 343, 344
Tuckman, J., 458
Tulving, F., 549
Turvey, M. T., 338
Tversky, A., 566, 575
Tynes, D. M., 268

Ulrich, S., 382
Ulvund, S. E., 264

Underwood, B., 13, 445, 451, 464, 468, 469, 471, 472, 473, 475, 476, 478

Valins, S., 187, 506
Vallance, M., 585
Van Egeren, L. F., 201
Van Hoesen, G. W., 141
Vaughn, B., 240
Vaughn, B. E., 291, 298
Velten, E., 570, 578
Velten, E. A., 89, 449, 453, 454, 455, 469, 472
Vine, I., 291
Viscusi, D., 467
von Hofsten, C., 145
von Holst, 76
von Wright, J., 506
Vygotsky, L., 370

Wada, J. A., 329
Waddington, C. H., 366
Waid, W. M., 506
Walk, R., 244
Walker, B. B., 78, 79
Walker, J. D., 84
Walker, J. P., 84
Wallon, H., 90, 97
Walster, E., 252
Warren, J. M., 322
Washburn, M. F., 89, 90
Waters, E., 237, 240, 244, 290, 291, 293, 297, 298, 346, 370, 371, 379, 384
Watson, J., 230, 232, 234, 255
Watson, J. B., 97, 266, 439
Watson, J. S., 268
Watson, T. R., 328
Wechsler, A. F., 328
Wedell-Monning, J., 383
Weerts, T. C., 201
Wehmer, G. M., 21, 22
Weimer, W. A., 338
Weinberger, A., 335, 336
Weinberger, D., 336
Weinberger, D. A., 351
Weiner, B., 10, 13, 167, 169, 170, 171, 172, 173, 174, 175, 176, 177, 178, 179, 181, 185, 450, 497
Weingertner, H., 554
Weiss, J. M., 143, 159
Weiss, P., 366
Weisz, J. R., 179
Weitzenhoffer, A. M., 548
Wellman, H. M., 440
Wells, G. L., 91
Wepman, J., 418
Werman, R., 329
Werner, H., 367, 395
Wessman, A. E., 468
Weyant, J. M., 454, 476

Whatmore, G. B., 89
Wheeler, L., 487
Whimbey, A. E., 325
White, R., 371
White, R. W., 458
Wickelgren, W. A., 83
Williams, C., 234
Williams, J. M. G., 454, 455
Williams, M., 252
Wilson, D. H., 139
Wilson, W. R., 91
Wing, L., 395
Wippman, J., 290, 384
Witkin, H. A., 149
Wittig, B., 394
Wolf, K., 237
Wolff, P., 239
Wolman, R., 411, 412, 424
Wolpe, J., 585
Wong, P. T. P., 167
Wong, R., 83
Woodworth, R., 230
Woolf, V. S., 517–23, 525–45
Wright, B., 419
Wright, W. F., 566
Wundt, W., 230, 234, 369
Wunsch, J., 372, 396
Wurtz, R. H., 141

Yakovlev, P. I., 346, 351
Yamaga, K., 325

Yeates, S., 395
Yeudall, L. T., 333
Yin, R. K., 88
Yochelson, S., 511n3
Yonas, A., 249
Young-Browne, G., 254
Younger, J. C., 491
Yozawitz, A., 333

Zahn-Waxler, C., 112, 116, 233, 387, 440
Zajonc, R. B., 9, 18, 19, 22, 23, 33, 73, 87,
    91, 92, 139, 186, 218, 245, 272, 273, 274,
    290, 311, 485, 494
Zanna, M. P., 492, 501
Zeigler, B. L., 146
Zeiss, A., 451, 465, 473
Zelazo, P., 59, 232, 255, 372
Zelko, F. A., 448
Zelner, B., 336
Zelniker, T., 149
Ziajka, A., 233
Zigler, E., 367, 372, 398
Zillmann, D., 493, 511n1, 578
Zimbardo, P. G., 186, 491, 493, 508, 549, 570
Zimmerberg, B., 323
Zinkin, S., 334
Ziven, G., 152
Zuckerman, M., 21, 31, 136, 137, 159, 508

Subject index

ability, causal attribution, 168, 169, 170, 171, 172, 176–7, 178–81
acceptance, 273
accessing, emotion prototype, 198–9, 200, 202, 211–14
acculturation, 580
acetylcholine, 146
acetylcholine projections, 135
achievement concerns, causal attribution, 168, 169–70, 171–2, 173, 174, 181, 183, 188
acoustic patterns, 239, 240
acting, 44
action: in emotions as motives, 272–3; hierarchical organization of, 146
action set(s): emotion as, 195–6, 198, 215–16, 217, 221, 222–3
action tendencies, 241, 252
activation, 4–5, 32, 320, 321; of emotional response, 199–200; facial feedback hypothesis of, 23–4, 31–2; of hypotheses, 267; meaning and, 217–19; in network theory of affect, 556, 565, 569, 571–4, 575, 576; of phobic prototype, 199; and sequence problem, 4–5; spreading, 80
active/passive, 416, 417, 419, 421
adaptation, 34; early development and, 367; emotion feeling basic to, 25–6; of infant to care-giver's affective responsiveness, 385; invariance of emotion feelings in, 27; position in dominance hierarchy and, 61
adaptive function of emotions, 18, 69, 230, 233, 242, 244, 256, 273, 355, 509; attention, 140; distress, anger, 31; hopelessness, 68; and perception, 246; social smile, 20; see also evolution
adjustment, 302
adolescence, 66–7, 111
adrenaline, 487, 505–6
adult temperament research, 153–60
adults: understanding of causes and consequences of emotional states, 438–63
affect(s), 230; as action and content, 195–6; assessment of (Minnesota Preschool

Project), 296–7; children's distinctions between, 412–14; in cognitive assessment, 371–3; continuity of, 545; development of, in childhood, 62–8; development of, first five years, 58–62; dimension-linked, 178–82; dimensions of, 194–5, 220; as epiphenomenal, 242; hard representation of, 76–80; hemispheric specialization and, 320–65; models of, 368–9; network theory of, 547–8, 571–85; as organizer of experience, 540–1, 544–5; preceding cognition, 18 (*see also* sequence issue); in psychoanalytic theory, 233; psychophysiological indices of, 3; regulation of, 336; relevance of emphatic distress model to, 127–30; representation of, 74–80; role of, in social competence, 289–319; in social interaction, 11–12; strangulated, 230; *see also* emotion(s)
affect/cognition interface, 73–102
affect modulation, 303, 305–6; social roots of, 293–4
affect terms; *see* emotion terms (words)
affect-cognition interaction, 9, 10; in atypical infants, 366–406; between infants and care givers, 378–84; in empathy, 10, 103–31; and hemispheric organization, 334, 352–6, 357; socialization of affect and, 384–90; *see also* emotion–cognition interactions
affection, 247; basic emotion, 229, 249
affective continuity: core of differentiated, 235, 256; invariant core of, 249
affective disorders, lateralized dysfunctions in, 329–34
affective expressions, 218, 346, 370; antecedents of, 300–1; and social behavior, 290, 291; and social competence, 298–9, 301–3, 308–10, 312; social roots of, 293–4; *see also* emotion expression
affective life, causal dimensions in, 172–3
affective patterns, in mother–infant dyad, 381–2
affective processing, 20
affective regulation, frontal lobe lesions effect on, 329

affective structures: development of, 579–81; preprogrammed, 20
affective-cognitive structures, 20, 24, 27, 33, 34, 138; open system of, 20
affective-motivational states, 150
affective-motivational systems, 10, 132, 161–2; in attention, 133, 140–2, 144–5, 153; primacy of, in temperament, 136
affiliative concerns, 168, 169
affordances, defined, 233
agency, in elicitation of emotion, 248
aggression: adaptive inhibition of, 62; children's understanding of, 452, 453; exercise-induced arousal, 493; as index of anger, 241; relation with frustration, 171
agoraphobia, 218, 220
Ainsworth's Strange Situation attachment assessments, 56, 294, 295
alpha power, 330, 332, 333
altruism, 252, 454, 496–7; differential effects of positive and negative emotions in, 13; effect of emotion on, 474–8, 480
amae, 39
ambient mood, 79
amino acids, 146
amphetamines, 323, 492
amygdala, 39, 140
anaclitic depression, 231
analogs, 94
anencephalic, 378
anger, 18, 188, 194, 213, 216–17, 273, 381; adults' understanding of, 447, 450, 454–5; autonomic reactions in, 241; basic (primary) emotion, 39, 137, 229, 249; causal attribution, 172, 176, 177, 178–81; children's understanding of, 442, 443, 449, 452; development of, 30–1, 183, 184; effect on infants, 387; effect on recall, 22, 23; effect on selective perception, 21, 23; elicitation of, 235, 236, 237–8, 248; emergence of, 28; evolutionary advantage of, 61; incentives for, 61; indexes of, 241; intensity of, 246; relevance of empathic distress theory to, 129
anger mechanism, 27
anger to frustration, 59
anger-rage (basic emotion), 580
anosognosia, 327
antecedents (emotions), 5, 7; adults' understanding of, 447–8; children's understanding of, 440–1, 442, 445; infants' emotions, 28; mood, 88–9
anterior cortical association region, 320, 326, 330, 345, 354–5, 357
anticipation, 144, 148, 183, 217; capacity for, 150; discrete circuitry for, 137
anticipatory guilt, 125, 126
anxiety, 53, 136, 194, 220, 241, 500; alterability of, 70; arousal of, 509;

complex emotion, 137, 151; indexes of, 57; measurement of, 54–5; moral value of, 69; in subjective phobic imagery, 201
anxiety to discrepancy, 58–9
anxiety to possible task failure, 60
apathy, 173, 194, 450
appraisal(s), 2, 5, 42, 234, 290; defined, 266; of emotional events, 583–4
appraisal theories, 266
appreciations, concept of, 234–5, 249, 252, 256
approach/avoidance, 18, 26, 194, 195, 266; as basis for asymmetry, 340–1, 353–4, 355, 356, 357
approach response, 147
approach system, 136, 138, 151, 152
appropriateness of affect, 293, 294, 305
Aristotle, 438
arm-pull response, 276, 277, 282, 283–4
arousal, 40, 79, 205, 216, 416, 429, 486, 494; in attribution theory, 186–7; causal role of, 135–6, 137; causes of, 500; children's understanding of, 411, 412; cognitive consequences of, 547–88; development of emotion attribution, 503; dimension of affect, 194, 195, 220, 221, 222; fear response, 196, 197; general, 509; high, 196; inhibitory, 502; intensity of, 245–6; misattribution, 501; narrows attention, 562, 565, 572; naturally induced, 492–3, 508, 511n1; and negative affect, 159, 508; response training and, 206–8; role of, in emotion theory, 484–5, 508–9; system (ARAS), 136; and temperament, 505–7; undifferentiated, 357n1; *see also* autonomic arousal; empathic arousal; peripheral arousal; psychological arousal
arousal balance, 509–10
arousal models, general, 133–6
arousal modes, 10
arousal modulation, 377–8, 380; *see also* modulation
arousal state, interpretation and evaluation of, 270, 271
articulation effects, 82–3
Ascending and Descending (artwork), 264
ascending reticular activating system, 133, 135
ascending reticular modulating system, 140–1
association, 230; emotional processing and, 210; *see also* free associations
associative network(s), 196, 197–8, 199, 200, 206, 219, 221
associative network model, 14
associative structures, 73, 74; representation as, 76, 79, 80
associative theories, 579–80

associative thinking, 559
attachment, 28, 53, 293; measurement of, 56,
    237; and social competence, 290–1, 295,
    300–1
attachment object, 60
attachment relationship, 393–4; in infant–
    care-giver dyad, 385–6
attack, 217, 323; as index of anger, 241
attending, 83
attention, 10, 79, 370, 581; affective-
    motivational systems in guidance of, 132,
    133, 139–44, 148–50, 151, 152–3; effect
    of emotion on, 13, 470–1; narrowed by
    increasing arousal, 562, 565, 574;
    obligatory, 148, 151; response parameters,
    144; selective, 18, 19, 24, 149, 560
attention control, 157, 159, 161, 162
attention focusing, 10, 34
attention rank, 291, 298, 299
attention shifting, 10, 159, 162
attentiveness, 58, 240, 371–2
attitudes, 22, 274; change in, 92, 492, 501,
    584; motor representations of, 90–2
attraction emotions, 416
attraction to others, 478–9
attribution, 23, 510; appropriate, 500–1; in
    cheating, 497–502; developmental
    perspectives re, 502–4; in emotion
    experience, 493–7, 510; interaction with
    schema activation, 499–501; in self-control
    with children, 493–7, 501–2; temperament
    and, 504–5; *see also* misattribution
attribution theory, 13, 14, 450, 466–7;
    problems in, 183–5; selective attention in,
    560
attribution-affect linkage, 184–5
attributional processes, 10, 167–91
audition, 86–7, 118, 381
auditory modality, lateralization and, 326
autism, 370, 393
autobiographical events, state-dependent
    recall of, 552–3, 555, 573–4
automatic processes, 581–3
autonomic arousal, 13, 134, 135, 231; in
    network theory of affect, 578
autonomic discrimination of emotions, 357n1
autonomic nervous system activation, 3
autonomic patterns, measurement of, 240–1
autonomic reactions, 247, 271
autonomic system, 17, 135, 136, 147;
    representational and mnestic function, 78;
    and temperament, 132, 135, 137, 142, 143,
    153
autonomy, 540
availability, 465–6, 479–80, 566–7
aversive conditioning, 585
aversive empathic distress, 124
avoidance, 241; of punished errors, 487–8,
    500; *see also* approach/avoidance

avoidance response, 147
avoidance system, 138, 151, 152
awareness, 581; emotion at conscious level is
    special kind of, 24, 27, 28

basal forebrain, 135
basic emotions, 484; characteristic facial
    expressions for, 578–9, 580; as family of
    related emotions, 249, 250T; genetically
    prespecified, 580; innate, 575
basic trust, 540
Bayley Mental Development Index, 295
Bayley scales, 372, 391
Beauvoir, Simone de, 523
Beck Depression Inventory (BDI), 330–1
behavior, 53, 139, 142, 220, 230, 285;
    adaptive/maladaptive, 368; affects
    influencing, 9, 371; effect of feeling states
    on, 451–3; innate, 580; in network theory
    of affect, 578–9
behavior genetics, 134, 153
behavior streams, 275–6
behavioral act(s), 195
behavioral consequences, 456–9; self-
    oriented, 468–74
behavioral inhibition system, 136
behavioral systems, 367
behavioral therapists, 218
behavioral-expressive level, interaction of
    emotion and cognition at, 19–21
behaviorism, 369, 516; emotions in, 230
belief in God, 67
beliefs, 67–8
beta activity, 330
bioelectric recording, 215–16, 222
biological change, 38; detected/undetected,
    41–2, 43, 50–1; *see also* physiological
    change
biological necessity, 268, 273
birdsong, 322–3
blaming the victim, 122–3
blind infants, 375, 379–80, 386, 387, 388,
    389–90
blocking of a goal, 53
bodily changes: awareness of, 1–2; patterned,
    34–5
body language, 91
Bohr's principle of complementarity, 43
boredom, 247, 267, 372; and depression, 447
brain, 17–18, 19, 44, 217; activation
    asymmetries, 355; development of, 144;
    homunculoid functions, 220; *see also*
    hemispheric specialization
brain activation, 330, 332, 333, 334, 341
brain damage, 378, 395
brain lesions, 234
brain organization, 352–6; in neonates, 346–
    7, 350–1
brainstem, 25, 135, 378

brainwashing, 92
breathers, 582
Breuer, 230

cardiovascular system, 135, 143;
   representational function of, 78–9
care giver, 32, 384–90; *see also* infant–care-
   giver dyad
care-giving environment, 367
Carmichael's Manual of Child Psychology,
   231
Carnegie-Mellon University, 232
case study, in developmental research, 516–7
catastrophic reaction, 327, 328
catecholamines, 324, 505–6
categories, 75
categorization, 95; dimensions of, 64–5
causal antecedents, children's understanding
   of, 409, 410, 412–13, 415, 417, 423, 424,
   428, 430
causal ascriptions, 175–6, 188; and
   emotions, 171–3
causal attributions, 167–70, 184; in empathy,
   10, 103, 122–5, 127; and guilt feeling, 125
causal consequences, children's
   understanding of, 409, 410, 412–13, 415,
   417, 423, 429, 430
causal dimensions, 168–70, 173;
   development of, 182–3; in dimension
   linked affects, 179
causal relationships, 13, 440; arousal and
   emotion, 135–6
causal search, 167–8
causal stability, 169, 170, 173
causality: attribution of, 248 (*see also* causal
   attributions); dimensions of, 10; self-
   attribution of, 466–7
causes, of emotional states, 438–63
central nervous system, 132, 135, 137, 487,
   572; maturation of, 44, 147; stimulants and
   tranquilizers, 492, 493, 508
cerebral arousal, 487
cerebral asymmetry(ies), 320–1, 322; affect-
   cognition interaction and, 352–6; for
   affective processes in adult humans, 326–
   45, 356; species-consistent functional,
   322–6, 356
cerebral hemispheres, 12; *see also*
   hemispheric specialization
cerebral lesions, 327–9; *see also* brain
   lesions
cerebral metabolism, 323–4
cerebral palsy, 375
cessation of play, 53, 57, 232
change: and alteration of appraisal, 584–5; in
   internal state, 38–9, 41–3, 51; *see also*
   attitudes, change in
character: literary, 515; psychological, 515,
   519

cheating, 487–91, 494, 497–502, 503, 507,
   510
cheerfulness, 89
child–care-giver dyad; *see* infant–care-giver
   dyad
childhood, development of affect in, 62–8
   (*see also* development)
children: effect of emotion on task
   performance of, 469; emotion attribution in
   self-control, 493–7, 501–2; understanding
   of causes and consequences of emotional
   states, 438–63; understanding of display
   rules, 457; understanding of emotions,
   409–37
chlorpromazine, 487, 494, 503
choice, 125; recognition of, 62
cholinergic mechanisms, 135
cholinergic pathways, 146
cingulate cortex, 141
clinical populations, cerebral asymmetries,
   326–7
close-loop theory, 78
cognition(s): assessment of, 215; as cause of
   emotion, 5; cold, 170, 232, 234, 256, 274,
   494; as conceptual information processing,
   221; control of emotions, 582–3; in
   emotion, 193–226; in emotion experience,
   167; emotions dependent on, 70; in
   empathic arousal, 104, 105, 106, 107, 112,
   114, 124, 126–7; goal-relevant, 234–5;
   hemispheric specialization, 320–65; hot, 3,
   127, 170, 234, 274; influence of emotion
   on, 138–44, 454; influence on emotion,
   170–1; information processing distinct
   from, 19–20; lateralization and, 325–6;
   problem of definition, 2, 7–8;
   representation of, 74; role of, in eliciting
   affect, 247; role of, in emotional response,
   578–9; role of hard representation in, 81–
   5; selectivity of, 138; serves affect, 290;
   and social competence, 310–12; software
   and hardware of, 9, 81–2; sufficient
   determinant of affect, 187–188; theoretical
   issues in, 2–9
cognition–emotion relation; *see* emotion–
   cognition interactions
cognitive behavior therapy, 582
cognitive consequences of affect: self-
   oriented, 465–8; *see also* consequences (of
   emotions)
cognitive development, 6, 69, 231–2, 369;
   assessment of, 370–1, 372–3;
   differentiation of emotional systems in,
   150, 151; and emotional (affective)
   development, 175, 183, 390–8; and
   expression of complex emotions, 264; and
   goal/events relevance, 252; necessary to
   coherent reactions, 60–2, 66–8
cognitive dissonance, 53, 272

cognitive epiphenomenalism, 396
cognitive functionalism, 168
cognitive mediation, 2, 19–20
cognitive process(es), 3; as antecedent of emotion, 5; effect of emotional arousal on, 546–88; effect of emotions on, 22, 34; emotion as regulator of, 244–6; inducing emotion, 34, 134; shallow, in empathy, 107
cognitive psychology, 1, 6, 7, 22, 153
cognitive representations, 75
cognitive science, 6, 19
cognitive sense of the other, 10; development of, 107–11, 112, 113–15, 117–18, 125, 126, 127, 129
cognitive sets, 6
cognitive style, 149; temperament and, 541
cognitive system, 17; and emotion system, 29
cognitive tasks, effect of self-esteem and induced emotion on, 21–2
cognitive theory, 73, 75, 76, 338
cognitive transformation of empathy, 115–26
cognitive-emotional fugue, 264–88; model of, 275–6; *see also* emotion–cognition interactions
cognitive-informational constructs, 371
coherence(s), 69, 70; of associative network, 199; discrete, 41, 50
coherent reactions, 57, 58–63, 66–8
commissural pathways, 351–2, 356
communication, 8–9; affective, in infancy, 242–3; complex, 356; emotional expression, 243–4; in infant–care-giver dyad, 378–9, 380, 381–2; interhemispheric, 12; understanding of emotional terms and, 428–9
communication potential, as classificatory scheme, 40
communication skills, 370
communicative role of affect, 292
comparisons, simultaneous, 267
compensatory mechanisms, 381, 383
competence, 273, 368, 446; effect on altruism, 474–5; *see also* social competence
complementarity (principle), 43, 54–7
complex emotions, 5, 137, 151, 248, 264; developmental change in, 249, 252; as patterns, 252, 253T
computer model, 81–2, 232
concept/data relationship, 1–2
conceptual-dependency theory, 579
concrete operations, 69
conditioned responses, 491–2, 501, 504
conditioning, 76, 118, 134, 195; classical, 104–5, 106, 107, 111
confidence, 65, 450
conscience, 511; *see also* resistance to temptation

consciousness, 24, 28, 141; contents of, 565, 573; emotion feelings in, 4–5, 32–3
consequences (of emotions), 7; adults' understanding of, 447–8, 453–5; children's understanding of, 441, 443, 445, 451–3; knowledge and beliefs re, 451–5; understanding of, 438–63
conservation of energy, 371
consistency, 66–8
constitutional differences, 132; *see also* individual differences
construct(s): defined, 236; emotion words as, 236–42
contempt (primary emotion), 39, 137
contempt-scorn (basic emotion), 580
content of emotions, 187–8, 521
context(s), 3, 216, 410, 417–18, 422–3, 429, 430; and emotion terms, 45–6, 47; knowledge of and experience in, 424–5; social, 5
context dependency, of emotions, 242–3, 244
contextual cues, 376; in children's understanding of emotion, 443–5
contingency awareness, 11
contingency experience, 268
continuation of looking, 241
control, 268, 447; in atypical infants, 386–7, 388; of emotions (moods), 581–3, 585; locus of, 169; sense of, 46
control (dominance), 194–5, 220, 221
controllability, 10, 450; as causal dimension, 169–70, 173, 179–83, 184, 185, 188
controlled processes, 581–5
co-occurrence of emotions, 424, 425, 428, 445
coordination (of emotion), in children, 428
coping behavior, 43, 321; repressive, 351, 356
coping response, 582–3; belief in lack of, 53; developmental change in, 249, 251–2
coping style(s), 149
copulation behavior, 323
corpus callosum, 351, 356
cortex, 135, 140; information processing in, 141; maturation of, 147
cortical arousal, 133, 134, 135, 150
cortical region (brain), 320
cortical response, 139
crawling, 251; and fear of heights, 244
creativity, 22
criminals, 511n3
crying, 61, 232; as index, 53, 57; pathological, 327–8; reactive, 104, 106, 107, 130n1
cues, 13; become conditioned stimuli, 104–5, of care givers, 387–8; in children's understanding of emotion, 443–4, contextual, 376, 443–5; in learning and recall, 549–50; salient, in empathy, 106–7, 120, 121, 127–8

culture: in causal attribution in empathy, 125; and commitment to beliefs, 68; emotion terms in, 44–7; influence on emotion expression, 31
curare studies, 96–7
Cuvier, Georges, 70
cycloheximide, 323

Dahl's theory, 415–16
Darwin, Charles, 57, 484
deaf infants, 375, 377, 381, 383, 385–6, 387, 388, 389–90
deafferentiation, 78
decentration, 411, 442
deep structure, of prototype, 198, 200, 202, 208, 216, 221
defense, 18
defiance, 152
deintensification, 456
delay of gratification, 13, 152, 272, 473–4, 480, 503
demand compliance, 547, 548, 569–71
dependency, 152, 247
depersonalization, 194
depictions, 566, 575
depression, 68, 137, 173, 175, 370, 450, 466, 511n2; childhood affective traits and vulnerability to, 545; complex emotion, 137; development of, 183; expressive dampening in, 234; guilt in, 504; hemispheric specialization and, 328, 329, 330–5, 345, 354–6, 357; knowledge/ beliefs re, 447; to loss of familiar object, 60; motor expression of, 89; neurotic, 136; predisposes toward negative feedback, 467; self-reward, 472–3; theories re, 143
desensitization, 214, 585
destruction, 273
detection, 42, 43
determinants (of emotion): adults' understanding of, 446–50; children's understanding of, 440–6, 459; cognitive and facial, 579
development: of affective structures, 579–81; in altruism, 476; analysis of, in V. Woolf, 519–46; atypical, 370–1; of causal dimensions, 182–3; of children's understanding of emotions, 441–6, 448–9, 452–3, 459; of emotion attribution, 502–5; in hemispheric specialization, 345–52; measurement of, 397–8; of moral socialization, 510–11; normal/deviant, 366–8, 372–3, 377, 379, 381–2, 384–5; and semantic distinctions, 424–8; of temperament, 144–53, 160–1; of understanding of emotions, 411–15, 424–30
developmental psychology, 1, 6, 153, 371; emotions in, 231–2

developmental research, use of case study in, 516–17
developmental theory, 272
Differential Emotions Scale, 552
differential emotions theory, 17, 19, 20, 23, 25, 27, 30, 552, 565, 574
differentiation, 151, 152, 173–4, 188; primitive emotions, 580–1
dimensional theory, 484–5, 486–7; *see also* peripheral-dimensional theory
direct affect, 129–30
direct association, 105, 106
direction (emotion), 13, 416, 417–24, 425, 429, 430
discharge, 79
discrepancy, 53, 371
discrepancy theories, 247, 266–9
discrepant events, 49–50, 51, 58–60, 61
discrete emotion theory, 484–5, 508, 509
discrete emotions, 374, 376
disease analogy, 42–3
disgust, 25, 194, 273; basic (primary) emotion, 39, 137, 229; in brain-damaged infants, 378; elicitation of, 238, 239; feedback in, 509; in neonates, 345, 347, 350, 356
disgust-revulsion (basic emotion), 580
dishonesty, 441, 448–9
display rules, 251, 375, 456–9
disposition–situation distinction, 169
dispositions, 214
dissonance research, 492, 501, 508
distancing, 121–2
distinctive dimension, in choice of referent, 64–5
distress, 25, 248, 381; adults' understanding of, 448; development of, 30, 31; early, 151; fundamental emotion, 137; heart rate in, 240; in neonates, 346, 347; to physical privation, 58; response to discrepancy, 372; *see also* empathic distress
distress-anguish (basic emotion), 580
divorce, 458
doctor–patient relationship, 244
dominance, 194–5; low, 196; *see also* control (dominance)
dominance hierarchy, 61, 63, 66
dopamine, 137, 143, 146, 323, 324
Down's syndrome, 12, 285, 370, 375, 376, 377–8, 379, 380, 383; affect/cognition relation in, 390–3, 395–6; attachment behavior, 386–7; emotional language, 388–90
Dreiser, Theodore, 516
drive, 187
drive reduction, 137, 371
drive tension, 368–9
drugs, 486–7

duration: of emotion, 32; of outcome-dependent affects, 175
dyadic relationships, 232–3; *see also* infant–care-giver dyad

Ebbinghaus, 516
Edinburgh Inventory, 332
effector systems, 136
efferent leakage, 222
efferent patterning, 200–10
efferent programs, 196, 200, 215, 216, 217, 219, 221
effort, in causal attribution, 169, 170, 171–2, 174, 176–7, 178–81
ego, 368
ego identity (concept), 110–11, 182
egocentric emotions, 477, 480
egocentric empathy, 113, 117, 128
egocentrism, 108, 411, 413–14
egoistic drift, 119, 129
electrodermal response (EDRec), 139, 507
electrodermal system, 135, 143
electroencephalograph (EEG), 234, 330–2, 341–2, 347, 354, 355
electrophysiological studies, hemispheric asymmetries, 330–45
elicitation of emotion, 234–5, 236, 237–8, 391, 583–4; goals and, 247–8; prediction of, 250T, 253T; studies of, 246–7
elicitor, 271; defined, 265, 322; role of cognition at level of, 266–8
embarrassment, 240
embedded figures task, 52
emogen processing units, 139
emotion(s): advantages of early, 61–2; analyzing definitions of, 2–4; as antecedent of cognition, 264, 272–5, 276; attribution-dependent, 174, 175–8, 188; automatic vs. controlled processes in, 581–5; basic, 137–8, 229; causal ascriptions and, 171–3; central role in unified representation of mind, 575–6; children's understanding of, 409–37; classification of, 39–51, 53–4; cognition in, 193–226; components of, 3, 265; conceptualization of, 217–18, 428–9; concomitants of, 7; conscious aspect of, 230; as consequence of cognition, 264, 265–72, 275, 276; context-dependent, 429; criteria identifying, 229; defined, 13, 24–5, 27, 321–2, 373–4, 416, 438–9, 464, 485–6; dependent on cognition, 70; development of, 28, 69, 229–63 (*see also* emotional development); emergence of, 28–9; as epiphenomenal, 231, 242, 396; events defining, 38; factor in information processing, 6; function of in early life forms, 18; functional at birth, 25; generation of, 2, 134; genuine, activated

by simulated emotion experience, 21; in human development, 24–33, 38–72; indexing of, 10; influence of, on arousal and cognition, 135–6, 137; influence of, on cognition, 138–44; influence of, on reaction to self and others, 464–83; as information, 196–200; innate, 229; issues in study of, 185–8; as motivators and organizers, 32, 256, 290; number of, limitless, 39; outcome-dependent, 173–5, 184, 188; pervasiveness of, 480; preprogrammed, 28–9; primacy of, 22, 24; primal, 34; problem of definition of, 1, 2–4, 6, 7; as process coordinating sensation and response, 162; pure, 485; quality of, 508; as regulators of social behavior, 11, 12; relation with learning, 276–85; role of, in moral socialization, 484–514; and sensory regulation, 138–44; shadings of, 577–8, 581; shifts in attitudes re, 229–35; simple, 248; social functions of, 18; study of, 1, 5–6; as superordinate term, 40–1, 42; as systems, 29–33; and temperament, 132–66; theoretical issues in, 2–9; types of studies of, 246–7; as units in associative network, 554, 555–6, 565, 571–4, 576, 578 (*see also* network theory of affect); *see also* basic emotions; complex emotions; consequences (of emotions)
emotion–cognition interactions, 2, 3–4, 5–6, 7, 8, 9, 11, 17–24, 234–5; attentional mechanisms in, 10; in atypical infants, 12; is bidirectional, 13; causal attribution in, 170–1; in character of V. Woolf, 515–46; dimension theory of 485; and human development, 17–37; interdependent and independent, 23–4; models of, 264–76; in network theory of affect, 578–9; separate systems of, 17–19, 22, 33–4, 396
emotion–cognition interrelationship, 485, 568–9
emotion concepts, 7–8
emotion experience, 4, 8, 75, 79–80; attribution in, 493–7, 510; children's understanding of, 412; cognition at level of, 270–2; defined, 265; early, 184; effects of cerebral insult on, 338; facial expressions identified with, 376–7; feeling as cue-providing, 24; meaning of, 508; meaning of, in temptation, 500, 501; role of feedback in, 509;
emotion expression, 5, 8, 11–12, 26, 75, 79–80; in atypical infants, 12, 378–9, 380, 381, 383–9, 389–90; basic emotions, 252; cognition at level of, 269–70, 285; defined, 265; development of, 372–3, 374–8, 384–5; of infants, 19–20; intensity of, 505; leads to emotion feeling, 33–4; learning and, 282–3; and quality of dyadic

emotion expression (cont.)
  relationship, 385; relation with affective
  experiences, 376–7; simulated, can
  activate genuine 21; species specific, 416
emotion expression/emotion experience
  relationship, developmental change in,
  249–51, 252
emotion feeling(s), activation of, 25; distinct
  from symbolized emotion, 33, 34;
  organizing and motivational force, 32–3,
  34; *see also* feeling state(s)
emotion processes, 187–8; central in moral
  choices, 494; primal in human behavior, 17
emotion system, 17; maturation of, 151;
  separate from cognitive system, 6, 9
emotion system models, discrete, 137–8;
  general, 136–7
emotion terms (words), 9, 44–7, 70, 409,
  411, 413–14, 415, 417, 428–9, 581; in
  case study of V. Woolf, 520–1, 522;
  children's understanding of, 440; as
  constructs, 235, 236–42; containing
  references to incentive, 58–63;
  differentiation of, 419; need for new,
  47–51
emotion theory, 73, 219–21, 232–5, 410,
  415, 438, 507–10, 578; dimensional/
  discrete distinction in, 484–5, 508;
  representation of affect in, 75–80
emotional change, media and, 211–14, 222
emotional development, 6, 10, 24–5, 29, 34,
  44, 302; attributional approach to, 167–91;
  at expressive level, 30–2; at
  neurophysiological level, 29–30; new
  perspective on, 248–55; postulates of, 11;
  at subjective-experimental level, 32–3; *see
  also* cognitive development; development
emotional phenomena, language of emotion
  and, 12–13; reality of, 11
emotional receptors, defined, 265
emotional resonance, 255
emotional states, 24, 222, 428, 430; altered
  by acquisition of information, 69–70;
  causes and consequences of, 13;
  classification of, 39–51; defined, 265, 269,
  285; effect of sodium amytal on, 329;
  facial expressions as origins of, 57; global,
  285; in infants, 58–62; inference of, 170–
  2, 443–5, 446, 459; isomorphic, 215–17;
  labels for, 429; measurement of, 160–1;
  self-monitoring of, 377–8; signs of, differ
  in centrality, 53; transient nature of, 43;
  understanding of, by children and adults,
  412–13, 438–63; valid indexes of, 57; *see
  also* feeling states
emotionality, scales for, 155, 157–9
emotion-attribution research, 491–3
empathic arousal, 115, 127–8, 129–30;
  modes of, 104–7, 111, 126

empathic distress, 103, 104, 105, 124, 128–
  9; guilt and, 125–6
empathic emotions, 477, 480; foster prosocial
  behavior, 24
empathy, 10, 33, 113, 233, 293, 311, 411;
  affect/cognition interaction in, 103–31;
  cognitive component of, 107–11, 126–7;
  cognitive transformation of, 115–26;
  defined, 103, 114, 127; development of,
  103–15, 128–9; measurement of, 54–5;
  moral value of, 69; precursors of, 112;
  self-reinforcing, 107; subjective experience
  of, 107–8
encoding, 139
endocrine system, 132, 135, 142, 143, 153
enhancement, 492–3; selective, 162
enjoyment, and learning, 279–80, 281, 283
enjoyment-joy (basic emotion), 580
ennui, 69
enthusiasm, 290
entorhinal cortex, 140
environment, 29
envy, 63–4
Escher, 264
euphoria, 327, 328, 329
evaluation, 47, 59, 69; absent in early
  infancy, 58; in classifying emotions, 43,
  46; coherence with incentives and
  physiological change, 52; symbolic, 63–8
evaluation mood, shift in, 584
event–emotion relationship, 13, 31
event–reaction relationship, 236
event-cognition relationship, 28–9
events, 42, 274; appraisals of, 583–4;
  attribution of meaning to, 51–2;
  combination of, creates emergent synthetic
  phenomenon, 51; meaning of, 311; as
  modulators of other behaviors, 582–3;
  monitoring of, 222
evolution: of affective expression, 371; and
  attribution-affect linkage, 185; in
  dimensions of affect, 195; emotions in, 18;
  function of emotions in, 61–2; gustation
  in, 26; of intellectual and expressive
  behaviors, 273; *see also* adaptive function
  of emotions
evolutionary biology, 1
excitability, 284, 285, 571–2
excitation transfer process, 578
excitement, 500; to assimilation, 58, 59–60;
  differentiation of, 173; evolutionary
  advantage of, 61; primary emotion, 39
exhaustion, 69
existential feeling, 33
expectancy(ies), 273; based on personal
  theory, 458; re consequence of emotions,
  452–3, 459; for personal outcomes, 456;
  self-attribution and, 466–7; violation of,
  267, 447

experience, 132, 195; early, effect on lateralization, 324, 325; organized and unified by affect, 541, 544–5; prior, 311; *see also* emotion experience
experiential level, interaction of emotion and cognition at, 21–4
Experimental Psychology (Woodworth and Schlosberg), 230–1
exploration, 273, 325
expressive level, emotional development at, 30–2
extraversion, 136, 138
eyewitness testimony studies, 232

face perception, 86–8
Facial Action Coding System, 145
facial electromyography, 3
facial expression(s), 32, 137, 229, 269, 345; affective information in, 20–1; blind infants, 380; characteristic across cultures, 578–9, 580; and children's understanding of emotion, 443; frontal lesions and, 329; as index, 3, 47; influence emotional reaction of infants, 242–3, 254–5; measurement of, 233–4, 238–9, 240, 276, 278–9, 369–70; of mother, 11; of neonates, 346–7; in network theory of affect, 578–9; ontogenesis of, 374–7; as origins of emotional states, 57; preprogrammed, 30; relation with internal state, 269–70; universal, 25, 374–5
facial feedback hypothesis, 23–4, 31–2, 508, 509
facial flushing, 241
facial muscles, 38, 138
facial wariness, as index, 53, 57
facilitation, 135
fago, 45
failure, 53, 172, 173, 441, 448, 449 450; attribution of, 175, 183; and delay of gratification, 473; effect on memory for interpersonal information, 470–1; as inducer of mood, 465; self-attribution and, 467; and self-reward, 471–2
family, 64–5
fantasies, 14, 274, 547, 570
fear, 12, 136, 151, 194, 247, 267, 273, 500; activation of, 11, 145; adults' understanding of, 454, 455; alterability of, 70; autonomic reactions in, 241; basic (primary) emotion, 39, 137, 229, 249; children's understanding of, 441, 442, 443, 449; discrete circuitry for, 137; Down syndrome infants, 377–8; effect on cognition, 80; elicitation of, 238, 239, 248; emergence of, 28, 348, 350; heart rate in, 240; of heights, 28, 244, 348; indexes of, 241; and learning, 281–2, 283–4; measurement of (infants), 160, 161; of

punishment, 252; relevance of empathic distress theory to, 129; response parameters, 143–4; to the unfamiliar, 58–9; of the unusual, 61
fear mechanism, 27, 29
fear prototype, 11
fear response, 197, 200
fear types, 222
fearful actions, 196
fear-terror (basic emotion), 580
feedback, 134; in emotion node hypothesis, 571; face to somatosensory system, 376; from facial expressions, 138, 508, 509; peripheral, 487, 490, 507; positive, 446; role in emotion experience, 509, 511
feedback-feedforward loop model, 5, 9, 13
feelings(s), 371; form cognitive representation, 76; leading to other emotional states, 448; quality of, 46, 47
feeling state(s), 3–4, 42; invariant across life-span, 26–7; motivational aspect of experience, 32–3, 34; naming of, 41, 44–51; negative, 449, 450; subjective report of, 54, 55–6; thought as consequence of, 272; variety in potential, 39; *see also* emotional states
feeling tone, 69; significance of detection of, 41–3
feelings of others, 113; *see also* empathy
field articulation, 149
field dependence–independence, 149
fluent aphasia, 356
focus, 521
focus of attention, 149, 476–7
force, in socialization, 494, 505
forebrain, 146
formal operations (stage), 66, 68, 69
frame(s), 42; objective/subjective, 54–7
free associations, 14; effect of emotion on, 245, 547, 559, 566, 569, 570, 575, 576
free recall, 274
freedom–constraint distinction, 169
Freud, Sigmund, 244–5, 368, 371; emotions in early theory of, 230
frontal cortex, 136, 323–4, 336
frontal lobe (brain), 328–9, 344
frontal region (brain), 320, 347, 348–9, 354–5, 356, 357
frustration, 136, 137, 447; and learning 276; measurement of, 160, 161; relation with aggression, 171
fun, capacity for, 292
fundamental emotions, 30–2; *see also* basic emotions
fussing (infants), 240

galvanic skin response (GSR) measures, 92
gastrointestinal system, 143
gating processes, 79

gaze patterns, 234
gender, 64
generalized empathic distress capacity, 114
generation of emotion, 76; components in,
  79–80
generosity, determinants of, 451, 453
genes, 20
genetics, in attribution-affect linkage, 185
gestural acts, expressions, 3, 229, 234; basic
  emotions, 252
glandular system, 78
global emotional states, 285
global empathy, 111–12
global self, 108, 116
goal attainment, 167–8; through effort, 53
goal/events relationship, 234, 235, 248, 252
goals (appetites), 416, 424, 425, 429; change
  in, 585; emotion elicitation and, 234, 235,
  247–8, 249, 256; prewired, 235
Gödel, Escher, Bach (Hofstadter), 264
gonadal hormones, 137
gratification, 290; *see also* delay of
  gratification
gratitude, 171, 174; causal attribution, 172
guilt, 5, 188, 500, 503, 504, 511n2; adults'
  understanding of, 450; affective and
  cognitive dimensions of, 125, 126, 127;
  alterability of, 70; causal attribution, 125,
  176, 178–81; cognitive antecedents of,
  183; concepts of, 130n3; development of,
  125–6, 184; elicitation of, 180–1, 248;
  emergence of, 29, 62; expression of, 252;
  over inaction, 125, 126; post-transgression,
  502; primary emotion, 39, 137; repressed,
  80
Gururumba, 46

habits, implicit, 582
habituation, 47, 50, 92, 214, 247; of
  orienting response, 283–4
happiness, 174; adults' understanding of,
  448, 449–50, 455; children's
  understanding of, 441, 442, 443, 444, 445,
  448, 449, 451; development of, 184; effect
  on learning, 562–5, 569, 574, 575; effect
  on reactions to others, 475, 478–80; effect
  on reactions to self, 464, 467, 468, 469,
  472, 473, 480
hard wire cognitive representations, 273–4
Harvard Group Scale of Hypnotic
  Susceptibility, Form A, 548
hearing, 377; *see also* audition
heart rate, 40; emotion response, 201, 205,
  206–7, 208, 212, 214; as index, 47, 48–9,
  50, 51, 52, 53; measurement of, 240
hedonic quality, 42
hedonic tone, 230, 268, 416
hedonic tradition, 272–3
helplessness, 68, 183

hemispheric specialization, 234, 320–65
heredity, 132
heretability, EDRec, 507
hierarchical organization (temperament), 138,
  139, 142–7, 149–50, 151–3, 160
hippocampus, 19, 140, 323–4
homeostatic perspective, re motivation, 17,
  150, 151, 161
hope, 136; elicitation of, 248
hopelessness, 173, 175, 449; adaptive
  function of, 68
hostility, complex emotion, 137, 151
human development: emotion-cognition
  relations and, 17–37; idea of emotion in,
  38–72; *see also* development
human ethology, 371
Hume, David, 46–7
humility, 47, 63
humor, 148
hydrocephaly, 375, 378
hyperactivity, 324; gross sympathetic, 194
hyperkinesis, 143, 149
hypnosis, 14, 34, 547, 548–9, 570–1, 578
hypnotherapy, 585
hypothalamic literature, 137
hypothalamus, 140, 141
hypotheses, unconfirmed, 232
hysterical syndrome, 92–4

Ifalukians, 39, 45–7
imagers, good, poor, 208–10, 212–13, 214,
  221–2
imagery, 34, 196, 222; bio-informational
  theory of, 221; cognitive representations in
  form of, 82; text processing and efferent
  patterning, 200-10; therapeutic, 202
imagination, 266; consequence of unfulfilled
  emotion state, 272
imagining oneself in another's place, 106,
  128
imitation, 87; neonatal, 255, 346; *see also*
  mimicry
impulse control, 152; *see also* control
impulsivity, 136
incentive(s), 44, 46, 47, 50, 53, 137;
  coherence with physiological change, 52;
  internally generated, 61; in reactions to
  other as referent, 63–4, 66; reference to,
  in emotion terms, 58–63; and response
  classes, 57
incongruity(ies), 150, 151, 266–7; *see also*
  discrepancy
incorporation, 273
indifference, 194, 327, 328
individual characteristics, 448–9
individual differences, 367, 373; in ability to
  access affective response codes, 221–2,
  233 (*see also* imagers, good, poor); in
  cognition/emotion relationship, 284–5; in

emotional development, 30–2; in forms of arousal, 509; and infant–care-giver relationship, 382–3; range of, 366; in regulation of affect, 293; in response to stressors, 236; in temperament, 132, 133, 134, 135, 137, 142, 143, 147, 149, 150–1, 152–3, 162
individual stereotype, 216
industry, 540
infancy, early, emotion in, 27–8
infant–care-giver dyad, 294, 295, 367; affect–cognition relation between, 378–84; attachment in, 371; disturbance in, 397; regulation of affect in, 293; socialization in, 385, 386, 387, 388–90
infant–mother relationship, 24, 31
infant temperament research, 160–1
infantile emotionality, 229; studies of, 242–3, 252–5
infants: contingency awareness in, 11; expressive emotional behavior of, 18; and need for new emotion terms, 47–51; premature, 382–3
infants, atypical, 12; affect–cognition relationship in, 366–406
inference, 46, 466, 567
inferiority, 63
inferotemporal visual cortex, 140
information: emotion as, 196–200, 220; emotions regulate flow of, 229; inhibitory, 351; interhemispheric transfer of, 342–3, 356; new, 584; as possibility of reaching goal, 267; preprogrammed, 20–1; about stimuli, 195
information network, in empathy, 114, 121, 127–8
information processing, 6, 7–8; cognition as, 2, 221; control of, by Limbic system, 141; distinct from cognition, 19–20; early, 264; in emotion, 216, 217, 220; empathic distress cues, 114–15, 127; hemispheric specialization and, 320; mood-dependent, 88–90; rate of, in Down syndrome infants, 375, 378, 380; role of emotion in, 73, 232; role of motor system in, 81–2, 85, 86, 87, 88, 91; semantic, 105–6, 107; in sensory systems, 147–8; *see also* response information, processing of
information structure(s), 196, 199–200, 202, 214, 217, 223
information-processing model, 18
inhibition, 29, 34, 135, 240, 583; evolutionary advantage of, 61; role in emotional expression, 377–8; to the unfamiliar, 49; *see also* behavioral inhibition system; resistance to temptation
inhibitory control, 351, 356
inhibitory maturation, 146
innate releaser, 20

instigators, emotions as, 274–5
instinct theory, 230
integration, 151-2, 173; *see also* organizational perspective
intellectual capacities, 234
intensification, 456
intensity, 5, 28, 32, 42, 132, 134, 143–4; appropriate, 580–1; as classificatory scheme, 40, 46; developmental change in, 29; of outcome-dependent emotions, 175; problem of, in network theory, 576–8; *see also* mood intensity
intention, 144, 146, 581; children's understanding of, 411; development of, 183
intentional system, 220
intentionality, 180, 184
interactionism, 346
interest, 18, 25, 151, 247, 311, 355, 372; elicitation of, 238; emergence of, 346, 356; fundamental emotion, 137; hemispheric specialization in, 327; and learning, 279–80, 281, 282, 283, 284; measurement of, 56–7; shadings of, 581
interest-excitement (basic emotion), 580
interference, 574; in recall, 550, 551, 557
internal representations, 579
internal states, 269–70, 550
internal tone, 42
interpersonal behavior, 446; emotion as organizer of, 11, 12, 232–3, 235, 242–6, 256; *see also* social behavior
interpretations, effect of mood on, 547, 559, 565, 566, 576; of imaginative stories, 245; rules for, 583–4
interruption of response routine, 59
intrapsychic processes, emotions as organizers of, 235, 242–6, 256
introspection, 230, 369, 439–40
introversion–extraversion, 133, 136
invariance in emotion feelings, 25–6, 34
inverted-U function, 133
IQ, 290, 334
It/Me emotions, 416, 417–18, 419, 423, 424, 425, 428, 429

James, William, 484
Japanese Buddhists, 39
jealousy, 5, 63–4
job burnout, 583
joy, 13, 231, 246, 273; basic (primary) emotion, 39, 137, 229, 249; capacity for, 290; development of, 184, 351; effect on perception, 21, 23; egocentric/empathic, 477; elicitation of, 238, 239, 248; heart rate in, 240; indexes of, 241; relevance of empathic distress theory to, 129; understanding of, 58

judgment(s), 559, 574–5, 576; effect of emotion on, 547, 576
justice, 183
justification, 423–4, 425–8, 447; in moral decisions, 494

Kant, Immanuel, 181
Kelly, George, 485–6
kinesthetic cues, 105
kinesthetic feedback, 74, 75, 76, 77, 78, 79, 80, 83, 91
knowledge/beliefs (re emotion), 438, 439–50, 451–5, 456–9

language, 74, 75, 322, 579, 581; acquisition of, 94, 113, 128; affective, 219–20; in development of emotion attribution, 503; emergence of, 356; emotional, 385–6, 388; in emotional development, 32–3; and emotional phenomena, 12–13; impact of, on empathy, 10, 103, 106, 117–20, 121, 128; natural, 200, 202, 207, 215, 217; nonverbal origins in human emotional interchange, 233; *see also* emotion terms (words)
language cues, 200–1
language-mediated association, 105–7
language production, 95
latency, 132, 143–4
lateral eye movements (LEMs), 336
lateral gaze shifts, 335–7
lateralization, phylogenetic antecedents of, 320, 322–6
lateralized dysfunctions, 329–34
lateralized electroconvulsive therapy (ECT), 334–5
lattice-hierarchical organization; *see* hierarchical organization
laughter, 160, 247, 375; Down syndrome infants, 378, 390–2; pathological, 327–8
leadership, in peer group, 289–90, 292, 312
learning, 7, 19, 195, 269; cultural, 580; effect of emotions on, 7–8, 14, 22, 34, 276–85, 469, 547, 576; emotional communication in, 244; and emotional expression, 282–3; enhanced by positive feeling states, 451; mood intensity and, 9, 554, 555, 560, 561–7, 569; in network theory of affect, 573; and reinforcement, 273, 282; results of, 282–3; selective, 245, 547, 557–60, 565, 573
learning context, and recall, 549–50
leveling–sharpening, 149
life condition, and empathy, 121–2
limbic lobe, 38
limbic system, 19, 26, 33, 79, 134, 140; affective-motivational circuitry of, 140-1
limbic-centered emotional systems, 136
limbic-cortical integrative processing, 23
linear models, 5, 242, 275, 285, 367

linguistic representations, 214
locomotion, 28, 146
locus, 10, 45; in causality, 168–9, 170, 173, 181–2, 185; of control, 467
loss of control, 447
love, complex emotion, 137, 151
luck, 474–5; in causal attribution, 168, 169, 171–2

maltreated infants, 381–2, 387, 390, 393–4
markers, emotions as, 274
Marlowe-Crowne Scale of Social Desirability (MC), 331
masking, 456
mastery, 351
mastery smile, 372
matching: affective stimulus/expression, 341; analyzer, 198; of input information with information stored in prototype, 20, 148, 198, 200, 202, 211–14, 221–2; observer/experiencer affect in empathy, 114–15, 119, 121–2, 127, 128; simple pattern, 107; in S-R habits, 583–4
maturation, 69, 132; *see also* development
Maudsley Hospital, 201
Maximally Discriminative Facial Movement Coding System ("Max"), 278–9
Mead, Margaret, 523
meaning: and activation, 217–19; crucial in self-control, 510; defined, 412, 429, 430
meaning propositions, 197, 212, 218, 219, 221
measurement, 51–7, 233–4, 238–42; of attachment, 237; of emotional/cognitive development, 397–8; errors in, 241–2; of facial movements, 3; indices for, 41, 47, 51–7; reliability of, 194, 220
media, and emotional change, 211–14
medial forebrain bundle, 136
medulla, 26
medullary cardiovascular centers, 146
memory, 8, 19, 46, 201, 210, 231–2, 274, 440; as basis of appraisal, 266; development of, 59; effect of emotion on, 8, 14, 34, 465–6, 469–70, 471, 479–80, 547, 576; effect of mood-congruency on, 22; emotion information coded in, 196, 199–200, 214, 221, 223; immediate, 28; kinesthetic, 84–5; for locations task, 52; long-term, 210; mood and, 139–40; as product of information processing, 82; reappraisal of events from, 584–5; relation of emotions to, 244–5; rote, 22; selective, 575; short-term, 565, 574: stimulus–response, 82–3; theories of, 549–50
memory search: mood-biased, 573–4; restricted domain of, 576
mental age, 395–6
mental representation(s), 28; affect/cognition contact in, 73, 74–5, 77, 78, 79, 81, 82,

83, 85, 86, 94; cross-culturally constant, 25; distinct from symbolized emotion, 34; of infants, 372
mental retardation, 391–3, 395
meta-attributions, 176–8
meta-emotion, 438, 459
metagu, 45, 46
meta-memory, 440
microcephaly, 375
midbrain, 26
mimicry, 105, 111, 127, 129
minimization, 327
Minnesota Preschool Project, 294–310; checklist for, 299, 313–17
misattribution, 488–91, 494, 507–8, 510; and enhancement, 492–3; and extinction of conditioned responses, 491–2; and reduced attitude change in dissonance research, 492
mnestic function, 76, 77, 78, 79; of motor processes, 81, 82, 83, 85, 86, 94
mode, 521
models: of emotion/cognition relationship, 265–76; role of emotions in self/other response, 464; *see also* linear models
modulation, 135, 141, 162, 351; sensory/response, 141–2, 145
monoamine afferents, 136
monoamine oxidase, 137
monoamine projections, 135, 161
monoamine systems, 146
mood(s), 70, 88–9, 95, 321, 450; causal attribution, 169; change in, 584; effect on recognition memory, 554–5, 574; impact of drugs on, 486–7; and memory, 139–40; and reactions to self, 465–74; and social judgments, 567–8, 569, 570, 575; in state-dependent recall, 550–2
mood bias, 547, 553–4, 555, 566, 567, 568, 569, 575
mood intensity, and learning, 560, 561–7, 569, 574, 575–6; and recall, 555, 569
mood intensity hypothesis, 547, 549, 561–7
mood-congruity hypothesis, 22, 547, 549, 557–60, 569, 570, 573
Moog synthesizer, 239
moral decisions, role of emotion in, 487–91
moral development, 174, 233
moral judgment, 109; preoperational children, 180–1
moral socialization, 13–14; role of emotion in, 484–514
moral standards, universal, 69
morality, population distribution of, 505
mother, permanent image of, 232
mother–infant attachment, 24, 31
mother–infant dyads, 12; *see also* infant–care-giver dyad
motivated behavior, 138, 141, 144, 151
motivation, 18, 24, 52, 248, 275, 371; arousal in, 133, 187; causal attribution,

169; in definition of emotion, 486; emotions as, 26, 27, 33; intrinsic–extrinsic, 169; maturation of, 147–8; perceived change in feeling state as, 42; social, 167, 217
motivational systems, 136, 138, 150–3; individual differences in, 143; self-regulatory, 142
motive(s), 40, 44, 46, 416; emotions as, 272–4; in empathy, 116–17, 127; in It emotions, 416; primary, 540
motor activity, 240
motor cortex, 42
motor cues, 9; in mood-dependent information processing, 88–90
motor mimicry, 105
motor patterns, preprogrammed, 20
motor processes: representational function of, 76–80, 81–97; role in cognition, 81–5
motor programs, 202; in emotion prototype, 211, 219; in emotional states, 216–17; link with response propositions, 222; regeneration of, 201
motor reactivity, 160
motor representations: of attitudes, 90–2; innate and universal, 25
motor reproducibility, of visual input and recognition memory, 86–8
motor skills, 348
motor specializations, 354
motor system, 17, 29, 142; in affective processes, 74, 76; as contact point of affect and cognition, 74, 76–80, 86–97; role of, in emotion and cognition, 9
motor theory, 97
motor-expressive level, 3, 34; emotion/cognition relationship, 33–4
muricide, 324–5
music, 239
myelination, 351, 356

naive theories, 410, 429
naklik, 39
National Science Foundation, 294
negative emotion, 12, 21–2, 157–9, 162, 171, 172, 369, 381; ability to express, 293, 305–7; children's understanding of, 412–13, 415, 419, 428, 430; in contingency experience, 268; effect on reactions to others, 475–6, 477, 480; effect on reactions to self, 465–6, 467–9, 471, 472, 473, 480; emergence of, 348; hemispheric specialization in, 323, 324, 325, 327, 328, 335, 336, 337, 340, 341–4, 345, 347, 348–50, 351, 353, 356, 357; and learning, 276, 280, 281, 284, 285; in moral discussion, 496–7; ontogenesis of, in Down syndrome infants, 392; and social competence, 300–1
negative feeling states, 451–3, 454

neocortical ablation, 324, 325
neonates: emotional expression/emotional
    experience relation in, 249–51; emotions
    in, 230; prewired goals in, 235; *see also*
    infant–care-giver dyad
nervour system mechanisms of emotion, 246;
    see also central nervous system
network theories, 555–6
network theory of affect, 547–8, 554, 555–6,
    566, 567, 568, 569, 570, 571–85; flaws in,
    576–9
neural antecedents, 77–8
neural structure, 29
neural substrates, 350; interaction between,
    33–4; maturation of, 28–9
neural systems, 17–18, 137
neurochemical process, of emotion, 25;
    maturation of, 150
neurochemical substrates, 24
neurochemical systems, 142
neurochemistry, 1
neuroendocrinology, 153
neurogenetics, 153
neuromuscular hypotonia, 375, 378
neuromusculature connections, 269
neurophysiological component, level, 2. 3,
    19, 30, 34; emotional development at,
    29–30
neurophysiologists, 230
neurophysiology, 1, 137, 153
neurotic extravert, 134
neurotic introvert, 134
neuroticism, 136, 506
neuroticism-stability, 134
neurotransmitters, 3
neutralization (emotion), 456
Newton, I., 51
nigrostriatal system, 323
Nin, Anais, 523
nonfluent aphasias, 328
nonreward, 136
nonsocial stimuli, 195
noradrenaline, 487, 505–6
norepinephrine, 135, 136, 137, 143, 161, 324
normal populations, hemispheric
    specialization research on, 335–45
novelty, 136
nurturance, 18, 441, 448

object permanence, 19, 28, 108, 234
objective frames, 54–7
obsessional syndrome, 92–4
ontogenesis, 366
ontogeny, of hemispheric specialization,
    345–52, 356
open-field activity, 325
opinion change, 21–2
Opioid peptides, 137
opponent-process theory, 283
optimal level theory, 133–4

optimism, 183
orbital frontal cortex, 140
orbitofrontal cortex, 140
organism environment relationship, 217
organismic systems: integration of, through
    emotions, 33, 34; separate, 17
organisms, subsystems shared by affect and
    cognition, 73, 81
organizational constructs, emotions as, 235–
    48, 256
organizational perspective: of development,
    367–8, 373, 385, 397; in study of
    emotions, 12, 233, 235–48
orientation, 273
orienting reflex, 83, 283–4
origin–pawn distinction, 169
oscillators, 138
oscillatory factors, 150–1
other(s): in causal attribution, 168, 169, 172,
    174; cognitive sense of, 10, 107–11, 112,
    113–15, 117–18, 125, 126, 127, 129;
    concept of, 149; focus in empathy, 113–
    15, 118–20, 121; influence of emotions on
    reactions to, 474–9; as referent, 63–8
outcomes, 417, 423, 430, 449; causal
    attribution, 173; expectancies for, 456–9;
    unexpected, 167
overarousal, empathic, 124
overjustification theory, 494
overt acts, 196, 202, 219, 221

pain, 239
panic, 194; discrete circuitry for, 137
parallelism, 17, 396
parasympathetic system, 17
parents, 389–90; children's understanding of
    emotions felt by, 442; discipline by, 125;
    perception of their children, 54–5
parietal asymmetry, 332, 341, 343, 344, 347,
    349, 354–5, 356
parietal cortex, 141, 147
passive outdoor experiences, 446
pathology, 195; diagnosing of, in infancy,
    398
pattern recognition, 10
patterns, complex emotions as, 252
peer group social structure, 24, 63, 65, 289,
    294
peer status, 302, 303, 305, 312
perceived origin, 42
perception, 8, 46, 486; causal, 183; of
    control, 467–8, 479, 480; effect of
    emotions on, 21, 34, 245–6, 416, 479,
    547; effects of self-esteem and induced
    emotion on, 21–2; of emotional
    expressions, 75; emotions prototypic
    affordances in, 233; hemispheric
    specialization in, 338–40, 341; mood and,
    568; selectivity of, 138; of stimuli, 80
perceptual defense, 139, 140

perceptual discrimination capability, 10, 104, 107
perceptual imagery, 201, 208, 210
perceptual system, 17
perceptual theory, 97n3
performance, 134; effect of emotion on, 470–1
peripheral arousal, 487; misattribution of, 488–90, 508, 510
peripheral autonomic, facial, and skeletal expressions of emotion, 246
peripheral feedback, 246
peripheral-dimensional theory, 486–7, 491, 492, 493, 507–10
Perlman, Itzhak, 84
person–environment distinction, 169
person identity, 103, 110–11, 120–2
person permanence, 103, 108–9, 111, 112; and transformation of empathic to sympathetic children, 115–17
personal characteristics, in display rules, 456
personal feelings, children's understanding of, 411, 412, 415, 424, 428–9, 430
personality, 132; causal attribution, 123, 169, 172; emotions in, 7–8; and moral decisions, 505–7; parental, 389; as set of systems, 9, 17, 33, 137–8; shaped by affective-cognitive structures, 34; temperament and emotion thresholds as determinants of, 30
personality development, 14; facial feedback hypothesis and, 32
personality structure, 468, 480
personality theory, 153, 516, 540, 544–5
personality-clinical psychology, 1, 7
perspective taking, 109, 234
pessimism, 183, 327
phase sequences (theory), 247
phobia, 196, 209, 210, 214, 219, 221
phobia prototype, 196–9, 202
phylogenetic continuity, 195
phylogenetic descent, 40
phylogeny, 69; of lateralization, 322–6
physical attractiveness, and social interaction, 291, 307
physical discomfort, 446
physiological arousal, affective patterns of, 201–2
physiological change, 2; coherence with incentives and evaluations, 52; detected/undetected, 9; as index, 52; media and, 212-13; perception of, as emotion, 270, 271
physiological disposition, and moral decisions, 505–7
physiological factors: in causal attribution, 168, 169; in social emotions, 171
physiological perspective: in classifying emotions, 40, 41; influence of emotion on cognition, 140–2

physiology, expressive, 194, 221
Piaget, Jean, 66, 109; children as case studies, 516
Piagetian theory, 369, 411, 425, 440
pity, 171, 188; adults' understanding of, 450; causal attribution, 176, 178–81; development of, 183, 184
play, symbolic, 395–6
pleasant emotions, 12, 69
pleasant events, 446
pleasure, 372; lack of, 381
pleasure–displeasure, as classification axis, 40
pleasure/pain, 272
pleasure-joy system, 151, 152
polarity, 429
pons, 26
positive affect (emotion), 12, 21–2, 171, 172, 312, 369; children's distinctions between, 412–13, 415, 419, 428, 430; consequence and prerequisite for learning, 276, 278–9, 281, 285; in contingency experience, 268; differential lateralization (hypothesis), 325, 327, 336, 337, 340, 341–4, 345, 347, 348–50, 353, 355, 356, 357; effect on reactions to others, 475, 476, 477, 480; effect on reactions to self, 465–6, 467, 468–9, 471, 472, 473, 480; emergence of, in Down syndrome infants, 391–2; in moral decisions, 496–7; and social competence, 299, 300–1
positive feeling states, 450; effect on behavior, 451–3, 454
positive sensory feedback loops, 377
posterior cortical association region, 320, 326, 330, 334, 341, 345, 354–6, 357
postural behavior, 3, 241, 269, 578–9
postural sway test, 202
power concerns, causal attribution, 168
precedence issue, 285, 311; *see also* sequence issue
preconscious processes, 8
prediction, 183, 417, 547; mood and, 566–7, 569, 570, 575, 576
preference, 22, 91–2, 273
preliterate tribes, 238–9
premenstrual tension, 218
prewired connections, 269
pride, 5, 47, 63, 152, 171, 172, 174, 188, 450; causal attribution, 181–2; damaged, 447; development of, 183, 184, 185, 351
primary circular reaction, 10, 104, 106, 107, 377
primary emotions, 39, 50, 346, 552; *see also* basic emotions
primary epistemology of the subject, 54
primitive emotion, differentiation of, 580–1
proactive interference in memory, 54
probability, 248
process vs. content, attribution theory, 187–8

productions, 580, 583–4
projection, 452, 454, 458, 547
propositions, 75, 94; cognitive
    representations in form of, 81–2; emotion
    information organized in, 219, 221;
    meaning, 196–9, 200; stimulus and
    response, 196–9, 200, 202, 203, 206, 219,
    221; *see also* meaning propositions;
    response propositions
proprioceptive feedback, 74, 75, 76, 77, 80
prosocial behavior, 24, 33, 474, 475, 476
protection, 273
prototype(s): accessing, 211–14, 218, 221–2;
    deep structure, 198, 200, 202, 208, 216,
    221; emotion, 11, 196, 200, 202, 216,
    219, 221, 222; of phobia, 196–9, 210, 214
psychoanalysis, role of motor system in,
    92–3
psychoanalytic psychology, theory derived
    from cause in, 516
psychoanalytic theory, emotions in, 233
psychobiography, 516
psychological arousal, 488
psychological perspective, influence of
    emotion on cognition, 139–40
psychological theory, emotions in, 230
psychology, normal and atypical development
    in, 366–7
psychopathology, 370, 397; EDRec in, 506–7
psychophysiological correlates of emotion,
    370
psychophysiology(ists), 1, 134, 153, 241;
    response training and, 203–10, 214–19,
    222
psychotherapy, coping responses in, 582–3,
    585
punishment, 136, 169, 495, 504, 507; fear
    of, 501; harsh, 505; justified, 441, 448;
    unjustified, 448
punishment system, 137, 159
punishment-avoidance system, 137

Questionnaire on Mental Imagery (QMI),
    208, 209

rage, discrete circuitry for, 137
rage-anger system, 151
Rasch method, 419, 422
reaction formations, 458
reaction sets, 58–9
reactions, unconscious, repressed, 458
reactivity, 26, 133, 136, 137, 155, 583–4; of
    cortical processing units, 140–1; defined,
    132; determinants of, 439–46; individual
    differences in, 152–3; and individual
    differences in temperament, 143–4;
    measurement of, 160–1; modulation of,
    150; scales for, 153–5
reafference, 76

reappraisals, 584–5
reasoning ability, 46
recall, 210; effect of emotions on, 22;
    improved when emotional state matches
    learning state, 454, 480; state-dependent,
    548, 549–57, 573–4; *see also* memory
recall/learning match(es): mood, 551–2, 574;
    state, 550
receptivity to emotional expressions,
    developmental change in, 249, 252–5, 256
recognition memory: effect of mood on, 554–
    5, 574; motor reproducibility and, 86–8
recovery time, 132, 143–4, 153
reference emotion(s), 416, 417–18, 419–24,
    425, 429, 430
referent(s), 74–5; choice of, 64; other as,
    63–8
referential eye contact, 380
reflectivity–impulsivity, 149
reflex patterns, 145–6
reflexes, 138, 144
regret, 248
regulation, 33; in systems theory, 242
reinforcement, 137, 273, 282–3
reintegration, 273
rejection, 273
relaxation to gratification, 58
releasing perspective, 150, 151
relief, 136, 248
reminding, selective, 559–60
repetition of successful action, 241
representation(s), 9, 74–5; of affect
    according to theories of emotion, 75–80;
    central, 97; hard, 9, 76–80, 81–5, 86–97;
    hard wire cognitive, 273–4; innate,
    acquired, transformed, 97; linguistic, 214;
    soft, 9, 76, 79–80, 89–90, 91, 93, 94–5,
    96, 97; *see also* mental representation(s)
representational capacity, 148, 150; Down
    syndrome infants, 395
representational processes, 8
representational thought, 234
representativeness (principle), 566–7
repression, 351–2, 356
repression–sensitization, 149
reproduction, 273
repulsion emotions, 416
requests for help, 450
research perspectives, on temperament, 153–
    61
resignation, 173, 450
resistance to temptation, 152, 487–8, 490,
    495, 496, 498, 499–501, 502, 503, 509,
    510
respiration, 135, 241
response: to emotion as information, 196,
    197, 200, 214, 221; remembering, 82–3; in
    representational functions, 97
response categories, in emotion theory, 485

response dispositions, context-bound, 194–5, 196, 200, 206, 220, 221

response information, processing of, 196, 201, 202–3, 208, 209–10, 215, 216, 218

response learning, 580

response parameters, 132, 143–4, 153

response processes, emotions regulate flow of, 229, 241

response propositions, 197, 202, 203, 206, 219, 221; link with motor programs, 222; primary mediators of affective influence on memory, 210

response systems, 145–7, 162, 346; multiple, 321, 322

response training, 203–10, 212, 213, 218, 222

response-regulatory systems, 139, 145–7, 162

restorers, 582

retreat, 241

retrieval cue overload, 576

reward distribution, 477–8

reward system, 159; kinds of, 137

reward-approach system, 137

rise time, 42, 132, 143–4, 153

role taking, 10, 22, 106, 107; in empathy, 108, 111, 118–20

role taking competence, 109–10, 111, 113

rostral/caudal plane, 320, 335, 344

rotation behavior (rats), 323

rus, 45–6

sadness, 13, 152, 174, 238, 273, 381; adults' understanding of, 448, 449–50, 455; basic (primary) emotion, 39, 229, 249; children's understanding of, 441, 442, 443, 444, 445, 448, 451; complex emotion, 151, 159; effect on cognition, 80; effect on learning, 280, 281–2, 283, 563, 565, 569, 574, 575; effect on reactions to others, 475, 477, 478–80; effect on reactions to self, 464, 467–8, 469, 470, 472–3, 480; effect on recall, 22; effect on self-attribution, 467; indexes of, 241; infant, 372; to loss of attachment object, 60, 61

Safford, Truman Henry, 84

scanning patterns, 148

schema activation, 497–502

schema formation, 391

schema theory, 78

schemas, 232; affective, cognitive, 395; emergent, 231

schizophrenia, 143, 370

scripts (scenes), 521, 523, 541–4, 578; social, 580

secondary thought, 272

seizure disorders, 375

selectivity, 138, 390

self: autonomous, 392; influence of emotions on reactions to, 464–74; integrative system of, 8, 17, 18; symbolic evaluation of, 63–8

self–other differentiation, 116–17

self–other orientation, 13

self-assessment, 429

self-attribution, 466–7, 480

self-concept, 34, 149, 184, 468–9, 480; and arousal, 500; threat to, 53; transient, 13

self-confidence, 449

self-control, 459, 505; emotion attribution in, with children, 493–7, 501–2, 510; emotion-mediated, 510–11; influence of emotion in, 451, 453; procedures for, 582–3, 585

self-control studies, 495–6

self-description of emotions, 194–5, 220, 221

self-esteem, 173, 175, 181, 450, 468; damaged, 447; effects of, 21–2

self-focus in empathy, 118–20, 121

self-inference, 23

self-monitoring, 453; of vulnerability, 457, 459

self-perception (theory), 33–4, 75, 504

self-recognition, atypical infants, 392–4

self-reflection, 181

self-regulation, 25, 29, 34, 152, 153; capacity for, 293; in emotion/cognition investigation, 280–1, 283, 284; of infant, 161; role in inhibition, 377–8; scales for, 155; temperament as, 132, 142

self-report, 47; as index, 54, 55–6

self-reward, 451, 453, 471–3; effect of emotion on, 13, 473–4, 478, 480

semantic elaboration, 245

semantic features, 410, 413–15, 419–24, 428–9, 430; development and, 424–8

semantic memory, 149

semantic processing, 105–6, 107, 117–20, 128; in empathy, 10

semantic-memory theories, 579

sensation, 230

sensation seeking, 137

sensorimotor programs, 195

sensory data, 28

sensory feedback, 33–4

sensory pleasure, 53, 68

sensory regulation, 107; emotion and, 138–44

sensory systems, 86–7, 147–8

sensory-regulating systems, 148–50, 162

separation, 351, 372, 386

separation anxiety, 28, 231, 232

septal-hippocampal system, 136

sequence issue, 4–5, 10, 20, 264, 396, 445, 485; in attribution theory, 186

seriation, 63, 65, 183

serotonin, 135, 143, 146, 161

servomechanisms, 138

sex differences: in affect, 213, 217; in cheating, 489, 490–1
sexual ardor, 229, 240, 249
sexual arousal, 509
sexual excitement, 66
sexual incentives, 53
sexuality, 67–8, 493
sexually related actions, 446
shallowness, 381
shame, 62, 151, 152, 500, 503; development of, 183, 392; expression of, 252; fundamental emotion, 39, 137
shame-humiliation (basic emotion), 580
shared affect, 290, 292, 305
siblings, 63, 65
signaling, 381, 384; noise in, 375
signals, ambiguous, 584
similarities, in choice of referent, 64
situational state, 248
situational stereotypy, 216
skepticism, 138
skin conductance response: fear, 201, 205; and level of socialization, 506
skin resistance, 40; as index, 47
sleep–wake behavior, 144, 160–1
slips of the tongue, 93, 94
slumped posture, 241
smile, 291; in atypical infants, 379, 380; Down syndrome infants, 390-2; endogenous, 270; as index, 60; mastery, 372; measurement of (infants), 160; spontaneous, 57, 329, 346
snake phobia, 197, 206–7, 214
social adjustment, 505, 506
social anxiety, 206–7
social behavior, emotion as organizer of, 11, 12, 242–4
social class, 246
social communication, 32–3; emotions and, 252–5
social comparison, 466–7
social competence, 12; assessment of, Minnesota Preschool Project, 297–8; internalized rules for, 456–8, 459; role of affect in, 24, 289–319
social control, 8–9
social emotions, 171, 188
social factors (in emotions), 8–9
social interaction, 446; affect in, 11–12, 289–90, 291, 312; emotions as regulators of, 229, 233, 292; mood and, 478–9; voluntary expressions in, 34
social judgments, 14, 454, 547; mood and, 567–8, 569, 570
social learning, 31, 185
social perception, 274
social psychology, 1, 7, 167
social referencing, 11, 242–3, 387–8
social relationships, 18
social sensitivity, 290; capacity for, 413, 414

social smile, 20, 31, 231–2; in Down syndrome infants, 375
social stimuli, 195
social world, influence of temperament on, 152–3
social-cognitive development, 128–9
socialization, 8, 130n2, 134, 152, 459; and affective-cognitive interaction, 384–90; emotion as consequence of, 269, 270; and emotion attribution, 493–4, 495, 496, 500–1, 502–4, 511; of infants, 251; may shape emotion experiences, 34; motoric representation in, 25; *see also* moral socialization
sociometric status, 12; and attention rank, 298, 299, 301–3, 312
sociophilia, 478–9
sociophobia, 478–9
sodium amytal, 329
Solvay Congress, 1
somatic nervous system, 3; under voluntary control, 20–1
somatic responses, 74, 76, 155; representative and mnestic capacity, 79
somatic system, 17, 135; and temperament, 132, 137, 153
somatic theories of emotion, 75, 76
somatosensory system, 376
song, 39, 45
soothability, 284, 285
sorrow, 248
spatial cognition, 355
speech perception, 81, 87
speech perception/speech production relationship, 338, 341
stability, 10, 450; causal, 169, 170, 173, 182–3
stable extravert (sanguine), 134
stable introvert (phlegmatic), 134
standard: deviation from, 63, 66; meeting of, 53; violation of, 53, 60, 62, 68
Stanford Hypnotic Susceptibility Scale, Form C, 548
startle tendency, 160, 161
state dependent learning, 88–90
Stephen, Thoby (brother of V. Woolf), 529, 532, 537
Stephen, Vanessa (sister of V. Woolf), 517, 518, 533, 534, 537
stereotypes, 458, 459–60, 546; individual, 216
stimulation, 133, 391; infant's need for, 371; releasing aspects of, 150
stimulus(i): emotional significance of, 140; external, internal, 74; familiar, 245; prepared or prepotent, 195; remembering, 82–3; in representative function, 97
stimulus context, 217, 218; affect as, 195–6; of emotion, 196
stimulus generalization, 105

stimulus information, 219, 222; reprocessing of, 201
stimulus learning and differentiation, 580
stimulus properties, emotional expression, 25
stimulus propositions, 196, 197–9, 200, 202, 203, 206, 219, 221; and accessing prototype, 211–12
stimulus training, 213
stimulus-pattern recognition, 580, 583–4
Strachey, Lytton, 534
"Strange Situation," 386–7, 394
stranger anxiety, 231, 232
stranger fear, 28, 247, 348
stranger reactions, 243
stress, 175, 505, 506; and learning, 276
stress management, 583
strivings of individuals, 235, 246–8
stuttering, 93–4
subcortical sensory systems, 147
subjective frames, 54–7
subjective-experiential level, 3–4, 34, 322; emotion at, 27; emotional development at, 32–3
subjectivism, 567
success, 172, 441, 448, 449, 450; and altruism, 474–5; attribution in, 174, 181, 183, 188; and delay of gratification, 473; effect on memory for interpersonal information, 470–1; effect on reaction to others, 474; as inducer of mood, 465; self-attribution and, 466–7; and self-reward, 471–2
success-failure studies, 464, 465
superior temporal sulcus, 140
superiority, 63
suppression, 384
surprise, 148, 194, 247, 273; basic (primary) emotion, 39, 137, 229, 249; causal attribution, 172, 176–7; causal search, 167; elicitation of, 238, 239; indexes of, 241; and learning, 279–80, 281, 282; to the unexpected, 58, 59
surprise-startle (basic emotion), 580
surrender, 173
survival value of emotions, 26, 184, 273–4; of empathy, 107; *see also* adaptive function of emotions
sustainers, 582
swaddling, 235
sweating, 197
symbolic association, 10
symbolic communication, 233
symbolization, 5, 8, 33, 395, 503
sympathetic distress, 103, 115–17
sympathetic nervous system, 505, 506, 509
sympathetic system, 17
sympathy in dimension-linked affect, 178, 179
systems concept of personality, 9, 17, 33
systems theory, 6, 233; regulation in, 242

tachycardia, 197
tacit knowledge, 5
task completion, 60-1
task ease/difficulty, 168, 169
task failure, anticipated, 60
task performance, 13, 245–6, 469–70, 480, 582–3
taste aversion studies (rats), 324, 325
taste discrimination, 26–7, 347
taste hedonics, 27
taxonomic scholarship, 53–4
teacher rankings, social competence, 12, 290, 298–9, 301–3, 312
tears, 240
temperament, 7–8, 10, 132–66, 240, 284–5, 511; and cognitive style, 541; defined, 132; development of, 144–53, 160–1; in emotion attribution, 504–5; and infant–care-giver relationship, 382, 383, 390; research perspectives re, 29–30, 153–61
temperament scales, 154–5T, 156–7, 158T
temperament systems, regulatory organization of, 132–3
temperament theories, 133–8
temperament types, 134
temporal lobe (brain), 341
temporal region (brain), 354
temptation, 498, 502; responses to, 13; *see also* resistance to temptation
Tennessee Self-Concept Scale, 21
tension, 371, 378, 391, 492, 504, 507–8; role of, in dissonance, 501; in temptation, 498, 500, 503
testing contexts, 236
text processing, 211–12, 213, 214, 218–19, 222; emotional imagery, 200–10
thalamus, 79; nonspecific, 135
Thematic Apperception Test, 522
themes, in study of V. Woolf, 14, 522–45
theory, imperfect: guides research, 13; naive, 410, 429
therapy, 195, 214, 398
thinking, 44; about ongoing behavior, 466
thought(s), 19, 417; causal, 170–1, 176, 184, 186, 188; content of, 274; disordered, 370; effect of mood on, 566, 574–5; elaborated, 272; induce emotion, 449–50; in network theory of affect, 572
threat: anticipation of, 53; to physical integrity, 53
threshold, 8, 29, 30, 132, 143–4, 150
tics, 92–4
To/From, 416, 417, 419, 421
toddler period, 303
tranquilizer(s), 492, 493, 508
treatment: of phobia, 199; psychophysiology of emotions in, 215
"two-factor" theory, 578

uncertainty, 194, 267; moral value of, 69;
  resolution of, 59–60
understanding of emotions: by children, 12–
  13, 409–37; by children and adults, 438–
  63; defined, 410; development of, 424–30
unexpectedness, 248
unpleasant emotions, 12, 69
unpleasant events, 446
unpredictability, 381
Utku Eskimos, 39, 46
Uzgiris-Hunt scales, 372, 391

valence, 13, 194, 195, 216, 220, 221, 311,
  354, 416, 417; and co-occurrence of
  emotion, 445; differential lateralization in,
  341; differentiated, in social behavior,
  243–4; differentiation of, 418–19, 421–2,
  424, 425, 430; of experienced emotion
  determines valence of memories recalled,
  466, 480; hemispheric specialization and,
  338; negative, 196
value: change in, 584; in emotion elicitation,
  235
vasovagal fainting, 194
Vaughan, Emma, 529
Velten mood induction procedure, 89, 570
verbal behavior, 196, 197, 202–3, 214, 215,
  217, 219, 221, 222, 230
verbal cues, in emotional expression, 34, 377
verbal mediation of empathic affect, 128
verbal system, 152
vigilant, 49–50
visceral and somatic events, 196, 197, 198,
  199, 201–2, 205, 208, 216, 217, 218, 219
visceral functioning, sympathetic, 194
visual cliff, 348, 372, 392
visual discrimination learning, 323
visual feedback: impaired, 381; smiling
  behavior, 380

visual field, 246
visual field asymmetry, 337–41
visual imagery, 118
visual information, 140; selective
  enhancement of, 141
visual input, motor reproducibility of, 86–8
visual learning, 325
visualization, 78
visuospatial ability, 354, 355
vocal cues, 443
vocal expressions, 32, 269; influence
  emotional reactions in infants, 243
vocal intonation, 3
vocalic emotion, measurement of, 239–40,
  241
vocalization behavior, Down syndrome
  infants, 380
voice, 234
voluntarily controlled expression, 458

wariness, 148, 151–2, 240
wariness-fear system, 151
Watson, "Little Albert" case, 516
Wernicke's aphasics, 355, 357
wishes, 416, 417; violation of, 447
withdrawal, 381
Woolf, Leonard, 518, 534
Woolf, Virginia Stephen, 14, 515–46;
  biographical background, 517–19
words: emotion in recall of, 470, 471; *see
  also* emotion terms (words)
work failure, 446
work pressure, 446
worry, 69

Yerkes-Dodson Law, 245–6

zygote, 51